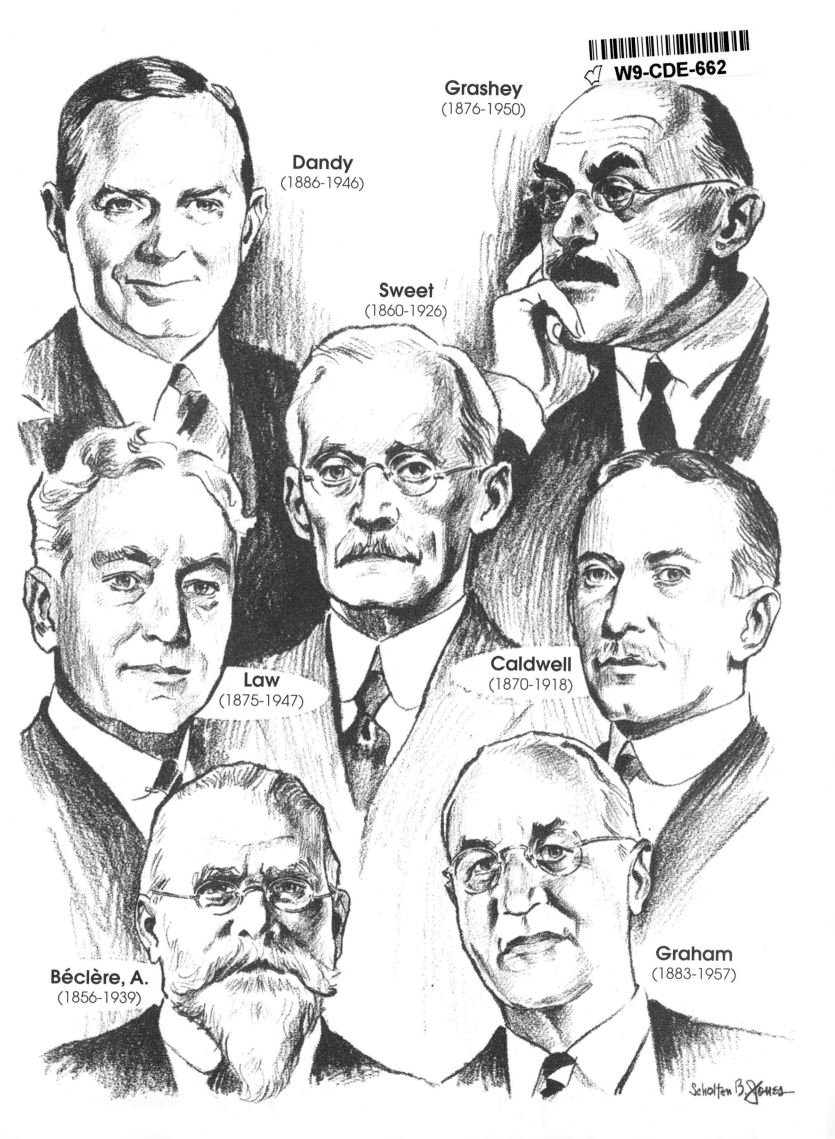

Grashey
(1876-1950)

Dandy
(1886-1946)

Sweet
(1860-1926)

Law
(1875-1947)

Caldwell
(1870-1918)

Béclère, A.
(1856-1939)

Graham
(1883-1957)

Scholten B. Jones

MERRILL'S ATLAS
of
RADIOGRAPHIC POSITIONS and RADIOLOGIC PROCEDURES

VOLUME THREE

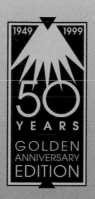

1949 — 1999

50 YEARS

GOLDEN ANNIVERSARY EDITION

MERRILL'S ATLAS

of

RADIOGRAPHIC POSITIONS and RADIOLOGIC PROCEDURES

VOLUME THREE

NINTH EDITION

Philip W. Ballinger,
MS, RT(R), FAERS

Assistant Professor Emeritus
Radiologic Technology Division
School of Allied Medical Professions
The Ohio State University
Columbus, Ohio

Eugene D. Frank,
MA, RT(R), FASRT

Director, Mayo Radiography Program
Department of Diagnostic Radiology
Mayo Clinic/Foundation
Assistant Professor of Radiology
Mayo Medical School
Rochester, Minnesota

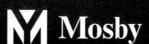 Mosby

St. Louis Baltimore Boston Carlsbad Chicago Minneapolis New York Philadelphia P

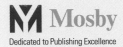

Publisher: Don E. Ladig
Executive Editor: Jeanne Rowland
Developmental Editor: Carole Glauser
Project Manager: Linda McKinley
Production Editors: René Spencer Saller, Cathy Comer, Barrett Schroeder
Designer: Renée Duenow
Manufacturing Manager: Betty Mueller

Composition and lithography by Graphic World, Inc.
Printing/binding by R.R. Donnelly & Sons Company

Mosby, Inc.
11830 Westline Industrial Drive
St. Louis, Missouri 63146

Library of Congress Cataloging in Publication Data

Ballinger, Philip W.
     Merrill's atlas of radiographic positions and radiologic
procedures. — 9th ed. / Philip W. Ballinger, Eugene D. Frank.
          p.   cm.
     Includes bibliographical references and index.
     ISBN 0-8151-2651-4 (alk. paper). — ISBN 0-8151-2652-2 (pbk.   :
alk. paper). — ISBN 0-8151-2653-0
     1.   Radiography, Medical—Positioning—Atlases.   I.   Frank, Eugene
D.   II.   Merrill, Vinita, 1905-   Atlas of roentgenographic positions
and standard radiologic procedures.   III. Title.   IV. Title: Atlas
of radiographic positions and radiologic procedures.   V.   Title:
Radiographic positions and radiologic procedures.
     [DNLM: 1.   Technology, Radiologic atlases.   2.   Diagnostic Imaging
atlases.   WN 17 B192m   1999]
RC78.4.B35   1999
616.07'572—dc21
DNLM/DLC
for Library of Congress

International Standard Book Number (Set): **0-8151-2650-6**
99   00   01   02   03   /   9   8   7   6   5   4   3   2   1

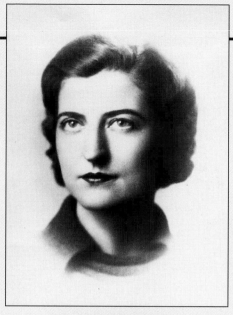

Vinita Merrill
1905-1977

Vinita Merrill had the foresight, talent, and knowledge to write the first edition of this atlas in 1949. The text she wrote became known as *Merrill's Atlas* in honor of the significant contribution she made to the profession of radiography and in acknowledgment of the benefit of her work to generations of students and practitioners.

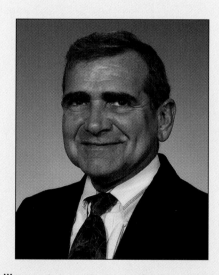

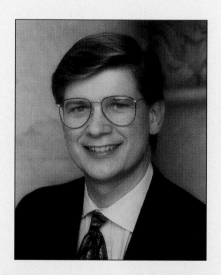

Philip Ballinger is now Assistant Professor Emeritus in the Radiologic Technology Division of the School of Allied Medical Professions at The Ohio State University in Columbus, Ohio. In 1995, he retired after a 25-year career as Radiography Program Director at The Ohio State University. Since his retirement, he has become more involved than ever in professional activities, such as speaking engagements at state, national, and international professional meetings. He began working on *Merrill's Atlas* in its fifth edition, which was published in 1982. The Golden Anniversary Edition is Phil's fifth as author of the atlas.

Eugene Frank is currently in his twenty-eighth year in radiography at the Mayo Clinic/Foundation in Rochester, Minnesota. For the last 8 years, he has been Director of the Mayo Radiography Program and Assistant Professor of Radiology in the Mayo Medical School. He frequently presents at professional gatherings throughout the world and has held leadership positions in state, national, and international professional organizations. He joins Philip Ballinger as co-author on this ninth edition of *Merrill's Atlas*.

ADVISORY BOARD

This edition of Merrill's benefits from the expertise of a special advisory board. The following board members have provided professional input and advice and have helped the authors make decisions about atlas content throughout the preparation of the ninth edition:

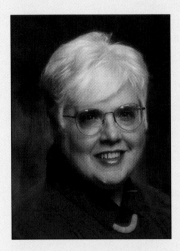

Joyce Ortego, MS, RT(R)
Program Coordinator,
   Radiologic Technology
Dona Ana Community
   College
Las Cruces, New Mexico

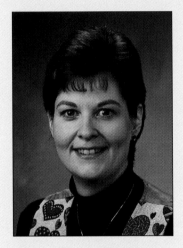

**Rita M. Oswald, BS, RT(R)
(CV)**
Clinical Instructor,
   Radiography Program
Mayo Clinic/Foundation
Rochester, Minnesota

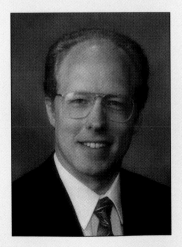

Curt L. Serbus, MEd, RT(R)
Radiologic Technology
   Educational Consultant
Indianapolis, Indiana

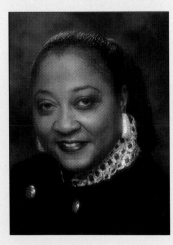

**Bettye Greene Wilson,
MA-Ed, RT(R)(CT),
RDMS**
Associate Professor,
   Division of Medical
   Imaging and Therapy
School of Health Related
   Professions
University of
   Alabama-Birmingham
   Birmingham, Alabama

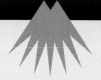

CONTRIBUTORS

Albert Aziza, BSc, MRT(R)
Hospital for Sick Children
Diagnostic Imaging
Toronto, Canada

Michael R. Bloyd, BSN, RN, RT(R)
Director of Educational Services
Taylor County Hospital
Greensburg, Kentucky

Barbara A. Blunt, MPH, RT(R), ARRT
Project Manager
Osteoporosis and Arthritis Research
    Group
University of California-San Francisco
San Francisco, California

Jeffrey A. Books, RT(R)
Director, Diagnostic Imaging
St Dominic-Jackson Memorial Hospital
Jackson, Mississippi

Michael G. Bruckner, BS, RT(R)(CV)
Angiographic Technologist and
    Clinical Instructor
The Ohio State University
Columbus, Ohio

Terri Bruckner, MA, RT(R)
Instructor, Radiologic Technology
    Division
The Ohio State University
Columbus, Ohio

Stewart C. Bushong, ScD, FACR, FACMP
Professor of Radiology
Baylor College of Medicine
Houston, Texas

Leila A. Bussman, BS, RT(R)(T)
Director, Radiation Therapy Program
Mayo Clinic/Foundation
Rochester, Minnesota

Luann J. Culbreth, MEd, RT(R)(MR)
MRI Manager
Baylor University Medical Center
Dallas, Texas

William F. Finney, MA, RT(R)
Assistant Professor, Radiography
    Program
The Ohio State University
Columbus, Ohio

Sandra Hagen-Ansert, BA, RDMS, RDCS
Program Director, Ultrasound
Baptist Memorial College of Health
    Science
Memphis, Tennessee

Richard D. Hichwa, PhD
Associate Professor
Director, PET Imaging Center
University of Iowa Hospitals
Iowa City, Iowa

Nancy L. Hockert, BS, ASCP, CNMT
Program Director, Nuclear Medicine
    Technology
Mayo Clinic/Foundation
Rochester, Minnesota

Jeffrey A. Huff, AS, RT(R)(CV), RCVT
Cardiac Catheterization Technologist
Kuakini Medical Center
Honolulu, Hawaii

Lorrie L. Kelley, MS, RT(R)(MR)(CT)
Associate Professor
Director CT/MRI Program
Boise State University
Boise, Idaho

Nina Kowalczyk, MS, RT(R)
Associate Director, Radiology
The Ohio State University
Columbus, Ohio

Deirdre Milne, MRT(R), ACR
ADAC Project Manager/Applications
    Specialist
Burlington, Ontario, Canada

Walter W. Peppler, PhD
Clinical Professor
University of Wisconsin-Madison
Madison, Wisconsin

Rex E. Profit, MA, RT(R)
Account Manager
Fuji Medical Systems, USA
Stamford, Connecticut

Terese McShane Roth, MS, RT(R)(M)
Assistant Professor, Radiology
Merritt College
Walnut Creek, California

Jane A. Van Valkenburg, PhD, RT(R)(N), FASRT
Department Chair, Radiologic
    Sciences
Weber State University
Ogden, Utah

Kari J. Wetterlin, MA, RT(R)
Unit Supervisor, Radiology
St. Mary's Hospital
Mayo Clinic/Foundation
Rochester, Minnesota

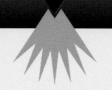

PREFACE

Welcome to the Golden Anniversary Edition of *Merrill's Atlas of Radiographic Positions and Radiologic Procedures*. The ninth edition continues the tradition of excellence begun in 1949, when Vinita Merrill wrote the first edition of what has become a classic text. Over the last 50 years, *Merrill's Atlas* has provided a strong foundation in anatomy and positioning for thousands of students who have gone on to successful careers as imaging technologists. *Merrill's Atlas* is also a mainstay for everyday reference in imaging departments all over the world. As the coauthors of this Golden Anniversary Edition, we are honored to follow in Vinita Merrill's footsteps.

Learning and Perfecting Positioning Skills

Merrill's Atlas has an established tradition of helping students learn and perfect their positioning skills. After covering preliminary steps in radiography, radiation protection, and terminology in introductory chapters, *Merrill's* then teaches anatomy and positioning in separate chapters for each bone group or organ system. The student learns to position the patient properly so that the resulting radiograph provides the information the physician needs to correctly diagnose the patient's problem. The atlas presents this information for commonly requested projections as well as those less commonly requested, making it the most comprehensive text and reference available.

The third volume of the atlas provides basic information about a variety of special imaging modalities, such as computed tomography, cardiac catheterization, magnetic resonance imaging, ultrasound, nuclear medicine technology, quality management, and radiation therapy.

Merrill's Atlas is not only a sound resource for students to learn from but also an indispensable reference as they move into the clinical environment and ultimately into their practice as imaging professionals.

New to This Edition

Since that first edition of *Merrill's Atlas* in 1949, many changes have occurred. This new edition incorporates many significant changes designed not only to reflect the technologic progress and advancements in the profession but also to meet the needs of today's radiography students. The major changes in this edition are highlighted below.

FULL COLOR THROUGHOUT!

The Golden Anniversary Edition of *Merrill's Atlas* will be the first-ever full-color anatomy and positioning text. As readers will quickly notice, full color greatly enhances the learning value of the anatomy illustrations and positioning photographs, making what has always been the best-illustrated anatomy and positioning text an even more effective learning tool.

NEW 3-D LINE ART

Over 45 three-dimensional line illustrations are new to this edition. Each is designed to clarify anatomy or projections that are difficult to visualize. New art appears in every chapter of Volumes 1 and 2.

NEW RADIOGRAPHS

Nearly every chapter contains new high-quality radiographs, including many that demonstrate pathology. With the addition of these new images, the ninth edition has the most comprehensive collection of high-quality radiographs available to students and practitioners in a text prepared for radiographers.

COMPUTED RADIOGRAPHY

Because of the rapid expansion and acceptance of computed radiography (CR), either selected positioning considerations and modifications or special instructions are indicated where necessary. A new icon

will alert the reader to CR notes. In addition, a newly revised chapter on CR (Chapter 33) will assist the reader in understanding the principles.

CLEARER TEXT WITH MORE BULLETED LISTS AND TABLES

The entire text has been carefully edited to present information, in particular descriptions of projections, more clearly and succinctly. Chapters 1 and 3 have been completely rewritten for clarity and the introduction of new material. More bulleted lists and tables than ever before help the reader organize information and focus quickly on the most important content.

NEW ORTHOPEDIC PROJECTIONS

New projections now commonly performed in imaging departments are presented for the first time in this edition. Among the new projections are the widely requested Robert projection of the thumb, the Rafert-Long scaphoid series, the Moore sternum, and standing projections of various joints.

SUMMARY OF PROJECTIONS

At the beginning of each procedural chapter is a new summary of all the projections described in the chapter. The projections and positions are organized by anatomic area. These summaries not only give a general overview of the chapter but also serve as a study guide for students.

ESSENTIAL PROJECTIONS

Essential projections are identified with the special icon shown here:

Essential projections are those most frequently performed and determined to be necessary for competency of entry-level practitioners. Of the over 400 projections described in this atlas, 192 have been identified as essential based on the results of two extensive surveys performed in the United States and Canada.[1]

OBSOLETE PROJECTIONS DELETED

Projections identified as obsolete by the authors and the advisory board have been deleted. A summary is provided at the beginning of any chapter containing deleted projections so that the reader may refer to previous editions for information.

NEW CHAPTERS AND CONTENT

An all-new, well-illustrated section on venipuncture (in Chapter 18) provides the theoretic basis and the procedural information needed to perform venipuncture.

Another entirely new chapter on mobile radiography (Chapter 30) describes the most frequently performed mobile projections, including for the first time anywhere detailed neonatal projections. The chapter includes an extensive introduction to mobile procedures and step-by-step instructions on how to perform each projection.

Also new to this edition is a chapter on bone mineral densitometry (Chapter 39), which discusses the relatively recent history, theoretic basis, equipment, and procedures for this technology. With the increased awareness and occurrence of osteoporosis and with radiographers performing these examinations in increasing numbers, this chapter is certainly a much-needed addition.

To reflect the continued rapid advancements in mammography, Chapter 24 has been entirely revised. It now includes all the American College of Radiology (ACR) recommended mammography projections along with all-new projection illustrations. This chapter, for the first time in radiologic technology, also details mammography as performed on the male patient. Chapter 42, on qual-

ity assurance, has also been expanded to include the latest ACR quality assurance procedures.

METRIC FILM SIZES

Because most radiographic film can no longer be purchased in English sizes, metric measurements are now used to state most film sizes. To ease the transition from English to metric, the English film size is parenthetically listed after the metric. For example, the traditional 14 × 17 inch film is now listed as 35 × 43 cm (14 × 17 in). Chapter 1 provides an introduction and discussion of the new metric sizes.

SUMMARY OF ANATOMY

At the beginning of each procedural chapter, the anatomic terms described and identified are succinctly summarized in a box. These boxes will enable readers, particularly students, to easily identify or study the anatomy described.

STANDARDIZED ANATOMY TERMINOLOGY

In the two previous editions of this atlas, the transition to new anatomic terminology was ongoing, with the more widely adopted anatomic term listed first, followed by the older term in parentheses (e.g., scaphoid [navicular]). In preparing this edition, we carefully reviewed the most widely used and adopted anatomy and physiology textbooks to identify the one anatomic term most commonly used in each case. After 8 years of printing dual anatomic terms, the secondary terms have been deleted from this edition.

Over 75 new anatomic terms have been introduced based on a comprehensive review of the widely used anatomy and physiology textbooks. The anatomy sections now present comprehensive anatomy equaling that of dedicated anatomy texts. An appendix at the end of volumes 1 and 2 contains a summary of the new and changed anatomic terms for this edition.

Learning Aids for the Student

POCKET GUIDE TO RADIOGRAPHY

A new edition of *Pocket Guide to Radiography* complements the revision of *Merrill's Atlas*. In addition to instruc-

tions for positioning the patient and the body part for all the essential projections, the new pocket guide includes information on computed radiography (CR) and automatic exposure control (AEC). Space is provided for writing department techniques specific to the user.

RADIOGRAPHIC ANATOMY, POSITIONING, AND PROCEDURES WORKBOOK BY STEVEN G. HAYES, SR.

The new edition of this two-volume workbook retains the features that made it so popular in its first edition: anatomy labeling exercises, positioning exercises, self-tests, and an answer key. The exercises include labeling of anatomy on drawings and radiographs, crossword puzzles, matching, short answers, and true/false. At the end of each chapter is a multiple-choice test to help students assess their comprehension of the whole chapter. New to this edition are more film evaluations to give students additional opportunities to evaluate images for proper positioning and more positioning questions to complement the workbook's strong anatomy review.

Teaching Aids for the Instructor

COMPUTERIZED TEST BANK BY EUGENE D. FRANK

An expanded, easy-to-use test bank of over 1200 questions, available electronically, facilitates test preparation. The test bank is on CD-ROM and can be used in both Mac and Windows environments.

MOSBY'S RADIOGRAPHIC INSTRUCTIONAL SERIES: RADIOGRAPHIC ANATOMY, POSITIONING, AND PROCEDURES

This multimedia program covers anatomy and the most commonly requested projections, with over 2200 images and over 20 hours of audio available in two formats: slides with audiotapes or CD-ROM for Windows. The program can be used for lecture support in the classroom or for self-directed learning and review by individual students in the media lab. The professionally recorded audio track discusses positioning of the patient and body part, central ray angle, and evaluation criteria.

[1]Ballinger PW, Glassner JL: Positioning competencies for radiography graduates, *Radiol Technol* 70:181-196, 1998.

RADIOGRAPHIC ANATOMY, POSITIONING, AND PROCEDURES INSTRUCTOR'S MANUAL REVISED BY CURT L. SERBUS, MEd, RT(R)

The Radiographic Anatomy, Positioning, and Procedures Instructor's Manual is available to help you enliven your teaching with *Merrill's Atlas* and the multimedia program, *Mosby's Radiographic Instructional Series: Radiographic Anatomy, Positioning, and Procedures*. The instructor's manual contains chapter outlines, teaching strategies, and a print version of the audio track from the multimedia program to aid in your planning.

We hope you will find this Golden Anniversary Edition of *Merrill's Atlas of Radiographic Positions and Radiologic Procedures* the best ever. Input from generations of readers has helped to keep the atlas strong through nine editions, and we welcome your comments and suggestions. We are constantly striving to build on Vinita Merrill's work, and we trust that she would be proud and pleased to know that the work she began 50 years ago is still so appreciated and valued by the imaging sciences community.

Philip W. Ballinger
Eugene D. Frank

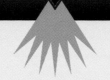

ACKNOWLEDGMENTS

As with any publication or project, those identified as the authors could never accomplish all that needs to be done without the help and support of others. The Golden Anniversary Edition of the atlas is the result of the work of many, many individuals who provided assistance along the way.

Advisory Board

In preparing for the ninth edition, our advisory board continually provided professional expertise and aid in decision making on the revision of this edition. The advisory board members are listed on page vi. We are most grateful for their input and contributions to this edition of the atlas.

Anatomy Summaries

The design and content of the new anatomy summaries seen in each procedural chapter were completed by Ellen Collins, MS, RT(R)(M), and Paula Maramonte, MEd, RT(R).

Contributors: Past and Current Editions

We are pleased to identify and credit those who served as contributing authors or who submitted high-quality radiographic images that have been published in the text over the years. We extend our heartfelt thanks to all of them for their significant contributions. These individuals are identified in special sections on pages xv-xvi.

Reviewers

The group of radiography professionals listed below extensively reviewed this edition of the atlas and made many insightful suggestions for strengthening the atlas. We are most appreciative of their willingness to lend their expertise.

Janice M. Blanchard, RT(R)
Sharyn D. Gibson, EdD, RT(R)
Robin Jones, MS, RT(R)
David Lindsay, PhD
Cynthia Liotta, MS, RT(R)
Beckey Miller, MS, RT(R)
Marsha M. Sortor, MHE, RT(R)(N)(M)
O. Scott Staley, MS, RT(R)
Beverly J. Tupper, BS, RT(R)(CV)
Rhonda Stadt Wahl, PhD
P.W.B. and E.D.F.

Special Acknowledgments, P.W.B

I wish to extend special thanks to **Eugene D. Frank.** Your efforts made this ninth edition possible. Gene's involvement in the eighth edition set the stage for his becoming a co-author on the ninth. Gene, I am pleased to welcome you to *Merrill's Atlas.*

This edition includes many new illustrations and radiographs. I want to thank **Mr. Harry Condry,** who kept track of my many photography orders. To **Theron Ellinger,** thanks for printing numerous illustrations used to replace those from the eighth and earlier editions. Thanks also to **Jennifer Torbert,** senior medical photographer, for many of the new photographs in this edition.

I have had the privilege of working with Mosby for nearly 20 years and during that time, I have worked with several editors. To my first editor and now publisher, **Don Ladig,** I thank you for your continuous support for nearly 20 years. To **Jeanne Rowland,** Executive Editor, I also thank you for your work over two editions. Sometimes we've missed a deadline, but in the end, we've always published on schedule. To **Carole Glauser,** Developmental Editor, and **Jennifer Genett,** Editorial Assistant, and to **René Saller** and **Barrett Schroeder,** Production Editors, thank you for keeping the project continually moving in the right direction.

To my family, where do I commence to say thank you? Your love and support have been ever-present. To my father-in-law, **L. Neil Hathaway** and his wife **Ruth,** thank you for your continuing love, support, and affection. Your understanding and acceptance are certainly appreciated.

To my parents, **D. W.** and **Mildred Ballinger,** too many times I could not, or did not, take the time to provide assistance and show my appreciation and love. I publicly thank you and acknowledge your support, commencing when I first announced three decades ago that I was going into "x-ray." To my sister, **Ms. Sandra Jameson** and her husband **Tom,** thank you for always being there to lighten up the situation.

To my registered nurse son, **Eric,** and professional baker and pastry chef daughter, **Monica,** wow, you grew up too fast. Too many times I was not available because I was at a professional meeting, making a presentation, or working on "the book," as it is described in our house. I love you both, and thank you for making me proud with your recent graduations.

To my wife, **Nancy,** our nearly 30 years of marriage have been a real trip—yes, many times going too fast and in too many directions. While I was out on book-related matters, you were always available to support the family. You also responded to my asking innumerable times, "Hey, Nanc, got a minute?" You were, and still are, my source for proofreading, ideas, and conceptual advice. Since my 1995 health challenge, your love and affection have been more apparent than ever, and for that I am extremely grateful. Thank you, Nancy.

Special Acknowledgments, E.D.F.

Preparation of a comprehensive textbook such as *Merrill's Atlas* requires the support of numerous individuals. **Phil Ballinger** served as my mentor during the past 3½ years of revising over 1600 pages of text and nearly 3000 illustrations. With your direct guidance, Phil, this monumental task was eventually completed. Thank you for "teaching me the ropes."

It is with great pleasure that I acknowledge the significant contributions of the following individuals from various departments of the Mayo Clinic. **David A. Factor,** medical illustrator, designed and created over 45 new anatomic line drawings that enhance every aspect of this edition. **Joseph M. Kane,** professional photographer, produced over 150 new color figures, including all the photography in the venipuncture, mobile, and mammography chapters. **Merlin K. Schrieber,** photographic printer, hand printed over 50 new radiographic images, including many that took hours to get just right. **Nancy J. Baker,** medical secretary, typed, formatted, and organized hundreds of pages of new and revised text. She also meticulously managed a database of every anatomic term and projection in the entire atlas for the new anatomy and projection summaries. **Susan K. Cosgrove,** medical secretary, and **Kevin C. Seisler, BA, RT(R),** Assistant Director of the Mayo Radiography Program, supported this entire project by keeping various aspects of the Radiography Program here at Mayo operational during my absences. Faculty members **Beverly J. Tupper, BS, RT(R)(CV), Janice M. Blanchard, RT(R), S. Jo Dean, RT(R),** and **Kari W. Wetterlin, MA, RT(R),** gathered all the new radiographs that are included in every chapter of this edition. Thank you all.

Steven G. Hayes, MEd, RT(R), author of the accompanying workbook, played a significant role in suggesting items for revision and helping to standardize various aspects of the atlas.

I am greatly indebted to the Advisory Board members, **Joyce Ortego, MS, RT(R), Rita M. Oswald, BS, RT(R)(CV), Curt L. Serbus, MEd, RT(R),** and **Bettye Wilson, MA, RT(R)(CT), RDMS,** who assisted in the major decisions regarding new text, illustrations, critical editing, and new chapters. They tackled every challenge with enthusiasm and enjoyed every challenging query. Thanks to this highly talented and experienced group of radiography educators, this edition of the atlas is technically the best it can be.

Medical illustrators **Jeanne Robertson** and **Nadine Sokol** did an excellent job of accurately colorizing every line drawing in the atlas—a monumental task.

Linda Wendling, of Wordbench, assisted in the initial organization of all the chapters and figures. Linda's enthusiastic approach to her part of the work launched the developmental process on a positive note.

My close friend **Kenneth L. Bontrager, MA, RT(R),** assisted in standardizing many terms, central ray angles, positioning techniques, and other technical aspects in both of our textbooks. Our goal was to reduce discrepancies in our textbooks and make learning easier for students.

My wife, **Jane Frank,** and children, **Matthew** and **Jillian Frank,** supported and encouraged me as I worked many long hours preparing this edition. Thank you for your support of all my professional work.

Lastly, I extend special thanks to **Jeanne Rowland,** Executive Editor, who invited me to co-author the atlas. Along with Jeanne, **Cathy Comer, Renée Duenow, Carole Glauser, Jennifer Genett, Linda McKinley, René Saller,** and **Barrett Schroeder** played significant roles in producing the Golden Anniversary Edition of the atlas. My experience with the entire Mosby editorial and production team has been very enjoyable, rewarding, and interestingly, "fun."

Contributors to Past Editions

For this fiftieth anniversary edition, we want to give credit to all those who have contributed specialty chapters to the atlas over its first eight editions. Because of the contributions of the professionals listed below, the atlas has presented the most current information available in not only general radiography but all the special imaging modalities.

Mel Allen
Albert Aziza*
Thomas J. Beck
Dr. David L. Benninghoff
Mary J. Blome
Michael R. Bloyd*
Barbara A. Blunt*
Dr. Carl R. Bogardus, Jr.
Steven J. Bollin, Sr.
Jeffrey A. Books*
Michael G. Bruckner*
Terri Bruckner*
Dr. Stewart C. Bushong*
Leila A. Bussman*
John Michael Chudik
Dorothea F. Cook
Luann J. Culbreth*
Barbara M. Curcio
Chris Democko
Dr. John P. Dorst
Paul Early
Dr. James H. Ellis
William F. Finney*
Joseph Fodor, III
Dr. Atis K. Freimanis
Sandra Hagen-Ansert*
H. Dale Hamilton

Dr. Marcus W. Hedgcock
Dr. Richard D. Hichwa*
Nancy L. Hockert*
Jeffrey A. Huff*
Keith R. Johnson
Kenneth C. Johnson
Joseph W. Kaplan
Lorrie L. Kelley*
Nina Kowalczyk*
Dr. Robert A. Kruger
Dr. Richard G. Lester
Jack C. Malott
Charles E. Marschke
Philip R. Maynard
Deirdre Milne*
Stephen T. Montelli
Dr. John O. Olsen
Richard C. Paskiet, Jr.
Dr. Walter W. Peppler*
Rex E. Profit*
Sheila Rosenfeld
Dr. Ronald J. Ross
Terese McShane Roth*
Dr. Alan H. Rowberg
Ann Hrica Seglinski
William J. Setlak
Dr. William H. Shehadi
Dr. Roy D. Strand
Donald L. Sucher
Carole A. Sullivan
Dwayne J. Termaat
Dr. Michael E. Van Aman
Dr. Jane A. Van Valkenburg*
Rome V. Wadlington
Dr. Ronald D. Weinstein
Kari J. Wetterlin*
Joan A. Wodarski

*Ninth edition contributors

Radiograph Contributions

The authors would like to extend a special note of gratitude to all those who have contributed radiographs to *Merrill's Atlas* over its nine editions. Thanks to them, the collection of radiographs in the atlas is judged the finest of any radiography positioning textbook. Thousands of radiography students, radiologic technologists, and physicians around the world who regularly use the atlas are able to learn more effectively from the high-quality radiographs.

To our readers, we continue to extend an invitation to send us any radiographs that you feel could be used in the atlas or any that are of better quality than those that now appear in the book. Our goal is to provide our profession with the finest collection of radiographs for learning and reference purposes.

Sidney Alexander
Marek Anderson
April S. Apple
Kim Bailey
Lois Baird
Dr. David H. Baker
Annette Baldwin
Steve Bargiel
Karen J. Bauer
Dr. Joshua A. Becker
Dr. Javier Beltran
Dr. David L. Benninghoff
Dr. Walter E. Berdon
Dr. David Bloom
Steven J. Bollin, Sr.
Dr. Jacques Boreau
Frank J. Brewster
Dr. Michael Burman
Kalma Butler
Fayette Capik
Beth Changet
Patti Chapman
Dianna Childs
Dr. K. Y. Chynn
Roland Clements
Dr. Arthur R. Clemett
Sharon A. Coffey
Dr. Constantine Cope
Carol Corder
Sylvia L. Cousins
Karen Cox
Karen Cubler
Julianne M. Curtin
Jeannie M. Danker
Dr. Howard P. Daub

Barbara Davis
Laurie Davis
Peter DeGraaf
Betsy Delzeith
Michael DeSalu
Terry Doherty
Carol Drobik
Dr. Albert A. Dunn
Kimberly Edgar
Dr. Milton Elkin
Dr. Bernard S. Epstein
Dr. John A. Evans
Gail A. Fisher
Michael Franklin
Dr. Robert H. Freiberger
Laurie Funk
Heide Galli
Dr. Francis H. Ghiselin
Colleen Gillespie
Delores Goodwin
Dr. John A. Goree
Edward F. Gunson
Norma Harmon
Dr. Robert Harris
Colleen Harty
Dr. Herbert F. Hempel
Timothy Hill
Robbie F. Hockenberry
Jana Hoffman
Paul T. Ichino
Dr. Harold G. Jacobson
Angelique Jacopin
Emelda James
Eva M. James
Dr. James Jerele
Dr. John C. Johnson
David M. Jones
Darla Kaikis
Ann Kay
Marilyn Knight
Jane Kober
Nina Kowalczyk
D. Peter Kuum
Carmela Kvas
Dr. Roger W. Lambie
Dr. Oswald S. Lowsley
Marigold Marsh
Dr. Richard H. Marshak
Charles McCartly
Judy McLaughlin
Deborah Meeker
Dr. Alan C. Merchant
Tom Meridith
Jonathan Miller
Dr. Lawson E. Miller, Jr.
Randy Miller
Dr. Roscoe E. Miller
Betty Jo Mixon
Martha Montalvo

Leon Montgomery
Stephen G. Moon
Carrol Moore
Susan M. Orlando
Javier Pagan
Eric Parsels
Nancy Patfield
Sharon Peterson
Dr. Raymond Pfeiffer
Dr. Robert L. Pinck
Dr. Etta Pisano
W. William Pollino
Dr. Michael Portnoff
M. G. Rauckis
Lynn Rhatigan
Brenda J. Rogers
Jeffrey L. Rowe
Stephen Rusk
Ammar Saadeh
Valerie Sasson
Deborah Saunders
David R. Schumick
Dr. William B. Seaman
Dr. William H. Shehadi
Keith Shipman
Holly Simmons
Daphne Smith
Dr. John Spellmeyer
Dr. Ramsay Spillman
Theresa Spotts
Dr. William Z. Stern
Cheryl Stillberger
Dr. Harold L. Stitt
Dr. Marcy L. Sussman
Cindy Swords
John Syring
Joyce Tarzewski
Rinette Tavitri
Tracy Taylor
James B. Temme
Ellen S. Titen
Lyn Van Dervort
Cindy Wedel
Dr. Solve Welin
Annette Wendt
Thomas White
Jennifer Wilkes
Dr. A. Justin Williams
Linda Willman
Dr. Hudson J. Wilson, Jr.
Dr. Hugh M. Wilson
Deborah Wolfenberger
Dr. Ernest H. Wood
Ross J. Wright
Dr. Martin Yaffe
Dr. Judah Zizmor
Elizabeth Zuffuto

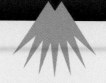

CONTENTS

MERRILL'S ATLAS

of

RADIOGRAPHIC POSITIONS

and

RADIOLOGIC PROCEDURES

VOLUME THREE

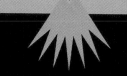

CENTRAL NERVOUS SYSTEM

NINA KOWALCZYK

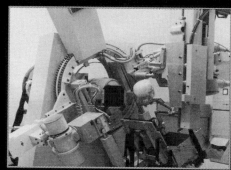

RIGHT: Somersault chair used for pneumoencephalography. In this procedure, holes were drilled in the patient's skull and air was injected into the ventricles. The patient was then somersaulted so that the air could rise to the highest point. Radiographs were taken to detect any space-occupying lesions of the brain.

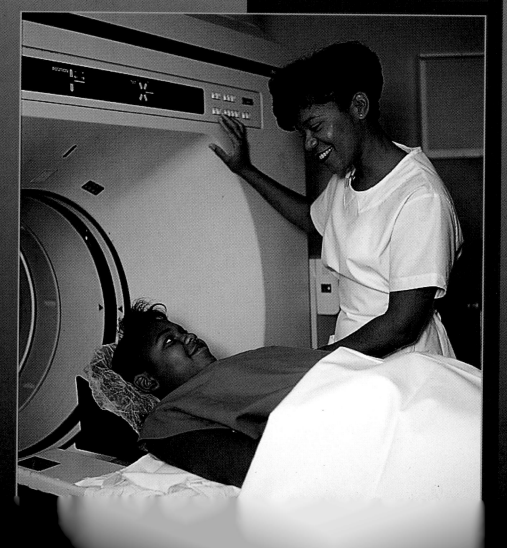

LEFT: Technologist preparing patient for computed tomography examination.

(From Kowalczyk N, Donnett K: *Integrated patient care for the imaging professional*, St Louis 1996 Mosby.)

For descriptive purposes, the central nervous system (CNS) is divided into two parts: (1) the *brain,* which occupies the cranial cavity, and (2) the *spinal cord,* which is suspended within the vertebral canal.

Brain

The brain is composed of an outer portion of gray matter called the *cortex* and an inner portion of *white matter.* The brain consists of the *cerebrum,* the *cerebellum,* and the *brainstem,* which is continuous with the spinal cord (Fig. 25-1). The brainstem consists of the *midbrain, pons,* and *medulla oblongata.*

The cerebrum is the largest part of the brain and is referred to as the *forebrain.* Its surface is convoluted by sulci and grooves that divide it into lobes and lobules. The stemlike portion that connects the cerebrum to the pons and cerebellum is termed the *midbrain.* The cerebellum, pons, and medulla oblongata make up the *hindbrain.*

A deep cleft, called the *longitudinal sulcus,* separates the cerebrum into *right* and *left hemispheres,* which are closely connected by bands of nerve fibers, or commissures. The main commissure between the cerebral hemispheres is the *corpus callosum.* Each cerebral hemisphere contains a fluid-filled cavity called a *lateral ventricle.* At the diencephalon, or second portion of the brain, the cerebral hemispheres surround the *third ventricle.* Extending inferiorly from the diencephalon is the *pituitary gland;* the endocrine gland resides in the hypophyseal fossa of the sella turcica.

The cerebellum, the largest part of the hindbrain, is separated from the cerebrum by a deep transverse cleft. The hemispheres of the cerebellum are connected by a median constricted area called the *vermis.* The surface of the cerebellum contains numerous transverse sulci that account for its laminated appearance. The tissues between the curved sulci are called *folia.* The pons, which forms the upper part of the hindbrain, is the commissure (coming together across the midline) between the cerebrum, cerebellum, and medulla. The medulla, which extends between the pons and spinal cord, forms the lower portion of the hindbrain.

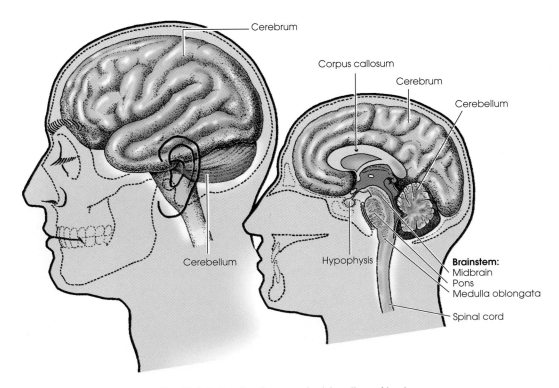

Fig. 25-1 Lateral surface and midsection of brain.

Spinal Cord

The *spinal cord* is a slender, elongated structure consisting of an inner, gray, cellular substance, which has an **H** shape on transverse section, and an outer, white, fibrous substance (Figs. 25-2 and 25-3). The cord extends from the brain, where it is connected to the medulla oblongata at the level of the foramen magnum, to the approximate level of the space between the first and second lumbar vertebrae. The spinal cord ends in a pointed extremity. A delicate, fibrous strand extending from the terminal tip attaches the cord to the upper coccygeal segment.

The spinal cord is connected to 31 pairs of spinal nerves, each arising from two roots at the sides of the spinal cord. The nerves are transmitted through the intervertebral and sacral foramina. Spinal nerves below the termination of the spinal cord extend inferiorly through the vertebral canal. These nerves resemble a horse's tail and are referred to as the *cauda equina.*

Meninges

The brain and spinal cord are enclosed in three continuous, protective membranes called *meninges.* The inner sheath, called the *pia mater* (Latin, "tender mother"), is highly vascular and closely adherent to the underlying brain and cord structure.

The delicate central sheath is called the *arachnoid.* This membrane is separated from the pia mater by a comparatively wide space called the *subarachnoid space,* which is widened in certain areas. These areas of increased width are called *cisternae.* The widest area is the cisterna cerebellomedullaris. This triangular cavity is situated at the posterosuperior part of the subarachnoid space between the base of the cerebellum and the dorsal surface of the medulla oblongata. The subarachnoid space is continuous with the ventricular system of the brain and communicates with it by way of the median aperture and by lateral apertures located between the cisterna cerebellomedullaris and the fourth ventricle. The ventricles of the brain and the subarachnoid space contain cerebrospinal fluid (CSF). The cisterna cerebellomedullaris is sometimes used as a point of entry into the subarachnoid space.

The outermost sheath, called the *dura mater* (Latin, "hard mother"), forms the strong, fibrous covering of the brain and spinal cord. The dura is separated from the arachnoid by the *subdural space* and from the vertebral periosteum by the *epidural space.* These spaces do not communicate with the ventricular system. The dura mater is composed of two layers throughout its cranial portion. The outer layer lines the cranial bones, thus serving as periosteum to their inner surface. The inner layer protects the brain and supports the blood vessels. The layer also has four partitions that provide support and protection for the various parts of the brain. The dura mater extends below the spinal cord (to the level of the second sacral segment) to enclose the spinal nerves, which are prolonged inferiorly from the cord to their respective exits. The lower portion of the dura mater is called the *dural sac.*

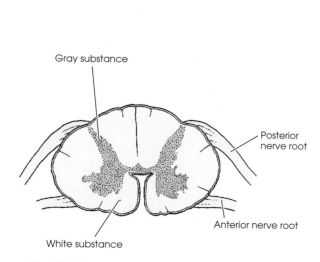

Fig. 25-2 Transverse section of spinal cord.

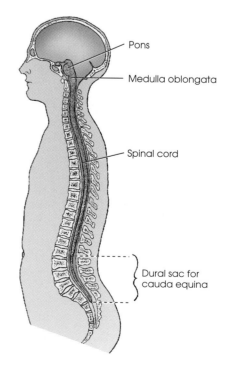

Fig. 25-3 Sagittal section showing spinal cord.

Ventricular System

The ventricular system of the brain consists of four irregular, fluid-containing cavities that communicate with one another through connecting channels (Figs. 25-4 to 25-6). The two upper cavities are an identical pair and are simply called the *right* and *left lateral ventricles*. They are situated, one on each side of the midsagittal plane, in the inferior medial part of the corresponding hemisphere of the cerebrum.

Each lateral ventricle consists of a central portion called the *body* of the cavity. The body is prolonged anteriorly, posteriorly, and inferiorly into hornlike portions that give the ventricle an approximate U shape. The prolonged portions are known as the *anterior, posterior,* and *inferior horns.* Each lateral ventricle is connected to the third ventricle by a channel called the *intraventricular foramen,* through which it communicates directly with the third ventricle and indirectly with the opposite lateral ventricle.

The *third ventricle* is a slitlike cavity with a somewhat quadrilateral shape. It is situated in the midsagittal plane just inferior to the level of the bodies of the lateral ventricles. This cavity extends anteroinferiorly from the pineal gland, which produces a recess in its posterior wall, to the optic chiasm, which produces a recess in its anteroinferior wall.

The interventricular foraminae, one from each lateral ventricle, open into the anterosuperior portion of the third ventricle. The cavity is continuous posteroinferiorly with the fourth ventricle by a passage known as the *cerebral aqueduct.*

The *fourth ventricle* is diamond shaped and is the cavity of the hindbrain. It is also a midline structure located anterior to the cerebellum and posterior to the pons and the upper portion of the medulla oblongata. The distal, pointed end of the fourth ventricle is continuous with the central canal of the medulla oblongata. The fourth ventricle communicates with the subarachnoid space via the *median aperture* and the *lateral apertures* (as discussed earlier in this chapter).

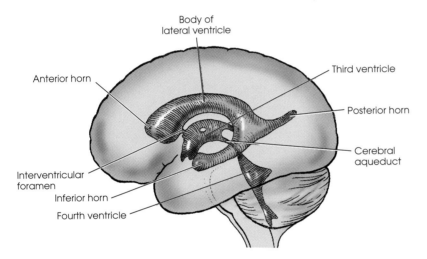

Fig. 25-4 Lateral aspect of cerebral ventricles in relation to surface of brain.

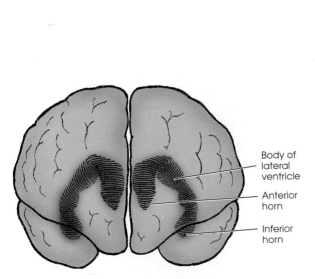

Fig. 25-5 Anterior aspect of lateral cerebral ventricles in relation to surface of brain.

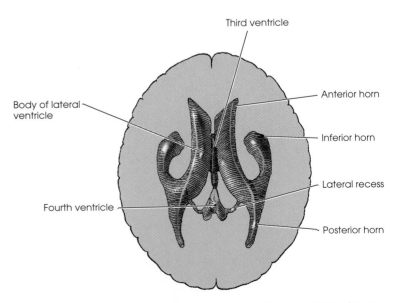

Fig. 25-6 Superior aspect of cerebral ventricles in relation to surface of brain.

Plain Radiographic Examination

Neuroradiologic assessment should begin with noninvasive imaging procedures. Radiographs of the cerebral and visceral cranium and the vertebral column may be employed to demonstrate bony anatomy. In traumatized patients, radiographs are obtained to detect bony injury, subluxation, or dislocation of the vertebral column and to determine the extent and stability of the bony injury.

For a traumatized patient with possible CNS involvement, a cross-table lateral cervical spine radiograph should be obtained first to rule out fracture or misalignment of the cervical spine. Approximately two thirds of significant pathologic conditions affecting the spine can be detected on this initial image. Care must be taken to demonstrate the entire cervical spine adequately, including the C7-T1 articulation. It may be necessary to employ the Twining (Swimmers) method (see Chapter 8) to demonstrate this anatomic region radiographically.

After the cross-table lateral radiograph has been checked and cleared by a physician, the following cervical spine projections should be obtained: an AP projection, bilateral AP oblique projections (trauma technique may be necessary), and an AP projection of the dens. A vertebral arch, or pillar image, of the cervical spine may provide additional information about the posterior portions of the cervical vertebrae (see Chapter 8). An upright lateral cervical spine radiograph may also be requested to better demonstrate alignment of the vertebrae and to assess the normal lordotic curvature of the spine.

Tomography may be used to supplement images of the spine for initial screening purposes (see Chapter 29). However, tomography has been largely replaced by computed tomography (CT) in many institutions (see Chapter 33). Tomography may be employed to demonstrate long, continuous areas of the spine; the use of CT for this purpose is restricted by the design and reconstruction limitations of the equipment. Disadvantages of tomography include the lack of soft tissue detail and the difficulty in positioning a traumatized patient for lateral tomographic radiographs.

Radiographs of the spine should always be obtained prior to myelography. Routine images of the vertebral column are helpful in assessing narrowed disk spaces because of degeneration of the disk, postoperative changes in the spine, and osteopetrosis of the vertebral column. Because the contrast agents used in myelography may obscure some anomalies, plain spinal images complement the myelographic examination and often provide additional information.

Routine skull images should be obtained when the possibility of a skull fracture exists. In trauma patients a cross-table lateral or upright lateral skull radiograph must be obtained to demonstrate air-fluid levels in the sphenoid sinus. In many instances these air-fluid levels may be the initial indication of a basilar skull fracture. In addition, skull images are helpful in diagnosing reactive bone formation and general alterations in the skull resulting from a variety of pathologic conditions, including Paget's disease, fibrous dysplasia, hemangiomas, and changes in the sella turcica.

Myelography

Myelography (Greek, *myelos*, "marrow; the spinal cord") is the general term applied to radiologic examination of the CNS structures situated within the vertebral canal. This examination is performed by introducing a contrast medium into the subarachnoid space by spinal puncture, most commonly at the L2-L3 or L3-L4 interspace or at the cisterna cerebellomedullaris.

Most myelograms are performed on an outpatient basis, with patients recovering for approximately 4 to 8 hours after the procedure before being released to return home. In many parts of the country, however, magnetic resonance imaging (MRI) has largely replaced myelography. Yet myelography continues to be the preferred examination method for assessing disk disease in patients with contraindications to MRI such as pacemakers or metallic posterior spinal fusion rods.

Myelography is employed to demonstrate extrinsic spinal cord compression caused by a herniated disk, bone fragments, or tumors, as well as spinal cord swelling resulting from traumatic injury. These encroachments appear radiographically as a deformity in the subarachnoid space or an obstruction of the passage of the column of contrast medium within the subarachnoid space. Myelography is also useful in identifying narrowing of the subarachnoid space by evaluating the dynamic flow patterns of the CSF.

CONTRAST MEDIA

A nonwater-soluble, iodinated ester (iophendylate [Pantopaque]) was introduced in 1942. It was used in myelography for many years but is no longer commercially available. The first water-soluble, nonionic, iodinated contrast agent, metrizamide, was introduced in the late 1970s. Thereafter, water-soluble contrast media quickly became the agents of choice. Nonionic, water-soluble contrast media provide good visualization of nerve roots (Fig. 25-7) and good enhancement for follow-up CT of the spine. In addition, these agents are readily absorbed by the body. One disadvantage of metrizamide was its tendency to be absorbed very quickly. Therefore radiographs must be produced promptly and accurately.

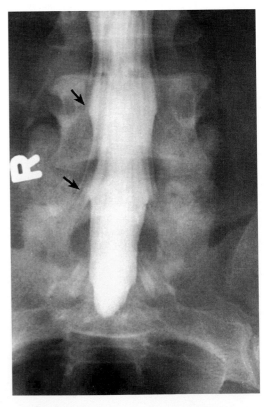

Fig. 25-7 Myelogram using water-soluble contrast medium (metrizamide). Nerve roots seen at arrows.

Further research led to the introduction of improved nonionic contrast agents such as iohexol, iopamidol, and ioversol in the mid 1980s. Improvements in nonionic contrast agents have resulted in fewer side effects. Consequently, they have become the preferred contrast media for both conventional and CT myelography (Fig. 25-8).

PREPARATION OF EXAMINING ROOM

One of the radiographer's responsibilities is to prepare the examining room before the patient's arrival. The radiographic equipment should be checked. Because the procedure involves aseptic technique, the table and overhead equipment must be cleaned. The footboard should be attached to the table, and the padded shoulder supports should be placed and ready for adjustment to the patient's height. The image intensifier should be locked so that it cannot accidentally come in contact with the spinal needle and/or sterile field.

The spinal puncture and contrast medium injection are performed in the radiology department. Under fluoroscopic observation, placement of the 20- to 22-gauge spinal needle in the subarachnoid space is verified, and the contrast medium is injected. The sterile tray and the non-sterile items required for this initial procedure should be ready for convenient placement.

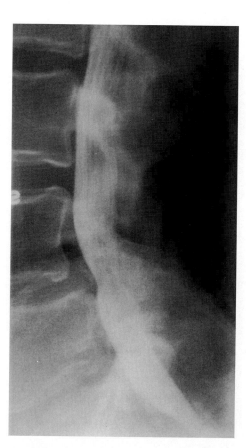

Fig. 25-8 Lateral projection of lumbar spine myelogram using water-soluble contrast medium (iohexol).

EXAMINATION PROCEDURE

Premedication of the patient for myelography is rarely necessary. The patient should be well hydrated, however, because a nonionic, water-soluble contrast medium is used. To reduce apprehension and prevent alarm at unexpected maneuvers during the procedure, the radiographer should explain the details of myelography to the patient before the examination begins. The patient should be informed that the angulation of the examining table will repeatedly and acutely change. The patient should also be told why the head must be maintained in a fully extended position when the table is tilted to the Trendelenburg position. The radiographer must provide assurance that the patient will be safe when the table is acutely angled and that everything possible will be done to avoid causing unnecessary discomfort.

Some physicians prefer to have the patient placed on the table in the prone position for the spinal puncture. Most, however, have the patient adjusted in the lateral position with the spine flexed to widen the interspinous spaces for easier introduction of the needle.

The physician usually withdraws CSF for laboratory analysis and injects approximately 9 to 12 ml of contrast medium. After completing the injection, the physician removes the spinal needle. Travel of the contrast medium column is observed fluoroscopically, and the direction of its flow is controlled by varying the angulation of the table. The radiographer obtains images at the level of any blockage or distortion in the outline of the contrast column. Conventional radiographic studies, with the central ray directed vertically or horizontally, may be performed as requested by the radiologist. Cross-table lateral radiographs are obtained with grid-front cassettes or a stationary grid; they must be closely collimated (Figs. 25-9 to 25-13).

The position of the patient's head must be guarded as the contrast column nears the cervical area to prevent the medium from passing into the cerebral ventricles. Acute extension of the head compresses the cisterna cerebellomedullaris and thus prevents further ascent of the medium. Because the cisterna cerebellomedullaris is situated posteriorly, neither forward nor lateral flexion of the head compresses the cisternal cavity.

After the procedure the patient must be monitored in an appropriate recovery area. Most physicians recommend that the patient's head and shoulders be elevated 30 to 45 degrees during recovery. The puncture site must be examined before the patient is released from the recovery area.

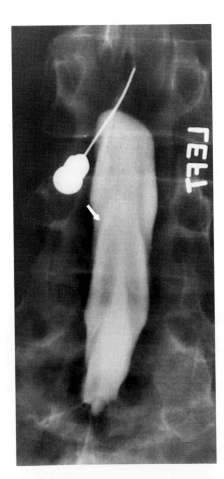

Fig. 25-9 Lumbar myelogram: AP projection with nonwater-soluble iodinated contrast medium, showing axillary pouches and corresponding nerve roots (*arrow*).

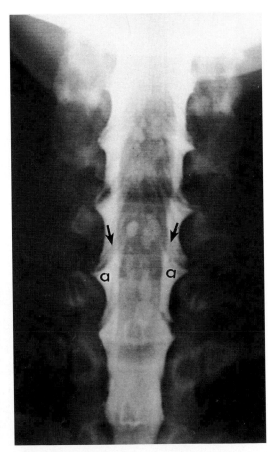

Fig. 25-10 Cervical myelogram: AP projection showing symmetric nerve roots (*arrows*) and axillary pouches (*a*) on both sides, as well as spinal cord.

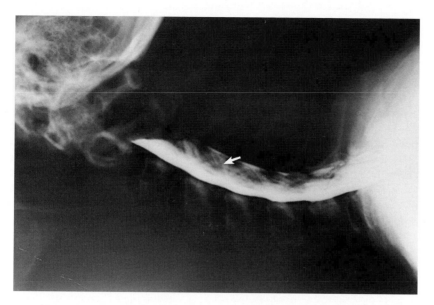

Fig. 25-11 Myelogram: prone cross-table lateral projection showing dentate ligament and posterior nerve roots *(arrow).*

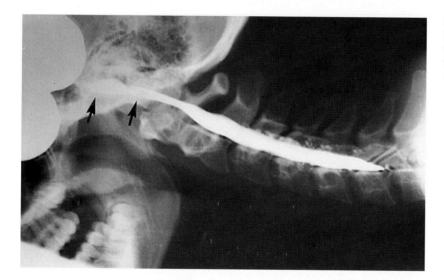

Fig. 25-12 Myelogram: prone, cross-table lateral projection showing contrast medium passing through foramen magnum and lying against lower clivus *(arrows).*

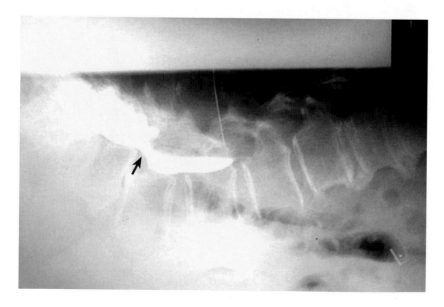

Fig. 25-13 Myelogram: cross-table lateral projection showing subarachnoid space narrowing *(arrow).*

Computed Tomography

CT is a rapid, noninvasive imaging technique that was first introduced for clinical use in the early 1970s. CT imaging of the head and spine expanded rapidly because of improvements in computer technology and this imaging modality's ability to demonstrate abnormalities with a precision never before possible.

A CT examination of the brain is commonly performed in an axial orientation with the gantry placed at an angle of 20 to 25 degrees to the orbitomeatal line, which allows the lowest slice to provide an image of both the upper cervical/foramen magnum and the roof of the orbit. Normally 12 to 14 slices are obtained, depending upon the size of the patient's head and the thickness of the CT image slices. Imaging continues superiorly until the entire head has been examined. Coronal images may also be obtained and are quite helpful in evaluating abnormalities of the pituitary gland and sella turcica. Axial slices may also be obtained during the imaging procedure, and the computer may be used to reconstruct and display the images in a variety of imaging planes.

CT scans of the brain are often obtained before and after IV injection of a nonionic, water-soluble contrast agent. These are often referred to as *preinfusion (C−)* and *postinfusion (C+)* scans. Common indications for scans with and without contrast agents include suspected primary neoplasms (Fig. 25-14); suspected metastatic disease; suspected arteriovenous malformation (AVM); demyelinating disease such as multiple sclerosis; seizure disorders; and bilateral, isodense hematomas. Common indications for CT of the brain without an IV infusion of contrast material include assessment of dementia, craniocerebral trauma, hydrocephalus, and acute infarcts. In addition, CT is often used for postevacuation follow-up examinations of hematomas.

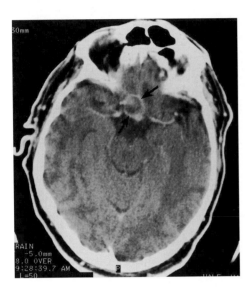

Fig. 25-14 Postinfusion (C+) CT scan of the brain, demonstrating a malignant neoplasm "highlighted" by the IV contrast material *(arrows)*.

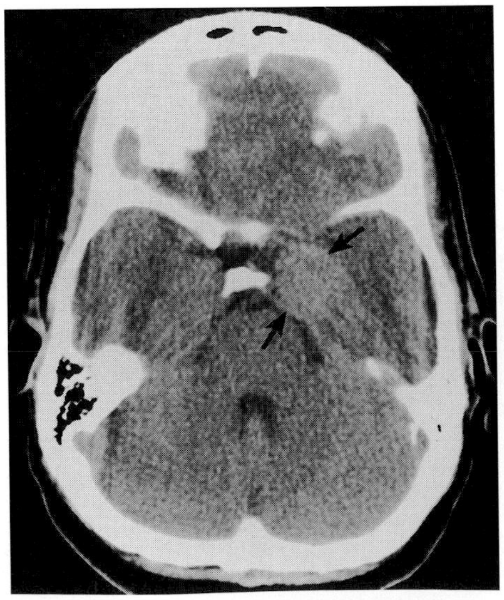

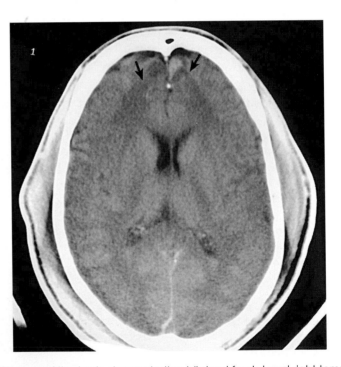

Fig. 25-16 CT scan of the brain demonstrating bilateral frontal and right temporal lobe brain contusions *(arrows)* subsequent to trauma.

Fig. 25-15 CT scan of the brain (C−) demonstrating a giant berry aneurysm *(arrows)* later confirmed by vascular imaging.

(Courtesy Brenda Dann, R.T.)

CT of the brain is particularly useful in demonstrating the size, location, and configuration of mass lesions, as well as surrounding edema. It is also quite helpful in assessing cerebral ventricle or cortical sulcus enlargement or lateral ventricle shifting resulting from the encroachment of a mass lesion, cerebral edema, or a hematoma. CT of the head is also the imaging modality of choice in evaluating hematomas, suspected aneurysms (Fig. 25-15), ischemic or hemorrhagic strokes, and acute infarcts within the brain. CT of the brain is the initial diagnostic procedure performed to assess craniocerebral trauma, because it provides a very accurate diagnosis of acute intracranial injuries, such as brain contusions (Fig. 25-16) and subarachnoid hemorrhage.

CT of the spine is helpful in diagnosing vertebral column hemangiomas and lumbar spinal stenosis. CT of the cervical spine following trauma is frequently performed to rule out fractures of the axis and atlas and to better demonstrate the lower cervical and upper thoracic vertebrae. This examination can clearly demonstrate the size, number, and location of fracture fragments in the cervical, thoracic, and lumbar spine. The information gained from the CT scans can greatly assist the surgeon (Fig. 25-17). Postoperatively, CT is used to assess the outcome of the surgical procedure.

Computed tomography myelography (CTM) involves CT examination of the vertebral column after the intrathecal injection of a water soluble contrast agent. The examination may be performed at any level of the vertebral column. Today most conventional myelograms are followed by CTM. Because CT has the ability to distinguish among relatively small differences in contrast, the contrast agent may be visualized up to 4 hours following the conventional myelogram. CTM demonstrates the size, shape, and position of the spinal cord and nerve roots (Fig. 25-18). It is extremely useful in patients with compressive injuries or in determining the extent of dural tears resulting in extravasation of the CSF. (CT is discussed further in Chapter 33.)

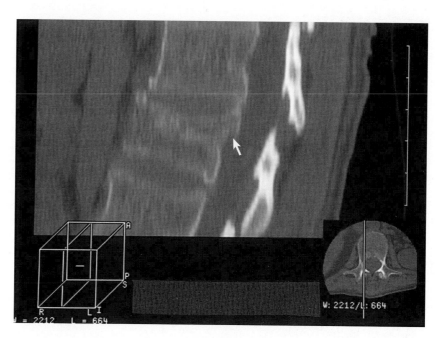

Fig. 25-17 Sagittal CT lumbar spine: reconstruction of axial images showing a compression fracture of L1 subsequent to trauma *(arrow)*.

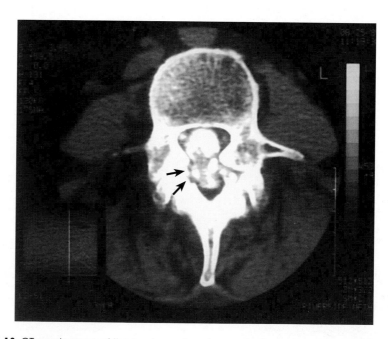

Fig. 25-18 CT myelogram of the lumbar spine demonstrating subarachnoid space narrowing *(arrows)*.

Magnetic Resonance Imaging

MRI was approved for clinical use in the early 1980s and quickly became the modality of choice for evaluating many anomalies of the brain and spinal cord. It is a noninvasive procedure that provides excellent anatomic detail of the brain, spinal cord, intervertebral disks, and CSF within the subarachnoid space. Furthermore, unlike conventional myelography, MRI of the spinal cord and subarachnoid space does not require intrathecal injection of a contrast agent.

Because MRIs are created primarily by the response of loosely bound hydrogen atoms to the magnetic field, this modality is basically "blind" to bone, unlike other conventional radiologic imaging modalities. Therefore, MRI allows clear visualization of areas of the CNS normally obscured by bone, such as the vertebral column or dense temporal bone; and in addition, the exact relationship between soft tissue structures and surrounding bony structures can be seen (Fig. 25-19). This makes MRI the preferred modality in evaluating the middle cranial fossa and posterior fossa of the brain. When these structures are imaged with CT, they are often obscured by artifacts. MRI is also the preferred modality for evaluating the spinal cord because it allows direct visualization of the cord, nerve roots, and surrounding CSF. In addition, MRI reconstruction may be performed in a variety of planes (sagittal, axial, and coronal) after acquisition (Figs. 25-20 and 25-21) to aid in the diagnosis and treatment of neurologic disorders. Both T1- and T2-weighted images are obtained to assist in the diagnosis, with a head coil used for the brain and cervical spine images and a body coil used in combination with a surface coil for the remainder of the spine.

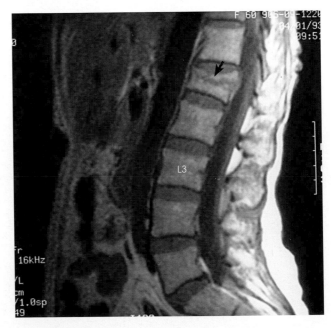

Fig. 25-19 Sagittal MRI section of the lumbar spine demonstrating a compression fracture of L1 subsequent to trauma *(arrow).*

MRI is very helpful in assessing demyelinating disease such as multiple sclerosis, spinal cord compression, paraspinal masses, postradiation therapy changes in spinal cord tumors, metastatic disease, herniated disks, and congenital anomalies of the vertebral column. In the brain, MRI is excellent for evaluating middle and posterior fossa abnormalities, acoustic neuromas, pituitary tumors, primary and metastatic neoplasms, hydrocephalus, AVMs, and brain atrophy.

Contraindications to MRI are primarily related to the use of a magnetic field. MRI should not be used in patients with pacemakers, ferromagnetic aneurysm clips, or metallic spinal fusion rods. In addition, MRI is of little value in assessing osseous bone abnormalities of the skull, intracerebral hematomas, and subarachnoid hemorrhage. CT provides better visualization of these pathologies. (Further discussion of MRI is presented in Chapter 36.)

Cardiovascular and Interventional Procedures

In general, cardiovascular and interventional procedures are performed after noninvasive evaluation techniques when it is necessary to obtain information about the vascular system or to perform an interventional technique. *Angiography* may be used to assess vascular supply to tumors, demonstrate the relationship between a mass lesion and intracerebral vessels, or illustrate anomalies of a vessel such as an aneurysm or a vascular occlusion. An angiographic procedure is performed in a specialized imaging suite under sterile conditions.

Cardiovascular and interventional imaging equipment requires biplane imaging and digital subtraction capabilities. Angiographic x-ray tubes should have a minimum focal spot size of 1.3 mm for routine imaging and a magnification focal spot size of 0.3 mm. The procedure requires the introduction of a catheter into the vascular system under fluoroscopic guidance. The image intensifier must be designed to move around the patient so that various tube angles may be obtained without moving the patient. The catheter is most commonly placed in the femoral artery; however, access may be gained using other arteries or veins, depending upon the patient's clinical history and the area of interest. After the catheter is placed in the appropriate vessel, a water-soluble contrast agent is injected into the vessels, and rapid-sequence images are obtained for evaluation.

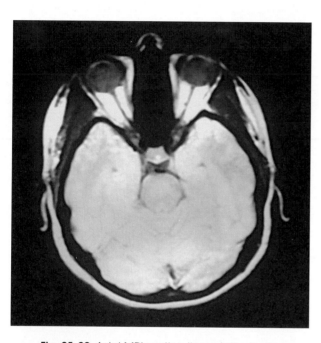

Fig. 25-20 Axial MRI section through the brain.

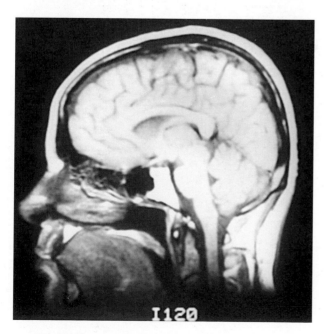

Fig. 25-21 Sagittal MRI section through the brain.

Angiography is helpful in assessing vascular abnormalities within the CNS such as AVMs, aneurysms (Fig. 25-22), subarachnoid hemorrhage, transient ischemic attacks, certain intracerebral hematomas, and cerebral venous thrombosis. It is also performed in combination with interventional techniques to assess the placement of devices before and after the procedures.

Interventional radiology involves the placement of various coils, medications, filters, or other devices to treat a particular problem or provide therapy. One type of interventional technique involves the introduction of small spheres, coils, or other materials into vessels to occlude blood flow. Embolization techniques are often performed to treat AVMs and aneurysms, and to decrease blood supply to various vascular tumors (Figs. 25-23 and 25-24). Other interventional techniques are used to open occluded vessels by the injection of specialized anticoagulant medications or by the inflation of small balloons within the vessel, as in the case of percutaneous angioplasty. In addition, therapeutic devices such as filters, stents, and shunts may be placed in the cardiovascular and interventional area, thereby eliminating the need for a more invasive surgical procedure. (Cardiovascular and interventional radiology is discussed in more detail in Chapter 26.)

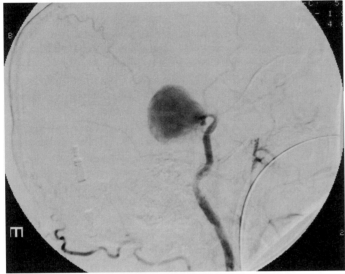

Fig. 25-22 Digital subtraction angiographic image demonstrating a large aneurysm of the right carotid artery.

(Courtesy Scott Chapman, R.T.)

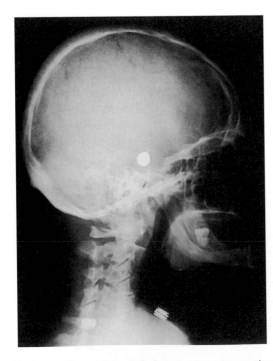

Fig. 25-23 Conventional lateral skull projection demonstrating an embolization coil placed just posterior and superior to the sella turcica.

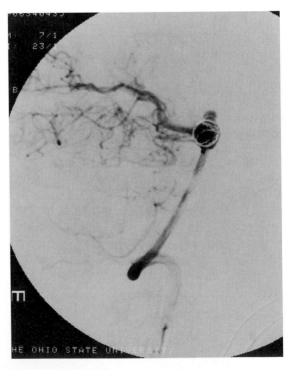

Fig. 25-24 Digital subtraction angiographic image demonstrating an embolization coil, which has been placed to treat a basilar tip aneurysm.

(Courtesy Jennifer Borucki, R.T.)

Other Neuroradiographic Procedures

Diskography and *nucleography* are terms used to denote the radiologic examination of individual intervertebral disks. The examination is performed with a small quantity of one of the water-soluble, iodinated media injected into the center of the disk by way of a double-needle entry. This procedure was introduced by Lindblom[1] in 1950, and it has been further detailed by Cloward and Buzaid,[2] Cloward,[3] and Butt.[4]

[1]Lindblom K: Technique and results in myelography and disc puncture, *Acta Radiol* 34:321, 1950.
[2]Cloward RB, Buzaid LL: Discography, *AJR* 68:552, 1952.
[3]Cloward RB: Cervical discography: a contribution to the etiology and mechanism of neck, shoulder, and arm pain, *Ann Surg* 150:1052, 1959.
[4]Butt WP: Discography—some interesting cases, *J Can Assoc Radiol* 17:167, 1966.

Diskography is used in the investigation of internal disk lesions, such as rupture of the nucleus pulposus, that cannot be demonstrated by myelographic examination (Fig. 25-25). Diskography may be performed separately, or it may be combined with myelography. Patients are given only a local anesthetic so that they remain fully conscious and therefore able to inform the physician about pain when the needles are inserted and the injection is made. MRI and CT myelography have largely replaced diskography. (More information on diskography is presented in Chapter 29 of the seventh edition of this atlas.)

A *radionuclide brain scan* is a nuclear medicine procedure used to demonstrate physiologic function and blood flow within the brain. CT and MRI have essentially eliminated the need for this procedure. Radionuclide brain scanning is now commonly used only in the assessment of brain death because the procedure clearly reveals the absence of intracranial blood flow.

Single photon emission computed tomography (SPECT) is another nuclear medicine procedure. It requires an IV injection of a radionuclide that is taken up in the brain tissue and studied by a specialized SPECT camera. As with most nuclear medicine studies, this examination also assesses physiologic function instead of anatomic detail. It is useful in diagnosing seizure activity and ischemic or hemorrhagic strokes. (Further discussion of nuclear medicine is presented in Chapter 38.)

Positron emission tomography (PET) uses a very specialized imaging unit in combination with IV injection of a radionuclide to evaluate brain function by demonstrating metabolic activity within the brain. Although PET is primarily used as a research tool, it is gaining popularity for the evaluation of patients with suspected Alzheimer's disease, Huntington's disease, schizophrenia, and cocaine abuse. (Further discussion of positron emission tomography is presented in Chapter 40.)

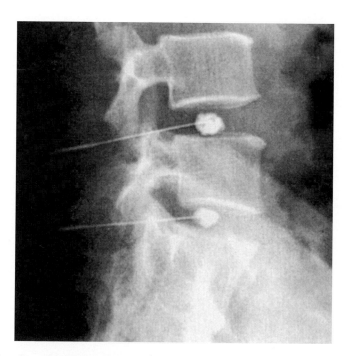

Fig. 25-25 Lumbar diskogram demonstrating normal nucleus pulposus of round contour type.

Magnetic resonance angiography (MRA) is a fairly new imaging technique that uses a conventional MRI unit to provide images of vessels within the body. Some clinicians believe that MRA is more accurate than conventional digital subtraction angiography in evaluating the carotid arteries and the circle of Willis within the brain. MRA does not require catheterization of a vessel or the injection of contrast material. Either venous or arterial vessels may be imaged. This technology takes advantage of the rapid laminar flow of blood within the vessels and is based on the intrinsic appearance of blood as it flows through the imaging slices. Blood travels so quickly that it does not stay in the scanning field long enough to return a signal back to the MRI coil. Using the correct MRI sequences results in a fairly clear image of the vessels of interest (Fig. 25-26). This imaging technique appears to be a promising tool for neuroradiology.

Stereotactic surgery and *stereotropic surgery* are terms used to denote a highly specialized neurosurgical therapeutic technique for the precise three-dimensional guidance of a slender surgical instrument through a burr hole in the cranium to a predetermined point deep within the brain. The first practical stereotactic instrument was introduced in the late 1940s for use with pneumoencephalography. Stereotactic surgery is used in the treatment of various diseases of the nervous system, some of which cause loss of control of body movement and some of which cause intractable pain. The most frequent use of this surgical technique may be for the treatment of Parkinson's disease. It is also used to obtain biopsy specimens from deep tumors within the brain and to drain abscesses. Stereotactic surgery is often the preferred technique for the treatment of these conditions because the diseased structure can be reached and surgically destroyed with the slender, specialized instrument, thus eliminating the need for open surgery.

The tip of the surgical instrument must be placed in the target area with an accuracy of 1-mm deviation from the target point. This precise placement requires a specialized instrument guidance system known as a *stereotactic frame* or *stereotactic device*. Numerous types of stereotactic devices are currently in use. Basically, they consist of a frame that the surgeon uses to immobilize the patient's head with attached fixation screws. The frame incorporates an external reference system and an adjustable instrument device.

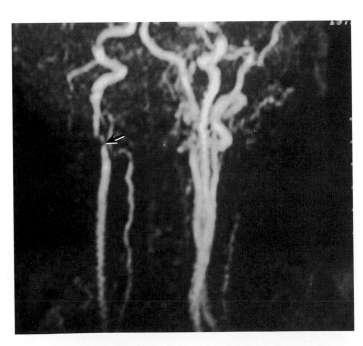

Fig. 25-26 Two-dimensional time-of-flight MRI image demonstrating high-grade stenosis of the right proximal internal carotid artery.

Stereotactic localization is currently performed with the assistance of CT. Early CT stereotactic devices used metal to fix the device to the skull, resulting in computer-generated artifacts on the CT image. Newer stereotactic devices contain carbon graphite posts and fine-metal skull pins surrounded by plastic bushings (Figs. 25-27 and 25-28). Computer programs are available that help to guide the needle for biopsy procedures. The data processing necessary to determine frame coordinates and probe depth can be performed with a programmable calculator. A software system transforms the two-dimensional coordinates obtained on the CT image to three-dimensional coordinates used by the surgeon. These coordinates are checked using a phantom simulator before the actual surgical procedure is performed.

For the procedure a metal head ring is fixed to the skull with an attached localizing system consisting of three sets of vertical and diagonal rods. These rods are visible on the CT images and are used to determine spatial relationships. After the CT examination the patient is transported to the operating room, where the localizing rods are removed and replaced by an arc-guidance system to allow passage of the surgical instruments. The stereotactic frame is removed after the surgical procedure, and a postoperative CT examination may be performed to check the biopsy site.

The use of MRI in conjunction with stereotactic surgery is still in its infancy. Stereotactic frames must have nonferromagnetic components, and they must be constructed so that eddy currents are not induced. The coordinate markers must be constructed of paramagnetic materials that are visualized on the MRI scans. MRI-assisted stereotactic procedures should prove useful for pathologic conditions that do not visualize well on CT images. Additional research on MRI applications is currently being conducted.

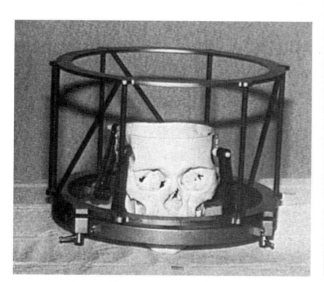

Fig. 25-27 Localizing system attached to head ring.

(From Haaga JR: *Computed tomography*, St Louis, 1983, Mosby.)

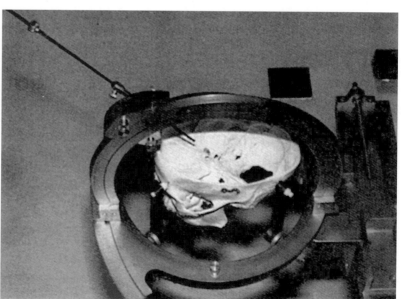

Fig. 25-28 Stereotactic instrument arc guidance system.

(From Haaga JR: *Computed tomography*, St Louis, 1983, Mosby.)

Selected bibliography

Brown RA, Roberts TS, Osborn AB: Stereotaxic frame and computer software for CT-directed neurosurgical localization, *Invest Radiol* 15:308, 1980.

Cooper PR, Cohen W: Evaluation of cervical spinal injuries with metrizamide myelography—CT scanning, *J Neurosurg* 61:281, 1984.

Donovon-Post MJ et al: Spinal infection: evaluation with MR imaging and interoperative ultrasound, *Radiology* 169:765, 1988.

Gehweiler JA, Osborn RL, Becker RF: *The radiology of vertebral trauma*, Philadelphia, 1980, WB Saunders.

Haaga JR, Alfidi RJ: *Computed tomography of the whole body*, ed 2, vols 1 and 2, St Louis, 1988, Mosby.

Javid MJ: Signs and symptoms after chemonucleolysis: a detailed evaluation of 214 worker's compensation and noncompensation patients, *Spine* 13:1428, 1988.

Katirji MB, Agrawal R, Kantra TA: The human cervical myotomes: an anatomical correlation between electromyography and CT/myelography, *Muscle Nerve* 11:1070, 1988.

Lemansky E: Contrast agents used for myelography: an historical perspective, *Radiol Technol* 60:489, 1989.

Maravilla KR, Cooper PR, Sklar FH: The influence of thin section tomography on the treatment of cervical spine injuries, *Radiology* 127:131, 1978.

Marymount JV, Shapiro WM: Vertebral hemangioma associated with spinal cord compression, *South Med J* 81:1586, 1988.

Osborn Anne, *Diagnostic Neuroradiology,* St Louis, 1994, Mosby.

Ramsey R: *Neuroradiology,* ed 3, Philadelphia, 1994, WB Saunders.

Russin LD, Guinto FC: Multidirectional tomography in cervical spine injury, *J Neurosurg* 45:9, 1976.

Stark D, Bradley W: *Magnetic resonance imaging*, ed 2, vols 1 and 2, St Louis, 1992, Mosby.

Woodruff W: *Fundamentals of neuroimaging,* Philadelphia, 1993, WB Saunders.

Zee CS et al: MR imaging of neurocysticercosis, *J Comput Assist Tomogr* 12:927, 1988.

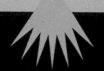

CIRCULATORY SYSTEM

MICHAEL G. BRUCKNER

RIGHT: Pneumatic injector powered by carbon dioxide cartridges (1960).

(From Amplatz K: A vascular injector with program selector, *Radiology* 75:955-956, 1960.)

BELOW: Modern biplane digital angiographic system.

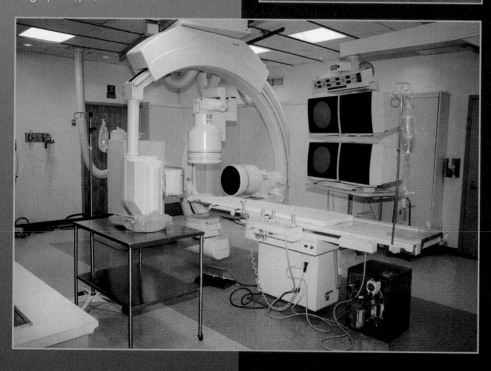

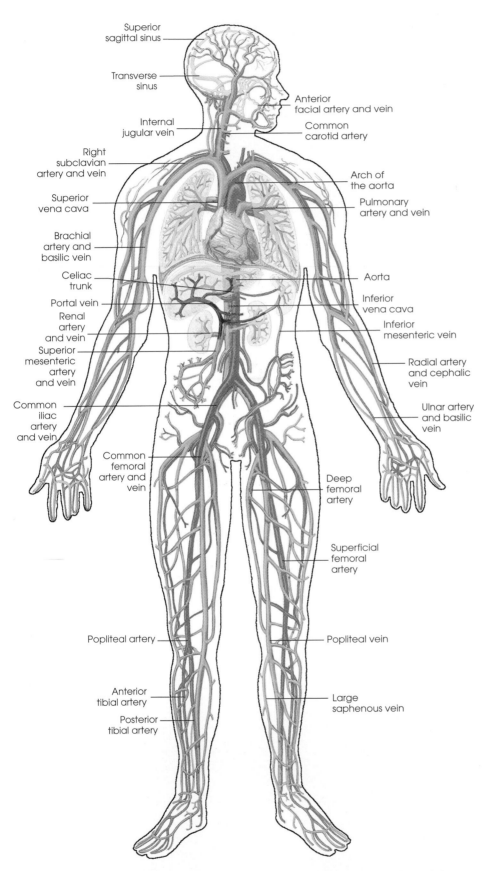

Superior
sagittal sinus

Transverse
sinus

Internal
jugular vein

Right
subclavian
artery and vein

Superior
vena cava

Brachial
artery and
basilic vein

Celiac
trunk

Portal vein

Renal
artery
and vein

Superior
mesenteric
artery
and vein

Common
iliac
artery
and vein

Common
femoral
artery and
vein

Popliteal artery

Anterior
tibial artery

Posterior
tibial artery

Anterior
facial artery and vein

Common
carotid artery

Arch of
the aorta

Pulmonary
artery and vein

Aorta

Inferior
vena cava

Inferior
mesenteric vein

Radial artery
and cephalic
vein

Ulnar artery
and basilic
vein

Deep
femoral
artery

Superficial
femoral
artery

Popliteal vein

Large
saphenous vein

Fig. 26-1 Major arteries and veins: *red,* arterial; *blue,* venous; *purple,* portal.

Circulatory System

The *circulatory system* has two complex systems of intimately associated vessels. Through these vessels, fluid is transported throughout the body in a continuous, unidirectional flow. The major portion of the circulatory system transports blood and is called the *blood-vascular system* (Fig. 26-1). The minor portion, called the *lymphatic system,* collects from the tissue spaces the fluid that is filtered out of the blood vessels and conveys it back to the blood-vascular system. The fluid conveyed by the lymphatic system is called *lymph.** Together the blood-vascular and lymphatic systems carry oxygen and nutritive material to the tissues. They also collect and transport carbon dioxide and other waste products of metabolism from the tissues to the organs of excretion: the skin, lungs, liver, and kidneys.

---

*Almost all italicized words on the succeeding pages are defined at the end of this chapter.

Blood-Vascular System

The blood-vascular system consists basically of the *heart, arteries, capillaries, and veins*. The *heart* serves as a pumping mechanism to keep the blood in constant circulation throughout the vast system of blood vessels. *Arteries* convey the blood *away* from the heart. *Veins* convey the blood *back* toward the heart for redistribution. Two circuits of arteries, capillaries, and veins branch out from and return blood back to the heart. One of these circuits traverses the lungs to discharge carbon dioxide and take up oxygen for delivery to the remainder of the body tissues; this circuit of vessels is known as *pulmonary circulation*. The second circuit branches throughout the body to the various organs and tissues and is called *systemic circulation*.

From the main trunk vessels arising at the heart—the pulmonary trunk for the pulmonary circulation and the *aorta* for the systemic circulation—the arteries progressively diminish in size as they divide and subdivide along their course, finally ending in minute branches called *arterioles*. The arterioles divide to form the capillary vessels, and the branching process is then reversed: the *capillaries* unite to form *venules*, the beginning branches of the veins, which in turn unite and reunite to form larger and larger vessels as they approach the heart. This joining of pulmonary veins ends with four veins opening into the left atrium of the heart (two trunk veins leading from each lung). The systemic veins are arranged in a superficial set and in a deep set with which the superficial veins communicate; both sets converge at a common trunk vein. The systemic veins end in two large vessels opening into the heart: the *superior vena cava* leads from the portion of the body above the diaphragm, and the *inferior vena cava* leads from below the level of the diaphragm.

The capillaries connect the arterioles and venules to form networks that pervade most organs and all other tissues supplied with blood. The capillary vessels have exceedingly thin walls through which the essential functions of the blood-vascular system take place—the blood constituents are filtered out and the waste products of cell activity are absorbed. The exchange takes place through the medium of tissue fluid, which is derived from the blood plasma and is drained off by the lymphatic system for return to the blood-vascular system. The tissue fluid undergoes modification in the lymphatic system. As soon as this tissue fluid enters the lymphatic capillaries, it is called *lymph*.

The *heart* is the central organ of the blood-vascular system and functions solely as a pump to keep the blood in circulation. It is shaped somewhat like a cone and measures approximately $4\frac{3}{4}$ inches (12 cm) in length, $3\frac{1}{2}$ inches (9 cm) in width, and $2\frac{1}{2}$ inches (6 cm) in depth. The heart is situated obliquely in the middle mediastinum, largely to the left of the midsagittal plane. The base of the heart is directed superiorly, posteriorly, and to the right. (Note that left and right are from the point of view of the person with the heart.) The apex of the heart rests on the diaphragm and against the anterior chest wall and is directed anteriorly, inferiorly, and to the left.

The muscular wall of the heart is called the *myocardium*. Because of the force required to drive blood through the extensive systemic vessels, the myocardium is about three times as thick on the left side as on the right. The membrane that lines the interior of the heart is called the *endocardium*. The heart is enclosed in the double-walled *pericardial sac*. The exterior wall of this sac is fibrous. The thin, closely adherent membrane that covers the heart is referred to as the *epicardium* or, because it also serves as the serous inner wall of the pericardial sac, the *visceral pericardium*. The narrow, fluid-containing space between the two walls of the sac is called the *pericardial cavity*.

The heart is divided by septa into right and left halves, with each half subdivided by a constriction into two cavities, or chambers. The two upper chambers are called *atria*, and each atrium consists of a principal cavity and of a lesser one called the *auricle*. The two lower chambers of the heart are called *ventricles*. The opening between the right atrium and right ventricle is controlled by the right atrioventricular (tricuspid) valve, and the opening between the left atrium and left ventricle is controlled by the left atrioventricular (mitral or bicuspid) valve.

The atria function as receiving chambers, and the ventricles function as distributing chambers. The right side of the heart handles the venous, or deoxygenated, blood, and the left side handles the arterial, or oxygenated, blood. The left ventricle pumps oxygenated blood through the aortic valve into the aorta. The right ventricle pumps deoxygenated blood through the pulmonary valve into the pulmonary trunk. The two right and left pulmonary veins open into the left atrium. The superior and inferior venae cavae open into the right atrium (Fig. 26-2).

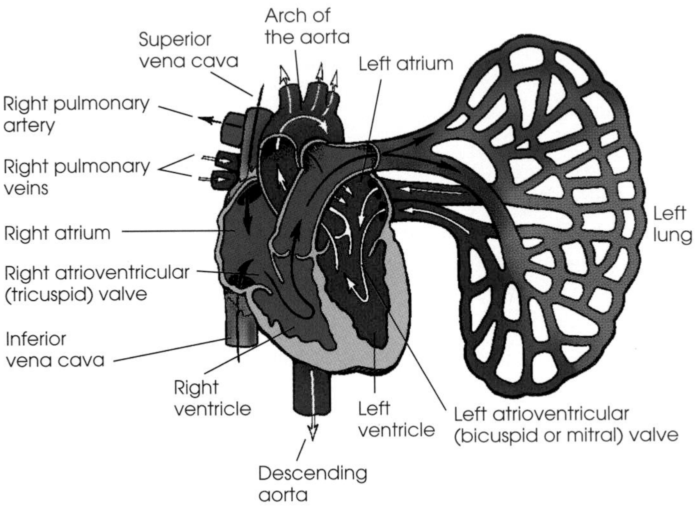

Blood is supplied to the myocardium by the right and left coronary arteries. These vessels arise in the aortic sinus immediately superior to the aortic valve. Most of the cardiac veins drain into the coronary sinus on the posterior aspect of the heart, and this sinus drains into the right atrium (Figs. 26-3 and 26-4).

The ascending aorta arises from the superior portion of the left ventricle and passes superiorly and to the right for a short distance. It then arches posteriorly and to the left and descends along the left side of the vertebral column to the level of L4, where it divides into the right and left common iliac arteries. The common iliac arteries diverge from each other as they pass to the level of the lumbosacral junction, where each ends by dividing into the internal iliac, or hypogastric, artery and the external iliac artery. The internal iliac artery passes into the pelvis. The external iliac artery passes to a point about midway between the anterior superior iliac spine (ASIS) and pubic symphysis and then enters the thigh to become the femoral artery.

The arteries are usually named according to their location. The three major portions of the aorta—the ascending aorta, the arch of the aorta, and the descending aorta—are described according to direction. The last division, the descending aorta, has thoracic and abdominal portions. The *systemic arteries* branch out, treelike, from the aorta to all parts of the body. The systemic veins usually lie parallel to their respective arteries and are given the same names.

Fig. 26-2 Heart and great vessels: deoxygenated blood flow *(black arrows)*; oxygenated blood flow *(white arrows)*.

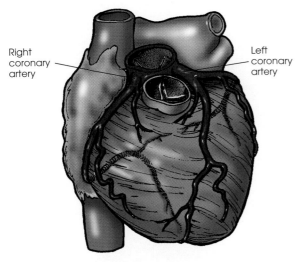

Fig. 26-3 Anterior view of coronary arteries.

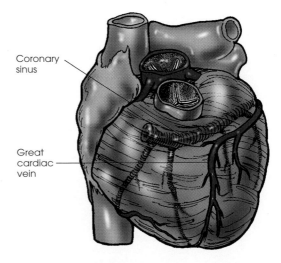

Fig. 26-4 Anterior view of coronary veins.

Every organ has its own vascular circuit that arises from the trunk artery and leads back to the trunk vein for return to the heart. The veins returning blood from the abdominal viscera do not join the systemic venous system directly; instead, they join to form the portal vein, which drains into the liver. After the blood is processed in the liver, it flows through the hepatic veins into the inferior vena cava.

The pulmonary trunk arises from the right ventricle of the heart, passes superiorly and posteriorly for a distance of about 2 inches (5 cm), and then divides into two branches, the right and left pulmonary arteries. These vessels enter the root of the respective lung and, following the course of the bronchi, divide and subdivide to form a dense network of capillaries surrounding the alveoli of the lungs. Through the thin walls of the capillaries, the blood discharges carbon dioxide and absorbs oxygen from the air contained in the alveoli. The oxygenated blood passes onward through the pulmonary veins for return to the heart. In the pulmonary circulation the deoxygenated blood is transported by the arteries, and the oxygenated blood is transported by the veins.

As shown in Fig. 26-5, the oxygenated (arterial) blood leaves the left ventricle by way of the aorta and is carried through the arteries to all parts of the body. The deoxygenated (venous) blood is collected by the veins and returned to the right atrium through the superior vena cava from the upper part of the body and through the inferior vena cava from the lower part of the body. This circuit, from the left ventricle to the right atrium, is called the *systemic circulation*. The venous blood passes from the right atrium into the right ventricle and out through the pulmonary artery and its branches to the lungs. After being oxygenated in the capillaries of the lungs, the blood is conveyed to the left atrium of the heart through the pulmonary veins. The circuit from the right ventricle to the left atrium is called the *pulmonary circulation*. The pathway of venous drainage from the abdominal viscera to the liver is called the *portal system*. Unlike the systemic and pulmonary circuits, which begin and end at the heart, the portal system begins in the capillaries of the abdominal viscera and ends in the capillaries of the liver.

The atria and ventricles separately contract *(systole)* in pumping blood and relax or dilate *(diastole)* in receiving blood. The atria precede the ventricles in contraction; therefore, while the atria are in systole, the ventricles are in diastole. One phase of contraction (referred to as the *heartbeat*) and one phase of dilation are called the cardiac cycle. In the average adult, one cardiac cycle lasts 0.8 second. However, the *heart rate*, or number of pulsations per minute, varies with size, age, and gender. Heart rate is faster in small persons, young individuals, and females. The heart rate is also increased with exercise, food, and emotional disturbances.

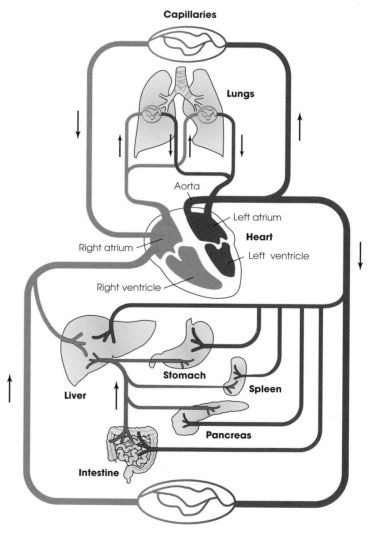

Fig. 26-5 Pulmonary, systemic, and portal circulation: oxygenated *(red)*, deoxygenated *(blue)*, and nutrient-rich *(purple)* blood.

The velocity of blood circulation varies with the rate and intensity of the heartbeat. Velocity also varies in the different portions of the circulatory system based on distance from the initial pressure of the intermittent waves of blood issuing from the heart. Therefore the speed of blood flow is highest in the large arteries arising at or near the heart because these vessels receive the full force of each wave of blood pumped out of the heart. The arterial walls expand with the pressure from each wave. The walls then rhythmically recoil, gradually diminishing the pressure of the advancing wave from point to point, until the flow of blood is normally reduced to a steady, nonpulsating stream through the capillaries and veins. The beat, or contraction and expansion of an artery, may be felt with the fingers at a number of points and is called the *pulse*.

Complete circulation of the blood through both the systemic and pulmonary circuits, from a given point and back again, requires about 23 seconds and an average of 27 heartbeats. In certain contrast examinations of the cardiovascular system, tests are conducted to determine the circulation time from the point of contrast medium injection to the site of interest. The circulation time is influenced by body position (i.e., upright or recumbent body position).

Lymphatic System

The lymphatic system consists of an elaborate arrangement of closed vessels that collect fluid from the tissue spaces and transport it to the blood-vascular system. Almost all lymphatic vessels are arranged in two sets: (1) a superficial set that lies immediately under the skin and accompanies the superficial veins and (2) a deep set that accompanies the deep blood vessels and with which the superficial lymphatics communicate (Fig. 26-6). The lymphatic system lacks a pumping mechanism such as the heart of the blood-vascular system. The lymphatic vessels are richly supplied with valves to prevent backflow, and the movement of the lymph through the system is believed to be maintained largely by extrinsic pressure from the surrounding organs and muscles.

The lymphatic system begins in complex networks of thin-walled, absorbent capillaries situated in the various organs and tissues. The capillaries unite to form larger vessels, which in turn form networks and unite to become still larger vessels as they approach the terminal collecting trunks. The terminal trunks communicate with the blood-vascular system.

The lymphatic vessels are small in caliber and have delicate, transparent walls. Along their course the collecting vessels pass through one or more nodular structures called *lymph nodes*. The nodes occur singly but are usually arranged in chains or groups of 2 to 20. The nodes are situated so that they form strategically placed centers toward which the conducting vessels converge. The nodes vary from the size of a pinhead to the size of an almond or larger. They may be spherical, oval, or kidney-shaped. Each node has a hilum through which the arteries enter and veins and efferent lymph vessels emerge; the afferent lymph vessels do not enter at the hilum. In addition to the lymphatic capillaries, blood vessels, and supporting structures, each lymph node contains masses, or follicles, of lymphocytes that are arranged around its circumference and from which cords of cells extend through the medullary portion of the node.

A number of conducting channels, here called *afferent lymph vessels*, enter the node opposite the hilum and break into wide capillaries that surround the lymph follicles and form a canal known as the *peripheral* or *marginal lymph sinus*. The network of capillaries continues into the medullary portion of the node, widens to form medullary sinuses, and then collects into several *efferent lymph vessels* that leave the node at the hilum. The conducting vessels may pass through several nodes along their course, each time undergoing the process of widening into sinuses. Lymphocytes, a variety of white blood cells formed in the lymph nodes, are added to the lymph while it is in the nodes. It is thought that a majority of the lymph is absorbed by the venous system from these nodes and only a small portion of the lymph is passed on through the conducting vessels.

The absorption and interchange of tissue fluids and cells take place through the thin walls of the capillaries. The lymph passes from the beginning capillaries through the conducting vessels, which eventually empty their contents into terminal lymph trunks for conveyance to the blood-vascular system. The main terminal trunk of the lymphatic system is called the *thoracic duct*. The lower, dilated portion of the duct is known as the *cisterna chyli*. The thoracic duct receives lymphatic drainage from all parts of the body below the diaphragm and from the left half of the body above the diaphragm. The thoracic duct extends from the level of L2 to the base of the neck, where it ends by opening into the venous system at the junction of the left subclavian and internal jugular veins.

Three terminal collecting trunks—the right jugular, the subclavian, and the bronchomediastinal trunks—receive the lymphatic drainage from the right half of the body above the diaphragm. These vessels open into the right subclavian vein separately or occasionally after uniting to form a common trunk called the right lymphatic duct.

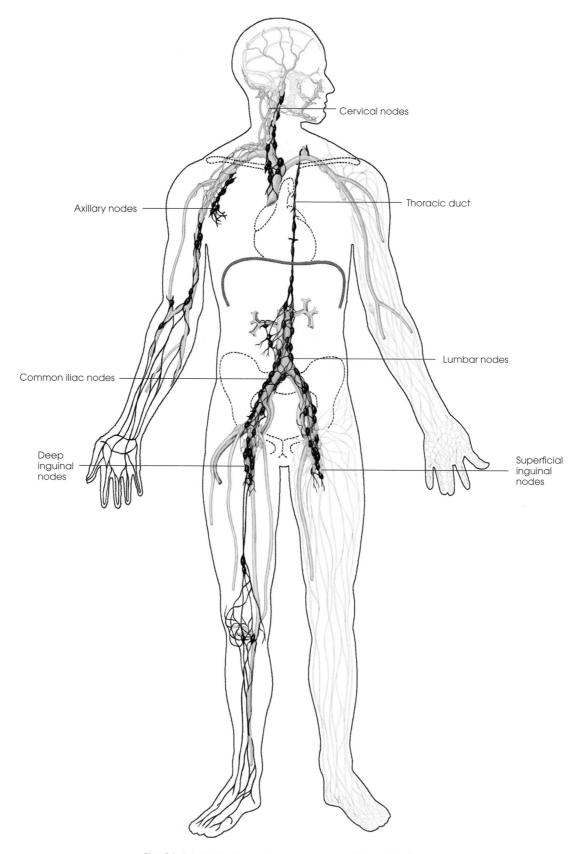

Cervical nodes

Axillary nodes

Thoracic duct

Lumbar nodes

Common iliac nodes

Deep inguinal nodes

Superficial inguinal nodes

Fig. 26-6 Lymphatic system: *green,* superficial; *black,* deep.

Definitions and Indications

Blood vessels are not normally visible in conventional radiography because no natural contrast exists between them and other soft tissues of the body. Therefore these vessels must be filled with a radiopaque contrast medium to delineate them for radiography. *Angiography* is a general term that describes the radiologic examination of vascular structures within the body after the introduction of an iodinated contrast medium.

The visceral and peripheral angiography procedures identified in this chapter can be categorized generally as either *arteriography* or *venography.* Examinations are more precisely named for the specific blood vessel opacified and the method of injection. For example, with IV digital vascular imaging of the right renal artery, a contrast medium is injected into a vein but images of the renal artery are obtained (see Chapter 35). Imaging of the right renal artery by injecting a contrast medium directly into the artery is accomplished by performing a selective right renal arteriogram.

Angiography is primarily used to identify the anatomy or pathologic process of blood vessels. For example, the lower limb *venogram,* probably the most common of all angiograms, is usually performed to determine if deep venous *thrombosis* is the cause of a patient's leg swelling or pain. Chronic cramping leg pain following physical exertion, a condition known as *claudication*, may prompt a physician to order an arteriogram of the lower limbs to determine if *atherosclerosis* is diminishing the blood supply to the leg muscles. Detection of a *stenosis,* most often caused by atherosclerosis, is the purpose of many arteriograms. Cerebral angiography is performed to detect and verify the existence and exact position of an *aneurysm.*

Although most angiographic examinations are performed to investigate anatomic variances, some evaluate the motion of the part. Certain cardiac catheterization procedures, for example, visualize the interior anatomy of the heart and the motion of the cardiac valves (see Chapter 31). Other vascular examinations evaluate suspected tumors by opacifying the organ of concern. Angiography for therapeutic rather than diagnostic purposes is discussed later in this chapter.

The broad term *angiography* also encompasses examinations involving other vessels of the body. For example, lymphangiography is discussed in this chapter, and cholangiography is described in Chapter 16.

Historical Development

In January 1896, just 10 weeks after the announcement of Roentgen's discovery, Haschek and Lindenthal announced that they had produced a radiograph demonstrating the blood vessels of an amputated hand using Teichman's mixture, a thick emulsion of chalk, as the contrast agent. This work heralded the beginning of angiography. The potential for this new type of examination to delineate vascular anatomy was immediately recognized. However, the advancement of angiography was hindered by the lack of suitable contrast media and low-risk techniques to deliver the media to the desired location. By the 1920s researchers were using sodium iodide as a contrast medium to produce lower limb studies comparable in quality to studies seen in modern angiography.

Yet limitations still existed. Until the 1950s, contrast medium was most commonly injected through a needle that punctured the vessel or through a ureteral catheter that passed into the body through a surgically exposed peripheral vessel. Then in 1952, shortly after the development of a flexible thin-walled catheter, Seldinger announced a *percutaneous* method of catheter introduction. The Seldinger technique eliminated the surgical risk associated with the exposure of tissues and made a much smaller wound (see p. 30).

Early angiograms consisted of single radiographs or the visualization of vessels by fluoroscopy. Because the advantage of *serial imaging* was recognized, cassette changers, roll film changers, cut film changers, and cine and serial spot-filming/digital devices were developed. Pumps to inject contrast media were also developed to allow more rapid and precise control of injection rates and volumes than was possible by hand. Early mechanical injectors were powered by pressurized gas, and the injection rate was a function of the pressure setting. (An early injector is shown on the title page of this chapter.) Electrically powered automatic injectors were subsequently developed that allowed the injection rate to be set directly.

Angiographic Studies

CONTRAST MEDIA

A wide variety of opaque contrast media are used in angiographic studies. All materials currently in use are organic iodine solutions. Although usually tolerated, the injection of iodinated contrast medium causes undesirable consequences. The medium is filtered out of the bloodstream by the kidneys but is *nephrotoxic*. It causes physiologic cardiovascular side effects, including peripheral vasodilation, blood pressure decrease, and cardiotoxicity. It also produces nausea and an uncomfortable burning sensation in muscular artery branches in about 1 of 10 patients. Most significantly, the injection of iodinated contrast medium may invoke allergic reactions. These reactions may be minor (hives or slight difficulty in breathing) and not require any treatment, or they may be severe and require immediate medical intervention. Severe reactions are characterized by a state of shock in which the patient exhibits shallow breathing and a high pulse rate and may lose consciousness. Historically, 1 of every 14,000 patients suffers a severe allergic reaction. The administration of contrast medium is clearly one of the significant risks in angiography.

At the kilovolt (peak) (kVp) used in angiography, iodine is slightly more radiopaque, atom for atom, than lead. The iodine is incorporated into water-soluble molecules formed as triiodinated benzene rings. These molecules vary in exact composition. Some forms are organic salts that dissociate in solution and are therefore ionic. The iodinated anion is diatrizoate iothalamate or ioxaglate. The radiolucent cation is meglumine, sodium, or a combination of both. These ionic forms yield two particles in solution for every three iodine atoms (a 3:2 ratio) and are six to eight times as osmolar as plasma.

Other triiodinated benzene rings are created as nonionic molecules. These forms have three iodine atoms on each particle in solution (a 3:1 ratio) because they do not dissociate and are only two to three times as osmolar as plasma. Studies indicate that these properties of nonionic contrast media result in decreased chemotoxicity to the kidneys. Nonionic contrast media also cause fewer physiologic cardiovascular side effects, less intense sensations, and fewer allergic reactions. They are, however, much more expensive than ionic media.

One form of ionic contrast medium is a dimer; two benzene rings are bonded together as the anion. This results in six iodine atoms for every two particles in solution, which yields the same 3:1 ratio as a nonionic contrast medium. The ionic dimer has advantages over the ionic monomeric molecule but lacks some of the properties of the nonionic molecule.

All forms of iodinated contrast media are available in a variety of iodine concentrations. The agents of higher concentration are more opaque. Typically, 30% iodine concentrations are used for cerebral and limb arteriography, whereas 35% concentrations are used for visceral angiography. Peripheral venography may be performed with 30% or lower concentrations. The ionic agents of higher concentration and the nonionic agents are more viscous and produce greater resistance in the catheter during injection. The choice of contrast medium may vary with the patient and is usually made by the examining physician.

INJECTION TECHNIQUES

The contrast medium may be introduced into a vessel through a "direct stick," which is simply the process of placing a needle tip into the desired vessel and injecting the contrast agent through the needle. This technique is acceptable in limited situations. A flush injection through a catheter involves placing the catheter tip into a large proximal vessel so that the vessel and its major branches are opacified. In a selective injection the catheter tip is positioned into the orifice of a specific artery so that only the specific artery is injected. This has the advantage of more densely opacifying the vessel and limiting the superimposition of vessels.

A contrast medium may be injected by hand with a syringe, but ideally an automatic injector is used. The major advantage of automatic injectors is that a specific quantity of contrast medium can be injected during a predetermined period of time. Automatic injectors have controls to set the injection rate, injection volume, and maximum pressure to be allowed to occur inside a catheter or other injection pathway. Another useful feature is a control to set a time interval during which the injector gradually achieves the set injection rate. This may prevent a catheter or needle from being dislodged by whiplash.

Because the opacifying contrast medium is often carried away from the area of interest by blood flow, the injection and demonstration of opacified vessels usually occur simultaneously. Therefore the injector is often electronically connected to the rapid imaging equipment to coordinate the timing between the injector and the onset of imaging. In particular, accurate timing is required when the imaging commences slightly before or after the injection begins.

EQUIPMENT

Most angiograms record flowing contrast medium in a series of images, which requires rapid *film changers,* cinefluorography devices, or digital subtraction angiography (DSA) (see Chapter 35). Less complex angiographic procedures, such as peripheral arteriography and venography, may be performed with a conventional Bucky tray.

A number of rapid film changers are available from different manufacturers. All these devices move the film and permit exposures at intervals of a fraction of a second. One device is capable of changing as many as 12 films per second, although most film changers have a maximum speed of six films or fewer per second. These rapid film changers transport films from a supply magazine to a position between screens that come into close contact with the film during exposure and then retract so that the film can be transported into a receiving magazine. Cut-film changers that can move 20 or 30 35 × 35 cm (14 × 14 inch) films are common.

Lower limb angiograms are the most likely to be performed using specialized cassette changers. These devices move large cassettes containing 30 × 120 cm (11 × 48 inch) or 35 × 130 cm (14 × 51 inch) film, depending on the manufacturer, into and out of the exposure field. Because these devices move heavy objects, they operate at slower maximum speeds, usually one cassette per second.

Fluroscopy, cine, and DSA systems consist essentially of a camera that photographs the output phosphor of an image intensification system. Fluoroscopy and DSA employ a video camera. In DSA the fluoroscopic image is digitized into serial images that are stored by a computer. The computer subtracts an early image (before contrast medium enters the vessel) from a later image (after the vessel opacifies) and displays the difference, or subtraction image, on the fluoroscopy monitor (see Chapter 35). Almost all image intensification devices used for vascular procedures include television monitoring. Such equipment allows angiographic examinations to be viewed on a television screen in real time and simultaneously recorded.

A cine camera uses 16- or 35-mm roll film and usually can achieve sequential exposure rates of up to 60 frames or more per second. The result is true motion picture radiography. The photographic resolution achieved with cine units is not as great as that seen with rapid film changers. However, many more events can be photographed with the cine attachment, and dynamic function can be more satisfactorily evaluated with cinefluorography.

Imaging systems may be used either singularly or in combination at right angles to obtain simultaneous frontal and lateral images of the vascular system under investigation with one injection of contrast medium. This arrangement of units is called a *biplane* imaging system.

Rapid serial radiographic imaging requires large focal-spot x-ray tubes capable of withstanding a high heat load. Magnification studies, however, require fractional focus tubes with focal spot sizes of between 0.1 and 0.3 mm. X-ray tubes may have to be specialized to satisfy these extreme demands. Rapid serial imaging also necessitates radiographic generators with high-power output. Because short exposure times are needed to compensate for all patient motion, the generators must be capable of producing high-milliampere output. The combination of high kilowatt-rated generators and rare earth film-screen technology significantly aids in decreasing the radiation dose to the patient while producing radiographs of improved quality, with the added advantage of prolonging the life of the high-powered generators and x-ray tubes.

A comprehensive angiographic room contains a great amount of equipment other than specifically radiologic devices. Monitoring systems record patient electrocardiographic data and blood pressure readings from within vessels. Emergency equipment may include resuscitators, a defibrillator for the heart, and anesthesia apparatus. The radiographer must be familiar with the use of each piece of equipment (Fig. 26-7).

MAGNIFICATION

Magnification occurs both intentionally and unintentionally in angiographic imaging sequences. Intentional use of magnification can result in a significant increase in resolution of fine vessel recorded detail. Fractional focal spot tubes of 0.3 mm or less are necessary for direct radiographic magnification techniques. The selection of a fractional focal spot necessitates the use of low milliamperage. Short exposure time is maintained by the use of the air gap rather than the grid to control scatter radiation.

The formula for magnification is:

$$M = \frac{SID}{SOD} \quad or \quad \frac{SID}{SID - OID}$$

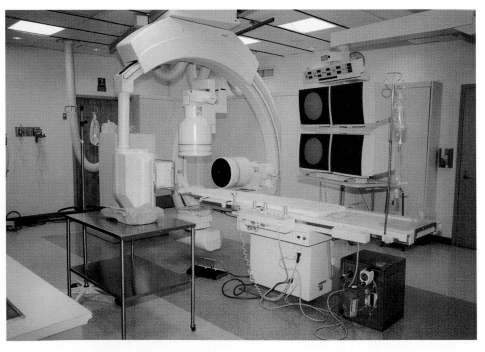

Fig. 26-7 Modern biplane digital angiographic suite.

The SID is the source-to-image receptor distance, the SOD is the source-to-object distance, and the OID is the object-to-image receptor distance. For a 2:1 magnification study using a SID of 40 inches (101 cm) both the focal spot and the image receptor are positioned 20 inches (50 cm) from the area of interest. A 3:1 magnification study using a 40-inch (101-cm) SID is accomplished by placing the focal spot 13 inches (33 cm) from the area of interest and the image receptor 27 inches (68 cm) from the area of interest (Figs. 26-8 to 26-10).

Unintentional magnification occurs when the area of interest cannot be placed in direct contact with the image receptor. This is particularly a problem in the bi-plane imaging sequence, in which the need to center the area of interest in the first plane may create some unavoidable distance of the body part to the image receptor in the second plane. Even in single plane imaging, vascular structures are separated from the image receptor by some distance. The magnification that occurs as a result of these circumstances is frequently 20% to 25%. For example, a 25% magnification occurs when a vessel within the body is 8 inches (20 cm) from the image receptor—an OID of 8 inches (20 cm)—and the SID is 40 inches (101 cm).

Angiographic images therefore do not represent vessels at their actual size. This must be taken into account when direct measurements are made from angiographic images. Unintentional magnification can be reduced by increasing the SID while maintaining the OID. Increasing the SID may not be an option, however, if the increase in technical factors would exceed tube output capacity or exposure time maximum.

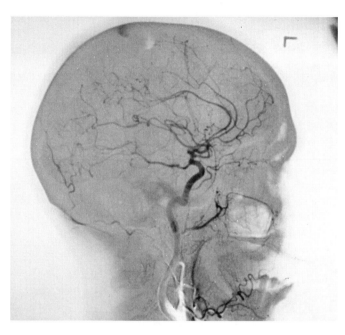

Fig. 26-8 Nonmagnified, photographically subtracted, lateral selective common carotid arteriogram.

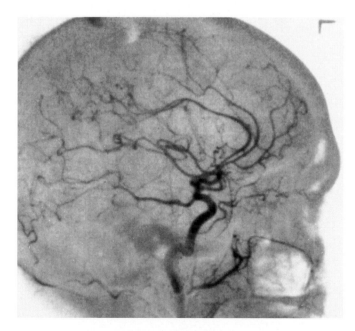

Fig. 26-9 2:1 magnified, photographically subtracted, lateral selective common carotid arteriogram.

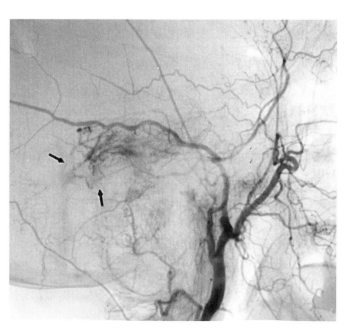

Fig. 26-10 3:1 magnified, photographically subtracted, lateral selective external carotid arteriogram. *Arrows* indicate visualization of fine tumor neovascularity.

FILM AND DIGITAL SUBTRACTION ANGIOGRAPHIC PROGRAMMING

Film programming is the task of controlling the rate and number of serial exposures made with a film changer. This is accomplished either through manipulation of the device intimately associated to the film changer, known as the *film programmer*, or through a combination of precisely patterning films in the film changer's supply magazine and setting the film programmer to operate the film changer at specific rates for specific amounts of time. Film programmers instruct the film changers to cycle at a specific rate, but every cycle does not necessarily transport and expose a film.

When two film changers operate together for simultaneous *biplane* imaging, exposures in both planes cannot be made at the same moment, because scatter radiation would fog the films. Yet, biplane changers must cycle exactly together so that synchronization can be electronically controlled. Therefore it is necessary to alternate the cycles that transport film in the two planes. In the first cycle, even though both changers are cycling, only one changer is allowed to transport and expose a film. In the second cycle the changer that transported film in the first cycle is allowed to cycle empty while the other changer transports and exposes a film. This process of changers alternating between transporting and not transporting film during opposite cycles must continue throughout the series. The maximum exposure rate of a film changer operated in the biplane mode is one half of its maximum cycle rate because only every other cycle transports and exposes a film.

The most sophisticated film programmers and all DSA systems (see Chapter 35) automatically control the alternation of images in the biplane mode. The radiographer selects single-plane or biplane mode and enters the number of exposures to be made in each second interval of the series. With less sophisticated film programming systems the radiographer has control of the cycle rate and rate duration but must manually select the cycles that will transport film. For a biplane program with manually loaded equipment, the film supply magazine for the AP changer is loaded with film in the odd-numbered spaces. The even-numbered spaces are left empty. The lateral film supply magazine is loaded in the even-numbered spaces. The film programmer must then be set to cycle the changers at a rate double to the film rate for each plane. The rate duration, however, remains the same. The time interval in which the film remains motionless for exposure must be known for every cycle rate so that a cycle rate with a motionless interval greater than the radiographic exposure time can be selected.

CATHETERIZATION

Catheterization for filling vessels with contrast media is a technique that is preferred over needle injection of the media. The advantages of catheterization are as follows:

1. The risk of *extravasation* is reduced.
2. Most body parts can be reached for selective injection.
3. The patient can be positioned as needed.
4. The catheter can be safely left in the body while radiographs are being examined.

The femoral, axillary, and brachial arteries are the ones most frequently catheterized. The femoral site is preferred because it is associated with the fewest risks.

The most widely used catheterization method is the modern Seldinger technique.[1] The steps of the technique are described in Fig. 26-11. The procedure is performed under sterile conditions. The catheterization site is suitably cleaned and then surgically draped. The conscious patient is given local anesthesia at the catheterization site.

With this percutaneous technique the arteriotomy or venotomy is no larger than the catheter itself. Therefore hemorrhage is minimized. Patients can usually resume normal activity within 24 hours after the examination. The risk of infection is lower than in surgical procedures because tissues are not exposed.

After a catheter is introduced into the blood-vascular system, it can be maneuvered by pushing, pulling, and turning the part of the catheter still outside the patient so that the part of the catheter inside the patient travels to a specific location. A wire is sometimes positioned inside the catheter to help manipulate and guide the catheter to the desired location. When the wire is removed from the catheter, the catheter is infused with sterile solution to help prevent clot formation. Infusing the catheter and assisting the physician in the catheterization process may be the radiographer's responsibility.

When the examination is complete, the catheter or needle is removed. Pressure is applied to the site until hemorrhage ceases, but blood flow through the vessel is maintained. The physician often prescribes complete patient bed rest and orders to be alert for the development of a *hematoma*.

When peripheral artery sites are unavailable, a catheter may sometimes be introduced into the aorta using the translumbar approach. For this technique the patient is positioned prone, and a special catheter introducer system is inserted percutaneously through the posterolateral aspect of the back and directed superiorly so that the catheter enters the aorta around the T11-T12 level. This method is used primarily for aortography and rarely for selective studies.

---

[1]Seldinger SF: Percutaneous selective angiography of the aorta: preliminary report, *Acta Radiol (Stockh)* 45:15, 1956.

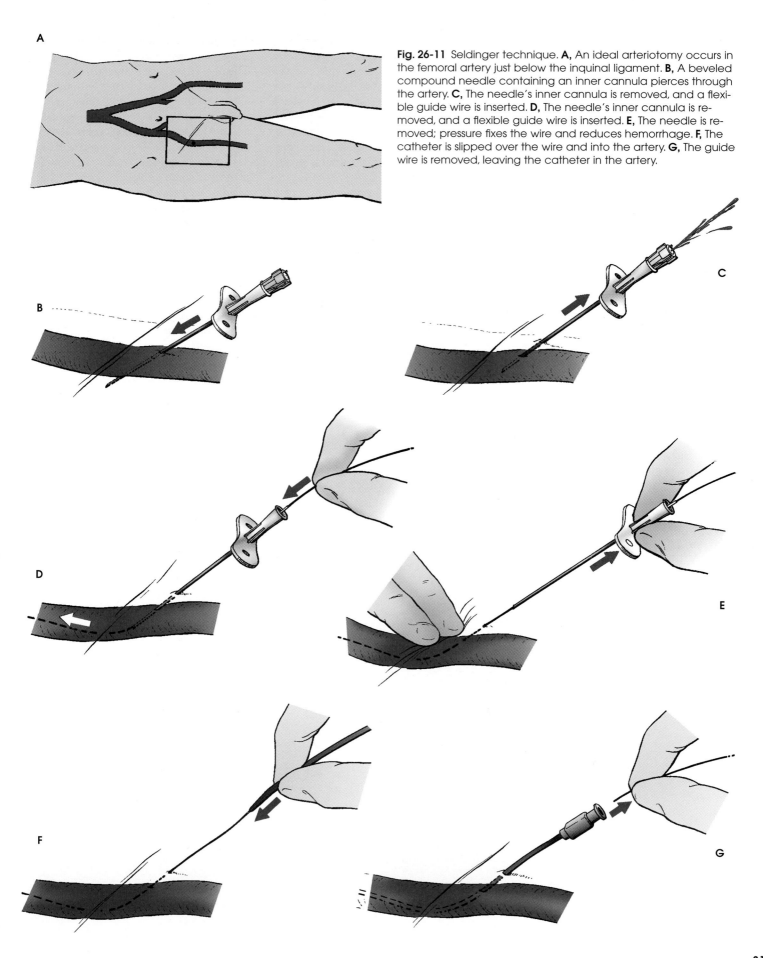

Fig. 26-11 Seldinger technique. **A,** An ideal arteriotomy occurs in the femoral artery just below the inquinal ligament. **B,** A beveled compound needle containing an inner cannula pierces through the artery. **C,** The needle's inner cannula is removed, and a flexible guide wire is inserted. **D,** The needle's inner cannula is removed, and a flexible guide wire is inserted. **E,** The needle is removed; pressure fixes the wire and reduces hemorrhage. **F,** The catheter is slipped over the wire and into the artery. **G,** The guide wire is removed, leaving the catheter in the artery.

Catheters are produced in various forms, each with a particular advantage in shape, maneuverability, or maximum injection rate (Fig. 26-12). Angiographic catheters are made of pliable plastic that allows them to straighten for insertion over the guide wire, also called a *wire guide*. They normally resume their original shape after the guide wire is withdrawn. The reverse-curve catheter, which has a bend of 180 degrees a few centimeters from the tip, usually requires manipulation from the angiographer to resume its original shape. Catheters with a bent tip are designed for maneuverability into artery origins for selective injections. They may have only an end hole, or they may have two additional side holes near the tip. The side holes stabilize the catheter tip by reducing the whiplash that occurs from the rapid ejection of contrast medium through the end hole. Some catheters have multiple side holes to facilitate high injection rates but are used only in large vascular structures for flush injections. A "pigtail" catheter is a special multiple side hole catheter that has a circular tip to further reduce the amount of contrast medium that exits the end hole. Common angiographic catheters range in size from 4 Fr (0.05 inch) to 7 Fr (0.09 inch), although even smaller or larger sizes may be used. Most have inner lumens that allow them to be inserted over guide wires ranging from 0.032 to 0.038 inches in size.

PATIENT CARE

Before the initiation of an angiographic procedure it is appropriate to explain the process and the potential complications to the patient. Written consent is often obtained after such an explanation. Potential complications include a vasovagal reaction; stroke; bleeding at the catheterization site; nerve, blood vessel, or tissue damage; and an allergic reaction to the contrast medium. Bleeding at the arteriotomy or venotomy site is usually easily controlled with pressure to the site. Blood vessel and tissue damage may require a surgical procedure. A vasovagal reaction is characterized by sweating and nausea caused by a drop in blood pressure. The patient's legs should be elevated, and IV fluids may be administered to help restore blood pressure. Minor allergic reactions to iodinated contrast media, such as hives and congestion, are usually controlled with medications and may not require treatment. Severe allergic reactions may result in shock, which is characterized by shallow breathing, high pulse rate, and possibly loss of consciousness. The examining physician must be immediately notified of any change in patient status. Of course, angiography is performed only if the benefits of the examination outweigh the risks.

Patients are usually restricted to clear liquid intake and routine medications before undergoing angiography. Adequate hydration from liquid intake may minimize kidney damage caused by iodinated contrast media. Solid food intake is restricted to reduce the risk of aspiration related to the nausea that occurs in 10% of patients who receive iodinated contrast media. Contraindications to angiography are determined by physicians and include previous severe allergic reaction to iodinated contrast media, severely impaired renal function, impaired blood clotting factors, and inability to undergo a surgical procedure or general anesthesia.

Because the risks of general anesthesia are greater than those associated with most angiographic procedures, adult patients are usually conscious for the examination. Just before the procedure most patients are given a sedative to reduce anxiety and discomfort. Thoughtful communication from the radiographer and physician also calms and reassures the patient. The radiographer or physician should warn the patient about the sensations caused by the contrast medium and the noise produced by the imaging equipment. This information also reduces the patient's anxiety and helps ensure a good radiographic series with no patient motion.

ANGIOGRAPHIC TEAM

The angiographic team consists of the physician (usually a radiologist), the radiographer, and other specialists, such as an anesthetist and a nurse.

The radiographer often assists in performing procedures that require sterile technique and may be responsible for operating monitoring devices and emergency equipment, as well as the radiographic equipment. When required to operate the supporting apparatus, the radiographer must receive adequate directions for proper use of the equipment. Instruction in patient care techniques and sterile procedure is included in the basic preparation of the radiographer.

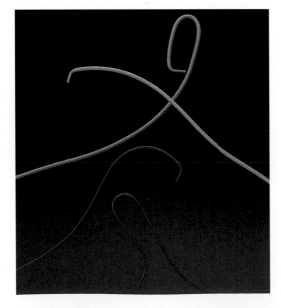

Fig. 26-12 Selected catheter shapes used for angiography.

(Courtesy Cook, Inc., Bloomington, Ind.)

Visceral Angiography

AORTOGRAPHY

The most satisfactory visualization of the aorta is achieved by placing a catheter into the aorta at the desired level. This is commonly accomplished with the Seldinger technique from the right or left femoral artery sites, using a catheter that has multiple side holes. Aortography is usually performed with the patient in the supine position for simultaneous frontal and lateral imaging with the central ray perpendicular to the imaging system. For translumbar catheter introduction, an alternative for aortography, the patient must be in the prone position.

Thoracic aortography

Thoracic aortography may be performed to rule out an aortic aneurysm or to evaluate congenital or postsurgical conditions. The examination is also used in patients with *aortic dissection.* Biplane imaging is recommended so that AP or PA and lateral projections can be obtained with one contrast medium injection. The radiographer observes the following guidelines:

- For lateral projections, move the patient's arms superiorly so that they do not appear in the image.
- For best results, increase the lateral SID, usually to 60 inches (152 cm), so that magnification is reduced.
- If biplane equipment is not available, use a single-plane 45-degree right posterior oblique (RPO) or left anterior oblique (LAO) body position, which often produces an adequate study of the aorta.
- For all projections, direct the perpendicular central ray to the center of the chest at the level of T6. This should allow visualization of the entire thoracic aorta, including the proximal brachiocephalic, carotid, and subclavian vessels.

The contrast medium is injected at rates ranging from 25 to 35 ml/sec for a total volume of 50 to 70 ml. The radiographer then performs the following steps:

- Begin imaging simultaneously with injection of the contrast material.
- Make exposures in each plane at rates ranging from one and one-half to three exposures per second for 3 to 4 seconds; exposures may then slow to one image or less per second for an additional 3 to 5 seconds.
- Make the exposures at the end of suspended inspiration (Figs. 26-13 and 26-14).

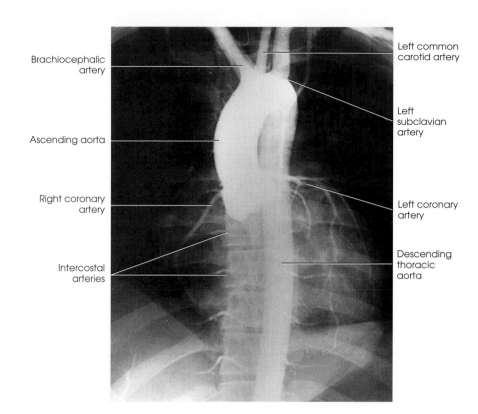

Fig. 26-13 AP thoracic aorta that also demonstrates right and left coronary arteries.

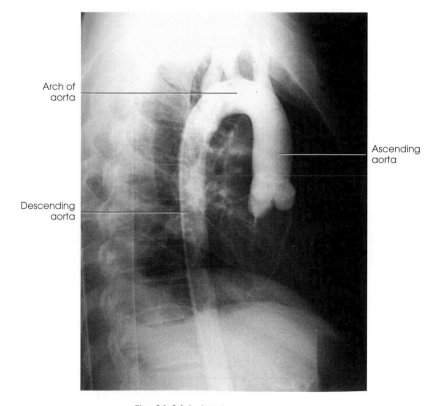

Fig. 26-14 Lateral thoracic aorta.

Abdominal aortography

Abdominal aortography may be performed to evaluate abdominal aortic aneurysm, occlusion, or atherosclerotic disease. Simultaneous AP and lateral projections are recommended. The radiographer observes the following guidelines:

- For the lateral projection, move the patient's arms superiorly so that they are out of the image field.
- Usually, collimate the field in the AP aspect of the lateral projection.
- Direct the perpendicular central ray at the level of L2 so that the aorta is visualized from the diaphragm to the aortic bifurcation. The AP projection best demonstrates the renal artery origins, the aortic bifurcation, and the course and general condition of all abdominal visceral branches. The lateral projection best demonstrates the origins of the celiac and superior mesenteric arteries because these vessels arise from the anterior abdominal aorta.
- Make the exposures. Representative injection and imaging programs are 25 ml/sec for a 60-ml total volume of contrast medium and two images per second for 4 seconds followed by one image per second for 4 seconds in each plane.
- Begin making the exposures simultaneously with the beginning of the injection and the end of suspended expiration (Figs. 26-15 and 26-16).

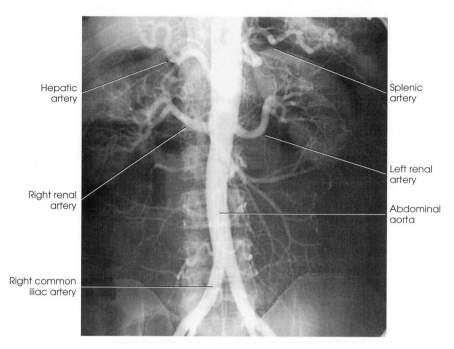

Hepatic artery

Right renal artery

Right common iliac artery

Splenic artery

Left renal artery

Abdominal aorta

Fig. 26-15 AP abdominal aorta.

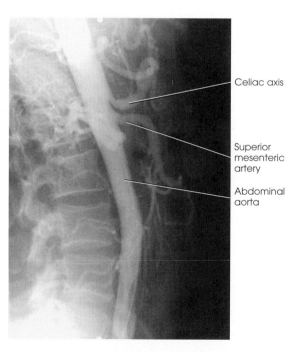

Celiac axis

Superior mesenteric artery

Abdominal aorta

Fig. 26-16 Lateral abdominal aorta.

Pulmonary Arteriography

Under fluoroscopic control, a catheter is passed from a peripheral vein through the vena cava and right side of the heart and into the pulmonary arteries. This technique is usually employed for a selective injection, and the examination is primarily performed for the evaluation of embolic disease.

Simultaneous AP and lateral projections of the supine patient are recommended for this procedure. The suggested SID for the lateral projection is 60 inches (152 cm). The radiographer observes the following guidelines:

- Move the patient's arms superiorly so that they are out of the field of view.
- When biplane projections are not possible, use a single-plane 35-degree RAO or LPO position. This approach usually achieves satisfactory results for both right and left pulmonary arteriograms.
- Direct the central ray perpendicular to the image receptor for all exposures.
- Use a compensating (trough) filter on the AP projection to obtain a radiograph with more uniform density between the vertebrae and the lungs if needed.
- In studies of the pulmonary arteries, lengthen the time of the imaging program to reveal the opacified left atrium, left ventricle, and thoracic aorta.
- Make the exposures. Representative injection and imaging programs are 25 ml/sec for a 50-ml total volume of contrast medium and two to four images per second for 4 seconds followed by one per second for an additional 4 seconds in each plane (Figs. 26-17 to 26-20).

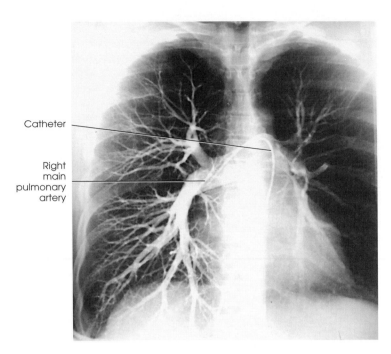

Fig. 26-17 AP right main pulmonary artery during early phase of injection.

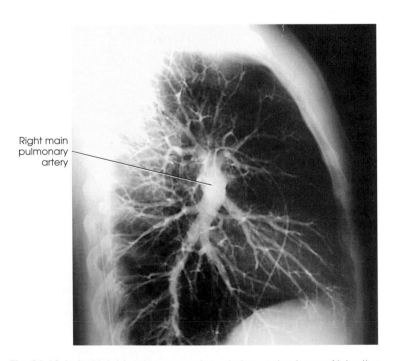

Fig. 26-18 Lateral right pulmonary artery during early phase of injection.

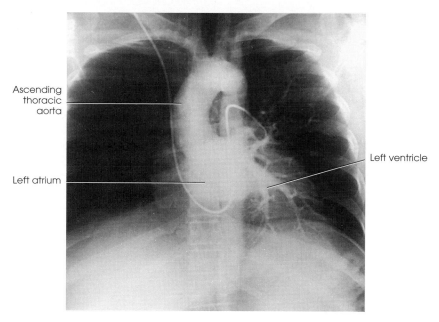

Ascending
thoracic
aorta

Left ventricle

Left atrium

Fig. 26-19 Late-phase AP pulmonary arteriogram demonstrating left atrium, left ventricle, and thoracic aorta.

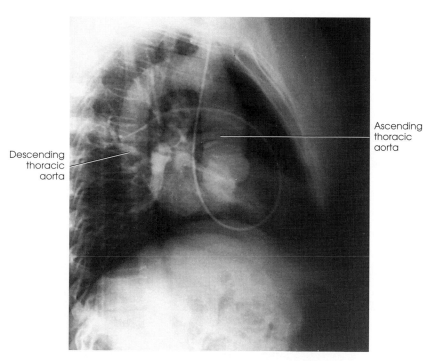

Ascending
thoracic
aorta

Descending
thoracic
aorta

Fig. 26-20 Late-phase lateral pulmonary artery injection showing aorta.

Selective Abdominal Visceral Arteriography

Abdominal visceral arteriographic studies are usually performed to visualize tumor vascularity or to rule out atherosclerotic disease, thrombosis, embolization, occlusion, and bleeding. The Seldinger technique is the preferred approach. An appropriately shaped catheter is introduced, usually at the femoral artery site, and advanced into the orifice of the desired artery. The radiographer observes the following steps:

- Perform all selective studies initially with the patient in the supine position for single-plane frontal images.
- Direct the central ray perpendicular to the image receptor.
- In most patients, obtain a preliminary radiograph to establish optimum exposure and positioning.
- If necessary, use oblique projections to improve visualization or avoid superimposition of vessels.
- For all abdominal visceral studies, obtain radiographs during suspended expiration.

Selective abdominal visceral arteriograms are described in the following sections.

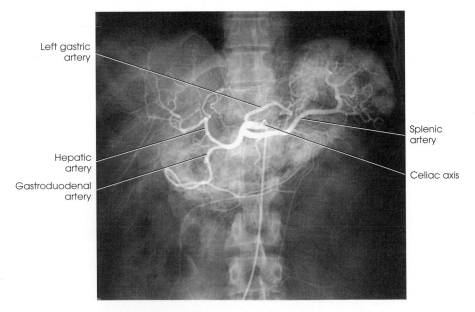

Left gastric artery

Hepatic artery

Gastroduodenal artery

Splenic artery

Celiac axis

Fig. 26-21 Selective AP celiac arteriogram.

CELIAC ARTERIOGRAM

The celiac artery normally arises from the aorta at the level of T12 and carries blood to the stomach, liver, spleen, and pancreas. These steps are followed:

- For the angiographic examination, center the patient to the image receptor.
- Direct the central ray to L1 (Fig. 26-21).
- Make the exposures. Representative injection and image programs are 10 ml/sec for a 40-ml total volume of contrast medium and two images per second for 5 seconds followed by one per second for 5 seconds.

HEPATIC ARTERIOGRAM

The common hepatic artery branches from the right side of the celiac artery and supplies circulation to the liver, stomach, duodenum, and pancreas. The radiographer follows these steps:

- Position the patient so that the upper and right margins of the liver are at the respective margins of the image receptor (Fig. 26-22).
- Make the exposures. Representative injection and imaging programs are 8 ml/sec for a 40-ml total volume of contrast medium and two images per second for 5 seconds followed by one per second for 5 seconds.

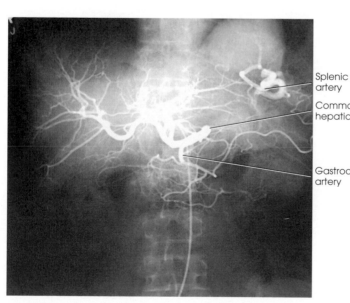

Splenic artery

Common hepatic artery

Gastroduodenal artery

Fig. 26-22 Superselective hepatic arteriogram with overflow into splenic artery.

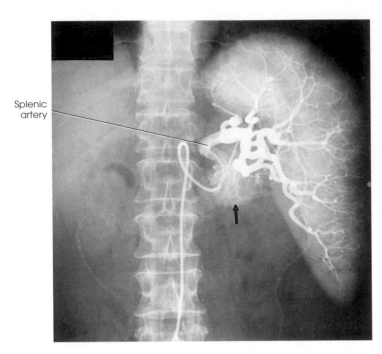

Splenic
artery

Fig. 26-23 Superselective splenic arteriogram with moderately enlarged spleen. Tail of pancreas (*arrow*).

SPLENIC ARTERIOGRAM

The splenic artery branches from the left side of the celiac artery and supplies blood to the spleen and pancreas. The steps are as follows:

- Position the patient to place the left and upper margins of the spleen at the respective margins of the image receptor (Figs. 26-23 and 26-24).
- Extend the length of the imaging sequence, which often allows adequate visualization of the portal system on the later radiographs. Splenic artery injection is, in fact, the common method of demonstrating the portal venous system.
- For demonstration of the portal vein, center the patient to the image receptor.
- Make the exposures. Representative injection and imaging programs for a standard splenic arteriogram are 8 ml/sec for a 40-ml total volume of contrast medium and two images per second for 5 seconds followed by one per second for 5 seconds. Representative programs for portal vein visualization are 8 ml/sec for an 80-ml total volume and one image per second for 20 seconds.

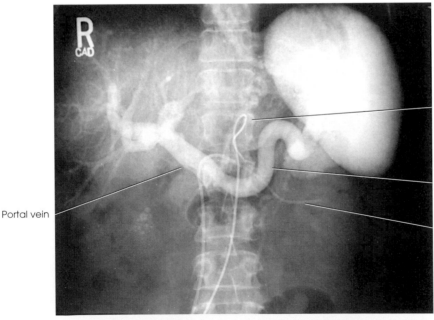

Portal vein

Splenic artery
catheter

Splenic vein

Catheter in left
renal vein

Fig. 26-24 Late-phase splenic arteriogram demonstrating portal system.

SUPERIOR MESENTERIC ARTERIOGRAM

The superior mesenteric artery (SMA) supplies blood to the small intestine and the ascending and transverse colon. It arises at about the level of L1 and descends to L5-S1. The radiographer follows these steps:

- To demonstrate the SMA, center the patient to the midline of the image receptor.
- Direct the central ray to the level of L3 (Fig. 26-25).
- Make the exposures. Representative injection and imaging programs are 8 ml/sec for a 40-ml total volume of contrast medium and two images per second for 5 seconds followed by one per second for 5 seconds.
- When attempting to visualize bleeding sites, conduct the imaging at one image per second for 18 seconds.
- Use an increased injection volume and an extended imaging sequence to optimize visualization of the mesenteric and portal veins.

INFERIOR MESENTERIC ARTERIOGRAM

The inferior mesenteric artery (IMA) supplies blood to the left colic flexure, descending colon, and rectosigmoid area. It arises from the left side of the aorta at about the level of L3 and descends into the pelvis. The steps are as follows:

- To best visualize the IMA, use a 15-degree right anterior oblique (RAO) or left posterior oblique (LPO) position that places the descending colon and rectum at the left and inferior margins of the image (Fig. 26-26).
- Make the exposures. A representative injection program is 3 ml/sec for a 15-ml total volume of contrast medium. The imaging is the same as that for the SMA.

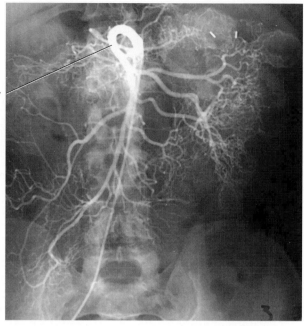

Superior mesenteric artery

Fig. 26-25 Selective superior mesenteric arteriogram.

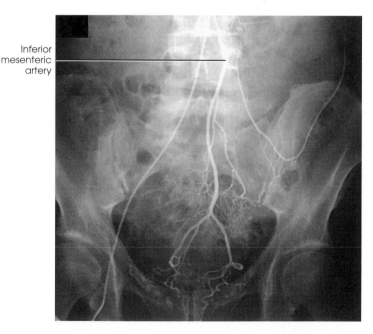

Inferior mesenteric artery

Fig. 26-26 Selective inferior mesenteric arteriogram.

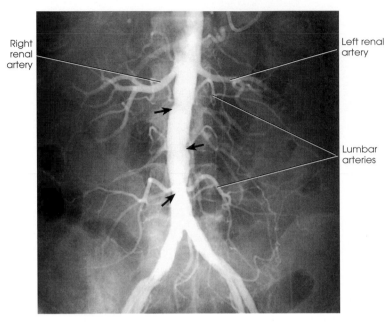

Right renal artery

Left renal artery

Lumbar arteries

Fig. 26-27 Renal flush arteriogram showing atherosclerotic changes in aorta *(arrows)*.

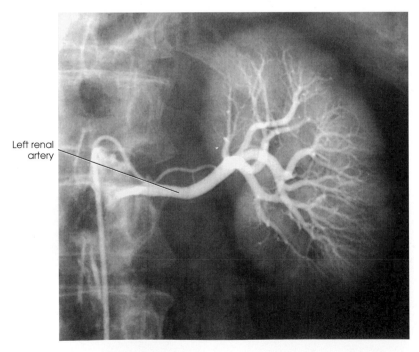

Left renal artery

Fig. 26-28 Selective left renal arteriogram in early arterial phase.

RENAL ARTERIOGRAM

The renal arteries arise from the right and left side of the aorta between L1 and L2 and supply blood to the respective kidney. The following steps are observed:

- Before performing this selective study, check the patient's IV urogram or renal flush arteriogram for the exact size and location of the kidneys. This step enables precise collimation to the kidney being studied and ensures exact centering of the patient and central ray.
- For a right renal arteriogram, position the patient so that the central ray enters at the level of L2 midway between the center of the spine and the patient's right side.
- For a selective left renal arteriogram, position the patient so that the central ray usually enters at the level of L1 and midway between the center of the spine and the patient's left side (Figs. 26-27 and 26-28).
- Make the exposures. A renal flush arteriogram may be accomplished by injecting 25 ml/sec for a 40-ml total volume of contrast medium through a multiple side hole catheter positioned in the aorta at the level of the renal arteries. A representative selective injection is 8 ml/sec for a 12-ml total volume. Imaging for both methods of injections is commonly three to six images per second for 2 to 3 seconds followed by perhaps only one or two nephrogram images made 5 to 10 seconds after the beginning of the injection.

OTHER ABDOMINAL ARTERIOGRAMS

Other arteries branching from the aorta may be selectively studied to demonstrate anatomy and possible pathologic condition. The positioning for these procedures depends on the area to be studied and the surrounding structures.

Central Venography

Blood in veins flows proximally. Injection into a central venous structure may not opacify the peripheral veins that *anastomose* to it. However, the position of peripheral veins can be indirectly documented by the filling defect from unopacified blood in the opacified central vein. The radiographer observes the following guidelines:

- Place the patient in the supine position for either a single-plane AP or PA projection or biplane projections. Move the patient's arms out of the field of view.
- Obtain lateral projections at increased SID, if possible, to reduce magnification.
- Remember that collimation to the long axis of the vena cava improves image quality but may prevent visualization of peripheral or *collateral* veins.

SUPERIOR VENACAVOGRAM

Venography of the superior vena cava is performed primarily to rule out the existence of thrombus or the occlusion of the superior vena cava. The contrast medium may be injected through a needle or an angiographic catheter introduced into a vein in an antecubital fossa, although superior opacification results from injection through a catheter positioned in the axillary or subclavian vein. Radiographs should include the opacified subclavian vein; the upper central chest, including the superior vena cava; and the right atrium (Fig. 26-29). The injection program depends mostly on whether a needle, an angiographic catheter, or a regular catheter is used. A representative program for a catheter injection is 10 to 15 ml/sec for a 30- to 50-ml total volume of contrast medium. Images are produced in both planes, if desired, at a rate of one or two images per second for 5 to 10 seconds and are made at the end of suspended inspiration.

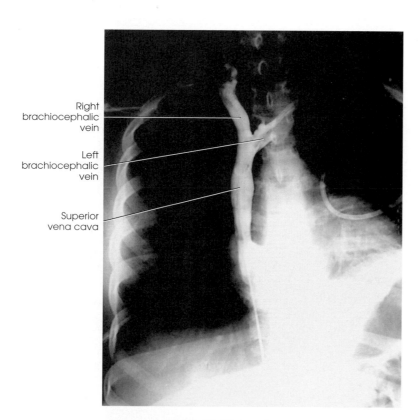

Right brachiocephalic vein

Left brachiocephalic vein

Superior vena cava

Fig. 26-29 AP superior vena cava.

INFERIOR VENACAVOGRAM

Venography of the inferior vena cava is performed primarily to rule out the existence of thrombus or the occlusion of the inferior vena cava. The contrast medium is injected through a multiple side hole catheter inserted through the femoral vein and positioned in the common iliac vein or the inferior aspect of the inferior vena cava. Radiographs may need to include the opacified vasculature from the catheter tip to the right atrium (Figs. 26-30 and 26-31). Representative injection and imaging programs are 25 ml/sec for a 50-ml total volume of contrast medium and two images per second for 4 to 8 seconds in both planes. Imaging begins at the end of suspended expiration.

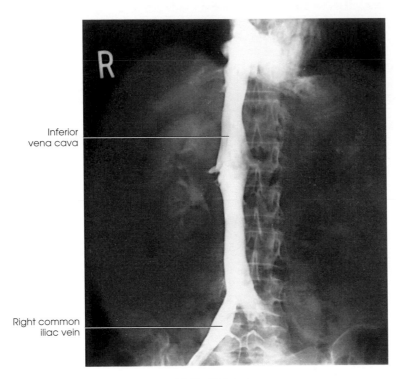

Inferior vena cava

Right common iliac vein

Fig. 26-30 AP inferior vena cava.

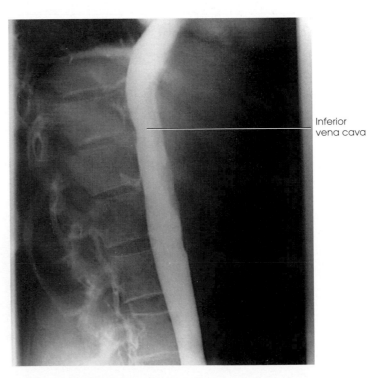

Inferior vena cava

Fig. 26-31 Lateral inferior vena cava.

Selective Visceral Venography

The visceral veins are often visualized by extending the imaging program of the corresponding visceral artery injection. For example, the veins that drain the small bowel are normally visualized by extending the imaging program of a superior mesenteric arteriogram. Portal venography can be performed by injecting the portal vein directly from a percutaneous anterior abdominal wall approach, but it is usually accomplished by late-phase imaging of a splenic artery injection. Some visceral veins are catheterized, however, for optimum visualization, blood sampling, or blood pressure measurements obtained through the catheter.

HEPATIC VENOGRAM

Hepatic venography is usually performed to rule out stenosis or thrombosis of the hepatic veins. These veins are also catheterized to obtain pressure measurements from the interior of the liver. The hepatic veins carry blood from the liver to the inferior vena cava. (The portal vein carries nutrient-rich blood from the other organs of digestion to the liver.) The hepatic veins are most easily catheterized from an upper limb vein approach, but a femoral vein approach may also be used. The radiographer follows these steps:

- Place the patient in the supine position for AP or PA projections that include the liver tissue and the extreme upper inferior vena cava (Fig. 26-32).
- Make the exposures. Representative injection and imaging programs are 10 ml/sec for a 30-ml total volume of contrast medium and one image per second for 8 seconds.
- Make exposures at the end of suspended expiration.

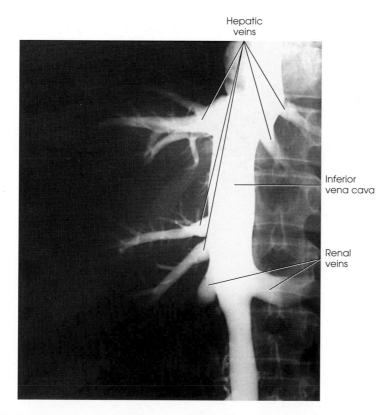

Hepatic veins

Inferior vena cava

Renal veins

Fig. 26-32 Hepatic vein visualization from inferior vena cava injection overflow.

RENAL VENOGRAM

Renal venography is usually performed to rule out thrombosis of the renal vein. The renal vein is also catheterized for blood sampling, usually to measure the production of renin, an enzyme produced by the kidney when it lacks adequate blood supply. The renal vein is most easily catheterized from an upper limb vein approach, but a femoral vein approach may also be used. The following steps are observed:

- Place the patient in the supine position for a single-plane AP or PA projection.

- Center the selected kidney to the image receptor, and collimate the field to include the kidney and area of the inferior vena cava (Fig. 26-33).
- Make the exposures. Representative injection and imaging programs are 8 ml/sec for a 16-ml total volume of contrast medium and two images per second for 4 seconds.
- Make exposures at the end of suspended expiration.

Peripheral Angiography
UPPER LIMB ANTERIOGRAMS

Upper limb arteriography is most often performed to evaluate traumatic injury or an arteriovenous shunt created for renal dialysis. The arteriograms are usually obtained by using the Seldinger technique to introduce a catheter, usually at a femoral artery site, and then positioning it for selective injection into the subclavian artery. The contrast medium may also be injected at a more distal site through a catheter or needle. The area to be radiographed may therefore be just a hand or other selected part of the arm, or it may include the entire upper limb and thorax.

Left renal veins

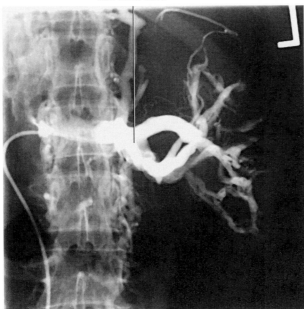

Fig. 26-33 Selective left renal venogram. AP projection.

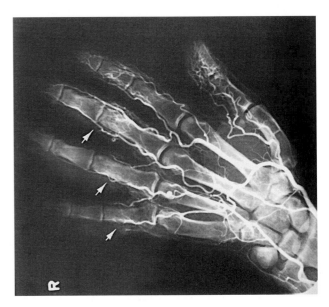

Fig. 26-34 Right hand arteriogram (2:1 magnification) showing severe arteriooclusive disease *(arrows)* affecting digits after cold-temperature injury.

The available equipment and the patient's condition control the imaging procedure. The recommended projection is a true AP projection with the arm extended and the hand supinated. Hand arteriograms may be obtained in the supine or prone arm position (Figs. 26-34 and 26-35). The injection and imaging programs depend on the equipment used. The injection varies from 3 or 4 ml/sec through a large needle positioned distally to 10 ml/sec through a proximally positioned catheter. Imaging using a long cassette changer may be performed with 1- or 2-second delays between exposures. A representative program for a rapid imaging system may be two films per second for 5 seconds followed by one per second for 5 seconds.

UPPER LIMB VENOGRAMS

Upper limb venography is most often performed to look for thrombosis. The contrast medium is injected through a needle or catheter into a superficial vein at the elbow or wrist. The radiographs should cover the vasculature from the wrist or elbow to the superior vena cava. The patient position selected may be determined by fluoroscopy, or the patient may be positioned for an AP projection with the hand supinated.

The projection and imaging sequence depend on the location of the injection site and the limitations and condition of the patient and equipment (Fig. 26-36). If the injection and filling of veins are observed with a fluoroscopic spot-film device, radiographs can be exposed as the vessels opacify. If a Bucky tray or rapid sequence imaging system is used, a series of images with a delay of a few seconds between exposures is normally obtained. Injections may be made by hand, or an automatic injector may be set to deliver a total of 40 to 80 ml at a rate of 1 to 4 ml/sec, depending on whether a needle or catheter is used. If the study is performed with the patient supine, tourniquets positioned proximal to the wrist and elbow are required to force the contrast medium into the deep veins.

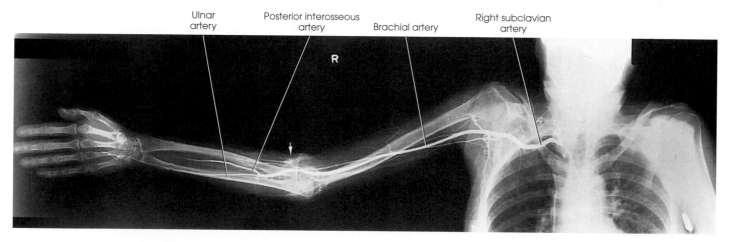

Ulnar artery   Posterior interosseous artery   Brachial artery   Right subclavian artery

Fig. 26-35 Right upper limb arteriogram showing iatrogenic occlusion of radial artery (*arrow*).

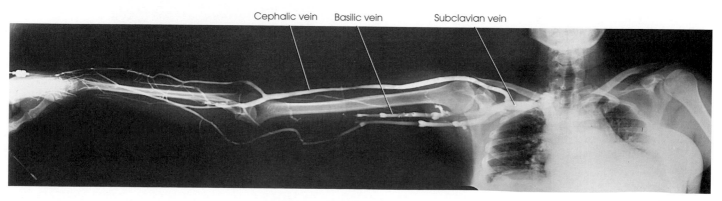

Cephalic vein   Basilic vein   Subclavian vein

Fig. 26-36 Normal right upper limb venogram.

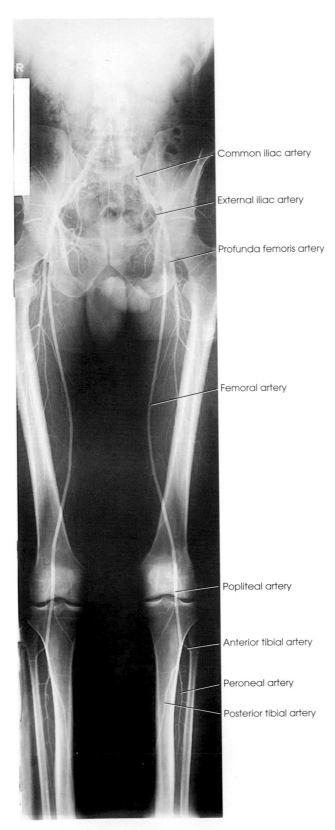

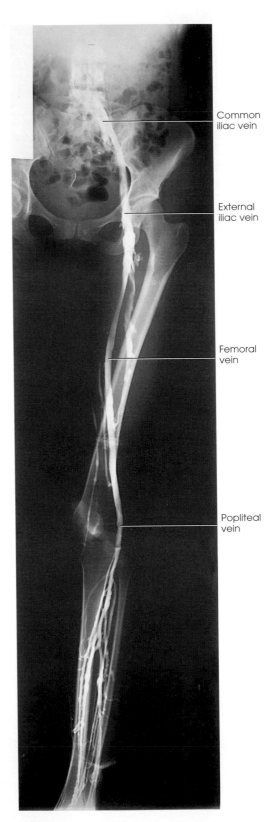

Common iliac artery

External iliac artery

Profunda femoris artery

Femoral artery

Popliteal artery

Anterior tibial artery

Peroneal artery

Posterior tibial artery

Common iliac vein

External iliac vein

Femoral vein

Popliteal vein

Fig. 26-37 Normal aortofemoral arteriogram in late arterial phase.

Fig. 26-38 Normal left lower limb venogram.

Aortofemoral arteriograms

Aortofemoral arteriography is usually performed to determine if atherosclerotic disease is the cause of *claudication*. A catheter is usually introduced into a femoral artery using the Seldinger technique. The catheter tip is positioned superior to the aortic bifurcation so that bilateral arteriograms are obtained simultaneously. When only one leg is to be examined, the catheter tip is placed below the bifurcation, or the contrast medium is injected through a needle placed in the femoral artery. The radiographer then observes the following guidelines:

- For a bilateral examination, place the patient in the supine position for single-plane AP projections and center the patient to the midline of the image receptor to include the area from the renal arteries to the ankles.
- Place the patient in the prone position for a translumbar catheterization if needed.
- For either patient position, internally rotate the legs 30 degrees.
- For best results, use a cassette changer with a length of 48 inches (122 cm).
- If the cassette changer is not available, have the cassettes overlap to ensure coverage of all vasculature. Overlapping cassettes can be produced automatically by "stepping" systems with moving tables or C-arms.
- Make exposures of the opacified lower abdominal aorta and aortic bifurcation with the patient in suspended expiration.

Imaging programs vary and are set based on the predicted rate of flow through the long arterial course of the lower limb. Flow through normal arteries may take as little as 10 seconds, whereas flow through severely diseased arteries may take 30 seconds or more. A representative injection program designed to create a long bolus of contrast medium is 13 ml/sec for an 80-ml total volume (Fig. 26-37).

Examinations of a specific area of the leg such as the popliteal fossa or foot are occasionally performed. For these procedures the preferred injection site is usually the femoral artery. AP, lateral, or both projections may be obtained with the patient centered to the designated area.

LOWER LIMB VENOGRAMS

Lower limb venography is common and is usually performed to rule out thrombosis of the deep veins of the leg. Venograms are usually obtained with contrast medium injected through a needle placed directly into a superficial vein in the foot. The radiographer then observes the following guidelines:

- Obtain radiographs with the patient on a tilt table in a semiupright position at a minimum angle of 45 degrees if possible.
- Begin imaging at the patient's ankle, and proceed superiorly to include the inferior vena cava as the injection continues.
- Without fluoroscopy, usually obtain AP projections with the leg internally rotated 30 degrees to include the entire area of interest (Fig. 26-38). Exact positioning is often determined with fluoroscopic direction.
- Perform lateral projections if needed.
- If imaging is performed with the patient supine, apply tourniquets just proximal to the ankle and knee to force filling of the deep veins in the leg.
- Usually, expose serial radiographs 5 to 10 seconds apart. Injections may be made by hand, or an automatic injector may be set to deliver 1 or 2 ml/sec for a total of 50 to 100 ml.

In all angiographic procedures, precise methods must be followed, and the sequence of imaging and injection must be determined in consultation with the physician. As in all surgical procedures, great care must be exercised to ensure that sterile techniques are strictly maintained. Precise positioning of the patient is also essential so that the desired body part is adequately demonstrated. Careful and complete cooperation among the physician, radiographer, and patient is essential to obtaining radiographs with the maximum amount of diagnostic information.

Angiography in the Future

Visceral and peripheral angiography is a dynamic area that challenges angiographers to keep abreast of new techniques and equipment. New diagnostic modalities that reduce or eliminate irradiation may be developed that may replace a number of current angiographic procedures. Some diagnostic information, however, can be obtained only through conventional angiographic methods. Consequently, angiography will continue to be used to examine vasculature and, through therapeutic procedures, to provide beneficial treatment.

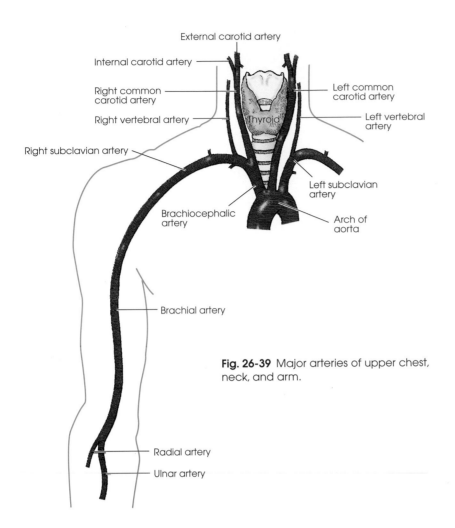

External carotid artery

Internal carotid artery

Right common carotid artery

Right vertebral artery

Right subclavian artery

Brachiocephalic artery

Thyroid

Left common carotid artery

Left vertebral artery

Left subclavian artery

Arch of aorta

Brachial artery

Radial artery

Ulnar artery

Fig. 26-39 Major arteries of upper chest, neck, and arm.

Cerebral Anatomy

Cerebral angiography is the term used to denote radiologic examinations of the blood vessels of the brain using injected radiopaque contrast medium. The procedure was introduced by Egas Moniz[1] in 1927. It is performed to investigate intracranial *aneurysms* or other vascular *lesions* and to demonstrate tumor masses, which are shown by displacement of the normal cerebrovascular pattern or by the tumor's circulation.

The brain is supplied by four trunk vessels: the right and left common carotid arteries, which supply the anterior circulation; and the right and left vertebral arteries, which supply the posterior circulation. These paired arteries branch from the arch of the aorta and ascend through the neck (Fig. 26-39).

[1]Egas Moniz AC: L'encéphalographie artérielle, son importance dans la localisation des tumeurs cérébrales, *Rev Neurol* 2:72, 1927.

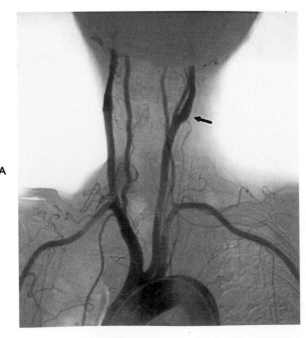

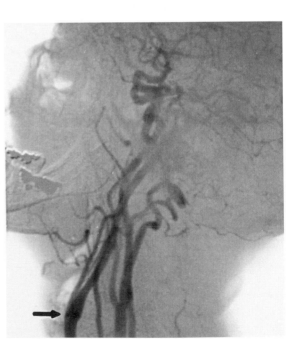

A

B

Fig. 26-40 Cerebral angiography, photographic subtraction technique: aortic arch. **A,** AP projection and **B,** AP oblique projection, RPO position. Excellent visualization of extracranial carotid and vertebral arteries is achieved. Normal left common carotid bifurcation is seen *(arrows).*

The left common carotid artery originates directly from the aortic arch. The right common carotid artery arises from the right subclavian artery about $1\frac{1}{2}$ inches (3.8 cm) higher at the *bifurcation* of the brachiocephalic artery (Fig. 26-40). The left subclavian artery originates directly from the arch of the aorta. The right and left vertebral arteries arise from the respective subclavian arteries. *Anomalies* in the origin of these vessels are common.

Each common carotid artery passes superiorly and somewhat laterally alongside the trachea and larynx to the level of C4. There each divides into internal and external carotid arteries. The external carotid artery contributes to the supply of the *meninges* but does not contribute to the intracerebral circulation. The internal carotid artery enters the cranium through the carotid foramen of the temporal bone and then bifurcates into the anterior and middle cerebral arteries. These vessels in turn branch and rebranch to supply the anterior circulation of the respective hemisphere of the brain (Fig. 26-41).

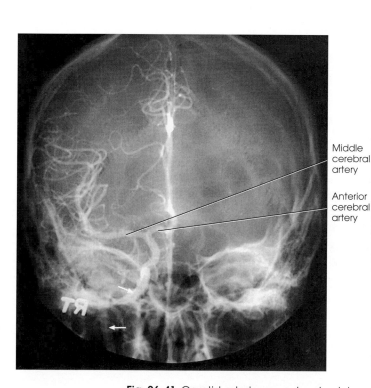

Fig. 26-41 Carotid arteriograms showing internal carotid artery *(arrows)* and anterior cerebral blood circulation.

The vertebral arteries ascend through the cervical transverse foramina and then pass medially to enter the cranium through the foramen magnum. The vertebral arteries unite to form the basilar artery, which, after a short superior course along the posterior surface of the dorsum sellae, bifurcates into the right and left posterior cerebral arteries. The blood supply to the posterior fossa (cerebellum) originates from the vertebral and basilar arteries (Fig. 26-42).

The anterior and posterior cerebral arteries are connected by communicating arteries at the level of the midbrain to form the *circle of Willis*. The anterior communicating artery forms an anastomosis between the anterior cerebral arteries. The right and left posterior communicating arteries each form an anastomosis between the internal carotid artery and the posterior cerebral artery on their side of the cerebral circulation.

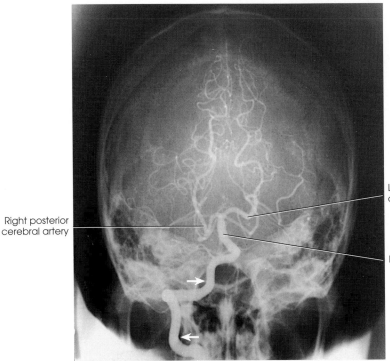

Right posterior cerebral artery

Left posterior cerebral artery

Basilar artery

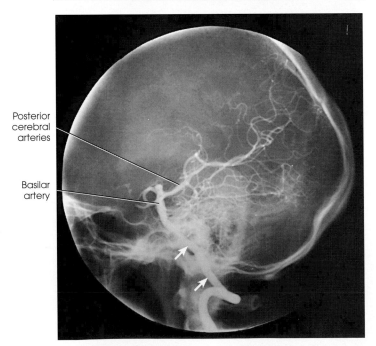

Posterior cerebral arteries

Basilar artery

Fig. 26-42 Vertebral arteriograms showing vertebral artery *(arrows)* and posterior cerebral blood circulation.

Cerebral Angiographic Studies

TECHNIQUE

Cerebral angiography should be performed only in facilities equipped to produce studies of high technical quality with minimal risk to the patient. The ability to obtain rapid-sequence biplane images with automatic injection represents the minimum standard. This equipment is available in all major medical centers and in most large community hospitals.

Access to the carotid, vertebral, and cerebral vessels is almost universally accomplished by catheterization from the femoral artery (Fig. 26-43). If this route is blocked by previous surgical procedures such as aortofemoral bypass grafting or intrinsic atherosclerotic disease, catheterization from a brachial or axillary artery approach is frequently employed. The entire intracerebral circulation can also be visualized by direct puncture and injection of the left common carotid artery and a right retrograde brachial artery injection. This technique is associated with a higher complication rate and significantly more discomfort to the patient. Selective catheterization techniques also allow the internal and external carotid circulations to be studied separately, which is useful in delineating the blood supply of some forms of cerebral tumors and vascular malformations.

The final position of the catheter depends on the information sought from the angiographic study. When atherosclerotic disease of the extracranial carotid, subclavian, and vertebral arteries is being evaluated, injection of the aortic arch with imaging of the extracranial portion of these vessels is an appropriate way to begin. Selective studies depend on fluoroscopic positioning of an appropriate catheter in a stable but *nonocclusive* position in the proximal segment of the carotid or vertebral artery of interest.

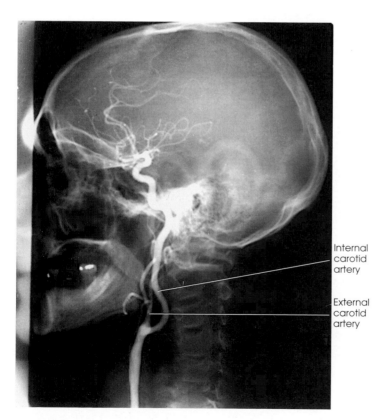

Internal carotid artery

External carotid artery

Fig. 26-43 Lateral intracranial and extracranial carotid arteriogram with catheter in right common carotid artery orifice by way of femoral artery catheterization.

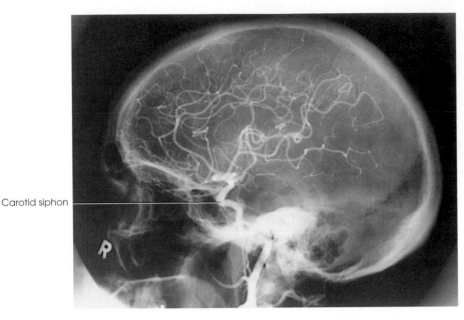

Carotid siphon

Fig. 26-44 Right lateral arteriogram showing arterial phase of circulation.

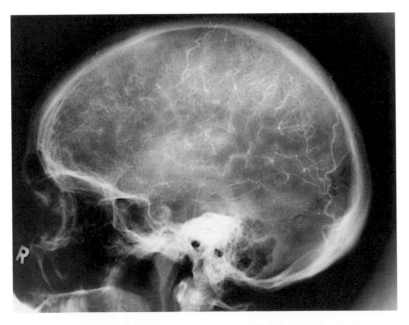

Fig. 26-45 Capillary phase of carotid circulation.

CIRCULATION TIME AND IMAGING PROGRAM

According to the estimation of Egas Moniz,[1] only 3 seconds is the usual time required for the blood to circulate from the internal carotid artery to the jugular vein, with the circulation time being slightly prolonged by the injected contrast solution. Greitz,[2] who measured the cerebral circulation time as "the time between the points of maximum concentration (of contrast medium) in the carotid siphon and in the parietal veins," found a normal mean value of 4.13 seconds. Thus time is a highly important factor in cerebral angiography.

Certain pathologic conditions significantly alter the cerebral circulation time. *Arteriovenous malformations (AVMs)* shorten the transit time, and increased intracranial pressure or arterial spasm may cause a considerable delay.

A standard radiographic program should include a radiograph taken before the arrival of contrast material to serve as a subtraction mask (see p. 86) and rapid-sequence images at one and one-half to three images per second in the AP and lateral projections during the early, or arterial, phase (first $1\frac{1}{2}$ to $2\frac{1}{2}$ seconds) of the arteriogram (Fig. 26-44). After the arterial phase, imaging may be slowed to one image per second for the capillary, or parenchymal, phase (Fig. 26-45) and maintained at one image per second or every other second for the venous phase (Fig. 26-46) of the angiogram. The entire program should cover 7 to 10 seconds, depending on the preference of the angiographer. The imaging program must be tailored to demonstrate the suspected pathologic condition.

Injection rates and volumes through the catheter are coupled with the imaging program, usually by automatic means. Injections at rates of 5 to 9 ml/sec for 1 to 2 seconds are most often employed in the cerebral vessels, with variations dependent on vessel size and the patient's circulatory status.

[1]Egas Moniz AC: *L'angiographie cérébrale,* Paris, 1934, Masson & Cie.
[2]Greitz T: A radiologic study of the brain circulation by rapid serial angiography of the carotid artery, *Acta Radiol Suppl* 140:Nov, 1956.

EQUIPMENT

Rapid-sequence biplane imaging with either film or DSA electronically coupled with an automatic injector is employed almost universally in cerebral angiography. Special instruction and experience are necessary to use this sophisticated and expensive equipment. The operational and imaging capabilities of cerebral angiographic units are diverse and vary considerably according to the manufacturer. However, routine maintenance of all equipment is essential to ensure reliable performance. Careful attention to maintenance and other details by technical and professional staff members is necessary to prevent unnecessary delays in completing studies as well as inconvenient downtime.

Collimating to the area of the head and neck is essential for improving image quality in the nonmagnified study. The standard tube collimator may be used for this purpose, or lead cutout diaphragms may also be positioned on the collimator. These diaphragms may have openings in the shape of a circle or a "keyhole." The keyhole diaphragm openings are rounded in the area of the cranium and taper inward in the area of the neck. The frontal and lateral keyhole diaphragms are each designed to resemble the shape of the head and neck in their respective images.

PREPARATION OF PATIENT

Other than withholding the preceding meal, preliminary preparation depends on the patient's condition and is accordingly determined by the radiologist and the referring physician. Whenever possible, adult patients are examined under local anesthesia in conjunction with sedation. Adequate sedation minimizes the intensity of the burning pain felt along the course of the vessel and the areas supplied by it during the rapid injections of iodinated medium. The sedative also lessens the possibility of a reaction resulting in reflex movement during initial arterial imaging at or before the end of each injection. It is imperative that conscious patients receive a careful explanation of what to expect during the examination and what is expected of them. This explanation is essential for the successful completion of the examination.

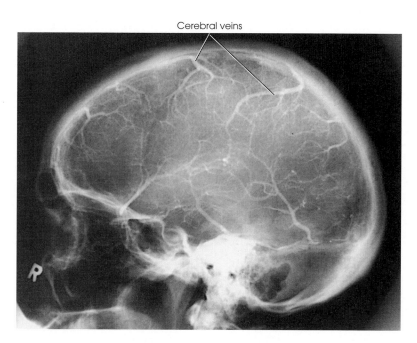

Cerebral veins

Fig. 26-46 Venous phase of circulation.

PREPARATION OF EXAMINING ROOM

It cannot be stated too often that the radiographic examining rooms and every item in it should be scrupulously clean. The room should be fully prepared, with every item needed or likely to be needed on hand before the patient is admitted. Cleanliness and advance preparation are of vital importance in examinations that must be carried out under aseptic conditions. The radiographer should observe the following guidelines in preparing the room:

- Check the radiographic machine and all working parts of the equipment, and adjust the controls for the exposure technique to be employed.
- Place identification markers and all accessories in a convenient location.
- Have compression and restraining bands ready for application.
- Adapt immobilization of the head (by suitable strapping) to the type of equipment employed.
- Make arrangements for immediate image processing as the examination proceeds.

The sterile and nonsterile items required for introduction of the contrast medium vary according to the method of injection. The supplies specified by the radiologist for each procedure should be listed in the angiographic procedure book. Sterile trays or packs, set up to specifications, can usually be obtained from the central sterile-supply room. Otherwise, it is the responsibility of a qualified member of the technologic staff to prepare them. Extra sterile supplies should always be on hand in case of an accident. Preparation of the room includes having life-supporting emergency equipment immediately available.

RADIATION PROTECTION

As in all radiographic examinations, the patient is protected by filtration totaling not less than 2.5 mm of aluminum, by sharp restriction of the beam of radiation to the area being examined, and by avoidance of repeat exposures. In angiography, each repeated exposure necessitates repeated injection of the iodinated compound. For this reason, only skilled and specifically educated radiographers should be assigned to take part in these examinations.

Angiography suites should be designed to allow observation of the patient at all times as well as to provide adequate protection to the physician and radiology personnel. These goals are usually accomplished with leaded glass observation windows.

POSITIONING FOR EXAMINATION
Position of patient

In positioning the patient, the radiographer observes the following steps:

- Place the patient in the supine position for the entire examination (as required by all cerebral angiographic injection methods).
- Regardless of whether the patient is awake, place suitable supports under points of strain (small of the back, knees, and ankles), and cover the patient according to room temperature.
- Apply wrist restraints and compression bands across the body as indicated by the patient's condition.
- Although the catheter is unlikely to be unseated during positioning, exercise care to prevent excessive patient motion, especially with extremely selective studies.

Position of head

The centering and angulation of the central ray required for demonstration of the anterior circulation differ from those required for demonstration of the posterior circulation. The same head position is used for the basic AP and lateral projections of both regions. The following steps are observed:

- For the initial right-angle studies, center the head to both the AP and lateral image receptors.
- Adjust the patient's head to place its midsagittal plane exactly perpendicular to the headrest and consequently exactly parallel with the laterally placed image receptor.
- Place the infraorbitomeatal line (IOML) perpendicular to the horizontal plane when positioning is manually accomplished.
- Angle the central ray for caudally inclined AP and AP oblique projections from the vertically placed IOML, or adjust the central ray so that it is parallel to the floor of the anterior fossa, as indicated by a line extending from the supraorbital margin to a point $\frac{3}{4}$ inch (1.9 cm) superior to the EAM.

In this chapter, head positioning is presented as if the image receptors were fixed in the horizontal and vertical planes. This necessitates the use of facial landmarks for precise positioning of the head in relation to the central ray to achieve certain projections. In some angiographic suites, however, fluoroscopy can be used to determine the final position of the head and the angulation of the central ray required to achieve the desired image.

Frontal projections are described in this section as AP projections, but equivalent PA projections also exist. Many angiographic imaging systems place the image receptor above the tabletop and the x-ray tube below. Because patients usually lie supine for cerebral angiography, the central ray, coming from below, enters the posterior cranium and exits the anterior cranium on its course to the image receptor. This results in PA projections equivalent to the AP projections described.

The literature on cerebral angiography contains numerous position variations concerning the degree of central ray angulation, the base from which the central ray should be angled or the line that it should parallel, and the degree of part rotation for oblique studies. This chapter discusses the most frequently employed images and reasonably standard specifications for obtaining them.

The number of radiographs required for satisfactory delineation of a lesion depends on the nature and location of the lesion. Oblique projections and/or variations in central ray angulation are used to separate the vessels that overlap in the basic positions and to evaluate any existing abnormality.

Aortic Arch Angiogram (for Cranial Vessels)

An aortic arch angiogram is most commonly obtained to visualize atherosclerotic or occlusive disease of the extracranial carotid, vertebral, and subclavian arteries. A multiple side hole catheter is positioned in the arch of the aorta so that the subsequent injection fills all of the vessels simultaneously.

SIMULTANEOUS BIPLANE OBLIQUE PROJECTIONS

For best results, simultaneous biplane oblique projections are produced so that superimposition of vessels is minimized. The radiographer observes the following steps:

- Place the patient in an RPO position on the tabletop, with the midsagittal plane of the head either perpendicular to the AP image receptor or in an RPO position. This patient position opens the arch of the aorta for the AP oblique projection and frees the carotid and vertebral arteries from superimposition for the lateral oblique projection.
- Raise the patient's chin to superimpose the inferior margin of the mandible onto the occiput so that as much of the neck as possible is exposed in the frontal radiograph.
- Move the patient's shoulders inferiorly so that they are removed as much as possible from the lateral image.
- If possible, use offset biplane imaging systems for this procedure.
- Position the lateral image receptor approximately 6 inches (15 cm) superior to the AP changer so that the lateral projection exposes the head and neck whereas the AP projection exposes the neck and upper chest.
- For the AP projection, direct the central ray perpendicular to the center of the image receptor to enter the patient at a level $1\frac{1}{4}$ inch (3 cm) superior to the sternal angle.
- For the lateral projection, direct the central ray perpendicular to the midline of the vertically oriented grid and to enter the patient a few centimeters inferior to the angle of the mandible.
- Collimate the lateral field in the AP aspect (see Fig. 26-40).

A representative injection program for an aortic arch examination is 30 to 35 ml/sec for a total volume of 60 to 70 ml. A representative imaging program is two to three images per second in each plane for 4 seconds. Because subtraction images are frequently produced from aortic arch angiograms, the initial images should be exposed before the injection begins. An alternative imaging program exposes one image in each plane, pauses 1 second as the injection begins, and then continues with two to three images per second for 3 seconds.

Anterior Circulation

LATERAL PROJECTION

The radiographer observes the following steps:

- Center the patient's head to the vertically placed image receptor.
- Extend the patient's head enough to place the IOML perpendicular to the horizontal.
- Adjust the patient's head to place the midsagittal plane vertical and thereby parallel with the plane of the image receptor.
- Adapt immobilization to the type of equipment being employed.
- Perform lateral projections of the anterior, or carotid, circulation with the central ray directed horizontally to a point slightly cranial to the auricle and midway between the forehead and the occiput. This centering allows for patient variation (Figs. 26-47 to 26-49).

NOTE: See Fig. 26-72 for assistance in identifying the cerebral vessels in radiographs.

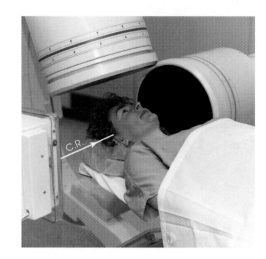

Fig. 26-47 Cerebral angiogram: lateral projection as part of a biplane setup.

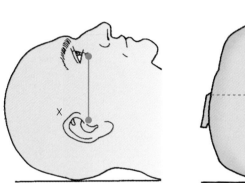

Fig. 26-48 Lateral projection.

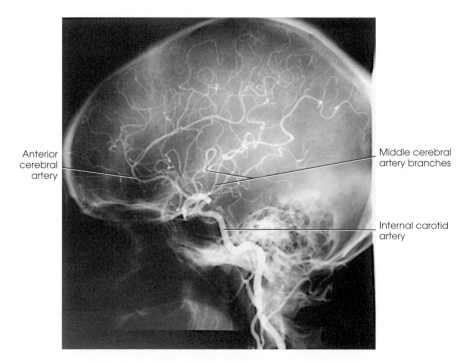

Anterior cerebral artery

Middle cerebral artery branches

Internal carotid artery

Fig. 26-49 Cerebral angiogram: lateral projection demonstrating anterior circulation.

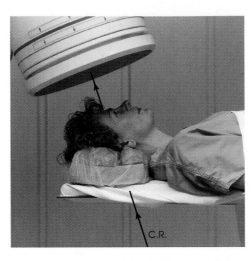

Fig. 26-50 Carotid angiogram: PA axial (supraorbital) projection.

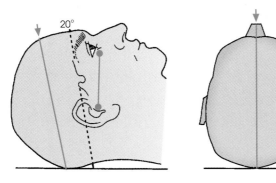

Fig. 26-51 AP axial (supraorbital).

AP AXIAL PROJECTION (SUPRAORBITAL)

The radiographer observes the following steps:

- Adjust the patient's head so that its midsagittal plane is centered over and perpendicular to the midline of the grid and so that it is extended enough to place the IOML vertical.
- Immobilize the patient's head.
- Keep in mind that achieving the goal in this radiograph requires superimposition of the supraorbital margins on the superior margin of the petrous ridges so that the vessels are projected above the floor of the anterior cranial fossa.
- To obtain this result in the majority of patients, direct the central ray 20 degrees caudal for the AP axial or 20 degrees cephalad for the PA axial projection along a line passing $^3/_4$ inch (1.9 cm) superior to and parallel with a line extending from the supraorbital margin to a point $^3/_4$ inch (1.9 cm) superior to the external acoustic meatus (EAM); the latter line coincides with the floor of the anterior fossa (Figs. 26-50 to 26-52).

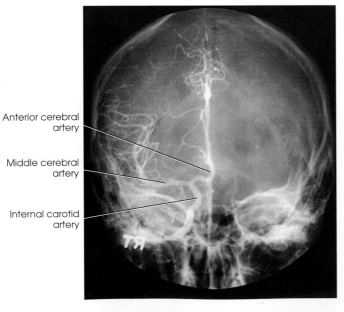

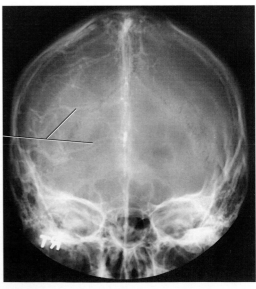

Anterior cerebral artery

Middle cerebral artery

Internal carotid artery

Cerebral veins

Fig. 26-52 Serial carotid angiograms: AP axial (supraorbital) projection. *Left,* Arterial phase of circulation. *Right,* Venous phases of circulation.

AP AXIAL OBLIQUE PROJECTION (SUPRAORBITAL)

The following steps are observed:

- For demonstration of the region of the anterior communicating artery, maintain the preceding position for the patient's head, but rotate the head approximately 30 degrees away from the injected side, or angle the central ray 30 degrees toward the injected side.
- Direct the central ray 20 degrees caudal (Figs. 26-53 and 26-54).

AP AXIAL PROJECTION (TRANSORBITAL)

The AP axial (transorbital) projection demonstrates the middle cerebral artery and its main branches within the orbit. The radiographer observes the following steps:

- Adjust the patient's head for the basic AP projection.

- Direct the central ray through the midorbits at an average angle of 20 degrees cephalad. The central ray should coincide with a line passing through the center of the orbit and a point about ¾ inch (1.9 cm) superior to the auricle of the ear (Figs. 26-55 and 26-56).

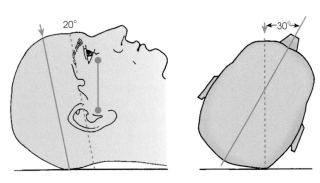

Fig. 26-53 AP axial oblique (supraorbital) projection.

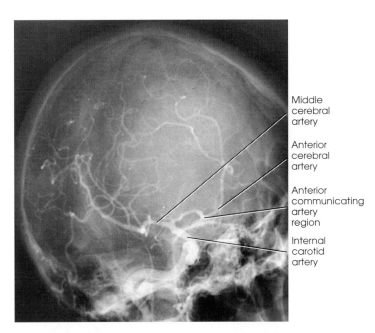

Fig. 26-54 Carotid arteriogram: AP axial oblique (supraorbital) projection.

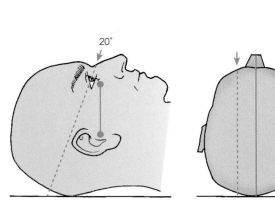

Fig. 26-55 AP axial (transorbital) projection.

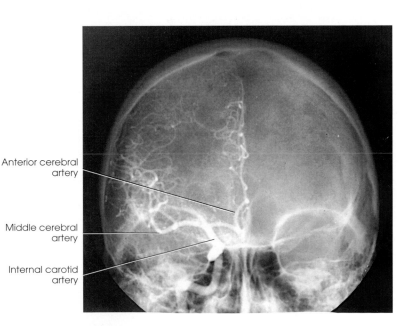

Fig. 26-56 Carotid arteriogram: AP axial (transorbital) projection.

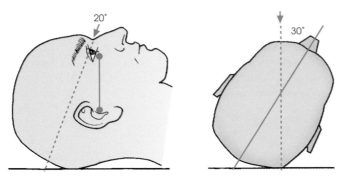

Fig. 26-57 AP axial oblique (transorbital) projection.

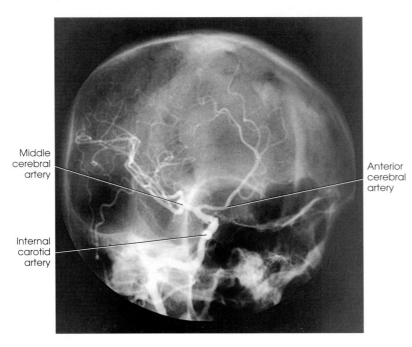

Middle cerebral artery

Anterior cerebral artery

Internal carotid artery

Fig. 26-58 Carotid angiogram: AP axial oblique (transorbital) projection.

AP AXIAL OBLIQUE PROJECTION (TRANSORBITAL)

The oblique transorbital projection demonstrates the internal carotid bifurcation and the anterior communicating and middle cerebral arteries within the orbital shadow. The steps are as follows:
- From the position for the basic AP transorbital projection, rotate the patient's head approximately 30 degrees away from the injected side, or angle the central ray 30 degrees toward the injected side.
- Angle the central ray 20 degrees cephalad and center it to the midorbit of the uppermost side (Figs. 26-57 and 26-58).

AP AXIAL AND AP OBLIQUE PROJECTIONS

AP axial and/or AP axial oblique projections are used in carotid angiography, when indicated, for further evaluation of vessel displacement or of aneurysms.

For an AP axial projection, the following steps are observed:
- Adjust the patient's head in the basic AP position.
- Direct the central ray to the region approximately $1\frac{1}{2}$ inches (3.8 cm) superior to the glabella at an average angle of 30 degrees caudad for the AP axial or 30 degrees cephalad for the PA axial projection. The central ray exits at the level of the EAM (Figs. 26-59 to 26-61).

For an AP axial oblique projection, the following steps are observed:
- Rotate the patient's head 35 to 45 degrees away from the injected side, or angle the central ray 35 to 45 degrees toward the injected side.
- Angle the central ray 30 degrees caudad (Figs. 26-62 and 26-63).

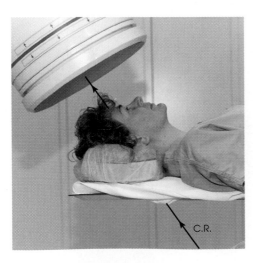

Fig. 26-59 PA axial projection.

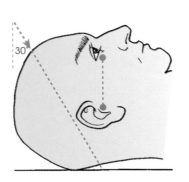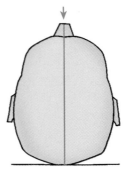

Fig. 26-60 AP axial projection.

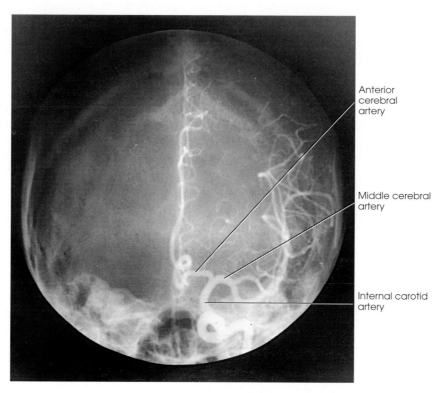

Anterior cerebral artery

Middle cerebral artery

Internal carotid artery

Fig. 26-61 Carotid angiogram: AP axial projection.

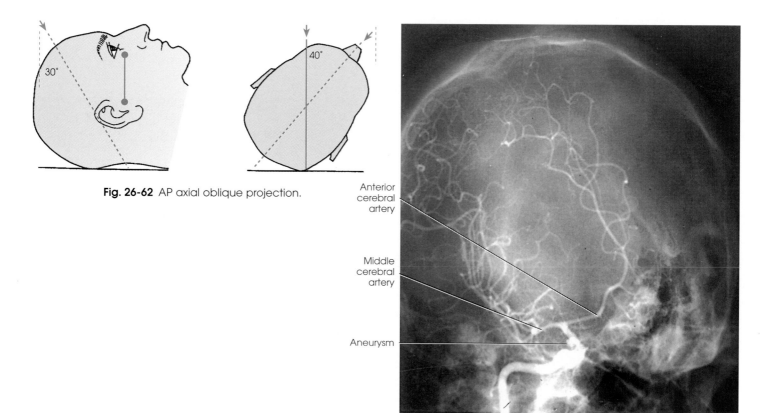

Fig. 26-62 AP axial oblique projection.

Anterior cerebral artery

Middle cerebral artery

Aneurysm

Fig. 26-63 Carotid angiogram: AP axial oblique projection showing small internal carotid artery aneurysm at posterior communicating junction.

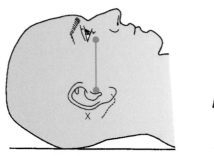
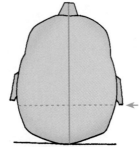

Fig. 26-64 Lateral projection for posterior circulation.

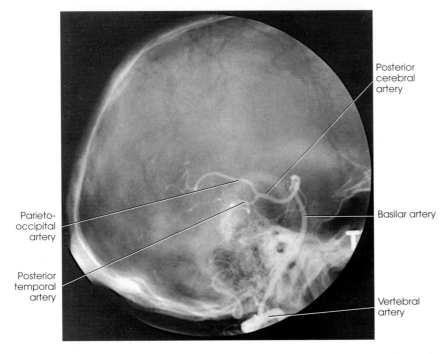

Posterior
cerebral
artery

Basilar artery

Parieto-
occipital
artery

Posterior
temporal
artery

Vertebral
artery

Fig. 26-65 Cerebral angiogram: lateral projection in early arterial phase showing vertebral artery and posterior vascular structures.

Posterior Circulation

LATERAL PROJECTION

The radiographer observes the following steps:

- Center the patient's head to the vertically placed image receptor.
- Extend the patient's head enough to place the IOML perpendicular to the horizontal plane, and then adjust the head to place the midsagittal plane vertical and thereby parallel with the plane of the image receptor.
- Rigidly immobilize the patient's head.
- Perform lateral projections of the posterior, or vertebral, circulation with the central ray directed horizontal to the mastoid process at a point about $\frac{3}{8}$ inch (1 cm) superior to and $\frac{3}{4}$ inch (1.9 cm) posterior to the EAM.
- Restrict the exposure field to the middle and posterior fossae for lateral studies of the posterior circulation (Figs. 26-64 to 26-67). Inclusion of the entire skull is neither necessary nor, from the standpoint of optimal technique, desirable.

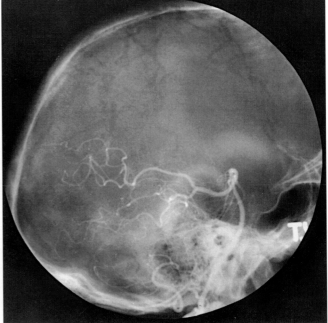

Fig. 26-66 Cerebral angiogram: lateral projection in arterial phase.

AP AXIAL PROJECTION

The following steps are observed:

- Adjust the patient's head so that its midsagittal plane is centered over and perpendicular to the midline of the grid, and extend the head enough so that the IOML is vertical.
- Immobilize the patient's head.
- Direct the central ray to the region approximately 1½ inches (3.8 cm) superior to the glabella at an angle of 30 to 35 degrees caudad. The central ray exits at the level of the EAM. For this projection the supraorbital margins are positioned approximately ¾ inch (1.9 cm) below the superior margins of the petrous ridges (Figs. 26-68 and 26-69).

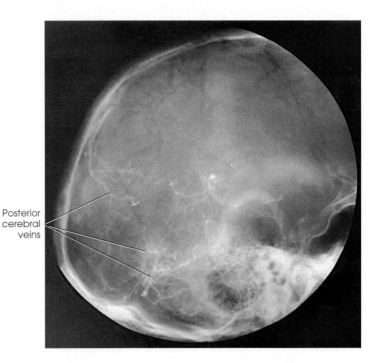

Fig. 26-67 Cerebral angiogram: lateral projection in venous phase. Contrast medium for the serial angiograms was introduced by percutaneous retrograde injection into left brachial artery.

Posterior cerebral veins

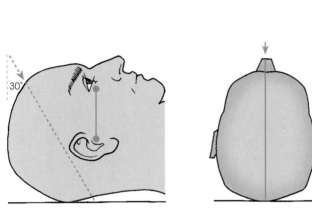

Fig. 26-68 AP axial projection for posterior circulation.

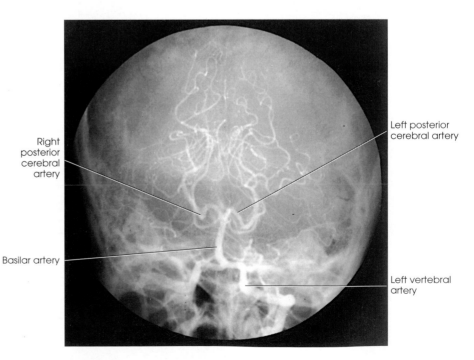

Right posterior cerebral artery

Basilar artery

Left posterior cerebral artery

Left vertebral artery

Fig. 26-69 AP axial projection: arterial phase of posterior circulation.

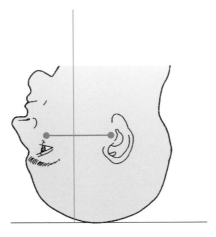

Fig. 26-70 SMV projection.

SUBMENTOVERTICAL PROJECTION

A modified submentovertical (SMV) projection is sometimes employed for the investigation of the posterior circulation. It is also used for the examination of the anterior circulation when a middle fossa lesion is suspected.

The success of this projection depends on the patient's ability to hyperextend the neck and maintain this hyperextension for the time required for an imaging sequence (Figs. 26-70 and 26-71). This body position may not be possible for elderly patients with cervical degenerative arthritis. A chart detailing intracerebral circulation is provided in Fig. 26-72.

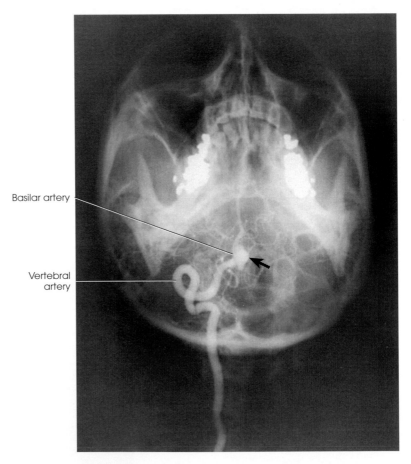

Basilar artery

Vertebral artery

Fig. 26-71 Transaxillary selective right SMV arteriogram showing excellent opacification of right vertebral artery and aneurysm *(arrow)* of vertebrobasilar junction.

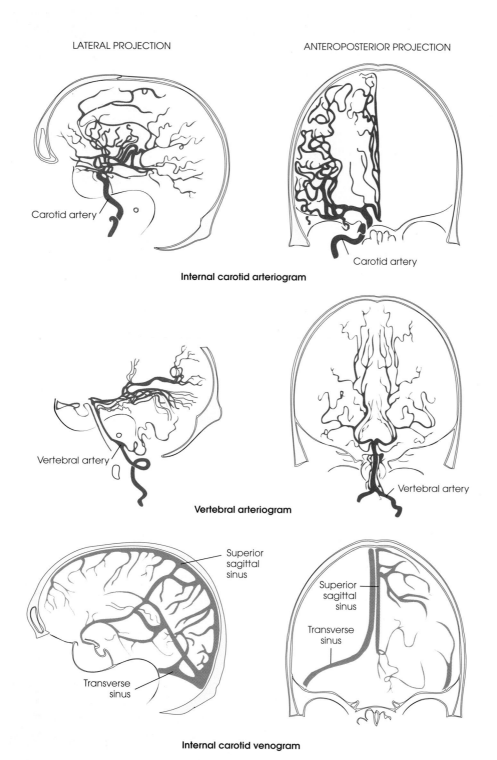

LATERAL PROJECTION

ANTEROPOSTERIOR PROJECTION

Carotid artery

Carotid artery

Internal carotid arteriogram

Vertebral artery

Vertebral artery

Vertebral arteriogram

Superior
sagittal
sinus

Superior
sagittal
sinus

Transverse
sinus

Transverse
sinus

Internal carotid venogram

Fig. 26-72 Intracerebral circulation.

(From Bean BC: A chart of the intracerebral circulation, ed 2, *Med Radiogr Photogr* 34:25, 1958; courtesy Dr. Berton C Bean and Eastman Kodak Co.)

Interventional radiology has a therapeutic rather than diagnostic purpose in that it intervenes in, or interferes with, the course of a disease process or other medical condition. Since the conception of this form of radiology in the early 1960s, its realm has become so vast and sophisticated that publishers of periodicals struggle to keep abreast of this rapidly advancing specialty.

Interventional radiology allows the angiographer to assume an important role in the management and treatment of disease in many patients. Interventional radiologic procedures reduce hospital stays in many patients and help some patients avoid surgery, with consequent reductions in medical costs.

Every interventional radiologic procedure must include two integral processes. The first is the interventional or medical side of the procedure, in which the highly skilled radiologist uses needles, catheters, and special medical devices (e.g., occluding coils, guide wires) to produce an improvement in the patient's status or condition. The second process involves the use of fluoroscopy and radiography to guide and document the progress of the steps taken during the first process. The radiographer must receive special education in the angiographic and interventional laboratory. This skilled radiographer has a very important role in assisting the angiographer in the interventional procedures.

The more frequently performed interventional procedures are described in the succeeding pages. Resources containing more detailed information are cited in the selected bibliography at the end of the chapter.

Percutaneous Transluminal Angioplasty

Percutaneous transluminal angioplasty (PTA) is a therapeutic radiologic procedure designed to dilate or reopen stenotic or occluded areas within a vessel using a catheter introduced by the Seldinger technique. PTA using a coaxial catheter method was first described by Dotter and Judkins[1] in 1964. First a guide wire is passed through the narrowed area of a vessel. Then a smaller catheter is passed over the guide wire through the stenosis to begin the dilation process. Finally, a larger catheter is passed over the smaller catheter to cause further dilation (Fig. 26-73). Although this method can achieve dilation of stenoses, it has the significant disadvantage of creating an *arteriotomy* as large as the dilating catheters.

[1]Dotter CT, Judkins MP: Transluminal treatment of arteriosclerotic obstruction: description of a new technique and preliminary report of its application, *Circulation* 30:654, 1964.

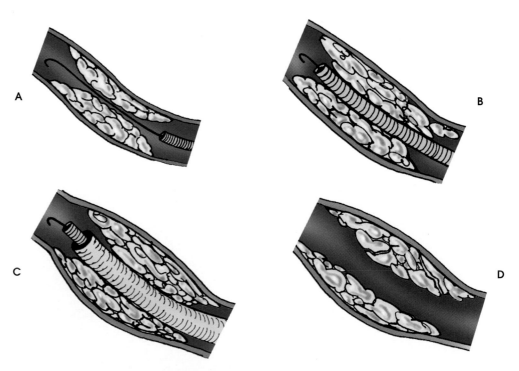

Fig. 26-73 Coaxial angioplasty of atherosclerotic stenosis. **A,** Guide wire advanced through stenosis. **B,** Small catheter advanced through stenosis. **C,** Large catheter advanced through stenosis. **D,** Postangioplasty stenotic area.

In 1974 Gruntzig and Hopff[2] introduced the double-lumen, balloon-tipped catheter. One lumen allows the passage of a guide wire and fluids through the catheter. The other lumen communicates with a balloon at the distal end of the catheter. When inflated, the balloon expands to a size much larger than the catheter. Double-lumen, balloon-tipped catheters are available in sizes ranging from 4.5 to 9 Fr, with attached balloons varying in length and expanding to diameters of 2 to 20 mm or more (Fig. 26-74).

Fig. 26-75 illustrates the process of *balloon angioplasty*. The stenosis is initially identified on a previously conducted angiogram. The balloon diameter used for a procedure is often the measured diameter of the normal artery adjacent to the stenosis. The angioplasty procedure is often conducted at the same time and through the same catheterization site as the initial diagnostic examination.

[2]Gruntzig A, Hopff H: Perkutane rekanalisation chronischer arterieller Verschlusse mit einem neuen dilatationskatheter; modifikation der Dotter-Technik, *Deutsch Med Wochenschr* 99:2502, 1974.

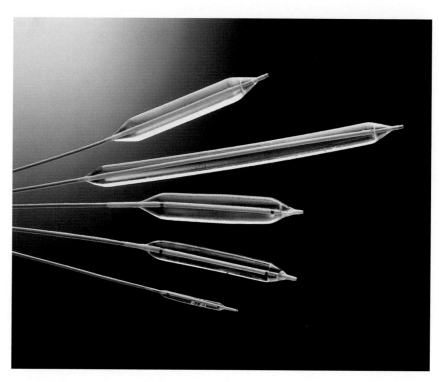

Fig. 26-74 Balloon angioplasty catheters with varied diameters and lengths.

(Courtesy Bard Radiology)

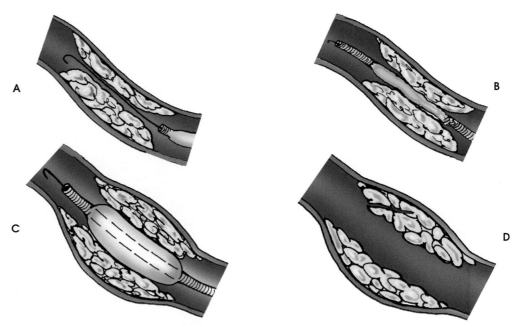

Fig. 26-75 Balloon angioplasty of atherosclerotic stenosis. **A,** Guide wire advanced through stenosis. **B,** Balloon across stenosis. **C,** Balloon inflated. **D,** Postangioplasty stenotic area.

After the guide wire is positioned across the stenosis, the angiographic catheter is removed over the wire. The balloon-tipped catheter is then introduced and directed through the stenosis by the guide wire. The balloon is usually inflated with a diluted contrast medium mixture for 15 to 45 seconds, depending on the degree of stenosis and the vessel being treated. The balloon is then deflated and repositioned or withdrawn from the lesion. Contrast medium can be injected through the angioplasty catheter for a repeat angiogram to determine whether or not the procedure was successful. The success of the angioplasty procedure may also be determined by comparing transcatheter blood pressure measurements from a location distal and a location proximal to the lesion site. Nearly equal pressures indicate a reopened stenosis.

Transluminal angioplasty can be performed in virtually any vessel that can be reached percutaneously with a catheter. The procedure is most commonly performed in the renal, iliac, and femoral arteries, and it is primarily used for therapy within an artery (Figs. 26-76 and 26-77). In 1978, however, Molnar and Stockum[1] described the use of balloon angioplasty for dilation of strictures within the biliary system (Fig. 26-78). Balloon angioplasty is also conducted in venous structures, ureters, and the gastrointestinal tract.

[1]Molnar W, Stockum AE: Transhepatic dilatation of choledochoenterostomy strictures, *Radiology* 129: 59, 1978.

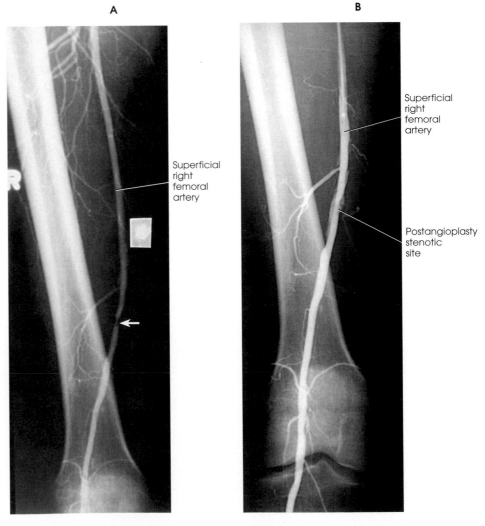

A

Superficial right femoral artery

B

Superficial right femoral artery

Postangioplasty stenotic site

Fig. 26-76 Femoral arteriograms. **A,** Stenosis *(arrow).* **B,** Postangioplasty femoral arteriogram.

A

B

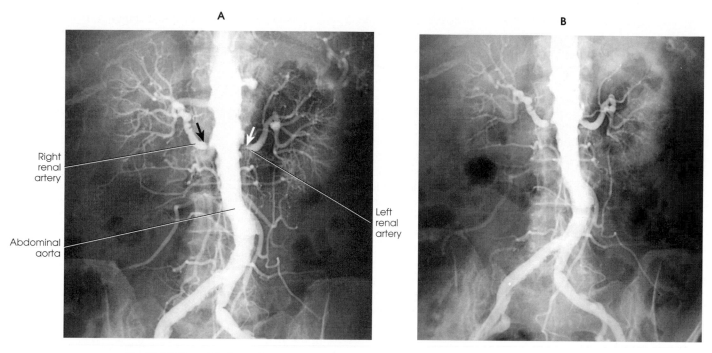

Right
renal
artery

Left
renal
artery

Abdominal
aorta

Fig. 26-77 Renal flush angiograms. **A,** Bilateral renal artery stenosis *(arrows).* **B,** Improved postangioplasty left renal artery.

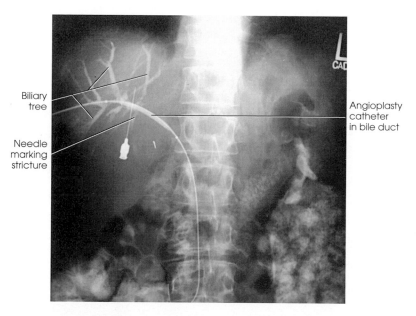

Biliary
tree

Angioplasty
catheter
in bile duct

Needle
marking
stricture

Fig. 26-78 Radiograph showing balloon catheter in common bile duct.

Balloon angioplasty has been used successfully to manage various diseases that cause arterial narrowing. The most common form of arterial stenosis treated by transluminal angioplasty is caused by atherosclerosis. Dotter and Judkins[1] speculated that this atheromatous material was soft and inelastic and therefore could be compressed against the artery wall. The success of coaxial and balloon method angioplasty was initially attributed to enlargement of the arterial lumen because of compression of the atherosclerotic plaque. Later research showed, however, that the plaque does not compress. If plaque surrounds the inner diameter of the artery, the plaque cracks at its thinnest portion as the arterial lumen is expanded. Continued expansion cracks the arterial wall's inner layer, the *intima,* then stretches and tears the middle layer, the *media,* and finally stretches the outer layer, the *adventitia.* The arterial lumen is increased by permanently enlarging the artery's outer diameter. Restenosis, when it occurs, is usually caused by deposits of new plaque, not arterial wall collapse.

In addition to balloon angioplasty, other angioplasty technologies are used to treat atherosclerotic disease. Some of these technologies involve the use of lasers. In *laser-tipped angioplasty,* laser energy is directed through a special catheter and pulsed at the atheromatous mass to vaporize it. This process leaves a smooth, carbonized surface up to 5 mm in diameter, which is somewhat larger than the catheter tip. In *thermal angioplasty* a laser-heated probe is advanced through an atheroma to recanalize the vessel lumen. Compared with balloon angioplasty, thermal angioplasty creates a smoother surface so that less restenosis occurs at the lesion site. Sometimes a balloon angioplasty procedure follows lumen recanalization to further expand the vessel lumen.

[1]Dotter CT, Judkins MP: Transluminal treatment of arteriosclerotic obstruction: description of a new technique and preliminary report of its application, *Circulation* 30:654, 1964.

Percutaneous atherectomy is an angioplasty technology that removes an atheroma by cutting it. Atherectomy catheter systems are either rotational or directional. A *rotational* catheter system has a blunt cam at the distal tip of the catheter that rotates at speeds up to 100,000 rpm. A fluid mixture is infused through the catheter as the cam rotates, creating a radial fluid spray. Together the rotating cam and fluid spray cut and recirculate atherosclerotic material until it is micropulverized, whereas normal tissue is spared. A balloon angioplasty procedure frequently follows lumen restoration by this method.

A *directional* atherectomy catheter system has, at its distal end, a cylindrically shaped chamber called the *housing* with an opening along one side called the *housing window.* Opposite the housing window is a balloon that, when inflated, presses the atheromatous mass into the window. A round, rotating cutter is then advanced through the housing to cut the atheroma, which is collected in the distal housing chamber. The balloon is then deflated, and the housing window is rotated 90 degrees in the vessel. The procedure is repeated until the atheroma has been removed circumferentially from the vessel lumen.

A final possibility for percutaneous treatment of vessel stenoses is the placement of vascular *stents.* A vascular stent is a wire or plastic cylinder that is introduced through a catheter system and positioned across a stenosis to keep the narrowed area spread apart. These devices permanently remain in the vessel (Fig. 26-79).

The success of PTA in the management of atherosclerosis has made it a significant alternative to surgical procedures in the treatment of this disease. PTA is not indicated in all cases, however. Long segments of occlusion, for example, may be best treated by surgery. PTA has a lower risk than surgery but is not totally without risk. Generally patients must be able to tolerate the surgical procedure that may be required to repair vessel damage that can be caused by PTA. Unsuccessful transluminal angioplasty procedures rarely prevent or complicate necessary subsequent surgery. In selected cases the procedure is effective and almost painless and can be repeated as often as necessary with no apparent increase in risk to the patient. The recovery time is often no longer than the time required to stabilize the arteriotomy site, usually a matter of hours, and general anesthesia is normally not required. Therefore the hospital stay and the cost to the patient are reduced.

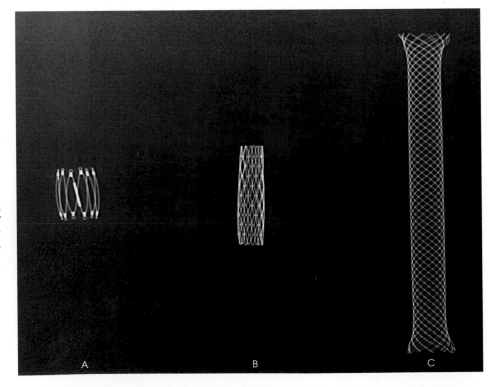

Fig. 26-79 Vascular stents. **A,** Gianturco-Rosch Biliary Z-stent; **B,** Palmaz; **C,** Wallstent.

Although most PTA procedures are conducted in the radiology angiographic laboratory, angioplasty involving the arteries of the heart is generally performed in a more specialized laboratory. *Percutaneous transluminal coronary angioplasty (PTCA)* takes place in the cardiac catheterization laboratory because of the possibility of potentially serious cardiac complications. Further information on PTCA is provided in Chapter 31.

BOX 26-1
Embolization Agents

Permanent
Ivalon (polyvinyl alcohol)
Silicone beads
Gianturco stainless-steel coils
Detachable balloons

Temporary
Gelfoam
Microfibrillar collagen (Avitene)
Vasoconstrictors such as
(vasopressin, (Pitressin))

Transcatheter Embolization

Transcatheter embolization was first discovered by Nusbaum and Baum[1] in 1963 when they found that active bleeding in various areas of the body could be demonstrated with angiography. *Extravasated* blood, when mixed with injected contrast media, appears as a collection of small "pools" at the bleeding site. They later discovered that this bleeding could be adequately managed using angiographic procedures.

Transcatheter embolization involves the therapeutic introduction of various substances to occlude or drastically reduce blood flow within a vessel. The three main purposes for embolization are (1) to stop active bleeding sites, (2) to end blood flow to diseased or malformed areas (e.g., tumors or AVMs), and (3) to stop or reduce blood flow to a particular area of the body before surgery.

[1]Nusbaum M, Baum S: Radiographic demonstration of unknown sites of gastrointestinal bleeding, *Surg Forum* 14:374, 1963.

The patient's condition and the situation must be considered when choosing an embolizing agent. The radiologist, in consultation with the attending physician, usually identifies the appropriate agent to be used. Embolizing agents must be administered with care to ensure that they flow to the predetermined vessel. Once given, *embolizing agents cannot be retrieved and their effects are irreversible.* Many embolizing agents are available, and the choice of agent depends on whether the occlusion is to be temporary or permanent. Box 26-1 lists some of the most widely used agents.

When the occlusion is to be temporary, as in the treatment of gastrointestinal bleeding, occlusion needs to be sustained only until adequate *hemostasis* occurs. Gelfoam* (the trade name for a sponge-like substance that can be formed into large or small *pledgets*) may be injected into the vessel. After each Gelfoam injection a contrast medium should be injected to check the progress of the occlusion. After satisfactory embolization occurs, the Gelfoam remains intact for a number of days.

Vasoconstricting drugs can be used to temporarily reduce blood flow. Vasoconstrictors such as vasopressin (Pitressin) drastically constrict vessels, resulting in hemostasis.

When permanent occlusion is desired, as in trauma to the pelvis that causes hemorrhage or when vascular tumors are supplied by large vessels, the Gianturco stainless-steel coil is most widely used. This coil (Fig. 26-80), which functions to produce *thrombogenesis*, is simply a looped segment of guide wire with dacron fibers attached to it. The coil is initially straight and is easily introduced into a catheter that has been placed into the desired vessel. The coil is then pushed out of the catheter tip with a guide wire. The coil assumes its looping shape immediately as it enters the bloodstream. It is important that the catheter tip be specifically placed in the vessel so that the coil springs precisely into the desired area. Numerous coils can be placed as needed to occlude the vessel.

*Gelfoam is the trademark for a sterile, absorbable, water-insoluble gelatin-base sponge that is used as a local hemostatic.

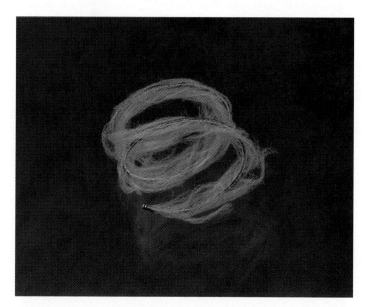

Fig. 26-80 Fibered Gianturco stainless-steel occluding coil (magnified).

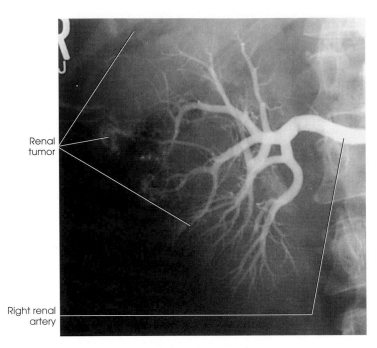

Renal
tumor

Right renal
artery

Fig. 26-81 Selective right renal arteriogram.

Fig. 26-81 presents an example of a situation in which transcatheter embolization is indicated. The arteriogram shows a large vascular tumor in the upper and middle portions of the right kidney. In a subsequent *nephrectomy* the significant reduction of surgical bleeding was attributed to the embolization therapy (Fig. 26-82).

Transcatheter embolization has also been used in the cerebral vasculature of the brain. AVMs within the cerebral vasculature can be managed using silicone beads or tissue adhesives. Very small catheters (2 or 3 Fr) are passed through a larger catheter that is positioned in the internal carotid artery. The smaller catheter is then manipulated into the appropriate cerebral vessel, and the embolic material is injected through it until sufficient embolization occurs.

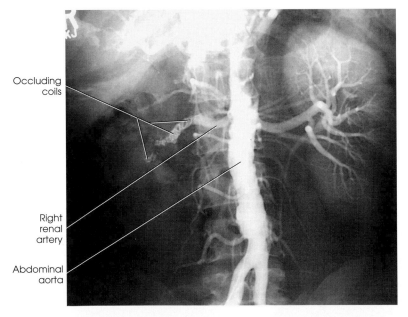

Occluding
coils

Right
renal
artery

Abdominal
aorta

Fig. 26-82 Postembolization renal flush angiogram in the same patient as in Fig. 26-81.

Percutaneous Nephrostomy Tube Placement and Related Procedures

Nephrostomy tube drainage is indicated in the patient who has some type of ureteral or bladder blockage that causes *hydronephrosis.* If urine is not eliminated from the kidney, renal failure with necrosis to the kidney will occur.

A nephrostomy tube is a catheter that has multiple side holes at the distal end through which urine can enter. The urine drains into a bag connected to the proximal end of the catheter outside the patient's body. These catheters range in size from 8 to 24 Fr and are usually about 12 inches (30 cm) in length. Nephrostomy tubes are also placed in patients with kidney stones to facilitate subsequent passage of ultrasonic lithotripsy catheters through the tract created by the nephrostomy tube from the flank to the renal pelvis.

The renal pelvis must be opacified to provide a target for percutaneous nephrostomy tube placement. Percutaneous nephrostography may be performed to accomplish this. For this procedure the patient is positioned prone or in an anterior oblique position on the tabletop. The patient's back and posterolateral aspect of the affected side are prepared and surgically draped. Following the administration of a local anesthetic, a 7-inch (17-cm) thin-wall cannula needle is passed through the back under fluoroscopic control and the cannula is removed. The needle is examined for drainage of urine. When urine returns through the needle, contrast medium is injected to opacify the renal pelvis.

A particular calyx of the opacified renal pelvis is often selected as the target for the nephrostomy tube placement. After a local anesthetic is administered, a 7-inch (17-cm) cannula needle is inserted through the posterolateral aspect of the back and directed toward the renal pelvis. A fluoroscopic C arm offers a distinct advantage for this process. The C arm can be obliqued to match the angle between the needle insertion site and the target. The needle can then be advanced directly toward the target visualized on the fluoroscopic monitor. The C arm is then angled obliquely 90 degrees to see if the needle tip has reached the renal pelvis or calyx.

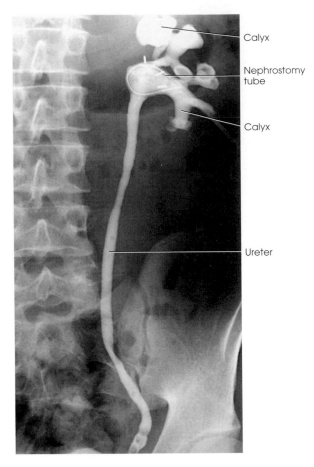

Calyx

Nephrostomy
tube

Calyx

Ureter

Fig. 26-83 Nephrostogram through Coop Loop drainage tube.

When the needle tip has entered the desired target, a guide wire is passed through the needle into the renal pelvis and is then maneuvered into the proximal ureter for additional support. The needle is then removed, the tract is dilated, and the drainage catheter is passed over the guide wire and into the renal pelvis. The pigtail end of the catheter must be placed well within the renal pelvis and not outside the kidney itself or in the proximal ureter (Figs. 26-83 and 26-84). The catheter's position is maintained by attaching it to a fixation disk or other device that is then sutured or taped to the body wall. A dressing is applied over the entry site. Either the fixation device or the dressing must prevent the catheter from becoming kinked, which would prevent the drainage of urine through the catheter. Periodic antegrade nephrostography may be performed by injecting the drainage catheter to evaluate anatomy and catheter function.

Nephrostomy tubes may be placed for temporary or permanent external drainage of urine. Nephrostomy tubes that are left in place for a long time need to be exchanged periodically for new ones. A guide wire is inserted through the existing catheter, and the catheter is removed, leaving the guide wire in place. A new nephrostomy tube is then passed over the guide wire and positioned in the renal pelvis. Nephrostomy tubes can be permanently removed by simply pulling them out. The tract from the body wall to the renal pelvis usually closes in a day or so without complication.

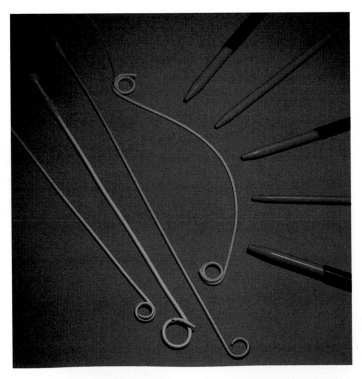

Fig. 26-84 Nephrostomy tubes *(left)* ureteral stent *(center)*, and dilators.

(Courtesy Cook, Inc., Bloomington, Ind.)

In addition to nephrostomy tube placement, other *uroradiologic* procedures are performed in the angiographic and interventional laboratory. *Percutaneous nephrolithotomy* is an alternative to surgical removal of relatively small kidney stones. Large stones may require surgery or ultrasonic lithotripsy for removal. The percutaneous nephrolithotomy procedure begins like a nephrostomy tube placement. After a wire is passed into the renal pelvis and ureter, a large tract is formed using dilators or a balloon-tipped catheter. Then a sheath large enough to facilitate removal of the stone is placed between the renal pelvis and the body wall. A stone basket or other retrieval catheter is introduced through the tract and manipulated to grasp the stone (Figs. 26-85 and 26-86). The stone is removed by withdrawing the retrieval catheter as it grasps the stone. The sheath is then withdrawn, and a nephrostomy tube is placed in the renal pelvis to drain urine and any blood resulting from trauma in the procedure. The nephrostomy tube is eventually removed.

Angioplasty of stenoses in the ureteral system, renal cyst puncture with drainage, and percutaneous antegrade ureteral stent placement are additional procedures. A ureteral stent is a double-ended pigtail catheter that is passed into the ureter and remains inside the body, with one end placed into the renal pelvis and the other into the bladder (Fig. 26-87). This catheter is used when a constriction of the ureter or ureterovesicular junction is blocking the drainage of urine from the renal pelvis. The multiple side holes at both pigtail ends allow urine to drain into one end of the stent and exit the other end. The stent provides an internal passageway for urine across the area of blockage. Usually a nephrostomy tube is initially placed to provide access to the renal pelvis and to allow a tract to form in the body. At a later time a guide wire is passed through the nephrostomy tube and down the ureter into the bladder. The nephrostomy tube is removed, and the stent is inserted over the guide wire using a catheter-like pusher. Usually the nephrostomy tube is replaced to provide external drainage until it is known that the stent is providing internal drainage. The stent can usually be removed through the urethra by a cystoscopic procedure.

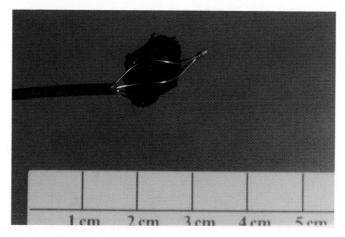

Fig. 26-85 Retrieval catheter and basket with large renal stone.

(Courtesy John R. Croyle.)

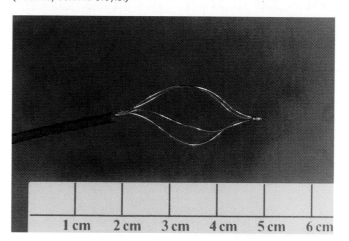

Fig. 26-86 Retrieval catheter with stone basket extended.

(Courtesy John R. Croyle.)

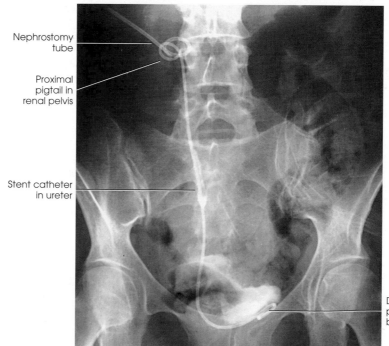

Nephrostomy tube

Proximal pigtail in renal pelvis

Stent catheter in ureter

Distal pigtail in bladder

Fig. 26-87 Postplacement radiograph of ureteral stent.

Inferior Vena Cava Filter Placement

As previously discussed in this chapter, pulmonary angiography primarily evaluates embolic disease of the lungs. A pulmonary embolus is usually a blood clot, but it does not form in the lungs. Instead, it commonly forms as a *thrombus,* usually in the deep veins of the leg (Fig. 26-88). When such a thrombus becomes dislodged and migrates, it is called an *embolus.* An embolus originating in the leg may migrate through the inferior vena cava and right side of the heart and finally lodge in the pulmonary arteries. A filter can be percutaneously placed in the inferior vena cava to trap such an embolus.

The idea of interrupting the pathway of an embolus is not a new one. Surgical interruption of the common femoral vein was first described in 1784, and surgical interruption of the inferior vena cava was described in 1868. These procedures and the partial surgical interruption procedures that evolved from them had a high rate of complications related not only to the surgical process but also to inadequate venous drainage from the lower limbs. Catheterization technology led to the development of detachable balloons for occluding the inferior vena cava, but that procedure also resulted in complications because of inadequate venous flow from the lower limbs.

The first true filter designed to trap emboli while maintaining vena cava *patency* was introduced in 1967 by Mobin-Uddin. It consisted of six metal struts joined at one end to form a conical shape that was covered by a perforated plastic canopy. The plastic canopy proved to be too occlusive, however, and the Mobin-Uddin filter is no longer in use. Because of this filter's striking resemblance to an open umbrella, vena cava filters of all types were for many years referred to as "umbrella filters."

Lower limb vein thrombosis is not necessarily an indication for inferior vena cava filter placement. Normally blood-thinning medications are administered to treat deep vein thrombosis. When anticoagulant therapy is contraindicated because of bleeding or the risk of hemorrhage, filter placement may be indicated. Filter placement itself has associated risks, including thrombosis of the vein through which the filter is introduced and thrombosis of the vena cava. However, these risks normally are not life-threatening. It is important to note that inferior vena cava filter placement is not a treatment for deep vein thrombosis of the leg but a therapy intended to reduce the chance of pulmonary embolism.

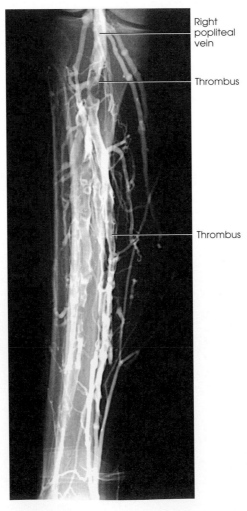

Right popliteal vein

Thrombus

Thrombus

Fig. 26-88 Lower limb venogram.

Inferior vena cava filters are available in a variety of forms. All of these filters are initially compact inside an introducer catheter device and assume their functional shape as they are released (Fig. 26-89). The introducers are passed through sheaths ranging in size from 9 to 29 Fr.

The filters are made of inert metals, and most are designed for permanent placement. The Kimray-Greenfield filter is composed of six wire struts joined at the apex to form a conical shape. Each strut has a hook on its end that engages the wall of the vena cava. The titanium Greenfield filter, a modification of the Kimray-Greenfield design, is introduced through a smaller venotomy. The Vena Tech filter also consists of six metal struts forming a cone, but each strut ends with a side rail that is parallel to the wall of the vena cava. The side rails have barbs to hold the filter in place. The Gianturco-Roehm Bird's Nest filter consists of a bundle of fine wire anchored on each end by a V-shaped hook wire strut. The Simon Nitinol filter is composed of wire that has thermal memory. This allows the device, which is very compact in its introducer, to achieve a completely different shape when placed in the body temperature environment of the vena cava. Inferiorly the device has six wire struts that form a cone, and superiorly it has seven overlapping loops of wire for additional clot-trapping capability.

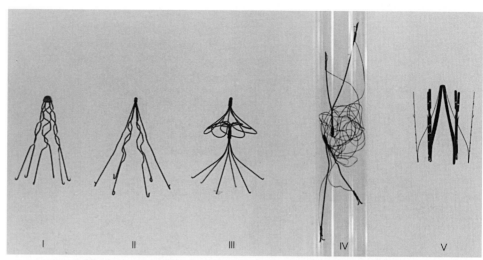

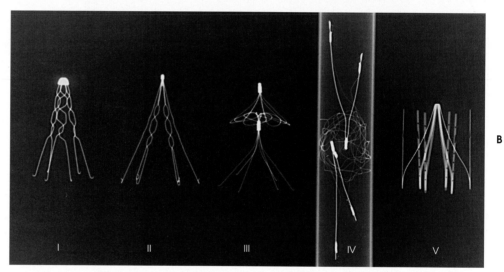

Fig. 26-89 Vena cava filters: *I,* Kimray-Greenfield; *II,* Titanium Greenfield; *III,* Simon Nitinol; *IV,* Gianturco-Roehm Bird's Nest; *V,* Vena Tech. **A,** Photographic image. **B,** Radiographic image.

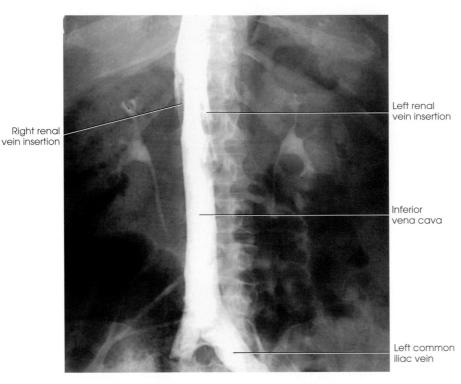

Right renal
vein insertion

Left renal
vein insertion

Inferior
vena cava

Left common
iliac vein

Fig. 26-90 Inferior vena cavogram.

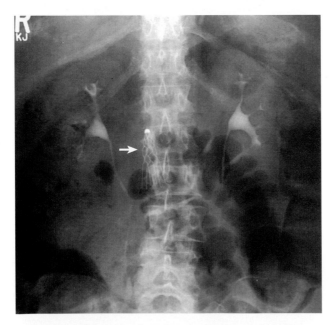

Fig. 26-91 Postplacement radiograph showing filter in place *(arrow)*.

Several filters are designed for temporary placement. They have a hook on the bottom that allows them to be grasped by a catheter snare device and removed percutaneously. One temporary filter remains attached to its introducer catheter, which is used to retrieve it. Some temporary filters must be removed within approximately 10 days or they become permanently attached to the vena cava endothelium. Various filter designs are in use in countries other than the United States. Inferior vena cava filter development continues, and new designs will certainly become available.

The filters are percutaneously inserted through a femoral, jugular, or antecubital vein, usually for placement in the inferior vena cava just inferior to the renal veins. Placement inferior to the renal veins is important to prevent renal vein thrombosis, which can occur if the vena cava is occluded superior to the level of the renal veins by a large thrombus in a filter. An inferior vena cavogram is performed using the Seldinger technique, usually from the right femoral vein approach because it provides the straightest course into the inferior vena cava. The inferior vena cavogram defines the anatomy, including the level of the renal veins, determines the diameter of the vena cava, and rules out the presence of a thrombus (Fig. 26-90). Filter insertion from the jugular or antecubital approach may be indicated if a thrombus is present in the inferior vena cava.

The diameter of the vena cava may influence the choice of filter, because each filter has a maximum diameter. The filter insertion site is dilated to accommodate the filter introducer. The filter remains sheathed until it reaches the desired level and is released from its introducer by the angiographer. The introducing system is then removed, and external compression is applied to the venotomy site until hemorrhage ceases. A postplacement plain radiograph is obtained to document the location of the filter (Fig. 26-91).

Transjugular Intrahepatic Portosystemic Shunt

The *portal circulation* drains blood from the digestive organs to the liver. The blood passes through the liver tissue and is returned to the inferior vena cava via the hepatic veins. Disease processes can increase the resistance of blood flow through the liver, elevating the portal circulation's blood pressure—a condition known as *portal hypertension*—and causing blood to flow instead through collateral veins to return to the systemic circulation. The *varices* that eventually result can be life-threatening if they bleed. The creation of a portosystemic shunt can decrease portal hypertension and the associated variceal bleeding by allowing the portal venous circulation to bypass its normal course through the liver. The percutaneous intervention for creating an artificial low pressure pathway between the portal and hepatic veins is called a *transjugular intrahepatic portosystemic shunt (TIPS)*.

Portography and hepatic venography are usually performed before a TIPS procedure to delineate anatomy and confirm *patency* of these vessels. Ultrasonography may be used for this purpose. Transcatheter blood pressure measurements may also confirm the existence of a pressure gradient between the portal and hepatic veins. An intravascular marker placed in the portal vein through a needle guided by CT may act as a target during the TIPS procedure.

To accommodate all of the catheter and needle manipulations during the TIPS procedure, a long sheath is passed from a right internal jugular venous puncture site to the middle or right hepatic vein. A hepatic venogram may be obtained at this time. A special long needle is passed into the hepatic vein and advanced through the liver tissue into the portal vein. The needle is exchanged for a balloon-tipped angioplasty catheter, and the tract through the liver tissue is dilated. An angiographic catheter may be passed through the tract and advanced into the splenic vein for a splenoportal venogram. An intravascular stent is positioned across the tract to maintain its patency (Fig. 26-92). The tract and stent may be further enlarged with balloon-tipped catheters until the desired reduction in pressure gradient between the portal and hepatic veins is achieved. The sheath is then removed from the internal jugular vein, and external pressure is applied until hemostasis at the venotomy occurs.

Other Procedures

When an angiogram demonstrates thrombosis, the procedure may be continued for thrombolytic therapy. Blood clot–dissolving medications can be infused through an angiographic catheter positioned against the thrombus. Special infusion catheters that have side holes may be manipulated directly into the clot. Periodic repeat *angiograms* evaluate the progress of *lysis* (dissolution). The catheter may have to be advanced under fluoroscopic control to keep it against or in the clot as lysis progresses.

Catheters can also be used to percutaneously remove foreign bodies, such as catheter fragments, from the vasculature. A variety of snares can be used for this purpose. A snare catheter introduced using the Seldinger technique is manipulated under fluoroscopic control to grasp the foreign body. Then the snare and foreign body are withdrawn as a unit.

Interventional radiologic procedures performed in the biliary system include biliary drainage and biliary stone removal (see Chapter 16).

Interventional Radiology: Present and Future

Interventional procedures bring therapeutic capabilities into the hands of the radiologist. Procedures that are done initially for diagnosis can be extended, using the same basic techniques, to perform therapeutic processes. New equipment is continually becoming available to improve techniques and broaden the scope of percutaneous intervention. Although use of the catheter for angiographic diagnosis may wane, its ability to provide therapy percutaneously ensures a future for angiography.

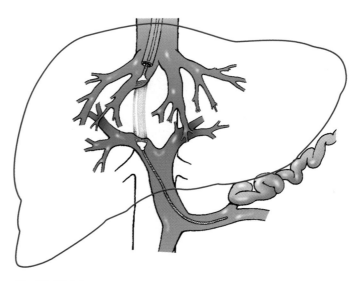

Fig. 26-92 Intravascular stent placement in a TIPS procedure.

Definitions and Indications

Lymphography is a general term applied to radiologic examinations of the lymph vessels and nodes after they have been opacified by an injected iodinated contrast medium (Figs. 26-93 and 26-94). The study of the lymph vessels, which may be called *lymphangiography,* is carried out within the first hour after injection of the contrast material. The study of the lymph nodes, which may be called *lymphadenography,* is performed 24 hours after injection of the contrast medium. The lymph vessels empty the contrast agent within a few hours. The nodes normally retain the contrast substance for 3 to 4 weeks. Abnormal nodes may retain the medium for several months, so delayed lymphadenograms may be made, as indicated, without further injection.

Lymphography is seldom performed in current practice because of the superior imaging capabilities of newer modalities. At present its primary purpose is to assess the clinical extent of lymphomas. Lymphography may also be indicated in patients who demonstrate clinical evidence of obstruction or other impairment of the lymphatic system. A more detailed description of lymphography is provided in previous editions of this text.

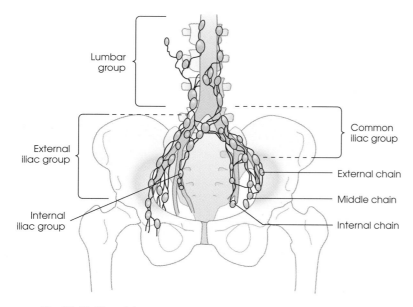

Fig. 26-93 Iliopelvic-aortic lymphatic system: anterior projection.

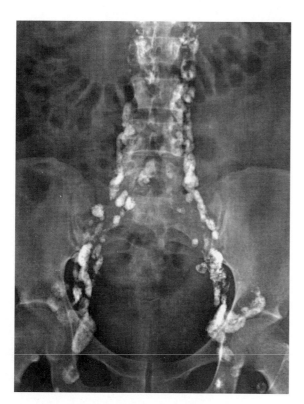

Fig. 26-94 AP projection of iliopelvic-abdominoaortic lymph nodes.

Procedures

INJECTION

Injections for lymphography are limited to easily accessible sites such as those of the hands and feet (Table 26-1). (Lymphatics of the feet are most commonly used.) For opacification of the lymphatic vessels and nodes, the vessels must be isolated and cannulated. Ordinarily the peripheral lymphatic vessels cannot be easily identified because of their small size and lack of color. For identification of the lymphatic vessels on the dorsum of the feet and hands, a blue dye that is selectively absorbed by the lymphatics is injected subcutaneously into the first and second interdigital web spaces about 15 minutes before the examination. (After patent blue violet is injected, the patient's urine and skin are tinted blue. This condition disappears within a few hours.)

A longitudinal incision is made on the dorsum of each hand or foot to locate the dye-filled lymphatic vessels. A 27- or 30-gauge needle is used to cannulate the isolated vessels. Iodinated oily contrast media is then slowly injected into the vessels over a 30-minute period. (As in any procedure involving the injection of foreign materials, untoward reactions must be anticipated. The patient must be observed closely, and appropriate medications and resuscitation equipment must be nearby.) Confirmation that the injection is intralymphatic is usually obtained fluoroscopically. After the injection, the needles are removed and the wounds sutured.

Injection of the feet provides visualization of the lymphatic structures of the lower limb (Fig. 26-95), groin, iliopelvic-abdominoaortic region, and thoracic duct. Injection of the lymphatics of the hands provides visualization of the upper limb (Fig. 26-96) and the axillary, infraclavicular, and supraclavicular regions.

IMAGING

For demonstration of the lymph vessels, radiographs are made within the first hour after the contrast agent is injected. A second series of radiographs is made 24 hours later to demonstrate the lymph nodes. The exposure factors employed for lymphographic studies are the same as those used for bone studies of the respective region. Table 26-1 summarizes the most common radiographic projections and the associated anatomic structures visualized.

TABLE 26-1

Projections and anatomy demonstrated with lymphography

Injection site	Projections	Anatomy demonstrated

Feet	AP abdomen
	RPO and LPO abdomen
	AP thorax
	Left lateral thorax
	Bilateral AP tibias
	Bilateral AP femora
	  (see Fig. 26-95)
	AP pelvis
		Iliopelvic and paraaortic
		  lymph nodes
		Thoracic duct
		
		Lower limb lymphatic vessels
		Inguinal lymph nodes

Hands	AP and lateral arm
	  (centered at elbow)
	AP and 45 degree AP
	  oblique shoulder
		Upper limb lymphatic vessels
		  and nodes (see Fig. 26-96)
		Axillary lymph nodes

AP, anteriorposterior; *RPO,* right posterior oblique; *LPO,* left posterior oblique.

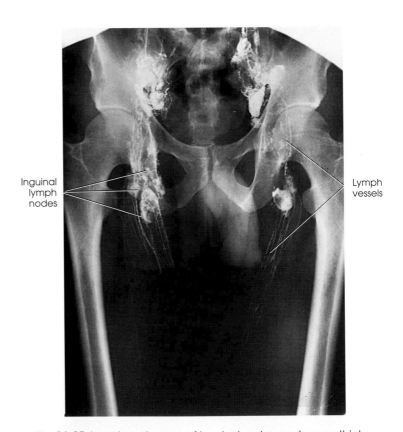

Fig. 26-95 Lymphangiogram of inguinal region and upper thighs.

Inguinal lymph nodes

Lymph vessels

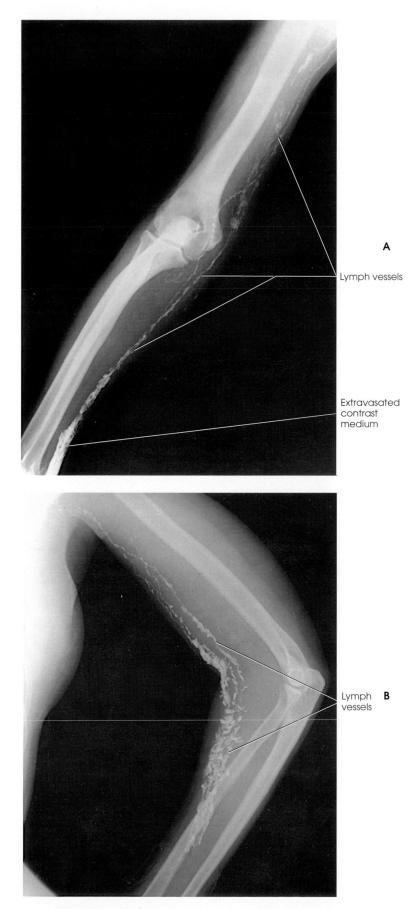

A

Lymph vessels

Extravasated
contrast
medium

Lymph
vessels   B

Fig. 26-96 Lymphangiograms. **A,** AP and **B,** lateral of upper limb, showing fluting of vessels and extravasation of contrast medium.

PHOTOGAPHIC SUBTRACTION TECHNIQUE

DONALD L. SUCHER*

Definitions and Indications

Photographic subtraction, introduced by Ziedses des Plantes,[1] is a technique by which bone structure images are subtracted, or canceled out, from a film of bones and opacified vessels, leaving an unobscured image of the vessels. The technique can be applied in all forms of angiography, wherever the vessels are superimposed in bone structures.

With the increasing popularity of digital subtraction angiography (see Chapter 35), the use of photographic subtraction has decreased in many institutions. However, photographic subtraction remains relatively widely used and is increasing in popularity in some situations. One such area of increasing frequency occurs in evaluation of joint replacements. (See the discussion of contrast arthrography in Chapter 12 of this atlas.)

*Visual Presentation Specialist, Department of Radiology, Children's Hospital, 300 Longwood Ave., Boston, MA 02114.
[1]Ziedses des Plantes BG: Subtraktion: eine roentgenographische Methode zur separaten Abbildung bestimmter Teile des Objekts, *Fortschr Roentgenstr* 52:69, 1935.

The purpose of subtraction in angiography and other specialized procedures is to fully define all vessels containing contrast material and at the same time eliminate the confusing overlying bone images. Following are a few terms that pertain to the subtraction technique:

registration Matching of one image over another so that bony landmarks are precisely superimposed. When so arranged, films are taped together to prevent slippage. Composites discussed herein may involve two or more films.

reversal film (also called a positive mask or diapositive) Reverse-tone duplicate of radiographic image, showing black changed to white and white to black. This positive transparency is obtained by exposing single-emulsion film through traditional radiographic film.

zero film or base film (also called control film) Film showing bone structures only, with no patient motion between it and subsequent contrast studies. For these reasons, zero film is exposed just before contrast medium is injected into vessels.

EQUIPMENT AND MATERIALS

Items needed for subtraction include the following:

1. A contact printer similar to the one illustrated in Fig. 26-97 (Several available units can also be used to duplicate radiographs.)
2. Radiographic processing facilities
3. A horizontally oriented illuminator for registration of images
4. Films—subtraction mask film for making the reversal masks and subtraction print film for making photographic prints of the final subtracted image

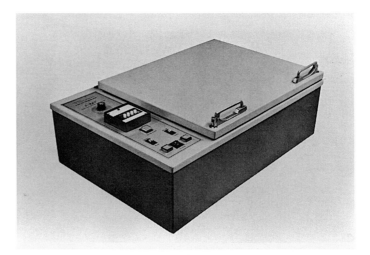

Fig. 26-97 Contract printer such as that used during exposure steps in producing subtraction prints.

First-Order Subtraction

The simplest method of photographic subtraction, called *first-order subtraction* (Fig. 26-98), consists of obtaining a positive mask, or reversal, of the first film (zero film) of the angiographic series (the one that does not contain contrast material). When the reversal mask is superimposed over a film in the series that contains contrast material, the positive and negative images of the bones tend to cancel each other out, and only the vessels are visible. The vessels are not canceled out because they were present on only one film—the one containing the contrast material. A contact printer makes a print of this combination of films.

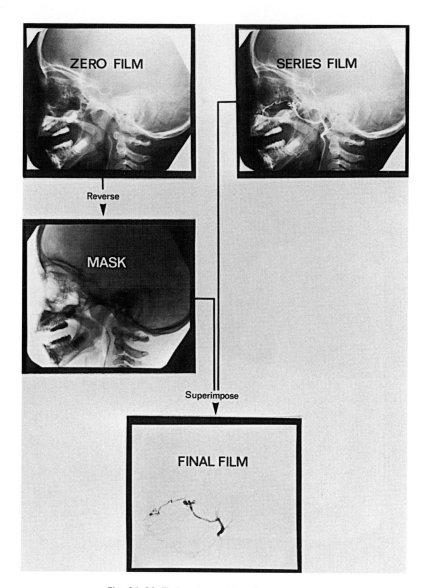

Fig. 26-98 First-order subtraction process.

FIRST-ORDER SUBTRACTION PROCEDURE

The following steps are observed:

- In a darkroom, place the nonemulsion side of the sheet of subtraction mask film in contact with the zero film, and expose it to light for approximately 5 seconds. When processed, this becomes the mask.*

*Exposure time varies according to equipment and material used.

- On a light box, carefully register the mask over the selected series film (Fig. 26-99), and tape the two securely together.
- In the darkroom, place the mask-series film combination in contact with the emulsion side of a sheet of subtraction print film, and expose it to light for approximately 5 seconds.* This produces the final subtraction image (Fig. 26-100).

Second-Order Subtraction

The reversal of the zero film obtained in the first-order subtraction is usually not the exact reversal of the density of the selected angiographic film; thus the subtraction result is imperfect. The imperfection can be corrected with second-order subtraction. This process involves producing another film, called a *secondary* or *correction mask*, which compensates for the slight differences. Hanafee and Shinno[1] led the way toward this improved subtraction method. Their method of second-order subtraction consists of superimposing the zero film on its own reversal mask. The additional print that results from the transmission of light through the two films, which in theory would be the exact opposite of each other, produces a faint radiographic image that corrects for the small "photographic mistake" between the first two. The reversal of the zero film, the correction film, and the film containing contrast material are carefully registered; this combination is then exposed to obtain the final subtraction print.

[1]Hanafee W, Shinno JM: Second-order subtraction with simultaneous bilateral carotid, internal carotid injections, *Radiology* 86:334, 1966.

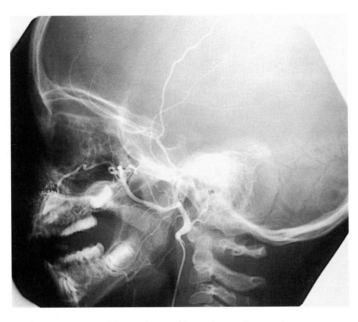

Fig. 26-99 Angiographic series radiograph.

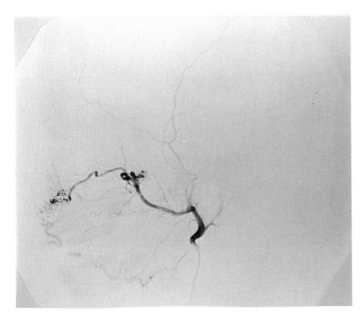

Fig. 26-100 First-order subtraction print.

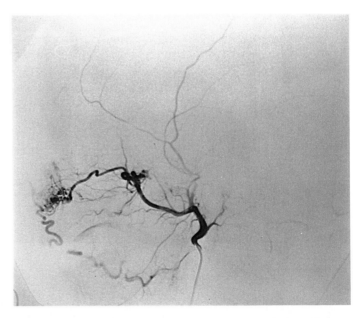

Fig. 26-101 Composite-mask, white-over-white technique. Bone has been completely removed, allowing improved visualization of vessels.

A further advancement toward the goal of complete subtraction was published by Sucher and Strand[1] in 1974. This second-order subtraction modification is called *composite-mask subtraction* or the *white-over-white technique*. When correctly applied, this technique almost totally eliminates both bony structures and soft tissues, leaving a display of the vessels in high-contrast reproduction (Fig. 26-101).

COMPOSITE-MASK SUBTRACTION PROCEDURE

The following steps are illustrated in Fig. 26-102:

1. In a darkroom, place the nonemulsion side of a sheet of subtraction mask film in contact with the zero film, and expose it to light for approximately 5 seconds.* When processed, this becomes the mask.

2. In a darkroom, place the emulsion side of a sheet of subtraction mask film in contact with the selected angiographic series film, which is then exposed to light. This process produces the series reversal film.

3. On a light box, carefully register the series reversal film with the zero film, and tape the two securely together.

4. In a darkroom, place the zero-series reversal film combination in contact with the emulsion side of a sheet of subtraction mask film, and expose it to light for approximately 20 seconds.* This process produces the secondary mask.

5. On a light box, carefully register the series film and the mask, and tape the two securely together. Carefully register and tape the secondary mask to this composite.

6. In a darkroom, place the series film–mask–secondary mask combination in contact with the emulsion side of a sheet of subtraction print film, and expose it to light for approximately 35 seconds.* The subtraction *final film* is thus produced.

---

[1]Sucher DL, Strand RD: Composite mask subtraction, white over white technique, *Radiology* 113:470, 1974.
*Exposure time varies according to the equipment and material used.

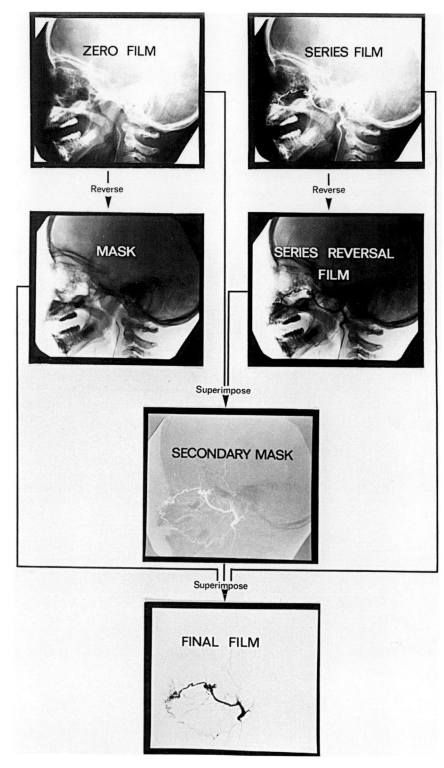

Fig. 26-102 Composite-mask subtraction process.

A comparison of second-order subtraction and composite-mask subtraction proves that the steps are almost identical. The only procedural difference is that in second-order subtraction the secondary mask is made by registering the zero film and the zero reversal mask. In composite-mask subtraction the zero film and the angiographic series reversal film are superimposed to produce the secondary mask. Although the procedures are similar, the composite-mask subtraction technique is recommended when increased resolution is required.

In recent years, marked advancement has been made in the production of films specifically designed for subtraction. In addition to the advantage of 90-second processing, these films often allow subtractions of adequate or even excellent quality to be made with the single-order subtraction technique. Composite-mask subtraction is recommended only when small structures require increased definition for visualization or when illustrations of high quality are needed for publications.

Definition of Terms

afferent lymph vessel Vessel carrying lymph toward a lymph vessel.

anastomose Join.

aneurysm Sac formed by local enlargement of a weakened artery wall.

angiography Radiographic study of vessels.

anomaly Variation from the normal pattern.

aortic dissection Tear in the inner lining of the aortic wall that allows blood to enter and track along the muscular coat.

arteriography Radiologic examination of arteries after the injection of a radiopaque contrast medium.

arteriole Very small arterial vessel.

arteriotomy Surgical opening of an artery.

arteriovenous malformation Abnormal anastomosis or communication between an artery and a vein.

artery Large blood vessel carrying blood away from the heart.

atherosclerosis Condition in which fibrous and fatty deposits on the luminal wall of an artery may cause obstruction of the vessel.

atrium One of the two upper chambers of the heart.

bifurcation Place where a structure divides into two branches.

biplane Two x-ray exposure planes 90 degrees from another, usually frontal and lateral.

capillary Tiny blood vessel through which blood and tissue cells exchange substances.

cerebral angiography Imaging of vascular system of the brain.

cinefluorography Same as cineradiography; the production of a motion picture record of successive images on a fluoroscopic screen.

claudication Cramping of the leg muscles after physical exertion because of chronically inadequate blood supply.

collateral Secondary or accessory.

diastole Relaxed phase of the atria or ventricles of the heart during which blood enters the chambers.

efferent lymph vessel Vessel carrying lymph away from a node.

embolus Foreign material, often thrombus, that detaches and moves freely in the bloodstream.

endocardium Interior lining of heart chambers.

epicardium Exterior layer of heart wall.

extravasation Escape of fluid from a vessel into the surrounding tissue.

film changer Device that transports radiographic films into and out of the exposure field for serial imaging.

hematoma Local swelling filled with effused blood.

hemostasis Stopping of blood flow or hemorrhage.

hydronephrosis Distention of the pelvis and calices of the kidney with urine, caused by ureteral obstruction.

iatrogenic Caused by a therapeutic or diagnostic procedure.

interventional Improving a condition; therapeutic.

lesion Injury or other damaging change to an organ or tissue.

lymph Body fluid circulated by the lymphatic vessels and filtered by the lymph nodes.

lymph vessels See **afferent** and/or **efferent lymph vessel.**

lymphadenography Radiographic study of the lymph nodes.

lymphangiography Radiographic study of the lymph vessels.

lymphography Radiographic evaluation of the lymphatic channels and lymph nodes.

meninges Three membranes that envelop the brain and spinal cord.

myocardium Muscular heart wall.

nephrectomy Surgical removal of the kidney.

nephrostomy Surgical opening into the kidney's collecting system.

nephrotoxic Chemically damaging to the kidney cells.

nonocclusive Not completely closed or shut; allowing blood flow.

patency State of being open or unobstructed.

percutaneous Introduced through the skin.

percutaneous nephrolithotomy Uroradiologic procedure performed to extract stones from within the kidney or proximal ureter.

percutaneous transluminal angioplasty (PTA) Surgical correction of a vessel from within the vessel using catheter technology.

pericardium Fibrous sac that surrounds the heart.

pledget Small piece of material used as a dressing or plug.

portal circulation System of vessels carrying blood from the organs of digestion to the liver.

pulmonary circulation System of vessels carrying blood from the heart to the lungs and back to the heart.

pulse Regular expansion and contraction of an artery that is produced by the ejection of blood from the heart.

serial imaging Acquisition of images in rapid succession.

stenosis Constriction or narrowing of a passage or an orifice.

stent Wire-mesh or plastic conduit placed to maintain flow.

systemic circulation System of vessels carrying blood from the heart out to the body (except the lungs) and back to the heart.

systole Contraction phase of the atria or ventricles of the heart during which blood is ejected from the chambers.

thrombogenesis Formation of a blood clot.

thrombosis Formation or existence of a blood clot.

thrombus Blood clot obstructing a blood vessel or cavity of the heart.

uroradiology Radiologic and interventional study of the urinary tract.

varices Irregularly swollen veins.

vein Vessel that carries blood from the capillaries to the heart.

venography Radiologic study of veins after the injection of radiopaque contrast medium.

ventricle One of two larger pumping chambers of the heart.

venule Any of the small blood vessels that collect blood from the capillaries and join to become veins.

Selected bibliography

Abrams HL: *Abrams angiography: vascular and interventional radiology,* ed 3, Boston, 1983, Little, Brown.

Ahn SS, Concepcion B: Current status of atherectomy for peripheral arterial occlusive disease, *World J Surg* 20:635, 1996.

Archer A, Horton K: Radiologic evaluation and treatment of gallbladder and biliary tree carcinoma, *Cancer Treat Res* 69:157, 1994.

Athanasoulis CA et al: *Interventional radiology,* Philadelphia, 1982, WB Saunders.

Beathard GA, Welch BR, Maidment HJ: Mechanical thrombolysis for the treatment of thrombosed hemodialysis access grafts, *Radiology* 200:711, 1996.

Cardella JF, Fox PS, Lawler JB: Interventional radiologic placement of peripherally inserted central catheters, *J Vasc Interv Radiol* 4:653, 1993.

Clouse ME, Wallace S: *Lymphatic imaging—lymphography, computed tomography and scintography,* ed 2, Baltimore, 1985, Williams & Wilkins.

Coldwell DM, Stokes KR, Yakes WF: Embolotherapy: agents, clinical applications, and techniques, *Radiographics* 14:623, 1994.

Comerota AJ, Aldridge SC: Thrombolytic therapy for deep venous thrombosis: a clinical review, *Can J Surg* 36:359, 1993.

Crain MR et al: Fibrin sleeve stripping for salvage of failing hemodialysis catheters: technique and initial results. *Radiology* 98:41, 1996.

Crystal KS et al: Utilization patterns with inferior vena cava filters: surgical versus percutaneous placement, *J Vasc Interv Radiol* 6:443, 1995.

D'Agostino R, Yucel EK: New method for simultaneous placement of antegrade ureteral stent and nephrostomy tube, *AJR Am J Roentgenol* 162:879, 1994.

Doherty MM, Carver DK: New relief for esophageal varices, *Am J Nurs* 93:58, 1993.

Dorffner R et al: Treatment of abdominal aortic aneurysms with transfemoral placement of stent-grafts: complications and secondary radiologic intervention, *Radiology* 204:79, 1997.

Dyet JF: Endovascular stents in the arterial system—current status, *Clin Radiol* 52:83, 1997.

Eustace S et al: Magnetic resonance angiography in transjugular intrahepatic portosystemic stenting: comparison with contrast hepatic and portal venography, *Eur J Radiol* 19:43, 1994.

Ferrucci JT et al: *Interventional radiology of the abdomen,* ed 2, Baltimore, 1985, Williams & Wilkins.

Fillmore DJ et al: Transjugular intrahepatic portosystemic shunt: midterm clinical and angiographic follow-up, *J Vas Interv Radiol* 7:255, 1996.

Fu WR: *Angiography of trauma,* Springfield, Ill, 1972, Charles C Thomas.

Gobin YP et al: Treatment of large and giant fusiform intracranial aneurysms with Guglielmi detachable coils, *J Neurosurg* 84:55, 1996.

Gupta S et al: Percutaneous nephrostomy with real-time sonographic guidance, *Acta Radiol* 38:454, 1997.

Hennequin LM et al: Superior vena cava stent placement: results with the Wallstent endoprosthesis, *Radiology* 196:353, 1995.

Higashida RT et al: Interventional neurovascular techniques for cerebral revascularization in the treatment of stroke, *AJR Am J Roentgenol* 163:793, 1994.

Johnsrude IS et al: *A practical approach to angiography,* ed 2, Boston, 1987, Little, Brown.

Kadir S: *Diagnostic angiography,* Philadelphia, 1986, WB Saunders.

Kandarpa K: *Handbook of cardiovascular and interventional radiologic procedures,* ed 2, Boston, 1996, Little, Brown.

Kandarpa K: Technical determinants of success in catheter-directed thrombolysis for peripheral arterial occlusions, *J Vasc Interv Radiol* 6(6 pt2 suppl):55S, 1995.

Kerlan RK Jr et al: Transjugular intrahepatic portosystemic shunts: current status, *AJR Am J Roentgenol* 164:1059, 1995.

Kerns SR, Hawkins IF Jr., Sabatelli FW: Current status of carbon dioxide angiography, *Radiol Clin North Am* 33:15, 1995.

Khabiri H et al: CT-guided localization of the portal vein before creation of a transjugular intrahepatic portosystemic shunt, *AJR Am J Roentgenol* 163:746, 1994.

Knelson MH et al: Functional restoration of occluded central venous catheters: new interventional techniques, *J Vasc Interv Radiol* 6:623, 1995.

Korogi Y, Hirai T, Takahashi M: Intravascular ultrasound imaging of peripheral arteries as an adjunct to balloon angioplasty and atherectomy, *Cardiovasc Interv Radiol* 19:1, 1996.

Krige JE, Beningfield SJ: Surgery and interventional radiology for benign bile duct strictures, *HPB Surgery* 7:94, 1993.

Lang EV et al: Percutaneous pulmonary thrombectomy, *J Vasc Interv Radiol* 8:427, 1997.

Laudicina P, Wean: *Applied angiography for radiographers,* Philadelphia, 1994, WB Saunders.

Matsui O et al: A new coaxial needle system, hepatic artery targeting wire, and biplane fluoroscopy to increase safety and efficacy of TIPS, *Cardiovasc Interv Radiol* 17:343, 1994.

Mickley V et al: Stenting of central venous stenoses in hemodialysis patients: long-term results, *Kidney Int* 51:277, 1997.

Muller-Hulsbeck S et al: Rheolytic thrombectomy of an acutely thrombosed transjugular intrahepatic portosystemic stent shunt, *Cardiovasc Intervent Radiol* 19:294, 1996.

Nazarian GK et al: Effect of transjugular intrahepatic portosystemic shunt on quality of life, *AJR Am J Roentgenol* 167:963, 1996.

Nelsen KM et al: Utilization pattern and efficacy of nonsurgical techniques to establish drainage for high biliary obstruction, *J Vasc Interv Radiol* 7:751, 1996.

Newton TH, Potts DG: *Radiology of the skull and brain—angiography,* vol 2, book 1, St Louis, 1974, Mosby.

Pentecost MJ: Transcatheter treatment of hepatic metastases, *AJR Am J Roentgenol* 160:1171, 1993.

Pieters PC, Miller WJ, DeMeo JH: Evaluation of the portal venous system: complementary roles of invasive and noninvasive imaging strategies, *Radiographics* 17:879, 1997.

Rees CR et al: Use of carbon dioxide as a contrast medium for transjugular intrahepatic portosystemic shunt procedures, *J Vasc Interv Radiol* 5:383, 1994.

Reuter SR et al: *Gastrointestinal angiography,* ed 3, Philadelphia, 1986, WB Saunders.

Ring EJ, McLean GK: *Interventional radiology: principals and techniques,* Boston, 1981, Little, Brown.

Rockall AG et al: Stripping of failing hemodialysis catheters using the Ampltaz gooseneck snare, *Clin Radiol* 52:616, 1997.

Rogers CG Jr, Paolini RM, O'Leary JP: Intrahepatic vascular shunting for portal hypertension: early experience with the transjugular intrahepatic porto-systemic shunt, *Am Surg* 60:114, 1994.

Roizental M et al: Portal vein: US-guided localization prior to transjugular intrahepatic portosystemic shunt placement, *Radiology* 196:868, 1995.

Savader SJ et al: Intraductal biliary biopsy: comparison of three techniques, *J Vasc Interv Radiol* 7:743, 1996.

Seldinger SI: Percutaneous selective angiography of the aorta: preliminary report, *Acta Radiol (Stockh)* 45:15, 1956.

Sharafuddin MJ et al: Percutaneous balloon-assisted aspiration thrombectomy of clotted hemodialysis access grafts, *J Vasc Interv Radiol* 7:177, 1996.

Snopek AM: *Fundamentals of special radiographic procedures,* ed 3, Philadelphia, 1992, WB Saunders.

Soulen MC: Chemoembolization of hepatic malignancies, *Oncology* 8:77, 1994.

Soulen MC et al: Mechanical declotting of thrombosed dialysis grafts: experience in 86 cases, *J Vasc Interv Radiol* 8:563, 1997.

Sticklin LA, Walkenstein M: Vena cava filters: a nursing perspective, *Oncol Nurs Forum* 20:507, 1993.

Tortorici MR, Apfel PJ: *Advanced radiographic and angiographic procedures with an introduction to specialized imaging,* Philadelphia, 1995, FA Davis.

Uflacker R, Wholey M: *Interventional radiology,* New York, 1991, McGraw-Hill.

Vinuela F, Duckwiler G, Mawad M: Guglielmi detachable coil embolization of acute intracranial aneurysm: perioperative anatomical and clinical outcome in 403 patients, *J Neurosurg* 86:475, 1997.

Von Sonnenberg E, Mueller PR: *Practical interventional radiology,* Philadelphia, 1989, WB Saunders.

Williams JA et al: Preirradiation osmotic blood-brain barrier disruption plus combination chemotherapy in gliomas: quantitation of tumor response to assess chemosensitivity, *Adv Exper Med Biol* 331: 273, 1993.

Wojtowycz M: *Handbook of interventional radiology and angiography,* ed 2, St Louis, 1995, Mosby.

Yamauchi T et al: Acute thrombosis of the inferior vena cava: treatment with saline-jet aspiration thrombectomy catheter, *AJR Am J Roentgenol* 161:405, 1993.

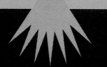

SECTIONAL ANATOMY FOR RADIOGRAPHERS

TERRI BRUCKNER

RIGHT: Early attempts to show body sections employed devices such as the one shown here. The patient was seated, and the x-ray tube and film moved in a coordinated fashion to blur out the unwanted layers of the body.

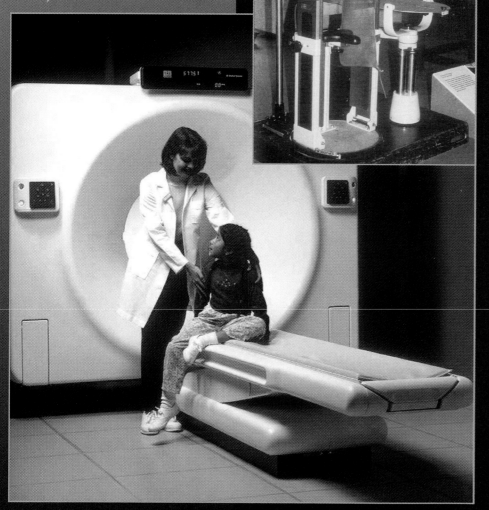

LEFT: Modern computed tomography equipment.

(Courtesy General Electric Medical Systems.)

Overview

An understanding of the relationships between visceral and skeletal structures is essential for the identification and localization of specific anatomic structures using computed imaging modalities. The trend in the development of new imaging methods is toward sectional reconstruction, whether using x-ray techniques, magnetic resonance imaging (MRI), or diagnostic medical sonography. The purpose of this chapter is to provide the radiographer who possesses a background in general anatomy with an orientation to sectional anatomy and correlate it with structures demonstrated on images from the various imaging modalities.

The cadaver sections were selected as being representative of major organ structures for each of the body regions and are *depicted from the inferior surface.* The major anatomic structures normally seen when using current imaging modalities are labeled. For each cadaver section presented, representative images are included to provide an orientation to anatomic structures normally seen using the available imaging modalities. The cadaver sections and diagnostic images do not match exactly; therefore some structures are seen on only one of the illustrations for each body region.

When *axial images* are viewed, it is useful to imagine standing at the patient's feet and looking toward the head. With this orientation the patient's right side is to the viewer's left and vice versa. The anterior aspect of the patient is usually at the top of the image, and the posterior is at the bottom. All relational terms in the following discussion refer to the body in normal anatomic position.

Cranial Region

The computed tomography (CT) localizer, or scout, image (Fig. 27-1) provides a lateral image of the cranium. CT imaging for the cranium may be performed with the gantry parallel to or angled 15 to 20 degrees to the orbitomeatal line (OML). MRI of the cranium generally results in images that are parallel to the orbitomeatal or infraorbitomeatal plane. More details on patient positioning for CT are provided in Chapter 33, and information on patient positioning for MRI is provided in Chapter 36. Because the imaging planes may be different for the cadaver sections and the CT and MRIs, some variation exists in the anatomic structures visualized on corresponding illustrations in this section.

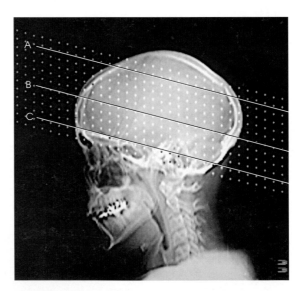

Fig. 27-1 CT localizer (scout) image of skull.

Three identifying lines represent the approximate levels for each of the labeled cadaver sections and images for this region. The cranial cadaver section seen in Fig. 27-2 is sectioned through the frontal and parietal bones. The *cortex,* or *outer layer of gray matter,* is clearly differentiated from the deeper *white matter.* The numerous *gyri,* or *convolutions,* and *sulci* are demonstrated. The *cerebral hemispheres* are separated by the *longitudinal cerebral fissure.* Invaginated in this fissure is a fold of *dura mater,* the *falx cerebri.* The *superior sagittal sinus* is a venous drainage system that runs through the superior margin of the falx and follows the contour of the superior skull margin. In cross section, the anterior and posterior aspects of this sinus can be seen in the midline deep to the bony plates. Two of the five *cerebral lobes* are seen (frontal and parietal). The division between these lobes is the *central sulcus.* The *corona radiata* is a tract of white matter that connects all parts of the cerebral hemisphere to the internal capsule.

Fig. 27-3 is a CT image demonstrating the same structures as the cadaver section in Fig. 27-2. However, the *superior sagittal sinus* appears white because of the introduction of contrast medium.

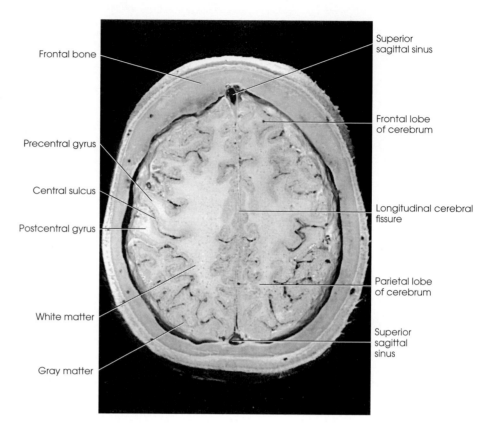

Fig. 27-2 Cadaver section corresponding to level *A* in Fig. 27-1.

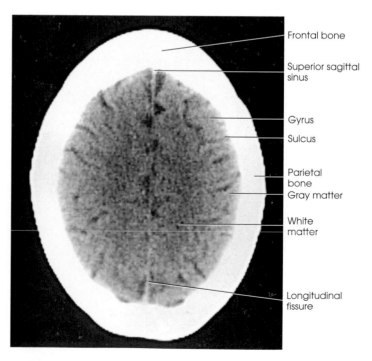

Fig. 27-3 CT image representing the anatomic structures located at level *A* in Fig. 27-1.

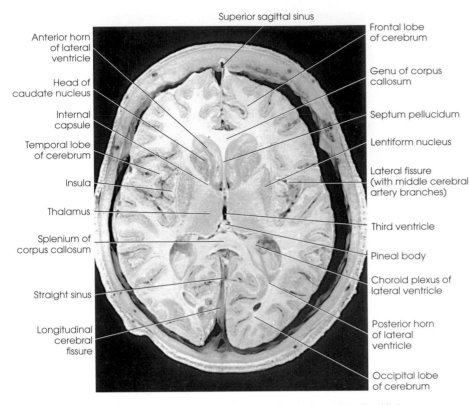

Superior sagittal sinus

Anterior horn of lateral ventricle

Head of caudate nucleus

Internal capsule

Temporal lobe of cerebrum

Insula

Thalamus

Splenium of corpus callosum

Straight sinus

Longitudinal cerebral fissure

Frontal lobe of cerebrum

Genu of corpus callosum

Septum pellucidum

Lentiform nucleus

Lateral fissure (with middle cerebral artery branches)

Third ventricle

Pineal body

Choroid plexus of lateral ventricle

Posterior horn of lateral ventricle

Occipital lobe of cerebrum

Fig. 27-4 Cadaver section corresponding to level *B* in Fig. 27-1.

The axial section through the midcranial region demonstrates many of the central structures of the cerebral hemispheres (Fig. 27-4). The falx cerebri is shown within the longitudinal fissure, with the superior sagittal sinus in the anterior and posterior margins. The hemispheres are joined by a tract of white fibers known as the *corpus callosum.* The corpus callosum is shaped like an inverted U; therefore in cross section at this level, only the anterior and posterior portions are seen. The anterior portion of the corpus callosum is called the *genu,* and the posterior portion is the *splenium.* In this section the *frontal, temporal,* and *occipital lobes* are visualized along with the *insula* (fifth lobe or island of Reil), which is deep to the temporal lobe at the lateral sulcus (lateral fissure).

At this level the *anterior* and *posterior horns* of the *lateral ventricles* are seen. The membranous layer of tissue between the anterior horns is the *septum pellucidum.* Within each posterior horn is a portion of the *choroid plexus,* a capillary network responsible for the formation of cerebrospinal fluid (CSF). Deep to the cortex, much of the cerebrum is composed of tracts of white matter. Several areas of gray matter are found deep within the white matter. These areas of gray matter relay and coordinate information and are known collectively as the *basal nuclei,* or "ganglia," or the cerebral nuclei. The major components of the basal nuclei seen at this level are (from lateral to medial) the *claustrum, lentiform nucleus* (composed of the putamen and globus pallidus), and the *caudate nucleus.* The lentiform nucleus is separated from the caudate nucleus and thalamus by a tract of white matter known as the *internal capsule.* The caudate nucleus is located lateral to the anterior horn of the lateral ventricle. The *midline third ventricle* is visualized at this level. The *thalamus,* which serves as a central relay station for sensory impulses to the cerebral cortex, forms the lateral walls of the third ventricle.

Between the third ventricle and the splenium of the corpus callosum is the *pineal body.* This is an important anatomic landmark because of its tendency to calcify in adults. Branches of the *anterior cerebral arteries* are found in the longitudinal cerebral fissure, just anterior to the genu of the corpus callosum. Branches of the *middle cerebral arteries* are found in the lateral fissure.

The MRI in Fig. 27-5 corresponds to the cadaver section discussed previously. In this T1-weighted image, bone cortex appears black because of a lack of signal return. The high content of fat in the marrow cavity appears white on these images. CSF within the ventricles appears dark. Note the differentiation between gray and white matter structures.

The cross section through the base of the cranium demonstrates the inferior portions of the cerebrum, brainstem, cerebellum, and associated major skeletal structures (Fig. 27-6). The *frontal sinuses* and the most inferior portions of the *frontal lobes* are seen in the anterior skull, along with the supraorbital fat. The *temporal lobes* are found in the middle cranial fossa between the *lesser wings* of the sphenoid bone and the *pars petrosa* of the temporal bone. The *pituitary gland* is located in the *hypophyseal fossa* of the *sella turcica,* in the body of the sphenoid bone. The *internal carotid arteries* lie lateral to the sella turcica between the anterior clinoid processes and the hypophysis cerebri. Posterior to the sphenoid bone is the *pons,* a portion of the brain that relays impulses between the *medulla oblongata* and *cerebrum.* Extending laterally and dorsally from the pons are the *middle cerebellar peduncles,* which transmit impulses between the pons and cerebellum. The *basilar artery* lies in the midline directly anterior to the pons. The major portion of the posterior fossa is occupied by the cerebellum.

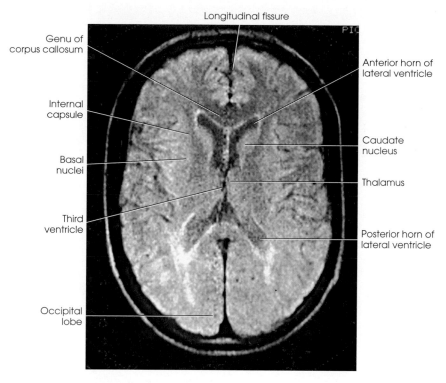

Fig. 27-5 MRI representing the structures located at level *B* in Fig. 27-1.

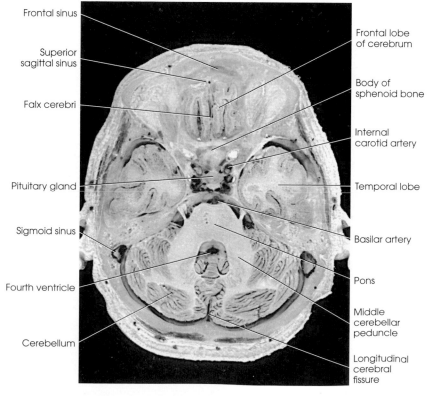

Fig. 27-6 Cadaver section corresponding to level *C* in Fig. 27-1.

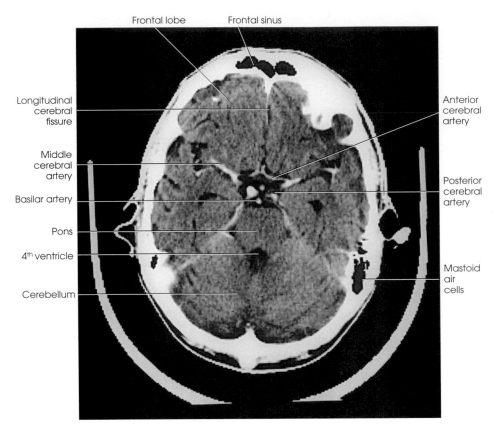

Fig. 27-7 CT image representing the anatomic structures located at level *C* in Fig. 27-1.

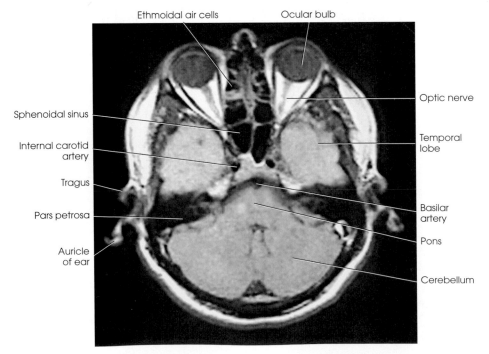

Fig. 27-8 MRI representing the anatomic structures located at level *C* in Fig. 27-1.

The *cerebellum* functions as a reflex center for coordinating skeletal muscle movements. It is divided into two hemispheres that are joined by the midline *vermis*. A fold of dura mater, the *falx cerebelli*, is found between the cerebellar hemispheres. The *fourth ventricle* is seen between the pons and cerebellum. Posterior to the cerebellum the *transverse dural venous sinuses* pass laterally in the margin of the *tentorium cerebelli*. As the transverse sinuses reach the pars petrosae, they change direction and are now called the *sigmoid sinuses*. The sigmoid sinuses ultimately exit the cranium via the *jugular foramina*, at which point they are known as the *internal jugular veins*.

Fig. 27-7 is a CT scan through the region of the *Circle of Willis,* pons, and cerebellum. Contrast medium makes the vascular structures visible on this image. The Circle of Willis encircles the *optic chiasm* and the stalk of the pituitary gland. It is the anastomosis of the anterior and posterior blood supply to the brain. The main vessels that make up the Circle of Willis are the anterior cerebral arteries, anterior communicating artery, posterior cerebral arteries, and posterior communicating arteries. The *anterior* and *middle cerebral arteries* are branches of the internal carotid artery; the *posterior cerebral arteries* are branches of the *basilar artery*, which is seen in the CT image directly anterior to the pons.

Fig. 27-8 is an MRI through the orbits and posterior fossa. (Note the difference in orientation to the orbitomeatal plane between this MRI and the preceding cadaver and CT images.) The *optic nerves* can be seen extending posteriorly from the eyeballs toward the optic chiasm. The *ethmoidal air cells* and *sphenoidal sinuses* are both visualized at this level. Posterior and lateral to the sphenoidal sinuses are the *internal carotid arteries* in the carotid canal. Posterior to the sphenoidal sinuses is the *clivus*, the junction of the dorsum sellae and the basilar portion of the occipital bone. Associated with the posterior clivus are the basilar artery and pons. The black areas of signal void lateral to the pons are the dense bony pars petrosae. The *tragi* and *auricles* of the ears are seen lateral to the petrous regions.

Fig. 27-9 is a cadaver section through C3. Visualized at this level is the *hyoid bone*, which serves as an attachment for the muscles of the tongue. The *submandibular (salivary) glands* are found lateral to the hyoid at this level. Immediately posterior to the submandibular glands are the *internal* and *external carotid arteries*. These arteries are enclosed in the carotid sheath along with the *internal jugular vein* and *vagus nerve*. The *vertebral arteries* can be seen in the neck within the *transverse foramina* of the cervical vertebrae. The *sternocleidomastoid muscles,* which attach to the mastoid processes and the sternum and clavicle, are visualized lateral to the internal jugular veins. Anterior to the vertebrae is the laryngeal portion of the *pharynx*. A portion of the epiglottic cartilage is seen in the anterior pharynx.

Fig. 27-10 is a CT image through the hyoid bone. This image is slightly inferior to the cadaver section and demonstrates the *symphysis* of the mandible anterior to the hyoid (with the suprahyoid muscles between). Deep to the hyoid bone is the *epiglottic cartilage.* The internal jugular vein and *common carotid arteries* are clearly visible because of contrast media enhancement for this particular scan.

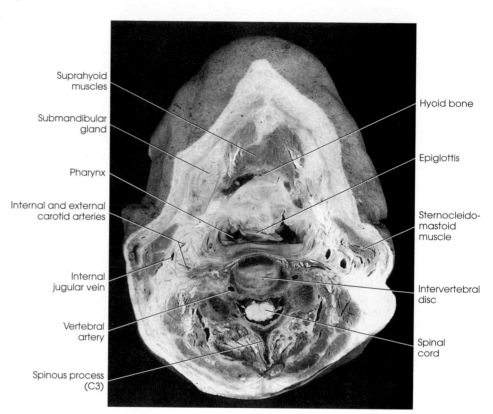

Fig. 27-9 Axial cadaver section through the C3.

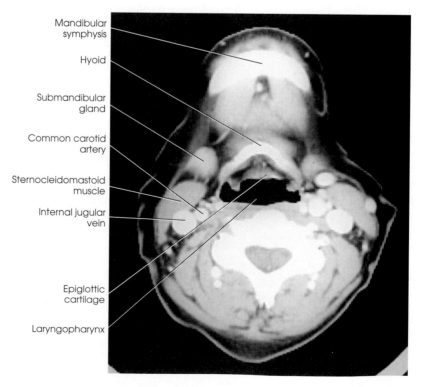

Fig. 27-10 CT image through the C4 corresponding to Fig. 27-9.

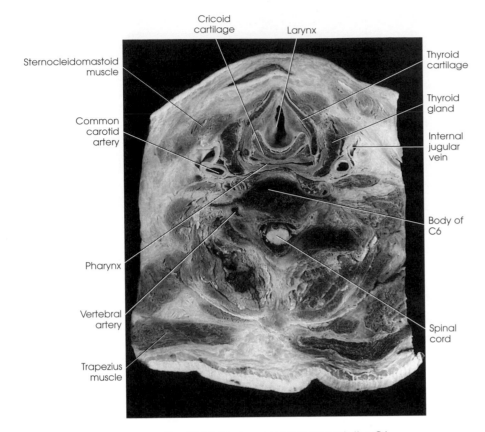

Fig. 27-11 Cadaver section through the C6.

The next cadaver section (Fig. 27-11) and CT image (Fig. 27-12) correspond to level of C6. The *thyroid cartilage* (Adam's apple) is the largest cartilage structure of the larynx and is seen surrounding the vocal cords. The cricoid cartilage is seen posterior to the vocal cords, and the *terminal laryngopharynx* is posterior to the *cricoid cartilage*. The *thyroid gland* has an H-shaped configuration with two lateral lobes connected by a horizontal portion *(isthmus)*. The lobes of the thyroid gland are found on the posterolateral aspects of the thyroid cartilage (and in lower sections lateral to the trachea) and appear highlighted on CT scans because of normal iodine content. At this level the common carotid artery, internal jugular vein, and vagus nerve are on each side of the pharynx and enclosed within the carotid sheath. The vagus nerve is not seen on these images. The vertebral arteries are noted again within the transverse foramina of C6. The sternocleidomastoid muscles lie anterior to the internal jugular veins and lateral to the thyroid cartilage at this level. The large posterior muscle masses lateral to the vertebral column are the *trapezius muscles.*

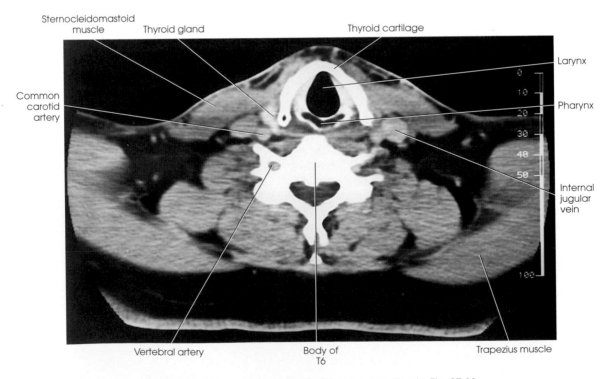

Fig. 27-12 CT image through the C6 corresponding to Fig. 27-11.

It is increasingly common to find images in sagittal, coronal, and oblique planes. CT scanners have the capability to obtain images in the axial and coronal planes and to reconstruct the information in alternate planes. MRI, on the other hand, is capable of direct axial, sagittal, oblique, and coronal imaging. Representative images have been selected in the sagittal and coronal planes to help interpret the anatomy demonstrated.

Fig. 27-13 is a midsagittal MRI of the cranium. The relationship between the cerebral hemisphere, cerebellum, and brainstem is demonstrated. In this image the frontal, parietal, and occipital lobes of the cerebrum are seen and correspond to the cranial bones. The corpus callosum is a white matter tract that connects the hemispheres and is found at the inferior aspect of the parietal lobe. CSF appears dark on this T1-weighted image, making it relatively easy to trace the ventricular system. The anterior horn of the lateral ventricle is inferior to the genu of the corpus callosum. The midline third ventricle receives CSF from each lateral ventricle by way of the *intraventricular foramen (of Monro)* and is not optimally visualized in this image. CSF drains from the third ventricle via the *cerebral aqueduct (of Sylvius),* which can be found within the midbrain (between the *corpora quadrigemina* and the *cerebral peduncles).* The *fourth ventricle* is also a midline structure and is situated between the pons and cerebellum. The large air-filled sphenoidal sinus is located anterior to the pons. Superior to this, the pituitary gland rests within hypophyseal fossa formed by the sella turcica. Directly superior to the pituitary gland is the optic chiasm.

Several vascular structures are well demonstrated in Fig. 27-13. The basilar artery appears between the clivus and pons. The *great cerebral vein (of Galen)* is posterior to the splenium of the corpus callosum. Between the cerebrum and cerebellum, the *straight sinus* (one of the dural venous sinuses) is noted within the tentorium cerebelli.

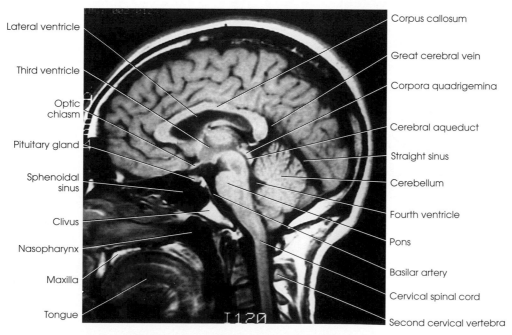

Fig. 27-13 MRI through midsagittal plane.

Lateral ventricle

Third ventricle

Optic chiasm

Pituitary gland

Sphenoidal sinus

Clivus

Nasopharynx

Maxilla

Tongue

Corpus callosum

Great cerebral vein

Corpora quadrigemina

Cerebral aqueduct

Straight sinus

Cerebellum

Fourth ventricle

Pons

Basilar artery

Cervical spinal cord

Second cervical vertebra

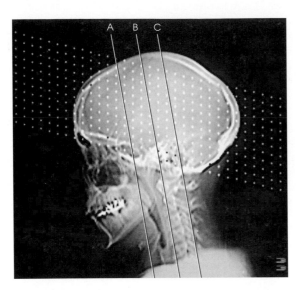

Fig. 27-14 CT localizer (scout) image of the skull.

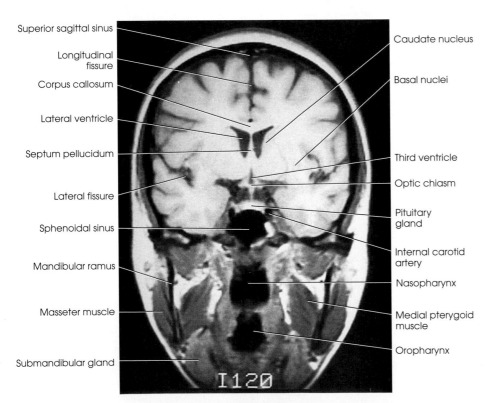

Superior sagittal sinus

Longitudinal fissure

Corpus callosum

Lateral ventricle

Septum pellucidum

Lateral fissure

Sphenoidal sinus

Mandibular ramus

Masseter muscle

Submandibular gland

Caudate nucleus

Basal nuclei

Third ventricle

Optic chiasm

Pituitary gland

Internal carotid artery

Nasopharynx

Medial pterygoid muscle

Oropharynx

Fig. 27-15 Coronal MRI corresponding to level *A* in Fig. 27-14.

A CT localizer, or scout, image (Fig. 27-14) is included as a reference for the next three coronal images. Fig. 27-15 is a coronal MRI through the anterior horns of the lateral ventricles and the pharyngeal structures. The anterior portions of the cerebral hemispheres are joined by the corpus callosum, which is immediately superior to the lateral ventricles. The membrane between the anterior horns of the lateral ventricles is the *septum pellucidum.* On the lateral aspect of each cerebral hemisphere is the *lateral fissure,* which divides the frontal lobe from the temporal lobe. The insula lies deep to this fissure.

Structures of the basal nuclei can again be identified. The caudate nucleus is seen lateral to the anterior horns. Inferolateral to the caudate nucleus are the *putamen* and *globus pallidus* (labeled basal nuclei because they are difficult to differentiate on the image). The anterior portion of the third ventricle is found in the midline inferior to the lateral ventricles. Inferior to the third ventricle are the optic chiasm and hypophysis cerebri. The *superior* and *inferior sagittal sinuses* occupy the margins of the falx cerebri in the longitudinal fissure between the hemispheres of the cerebrum. The internal carotid arteries occupy the *cavernous sinus* along with several cranial nerves and are found lateral to the hypophysis cerebri and sella turcica. Branches of the middle cerebral arteries occupy the lateral sulci of the cerebrum. Several air-filled structures are seen on this image; they are (from superior to inferior) the sphenoidal sinus, *nasopharynx,* and *oropharynx.* This image also demonstrates the *rami of the mandible* along with the *masseter* and *pterygoid muscles.* The submandibular glands, one set of salivary glands, are found deep to the *gonions* (angles) of the mandible.

Fig. 27-16 is a coronal MRI through the bodies of the lateral ventricles, the brainstem, and the bodies of the cervical vertebrae. The third ventricle is well demonstrated and bordered laterally by the thalamus. The cartilaginous structures of the *external ear* surround the *external acoustic meatus* and *canal*. The dark region (low signal return) medial to the external acoustic canal corresponds to the *petrous portion of the temporal bone.* Within this region the *seventh* and *eighth* (*facial* and *vestibulocochlear*) *cranial nerves* are found in the *internal acoustic canal.* The first three cervical vertebrae are detailed in this section with the *dens* of the *axis* (C2*)* seen between the lateral masses of the *atlas* (C1). The vertebral arteries are demonstrated within the transverse foramina, lateral to the bodies of cervical vertebrae. The internal carotid arteries are found more laterally in the neck between the sternocleidomastoid muscles and cervical spine. The large whitish masses inferior to the external acoustic canals are the *parotid glands.*

Fig. 27-17 shows a coronal MRI through the lateral ventricles, brainstem, and spinal cord. The splenium of the corpus callosum is found between the lateral ventricles. Inferior to the splenium is the midline pineal body. The cerebral aqueduct is also a midline structure found within the midbrain. On either side of the cerebral aqueduct are the *superior* and *inferior colliculi,* which are associated with visual and auditory reflexes. Two large white matter tracts are seen extending laterally, inferior to the colliculi. These are the middle cerebellar peduncles, which conduct impulses between the pons and cerebellum. Portions of the cerebellum are visualized superior and inferior to the middle cerebellar peduncles. The medulla oblongata is the most inferior segment of the brainstem and is continuous with the spinal cord as it passes through the foramen magnum. The large dark areas (signal void) lateral to the cerebellum correspond to the bony mastoid portions of the temporal bone.

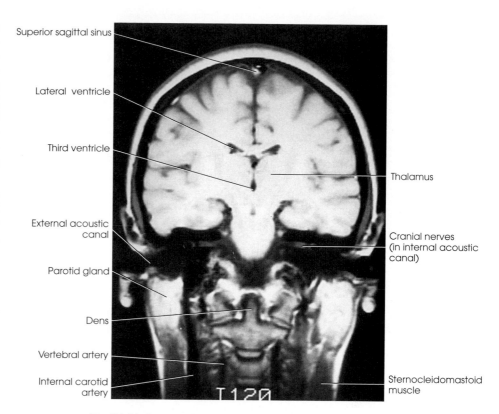

Fig. 27-16 Coronal MRI corresponding to level *B* in Fig. 27-14.

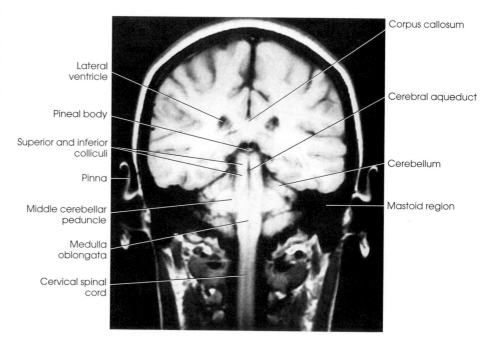

Fig. 27-17 Coronal MRI corresponding to level *C* in Fig. 27-14.

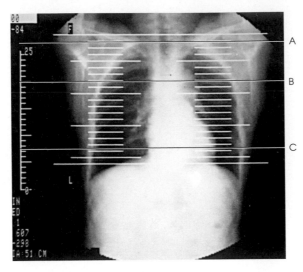

Fig. 27-18 CT localizer (scout) image of thorax.

Thoracic Region

The CT localizer, or scout, image represents an AP projection of the thoracic region with three identifying lines (Fig. 27-18). These lines demonstrate the approximate three levels for each of the labeled cadaver sections for this region.

Figs. 27-19 and 27-20 represent respectively a cadaver section and CT image at the level of T2 and demonstrate the relationship between the vertebral column, esophagus, and trachea. The inferior portion of the *thyroid gland,* which extends from C6 to T1, is positioned lateral to the *trachea* in the cadaver image. The *vertebral arteries* are positioned lateral to the vertebral column, and the *common carotid arteries* are found lateral to the trachea. At this level the *internal jugular veins* are anterior to the carotid arteries. The *apices of the lungs* are visualized along with the first two *ribs,* the *glenohumeral joint,* and the *sternal extremity of the clavicle.* The *trapezius, pectoral,* and *deltoid muscles* are clearly seen. The muscles of the *rotator cuff* (supraspinatus, infraspinatus, subscapularis, and teres minor) stabilize the glenohumeral joint. At this level the *supraspinatus,* which lies superior to the scapular spine, is visible on the cadaver section.

The CT scan at this level is slightly more inferior than the cadaver image. The five major vessels of the superior thorax are visualized posterior to the manubrium. The right and left *brachiocephalic veins* are formed by the junction of the *subclavian veins* and the internal jugular veins. These unite and form the *superior vena cava* at a more inferior level. The three branches of the *aortic arch* are also visualized on this image. From the patient's right to left they are the *brachiocephalic artery, left common carotid artery,* and *left subclavian artery.* The brachiocephalic artery gives rise to the right subclavian and right common carotid arteries, which are both seen in more superior sections of the thorax.

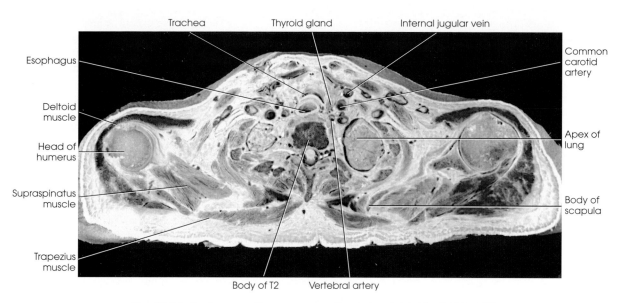

Trachea Thyroid gland Internal jugular vein

Esophagus

Common carotid artery

Deltoid muscle

Head of humerus

Apex of lung

Supraspinatus muscle

Body of scapula

Trapezius muscle

Body of T2 Vertebral artery

Fig. 27-19 Cadaver section corresponding to level *A* in Fig. 27-18 at T2.

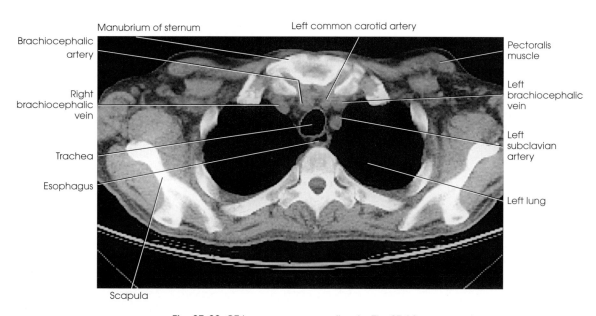

Manubrium of sternum Left common carotid artery

Brachiocephalic artery

Pectoralis muscle

Right brachiocephalic vein

Left brachiocephalic vein

Trachea

Left subclavian artery

Esophagus

Left lung

Scapula

Fig. 27-20 CT image corresponding to Fig. 27-19.

Figs. 27-21 and 27-22 represent respectively a cadaver section and CT image at the level of T5 and demonstrate the great vessels superior to the heart. (The heart is normally positioned between T7 and T11, with the majority of the organ lying left of the midline.) The *ascending aorta* is found anteriorly in the midline; the *descending aorta* is related to the left anterolateral surface of the vertebral bodies. (This relationship between the descending aorta and vertebral column is continuous through the thorax and abdomen.) The superior vena cava is located to the right of the ascending aorta, and the pulmonary trunk is located to the left of the ascending aorta at this level. The *pulmonary trunk* originates from the right ventricle of the heart and divides into the right and left pulmonary arteries, which carry deoxygenated blood to the lungs. In Figs. 27-21 and 27-22 the right and left *pulmonary arteries* are seen at the *hilum* of each lung. The *azygos vein,* which drains the thoracic and posterior abdominal walls, is positioned anterior and to the right of the vertebral column from its origination near the diaphragm until it arches anteriorly over the root of the right lung and empties into the superior vena cava at the level of T4 or T5. At the T5 level the trachea divides into the left and right *primary bronchi.* The *thoracic duct,* one of the major channels for lymphatic drainage, generally originates at T12 and ascends the thorax in the posterior mediastinum between the aorta and azygos vein. The duct ultimately empties into the venous blood system at the junction of the left subclavian and internal jugular veins.

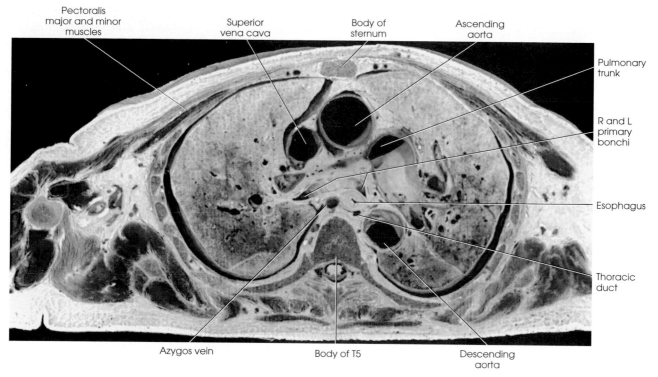

Pectoralis major and minor muscles

Superior vena cava

Body of sternum

Ascending aorta

Pulmonary trunk

R and L primary bonchi

Esophagus

Thoracic duct

Azygos vein

Body of T5

Descending aorta

Fig. 27-21 Cadaver section corresponding to level *B* of Fig. 27-18 at T5.

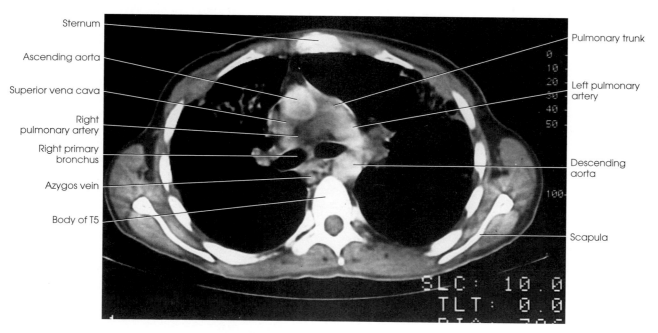

Sternum

Ascending aorta

Superior vena cava

Right pulmonary artery

Right primary bronchus

Azygos vein

Body of T5

Pulmonary trunk

Left pulmonary artery

Descending aorta

Scapula

SLC: 10.0
TLT: 0.0

Fig. 27-22 CT image corresponding to Fig. 27-21.

The cadaver section and CT image depicted respectively in Figs. 27-23 and 27-24 demonstrate the *lungs* and the midsection of the *heart*. Generally when the heart is imaged in cross section, the *left atrium* is the most superior structure encountered, and the *pulmonary veins* are seen emptying into it (not seen in these figures). The *right atrium* is seen lying the farthest toward the right side of the body, anterior and somewhat inferior to the left atrium. The *inferior vena cava (IVC)* may be seen at this level as it enters the right atrium. The *right ventricle* lies to the left of the right atrium and anterior to the more muscular *left ventricle*. The *interventricular septum* can be seen between the ventricles.

The lungs are divided into superior and inferior lobes by the diagonally oriented *oblique fissure*. The *superior lobes* lie superior and anterior to the inferior lobes. The *superior lobe* of the right lung is further divided by the *horizontal fissure,* with the lower portion termed the *middle lobe.* The left lung has no horizontal fissure. The inferior and anterior portion of the left lung (corresponding to the right middle lobe) is termed the *lingula.*

Muscular structures that can be seen at this level include the trapezius, *latissimus dorsi,* and *serratus anterior muscles.* The *esophagus* is normally seen anterior and slightly to the left of the vertebral column at this level as it veers toward the *esophageal hiatus* of the diaphragm. Fig. 27-24 demonstrates the superior portion of the liver bulging against the base of the right lung. The descending aorta normally lies along the left anterolateral surface of the vertebral column, and the azygos vein is normally on the right anterolateral surface. Because of patient pathology the azygos vein, esophagus, and aorta are abnormally displaced to the left in Figs. 27-23 and 27-24.

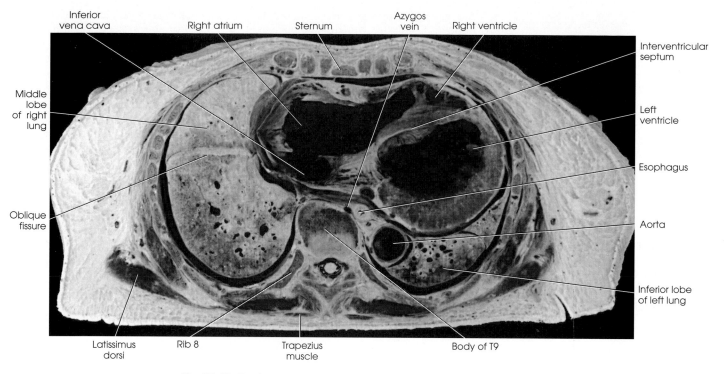

Fig. 27-23 Cadaver section corresponding to level *C* in Fig. 27-18 at T9.

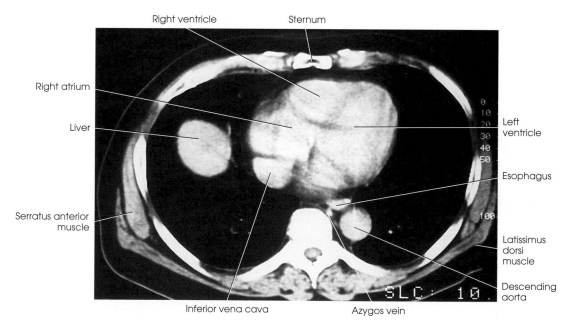

Fig. 27-24 CT image corresponding to Fig. 27-23.

Fig. 27-25 presents a sagittal MRI through the midline structures of the neck and upper thorax. The air-filled pharynx and trachea are easily identified. The cartilaginous flap within the laryngeal portion of the pharynx is the *epiglottis*. Spinal structures are clearly visible in this image, and the relationship between the *intervertebral disks* and *spinal cord* is demonstrated. The major blood vessels of the superior thorax are seen posterior to the *manubrium*. The most anterior of these vessels is the left brachiocephalic vein, which ultimately unites with the right brachiocephalic vein to form the superior vena cava. Posterior to the brachiocephalic vein is a portion of the aortic arch with the origin of the brachiocephalic artery. Inferior to the arch is the right pulmonary artery.

The coronal MRI in Fig. 27-26 is slightly posterior to the midcoronal plane and also demonstrates structures of the neck and superior thorax. The distal cervical and superior thoracic vertebrae are identifiable. On the patient's left side, the *humeral head, clavicle, acromion process,* and *acromioclavicular joint* are seen. The *tracheal bifurcation* is visualized on this image. The aortic arch and left pulmonary artery are found in close proximity to the left main bronchus. From the superior aspect of the arch extends the left subclavian artery. The heart and lungs are not ideally imaged in this scan because of motion artifacts. (Methods for overcoming this problem are discussed in Chapter 36.)

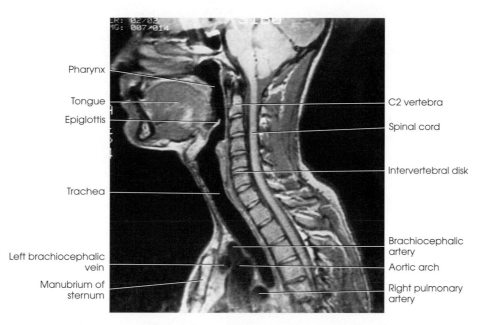

Fig. 27-25 Midline sagittal MRI through neck and upper thorax.

Pharynx

Tongue

Epiglottis

Trachea

Left brachiocephalic vein

Manubrium of sternum

C2 vertebra

Spinal cord

Intervertebral disk

Brachiocephalic artery

Aortic arch

Right pulmonary artery

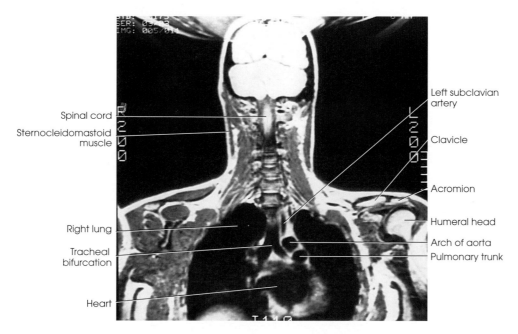

Fig. 27-26 MRI of neck and thorax through midcoronal plane.

Spinal cord

Sternocleidomastoid muscle

Right lung

Tracheal bifurcation

Heart

Left subclavian artery

Clavicle

Acromion

Humeral head

Arch of aorta

Pulmonary trunk

Abdominopelvic Region

Fig. 27-27 is a CT localizer, or scout, image representing an AP projection of the abdominopelvic region. It has six identifying lines demonstrating the levels for each of the labeled cadaver sections and images for this region.

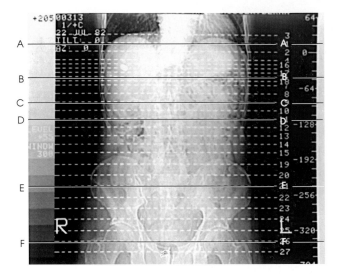

Fig. 27-27 CT localizer (scout) image of abdominopelvic region.

Figs. 27-28 and 27-29 represent structures seen at the T10-11 levels (corresponding to level *A* in the localizer image, Fig. 27-27). The cadaver section (Fig. 27-28) demonstrates the *right hemidiaphragm* surrounding the superior portion of the *liver* and the *left hemidiaphragm* in its entirety. (The multiple white spots in this patient's liver are pathologic.) The pericardial fat at the apex of the heart is seen to the left of the liver. The *esophagus,* posterior to the liver, has migrated toward the patient's left as it nears its entrance into the stomach. The *aorta* is in its normal position, anterior and slightly left of the vertebral body. The IVC appears embedded within the liver. Two of the *hepatic veins* are draining into the IVC at this level. The CT scan (see Fig. 27-29) is at a slightly more inferior level than the cadaver section. The lower lobes of both lungs are seen. The right hemidiaphragm surrounds the superior portion of the liver. The *spleen* and contrast-filled *stomach* are seen on the patient's left side, where they are surrounded by the left hemidiaphragm and lower lobe of the left lung. The esophagus still appears in the midline. The IVC is difficult to see in this image because of its proximity to the isodense liver tissue.

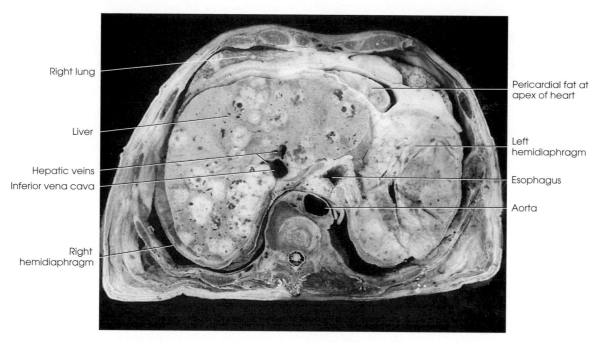

Right lung

Liver

Hepatic veins
Inferior vena cava

Right
hemidiaphragm

Pericardial fat at
apex of heart

Left
hemidiaphragm

Esophagus

Aorta

Fig. 27-28 Cadaver section corresponding to level *A* in Fig. 27-27 at T10.

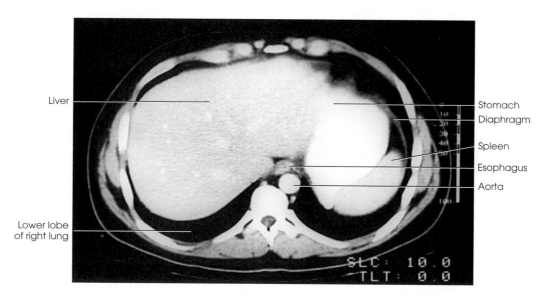

Liver

Lower lobe
of right lung

Stomach
Diaphragm

Spleen

Esophagus

Aorta

SLC: 10.0
TLT: 0.0

Fig. 27-29 CT image corresponding to Fig. 27-28.

The cadaver section and CT image at the level of T12 demonstrate the relationship between the liver, stomach, and spleen (Figs. 27-30 and 27-31). The cardiac portion of the stomach is located at approximately the T11 level in the anterior aspect of the left upper quadrant, and the *pyloric portion* normally lies anterior to L2. The spleen, located between the levels of T12 and L1, is in the posterolateral aspect of the left upper quadrant posterior to the *fundus* of the stomach. The liver is generally found between T11 and L3 and occupies the entire right upper quadrant. The right lobe of the liver has two small subdivisions, the *caudate* and *quadrate lobes,* which are bounded by the *gallbladder, ligamentum teres,* and IVC. The left lobe of liver stretches across the midline and into the left upper quadrant. The *suprarenal glands* are normally located superior to the kidney. The right suprarenal gland is found at this level between the liver and the right *diaphragmatic crus.* The *abdominal aorta* is positioned anterior and to the left of the vertebral column with the celiac trunk projecting anteriorly.

The three branches of the *celiac trunk* (hepatic, splenic, left gastric arteries) supply the liver, spleen, pancreas, and stomach with oxygen-rich blood. The *splenic artery* runs a very tortuous course and normally cannot be visualized in its entirety in axial sections. The IVC can be seen in its normal position anterior and to the right of the vertebral column. Branches of the portal vein are seen within the liver.

The muscles of the abdomen are located between the lower rib cage and the iliac crests. This group of muscles includes the *external oblique, internal oblique,* and *transverse abdominal muscles.* The two *rectus abdominis muscles* are located on the anterior aspect of the abdomen on either side of the midline and extend from the *pubic symphysis* to the *xiphoid process.* The *psoas muscles* originate from the body of T12 and the transverse processes of the lumbar vertebrae and descend the abdomen lateral to the vertebral bodies. The *quadratus lumborum muscles* are located posterolateral to the psoas muscles through the abdomen.

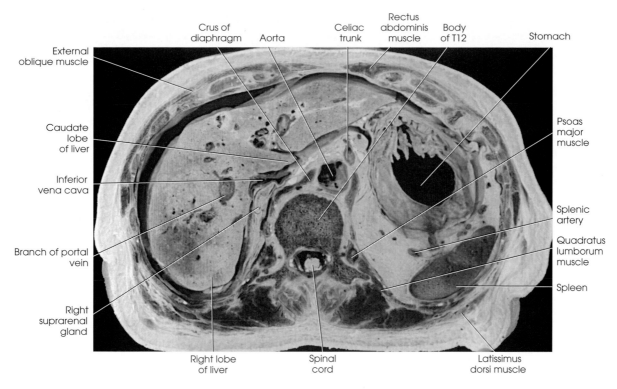

Fig. 27-30 Cadaver section corresponding to level *B* in Fig. 27-27 at T12.

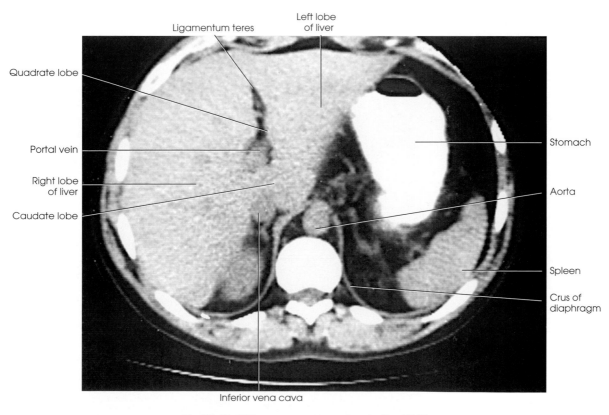

Fig. 27-31 CT image corresponding to Fig. 27-30.

The cadaver section and CT image at the level of L2 demonstrate the inferior aspect of the liver with the *porta hepatis* (Figs. 27-32 and 27-33). At the porta hepatis the vasculature of the liver can be seen in its normal configuration, with the *hepatic duct* lying anterior to the *hepatic artery* and the portal vein lying posterior to the hepatic artery. The superior pole of the *left kidney* is visualized along with the pylorus of the stomach. The *pancreas* lies essentially in a horizontal plane posterior to the stomach and liver. The head of the pancreas is near the liver and is surrounded by the *duodenum* (C-loop). The tail of the pancreas is slightly superior to the head and is located near the hilum of the spleen. The *transverse colon* arches posteriorly, then inferiorly, near the spleen at the *left colic flexure,* which is seen on the CT scan at this level. The junction of the *splenic vein* and *superior mesenteric vein* is visible posterior to the left lobe of the liver and the neck of the pancreas. This junction is the origin for the *portal vein.* The *superior mesenteric artery* lies anterior and slightly to the left of the aorta and can be seen originating from the aorta in the CT scan. The IVC is seen as the *left renal vein* empties into it.

Lateral to the vertebral body are the psoas muscles. The quadratus lumborum muscles are seen between the psoas muscles and the transverse processes of the *lumbar vertebrae.* The *spinal cord* normally terminates at the level of L1. Inferior to L1 the *spinal nerves,* known as *cauda equina,* are seen within the spinal canal.

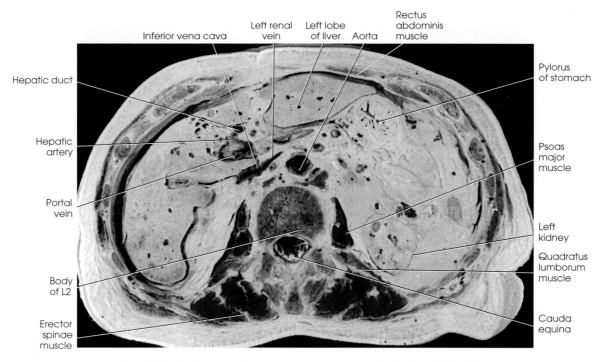

Inferior vena cava · Left renal vein · Left lobe of liver · Aorta · Rectus abdominis muscle

Hepatic duct

Hepatic artery

Portal vein

Body of L2

Erector spinae muscle

Pylorus of stomach

Psoas major muscle

Left kidney

Quadratus lumborum muscle

Cauda equina

Fig. 27-32 Cadaver section corresponding to level *C* in Fig. 27-27 at L2.

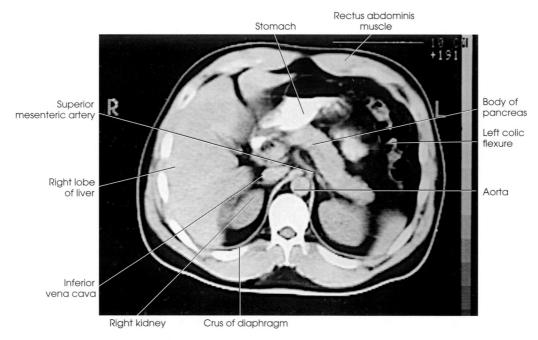

Stomach · Rectus abdominis muscle

Superior mesenteric artery

Right lobe of liver

Inferior vena cava

Right kidney · Crus of diaphragm

Body of pancreas

Left colic flexure

Aorta

Fig. 27-33 CT image corresponding to Fig. 27-32. Note the crus (tendinous origin) of the diaphragm surrounding the aorta.

Figs. 27-34 and 27-35 represent the level of the *intervertebral disk* between L2 and L3. At this level the gallbladder is seen lying against the inferior aspect of the liver. The pylorus of the stomach and the first, or horizontal, portion (bulb) of the duodenum are anterior in the abdomen. The *descending colon* is seen in the left posterior and lateral aspect of the abdomen. In Fig. 27-34 the *ascending colon* is seen lateral to the right kidney as it makes its anterior turn toward the transverse colon *(right colic flexure)*. This level demonstrates the *hilum* of each kidney and the head, neck, and body of the pancreas (across the midline). The IVC is seen behind the head of the pancreas with the *right renal vein* emptying into it. The superior mesenteric vessels and aorta are located posterior to the body of the pancreas.

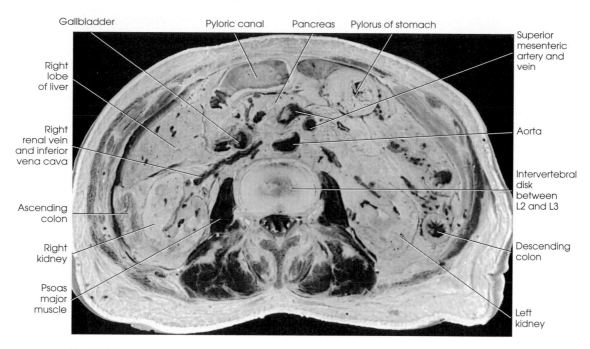

Gallbladder Pyloric canal Pancreas Pylorus of stomach

Right lobe of liver

Right renal vein and inferior vena cava

Ascending colon

Right kidney

Psoas major muscle

Superior mesenteric artery and vein

Aorta

Intervertebral disk between L2 and L3

Descending colon

Left kidney

Fig. 27-34 Cadaver section corresponding to level *D* in Fig. 27-27 at the interspace between L2 and L3.

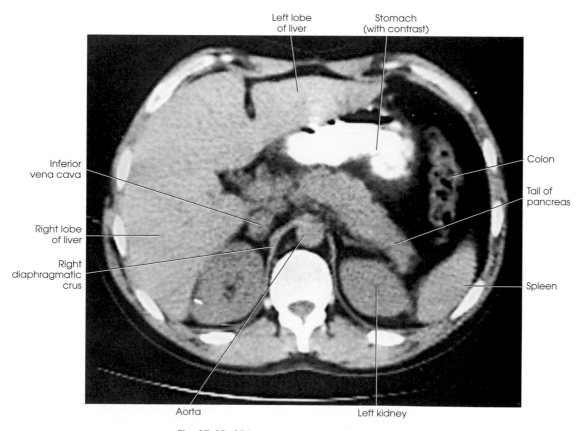

Left lobe of liver Stomach (with contrast)

Inferior vena cava

Right lobe of liver

Right diaphragmatic crus

Colon

Tail of pancreas

Spleen

Aorta Left kidney

Fig. 27-35 CT image corresponding to Fig. 27-34.

The cadaver section and CT image seen respectively in Figs. 27-36 and 27-37 are at the midsacral level and demonstrate the *wing* of the *ilium*, the *anterior superior iliac spine (ASIS)*, and the *sacroiliac joints*. At the posterolateral aspect of the ilium the three *gluteal muscles* are visible. The *iliacus muscle* is seen lining the internal aspect of the iliac wings near the psoas muscles. The two rectus abdominis muscles are found in the anterior abdomen on both sides of the midline. The *cecum* is found at the right anterior aspect of the pelvic cavity, and the descending colon is seen at the left lateral aspect. Multiple loops of *small intestine* are found throughout this level in the images. The abdominal aorta bifurcates at L4 into the *common iliac arteries*. Each common iliac artery divides at the level of the ASIS into *internal* and *external iliac arteries*. The internal iliac arteries tend to be located in the posterior pelvis and branch to feed the pelvic structures. The external iliac vessels are found progressively anterior in succeeding inferior sections to become the femoral vessels at the superior aspect of the thigh.

The *internal* and *external iliac veins* unite inferior to the ASIS to form the *common iliac veins,* and the IVC is formed anterior to L5 by the junction of the common iliac veins. The common iliac veins are positioned at the anterior aspects of the *sacrum* with the internal and external *iliac arteries* lateral to the veins in these images. Through the lower abdomen and at this level the *ureters* are located along the anterior aspect of the psoas muscles and can be seen filled with contrast medium in the CT image (see Fig. 27-37). In the female pelvis the *ovaries* are normally located laterally in the pelvis near the ASIS.

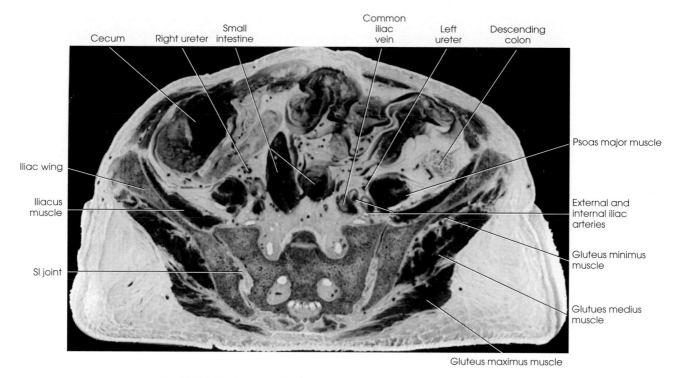

Fig. 27-36 Cadaver section corresponding to level *E* in Fig. 27-27 at the ASIS.

Labels in Fig. 27-36:
Cecum
Right ureter
Small intestine
Common iliac vein
Left ureter
Descending colon
Iliac wing
Iliacus muscle
SI joint
Psoas major muscle
External and internal iliac arteries
Gluteus minimus muscle
Glutues medius muscle
Gluteus maximus muscle

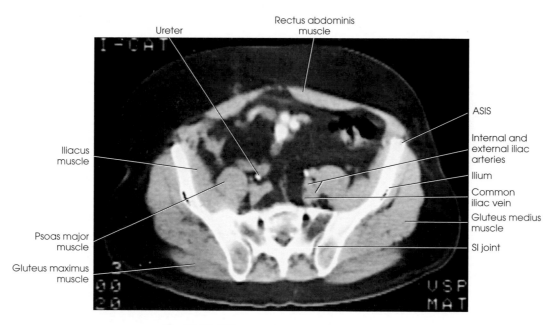

Fig. 27-37 CT image corresponding to Fig. 27-36.

Labels in Fig. 27-37:
Ureter
Rectus abdominis muscle
Iliacus muscle
Psoas major muscle
Gluteus maximus muscle
ASIS
Internal and external iliac arteries
Ilium
Common iliac vein
Gluteus medius muscle
SI joint

The cadaver section in Fig. 27-38 is at a level just superior to the *pubic symphysis.* The CT image in Fig. 27-39 is through the pubic symphysis. The *ischial spines, acetabula, femoral heads,* and *greater trochanters* are visualized. The *coccyx* is seen posterior to the *rectum* in Fig. 27-39. The relationship between the *rectum, vagina,* wall of the *bladder,* and superior aperture of the *urethra* is demonstrated from posterior to anterior in the pelvic region. The external iliac vessels are now referred to as the *femoral vessels,* with the name change occurring at the inguinal ligament, which is found between the pubic symphysis and the ASIS. The *iliopsoas muscles* (formed by the junction of the psoas and iliacus muscles) are found anterior to the femoral heads; the *obturator internus muscle,* with its characteristic right-angle bend, is found medial to the acetabulum.

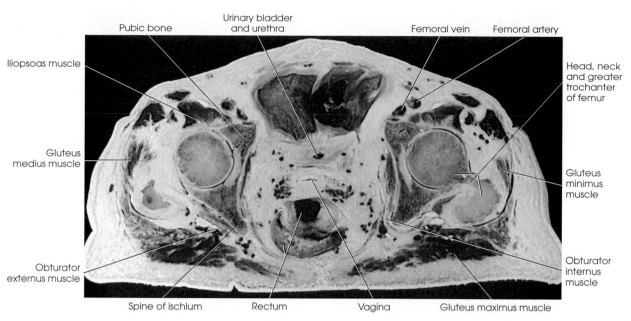

Fig. 27-38 Cadaver section corresponding to level *F* in Fig. 27-27 at the coccyx (female).

Iliopsoas muscle

Pubic bone

Urinary bladder and urethra

Femoral vein

Femoral artery

Head, neck and greater trochanter of femur

Gluteus medius muscle

Gluteus minimus muscle

Obturator externus muscle

Obturator internus muscle

Spine of ischium

Rectum

Vagina

Gluteus maximus muscle

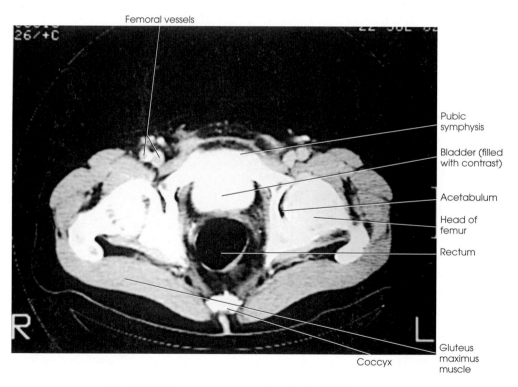

Fig. 27-39 CT image corresponding to Fig. 27-38.

Femoral vessels

Pubic symphysis

Bladder (filled with contrast)

Acetabulum

Head of femur

Rectum

Coccyx

Gluteus maximus muscle

Figs. 27-40 and 27-41 are respectively a male pelvic cadaver section and a corresponding MRI. These figures highlight structures of the male reproductive system. At this level the relationship between the rectum, *prostate gland,* and pubic symphysis is noted. The prostatic portion of the urethra is seen within the prostate. Posterior to the prostate are the *prostatic venous plexus* and *ductus deferens.* The *spermatic cord* contains the ductus deferens and *testicular vessels,* and it is found superficial and lateral to the pubic symphysis. The circular opening formed by the rami of the pubic and ischial bones is the *obturator foramen.* It is bounded by the *obturator externus* and *obturator internus muscles.* The muscles of the lower limb are anterior to the femur.

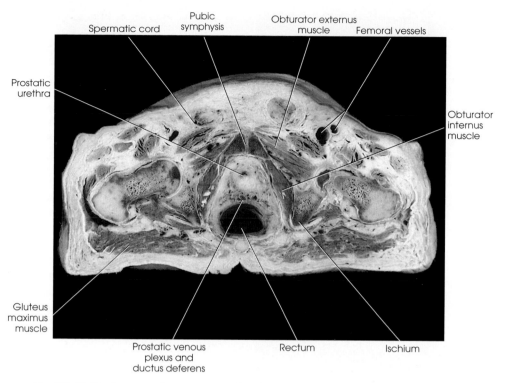

Fig. 27-40 Cadaver section corresponding to level *F* of Fig. 27-27 at the coccyx (male).

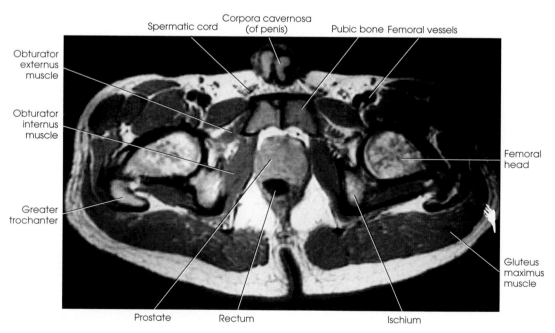

Fig. 27-41 MRI corresponding to Fig. 27-40.

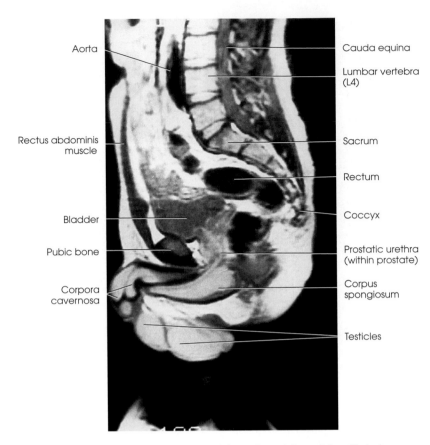

Aorta

Rectus abdominis muscle

Bladder

Pubic bone

Corpora cavernosa

Cauda equina

Lumbar vertebra (L4)

Sacrum

Rectum

Coccyx

Prostatic urethra (within prostate)

Corpus spongiosum

Testicles

Fig. 27-42 MRI of the abdominopelvic region at the midsagittal plane.

Fig. 27-42 is a sagittal MRI of the structures of the abdomen and pelvis near the midline. L3 through L5, the sacrum, and the coccyx are visualized. The cauda equina is seen descending the spinal canal. Anterior to the vertebral bodies is the distal portion of the abdominal aorta. At the level of L4, the aorta bifurcates to form the right and left common iliac arteries. The large areas of signal void anterior to the sacrum represent the rectum. The bladder is anterior to the rectum and superior to the prostate. The urethra appears faintly, traversing the prostate. The *corpus spongiosum* and *corpora cavernosa* of the penis are inferior and anterior to the pubic symphysis. The right and left *testes* are seen inferior to the *penile* structures. The rectus abdominis muscle extends superiorly from the pubis in the anterior abdominal wall.

A coronal MRI through the femoral heads and greater trochanters is presented in Fig. 27-43. The femoral heads are demonstrated within the *acetabula*. The crests of the ilia are visualized with their associated musculature. The internal surface of the iliac bone is lined by the iliacus muscle. In this image the psoas muscles are seen joining the iliacus muscles to form the iliopsoas muscles. (Iliopsoas muscles are visualized on more anterior sections of the pelvis.) *Gluteus medius* and *minimus* muscles are found external to the iliac bones. The bladder and prostate are seen within the pelvic cavity. Superior to the bladder is a portion of the *sigmoid colon*. The right ductus deferens is found lateral to the neck of the bladder. Between the rami of the pubic bones are the corpus spongiosum and corpora cavernosa. The *scrotum* is seen inferior to the *penis* and between the *gracilis muscles* of the thighs.

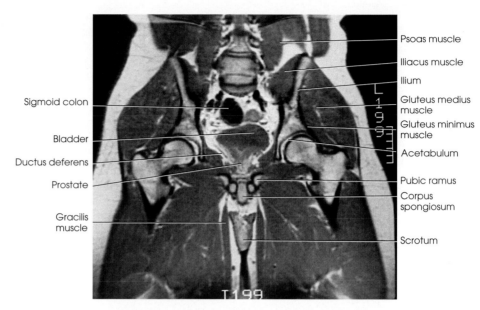

Fig. 27-43 MRI of the abdominopelvic region at the midcoronal plane.

SUMMARY OF ANATOMY*

Cranial region
Bony structures
parietal bones
frontal bone
  frontal sinuses
  orbital roof
occipital bone
  inion
  internal occipital
    protuberance
  foramen magnum
temporal bones
  mastoid air cells
  petrous ridges
  external acoustic
    meatus (EAM)
  internal auditory
    canal
sphenoid bone
  greater and lesser
    wings
  sella turcica
  optic canal
  clivus
  sphenoidal sinuses
  anterior and
    posterior
    clinoids
ethmoid bone
  crista galli
  ethmoidal air cells
  perpendicular
    plate
  cribriform plate
  labyrinths
zygomatic/malar
  bones
nasal bones
maxillae
  maxillary sinuses
vomer
mandible
  coronoid and
    condyloid
    processes
  neck
  rami

Cranial region—cont'd
Vasculature
dural venous sinuses
  superior sagittal
  inferior sagittal
  straight
  transverse
  cavernous
  confluence of
    sinuses
internal jugular veins
arterial system
  internal carotid
    artery
  middle cerebral
    arteries
  anterior cerebral
    arteries
  basilar artery
  vertebral arteries
  circle of Willis

Neurologic structures
cranial nerves
  optic
  olfactory
  trigeminal
  acoustic
brain
lobes (frontal,
    parietal, temporal,
    occipital, insula)
ventricular system
  lateral ventricles
  third ventricle
  fourth ventricle
  interventricular
    foramen
  cerebral aqueduct
cortex, gyri, sulci
thalamus
pituitary gland
basal nuclei
lateral fissure
longitudinal fissure
caudate nucleus
falx cerebri and falx
  cerebelli
tentorium cerebelli
pineal gland
midbrain
pons
medulla oblongata
cerebellum
  vermis
  arbor vitae

Lower face and neck
**Bony and
cartilaginous
structures**
mandible
cervical vertebrae
thyroid cartilage
cricoid cartilage

Vasculature
internal and external
  carotid arteries
common carotid
  arteries
vertebral arteries
internal jugular veins

Musculature
sternocleidomastoid
  muscles
masseter muscles
trapezius muscles
levator scapulae
  muscles

Viscera
salivary glands
  (parotid,
  submandibular,
  sublingual)
tongue
pharynx
larynx
epiglottis
thyroid gland
trachea
esophagus

*The author of this chapter considers the anatomic terms included in this table to be the most significant for identification. The list may be modified as judged appropriate.

SUMMARY OF ANATOMY*

Thorax
Bony structures
ribs
scapula
  coracoid process
  acromion
  spine
clavicle
thoracic vertebrae
sternum
superior humerus

Vasculature
common carotid
  arteries
internal jugular veins
subclavian arteries
  and veins
brachiocephalic
  artery and veins
aorta
superior and inferior
  vena cavae
pulmonary arteries
  and veins
azygos vein

Musculature
pectoralis major and
  minor
trapezius
latissimus dorsi
serratus anterior
diaphragm

Viscera
trachea
  carina
lungs
  lobes
  apices and bases
  hila
  main bronchi
heart
  atria
  ventricles
  valves
esophagus
thymus

Abdomen and pelvis
Bony structures
lumbar vertebrae
sacrum
coccyx
hip bones
  ilium
  ischium
  pubis
  pubic symphysis

Vasculature
aorta
  aortic bifurcation
celiac trunk
superior mesenteric
  artery and vein
inferior mesenteric
  artery and vein
renal arteries and
  veins
common iliac
  arteries and veins
external iliac arteries
  and veins
femoral arteries and
  veins
portal vein
inferior vena cava

Musculature
diaphragm
  crura
external and internal
  oblique muscles
transverse abdominis
  muscles
rectus abdominis
  muscles
psoas major muscles
iliacus muscles
gluteal muscles
  (maximus, medius,
  minimus)

Abdomen and pelvis—cont'd
Viscera
liver
  lobes (left, right,
    caudate,
    quadrate)
  porta hepatis
spleen
  hilum
stomach
  fundus
  cardia
  body
  pyloric antrum
kidneys
  hila
  cortex
  medulla
  perirenal fat
  suprarenal glands
  ureters
pancreas
  head
  body
  tail
gallbladder
small intestine
  duodenum (bulb
    and C-loop)
  jejunum
  ileum (ileocecal
    junction)
large intestine
  cecum
  ascending and
    descending
    colon
  right and left
    flexures
  sigmoid and
    rectum
bladder
  urethra
male reproductive
  organs
  prostate
  seminal vesicles
female reproductive
  organs
  uterus
  vagina

Selected bibliography

Bo WJ et al: *Basic atlas of cross sectional anatomy,* ed 2, Philadelphia, 1990, WB Saunders.

Cahill DR: *Atlas of human cross sectional anatomy,* Philadelphia, 1984, Lea & Febiger.

Cahill DR, Fisher DR, Miller GM: Sectional anatomy using the personal computer, *J Digit Imaging* 10:227, 1997.

Carter BL et al: *Cross sectional anatomy: computed tomography and ultrasound correlation,* Englewood Cliffs, NJ, 1977, Appleton-Century-Crofts.

Chiu L, Lipcamon J, Yiu-Chiu V: *Clinical computed tomography,* Rockville, Md, 1986, Aspen.

Christoforidis A: *Atlas of axial, sagittal, and coronal anatomy,* Philadelphia, 1988, WB Saunders.

El-Khoury GY, Bergman RA, Montgomery WJ: *Sectional anatomy by MRI/CT,* New York, 1990, Churchill Livingstone.

Ellis H et al: *Human cross sectional anatomy: atlas of body sections and CT images,* Oxford, 1991, Butterworth-Heinemann.

Elster A, Goldman A, Handel S: *Magnetic resonance imaging,* Philadelphia, 1987, Lippincott.

Hagen-Ansert S: *The anatomy workbook,* Philadelphia, 1986, Lippincott.

Hayran M et al: Evaluation of the temporal bone by anatomic sections and computed tomography, *Surg Radiol Anat* 14:169, 1992.

Karssemeijer N et al: Recognition of organs in CT-image sequences: a model guided approach, *Comput Biomed Res* 21:434, 1988.

Keiffer S, Heitzman E: *An atlas of cross sectional anatomy,* Hagerstown, Md, 1979, Harper & Row.

Kelley LL, Peterson CM: *Sectional anatomy for imaging professionals,* St Louis, 1996, Mosby.

Koritke J, Sick H: *Atlas of sectional human anatomy,* Germany, 1988, Urban & Schwarzenberg.

Ledley RS, Huang HK, Mazziotta JC: *Cross sectional anatomy: an atlas for computerized tomography,* Baltimore, 1977, Williams & Wilkins.

Metrewelli C: *Practical abdominal ultrasound,* St Louis, 1978, Mosby.

National Institute of Health: The Visible Human Project, http://www.nlm.nih.gov/research/visible/visible_human.html

Novelline R, Squire L: *Living anatomy: a working atlas using computed tomography, magnetic resonance and angiography images,* St Louis, 1986, Mosby.

Peterson R: *A cross sectional approach to anatomy,* St Louis, 1978, Mosby.

Spitzer VM, Whitlock AG: *Atlas of the visible human male,* Sudsbury, Mass, 1998, Jones and Bartlett.

Taylor K: *Atlas of gray scale ultrasonography,* New York, 1978, Churchill Livingstone.

Wagner M, Lawson TL: *Segmental anatomy,* New York, 1982, Macmillan.

Wicke L: *Atlas of radiologic anatomy,* ed 6, Baltimore, 1998, Urban & Schwarzenberg.

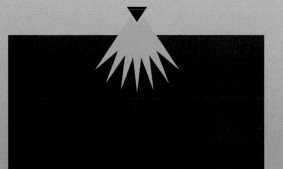

PEDIATRIC IMAGING

DEIRDRE A. MILNE

ALBERT AZIZA

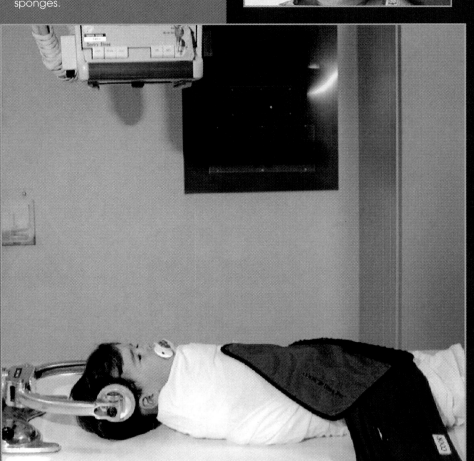

RIGHT: Pediatric patient positioned with old 1949 head clamps for an AP skull projection. If a head clamp was not available, the parent might hold the child's head between two large sponges.

Patient positioned with modern
head clamps.

Principles of Pediatric Imaging

Understanding that *children are not just small adults* and appreciating that they need to be approached on their level are essential ingredients for successful encounters with children in the imaging department. Many good cooks agree that simply being able to read does not make one a great chef. As with any challenging recipe, the basic steps of pediatric radiography can be explained, but they must also be practiced. Radiographers often lack confidence in two main areas of pediatric radiography—pediatric communication skills and immobilization techniques.

Although pediatric imaging and adult radiography have many similarities, including basic positioning and image quality assessment, some significant differences remain. The way to *approach* the child tops the list of differences. It may help novice pediatric radiographers to think about children of various ages whom they know and to imagine how they would explain a particular radiographic examination to those children. This strategy, along with the descriptions that follow, will prove quite effective. Working successfully with children requires an open mind, patience, creativity, the willingness to learn, and the ability to look at the world through the eyes of a child.

Atmosphere

The environment in which patients are treated and recover plays a significant role in the recovery process. Research studies have compared the recovery course of patients whose hospital rooms looked out over parks with the recovery course of those whose view was a brick wall. The patients who faced the park had a much shorter hospital stay than the other patients, and they required considerably fewer pain killers. With these differences in mind, the patient care center at the Hospital for Sick Children (Toronto) was designed and built as an atrium (Fig. 28-1). Each patient room receives natural light, either by facing outside or overlooking the atrium, which receives natural light from the glass roof. Although it is easy to see how children can be amused by Miss Piggy and the barnyard animals that fly across the atrium, the environment does not have to be this elaborate to be appreciated by children. Small measures can be taken at relatively little cost to make a child's hospital stay more comfortable.

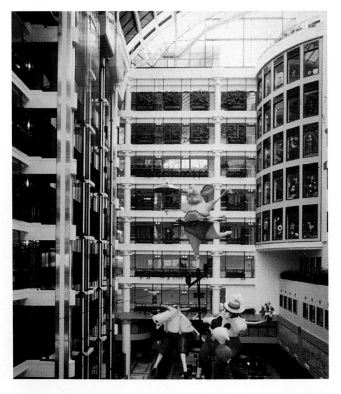

Fig. 28-1 Atrium of the Hospital for Sick Children (Toronto), which provides inpatient care and directly related support services.

WAITING ROOM

Parents of pediatric patients often arrive at the reception desk feeling anxious. They may be worried about what is involved in a procedure because they have not had the specifics explained to them or because they *did not hear* all that was explained to them. They also may be worried about the amount of time the care of their child will take, not to mention the outcome.

Feelings of anxiousness and tension are often transferred from parent to child—the child senses a parent's tension through the parent's tone of voice or actions. A well-equipped waiting room (this does not have to be expensive) can reduce this tension. Children are attracted to and amused by the toys, leaving the parents free to check in or register and ask pertinent questions.

Gender-neutral toys or activities such as a small table and chairs with crayons and coloring pages are most appropriate. (Children should be supervised to prevent them from putting the crayons in their mouths.) Books or magazines for older children are also good investments. The child life department of the hospital can provide advice and recommendations (Fig. 28-2).

IMAGING ROOM

Time can pass quickly for lengthy procedures if age-appropriate music or videos are available. A child who is absorbed in a video often requires little or no immobilization (other than the usual safety precautions designed to prevent the child from rolling off the table). Charitable and fund-raising organizations are often happy to donate televisions and videocassette recorders (VCRs) for this purpose on request.

Experience has shown that children are less likely to become upset or agitated if they are brought into a room that has been prepared before they enter. This preparation should include placement of the cassette, approximate centering of the tube to the cassette, and placement of all immobilization tools likely to be needed at one end of the table.

Young children are often afraid of the dark. They dislike having the lights turned out but are often comfortable with low levels of illumination. Dimming the lights enough to see the collimator light before the child enters can prevent the need to explain why the lights have to be dimmed. Busy radiographers often turn the lights down without explanation, causing unnecessary anxiety.

After the procedure is complete, the radiographer or other imaging professional should take a moment to emphasize, *even overemphasize,* how helpful the child was and to explain where the child should wait or what the child should do next, *ensuring that the parent is comprehending the instructions.*

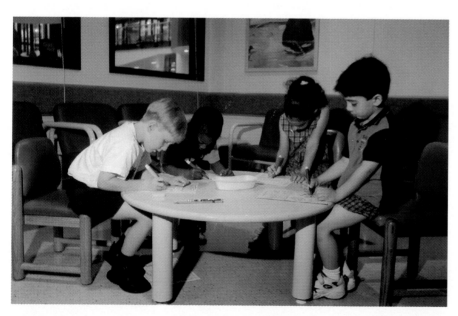

Fig. 28-2 Children in waiting area enjoying *normal* activity before being radiographed.

Approach

APPROACHING THE PARENT

No discussion of dealing with children is complete without mentioning ways to approach the parent(s). Although children are sometimes brought for medical care by someone other than the parents, for the purposes of this discussion the caregiver is referred to as the *parent*.

In many cases, radiographers find that they are dealing with two patients—the child and the parent. They may wonder to whom they should primarily speak. The answer, however, is easy:

- If the child is capable of understanding, direct the explanation to the child but use age-appropriate language (discussed later). The parents will listen and consequently understand what is expected. Communicating in this way puts the parents more at ease and increases their confidence in the radiographer's skills. They appreciate the fact that their child has been made the focus of attention.

- If the child is too young to comprehend, direct the explanation to the parent, explaining in simple sentences what is going to happen and what is expected of the parent. The importance and value of simple sentences cannot be emphasized enough. People in stress-filled situations do not think as clearly as they normally do, and many parents in this setting are under stress. Successful communication involves the use of short sentences repeated once or twice in a soothing tone.

Dealing with the agitated parent

When approaching the agitated parent, the radiographer should observe the following guidelines:

- Remain calm and speak in an even tone, remembering that fear and frustration may be the cause of the agitation.
- Use phrases such as "My name is. . . . I can identify with how you must be feeling and can appreciate your concern," followed by "Let me explain to you what is happening."
- If possible, escort the parent to a nearby room or office to continue the explanation. This can avoid an unwanted scene in the waiting room.

Parent participation

The degree of parent participation depends on several factors:
1. The general philosophy of the department
2. The wishes of the parent and patient
3. The laws of the province or state regarding radiation protection

The advantages of parental participation can be great for everyone concerned—patients, parents, radiographers, and departmental administrators. Experience has shown that both parents should have the basic procedure explained to them. However, it is advisable that only *one* parent be present in the imaging room. The presence of both parents often causes the room to become crowded; moreover, it is distracting and can actually lengthen the procedure. Many provincial or state laws permit only one additional person in the room, and this serves nicely as a rationale when the radiographer explains the policy to parents. Posting signs to this effect in strategic locations also can be helpful.

Parental participation is insisted on by many parents and advocated by many pediatric radiographers for the following reasons:
1. The parent can watch the child if the attention of the radiographer or radiologist is directed to the equipment or the fluoroscopic monitor.
2. The radiographer may need to leave the room.
3. The parent can assist with immobilization if needed (where permitted).
4. The parent who witnesses an entire procedure has little room for doubt about professional conduct.

This last point illustrates a benefit to parents, as well as medical personnel. The parent's presence ensures that no action, explanation, or question is misinterpreted by the child or adolescent. At the same time, the parent can take comfort in seeing that the child is being cared for in a professional manner. Although parental participation is perhaps less controversial now than it was in the past, radiographers can put the situation in perspective by imagining themselves in the position of parents and asking whether they would want to be present. With increasing public knowledge and the ever-present threat of litigation, parents are participating in more procedures.

Informed parents, whether physically present in the imaging room or not, can usually help to explain the procedure to the child. Some hospitals and commercial organizations have prepared pamphlets describing procedures and answering many commonly asked questions.

In some situations, parental presence is not advised. For example, some children are further agitated by their parents' presence, or some parents may find certain procedures too disturbing, such as those performed in the angio/interventional suites.

Whenever parents are in the room during a radiographic exposure, they should be protected from scatter radiation. They should also be given lead gloves if their hands will be near the primary radiation beam.

APPROACHING THE CHILD

Naturally, good communication is essential to obtaining maximum cooperation. Thus children should be spoken to at their level in words that they can understand. Fortunately, this is not as difficult as learning a new language, and it can be made even easier if the radiographer keeps a few strategies in mind:

- Have the room prepared beforehand, and greet the patient and parent in the waiting area with a smile.
- Bend down to talk to the child at the child's eye level.
- Take a moment to *introduce yourself and ensure that you have the correct patient*; then state briefly what you are going to do.
- Suggest, rather than ask, the child to come and *help* you with some pictures. This *firm, yet gentle* approach avoids creating the idea that the child has a choice. After all, the patient may be tempted to be emphatic and say *no*.
- Use sincere *praise*. This is a powerful motivator, no matter what the age of the patient. Praise for young children (3 to 7 years old) should be immediate. Children have short attention spans and often expect to receive rewards immediately. The reward should be linked directly to the task that has been well done. Use phrases such as "You sat very still for me, thank you" or "You took a nice, big breath in for that picture, and I am going to ask you to do it again for the next one."
- When the outcome will be the same, *give children an option*: "Would you like Mom to help lift you up on the table, or can I help you?" or "We have two pictures to do. Which would you like first—the one with you sitting down or the one with you lying down?"

- Employ distraction techniques. As radiographers develop confidence in basic radiography skills and adapting these skills for children, they find themselves able to engage in *chatter* and *distraction techniques,* thus making the experience as pleasant as possible for the child. Ask the child about brothers, sisters, pets, school, or friends—the topics are limitless. As homework, watch a few popular children's cartoons. Communication is improved when the radiographer can build rapport with a child, and learning a few more distraction techniques is helpful.
- Answer all questions truthfully—regardless of their nature. Maintaining honesty is crucial in all communications with children. Confidence and credibility built by the previous strategies can be lost if the truth is withheld. The secret is not to volunteer information too early or dwell on unpleasantries.

The child's age should greatly influence the approach. Children are unique individuals with unique social styles, of course, but the following guidelines may still prove helpful.

Infants

The basic needs of infants to the age of 6 months are warmth, security, and, of course, nourishment. They do not make an appreciable distinction among caregivers. They are often calmed by the use of a pacifier or soother. As they get older, they become attached to familiar objects, which they should be allowed to keep with them. Because infants are easily startled, care should be taken to minimize loud stimuli.

Children 6 months to 2 years old

Children between 6 months and 2 years of age are particularly fearful of pain, separation from their parents, and limitation of their freedom of movement. This helps to explain why they are very disturbed by immobilization. Unfortunately, children in this age group usually require the most assertive immobilization techniques. Experience has shown it is less disturbing to children to be well immobilized than to have a number of adults in lead aprons trying to hold them in the correct positions.

Although radiographers should be knowledgeable in the art of immobilization for children in this age group (particularly 2-year-olds), one of the most valuable forms of immobilization is natural sleep. The challenge, of course, is to complete the entire radiographic sequence without waking the child. This can be done by carefully transferring the child to the table and taking care to maintain warmth, comfort, and safety.

Parental participation is especially valuable with this age group, as it is with children between the ages of 2 and 4 years. Radiographers can easily pick up tips for communicating with children by taking cues from parents as they explain procedures to their children. Parents are also helpful because they can act as "baby-sitters" during the procedure.

NOTE: Chest radiography must be performed while children are awake. Because respirations are generally shallow during sleep, it is not possible to obtain an adequate degree of inspiration.

Children 2 to 4 years old

Preschoolers can test the power of the radiographer's imagination. They are extremely curious—their favorite question is "Why?" They enjoy fantasy and may readily cooperate if the situation is treated like a game or distraction techniques are used. The following strategies can be useful:

- Give explanations at the child's eye level by bending down or by sitting the child on the radiographic or scanner table.
- Take a moment to show the child how the collimator light works and let the child turn it on (Fig. 28-3)—for a child this is as much fun as pressing the buttons in an elevator.
- Use the camera analogy to describe the x-ray tube, taking care to explain that the tube may move sideways but will never come down and touch the child.
- Avoid any unnecessary equipment manipulation.
- Encourage the child gently as the child attempts to cooperate—then praise the cooperation.

Children between 2 and 4 years of age can be verbally and physically aggressive. A child who is having a tantrum will not respond to games and distraction techniques. Making the procedure as short as possible through the use of practiced and kind, yet effective, immobilization techniques is the best approach. Young patients generally calm down quickly when they are back in their parents' arms or resume the activity they were involved in before the examination.

The 5-year-old

The 5-year-old has typically reached a time that is rich in new experiences. Reactions can differ widely, depending on how at ease the child feels with a given environment. Children in this age group generally want to perform tasks correctly, and they enjoy mimicking adults. When a 5-year-old feels confident, that child will act like a 6-, 7-, or 8-year-old; however, when afraid or worried, that same child may cling to parents and become reticent and uncooperative. Constant reassurance and simple explanations help in such moments.

School-age children 6 to 8 years old

For the radiographer who is not accustomed to working with children, the perfect group to start with is the 6- to 8-year-olds. These children are generally accommodating and eager to please. They are modest and embarrass easily, so their privacy should be protected. These children are the easiest age group with which to communicate; they appreciate being talked through the procedure, which gives them less time to worry about their surroundings or the procedure itself. Anatomic landmarks are easy to locate for positioning, and body habitus evens out nicely—the "big belly" of the toddler disappears. From an imaging standpoint, the bones are maturing, with the increased calcium content enhancing subject contrast (Fig. 28-4).

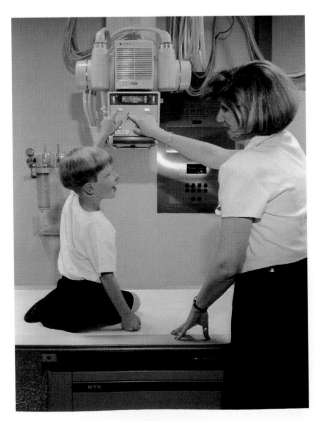

Fig. 28-3 The radiographer should make an introduction to the child and show the child how the collimator light is used. The child can be allowed to turn on the light.

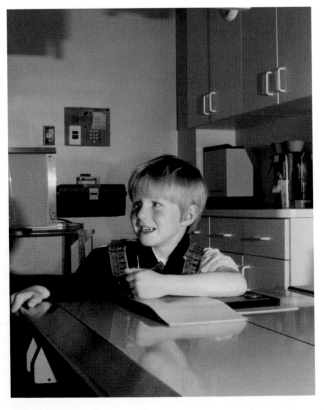

Fig. 28-4 Child properly positioned and shielded for a lateral elbow radiograph.

Adolescents

Image is important to preteens and adolescents. Although they are better able to understand the need for hospitalization, they are upset by interference in their social and school activities. They are particularly concerned that as a result of the injury they may not be able to return to their preinjury state. These patients require, and often demand, explicit explanations. Health care workers should not be surprised by the frankness of their questions and should be prepared for some discussion.[1]

Adolescents want to be treated as adults, and the radiographer must exercise judgment in assessing the patient's degree of maturity. The radiographer should become familiar with the local statutes regarding consent in order to understand when children are deemed to be responsible for themselves.[2]

Sensitive issues, such as the possibility of pregnancy in the postpubescent girl, must be approached discreetly. Honest responses are more likely to be elicited if the girl is alone with the radiographer (i.e., the parent is not present), and the following guidelines are observed:

- Preface the questioning by stating that information of a sensitive nature needs to be obtained for radiation safety.
- Ask the 10-, 11-, 12-, or 13-year-old girl if she has started menstruating. If the response is affirmative, continue by saying that a slightly more sensitive question needs to be asked. Then ask if there is any possibility of pregnancy.
- Simply but tactfully ask girls 14 years and older if there is any chance of pregnancy. Judging from the patient's expression and response, decide how to continue.
- Differing levels of maturity call for different explanations. If necessary, apologize for the need to ask sensitive questions and assure the patient that the same questions are asked of all girls of this age.
- Follow the questioning with an explanation that it is unsafe for unborn babies to receive radiation.
- If possible, have the questioning performed by a female.

[1]Wilmot DM, Sharko GA: *Pediatric imaging for the technologist,* New York, 1987, Springer-Verlag.
[2]Torres LS: *Basic medical techniques and patient care in imaging technology,* ed 5, Philadelphia, 1997, Lippincott-Raven.

APPROACHING PATIENTS WITH SPECIAL NEEDS

Children with physical and mental disabilities

The radiographer should consider age when approaching children with physical and mental disabilities. Children over 8 years old with disabilities strive to achieve as much autonomy and independence as possible. They are sensitive to the fact that they are less independent than their peers. The radiographer should observe the following guidelines:

- Direct communication toward the child first. All children appreciate being given the opportunity to listen and respond. Like any patients, these children also want to be talked to rather than talked about.
- If this approach proves ineffective, turn to the parents. As a general rule the parents of these patients are present and can be very helpful. In strange environments younger children may trust only one person—the parent. In that case the medical team can gain cooperation from the child by communicating through the parent. Parents often know the best way to lift and transfer the child from the wheelchair or stretcher to the table. Children with physical disabilities often have a fear of falling and may want only a parent's assistance.
- After introducing yourself, briefly explain the procedure to the child.
- Place the wheelchair or stretcher parallel to the imaging table, taking care to explain that you have locked the wheelchair or stretcher and will be getting help for the transfer. These children often know the way they should be lifted—*ask them.* They can tell you which areas to support and which actions they prefer to do themselves.

Finally, children with spastic contractions are often frustrated by muscle movements that are counterproductive to the intended action. Gentle massage should be used to help relax the muscle, and a compression band should be applied to maintain the position.

Communicating with a child who has a mental disability can be difficult, depending on the severity of the disability. Some patients react to verbal stimuli. Loud or abrupt phrases can startle and consequently agitate them.

Patient Care: Psychologic Considerations

Although pediatric patients have many of the same psychologic characteristics as adults, some factors are worthy of mention to better prepare the radiographer for interactions with children and their parents.

EMERGENCY PATIENT

When an accident happens, emotions run high, thought processes are clouded, and the ability to rationalize is often lost. For the parents of the child who has been injured, another powerful factor is often involved—guilt. As parents try to absorb information about the child's condition, they also ask themselves how they could have let the accident happen. Dealing with these questions often prevents parents from hearing or understanding all that is being explained. In addition, fearing that permanent damage has been done, the child can feel extremely traumatized by a relatively minor injury. The radiographer should observe the following guidelines in dealing with emergency patients and their parents:

- Greet the patient and parents, and then describe the procedure using short, simple, and often-repeated sentences.
- Remember that when patients and parents speak with a tone of urgency and frustration, this usually stems from fear. Maintaining a calm perspective in these situations can ensure a smooth examination.
- Increase the level of confidence the parents and child have in your abilities with frequent reassurance presented in a calming tone. (The *reassurance* referred to here is reassurance that the radiographer knows how to approach the situation, not reassurance that all will be well with respect to the injury.)
- In emergency examinations, as with any other examination, ensure that only one caregiver is giving the child instructions and explanations. (Caregivers include parents, nurses, doctors, and radiographers, all of whom may be present.) Much greater success is achieved when only one person speaks to the child.
- After completing the procedure, ensure that you have the parents' attention. Speaking slowly, give clear instructions about where to wait and what to expect.

OUTPATIENT

Generally speaking, outpatients and their parents are easier to approach than inpatients. For the radiographer who has had little experience with children, these are among the best patients with whom to begin. Outpatient visits are frequently a form of progress report, and patients are usually ambulatory and relatively healthy. For the most part, parents are calm because they are not dealing with the emotions of an emergency situation or perhaps the tension or fear that the parents of inpatients can experience. However, they can become agitated if kept waiting too long, which unfortunately happens often in the outpatient clinical setting.

INPATIENT

A child must usually be very sick to be admitted to a hospital. Children often become acutely ill in a much shorter period than adults. However, they generally heal quicker than adults, which decreases the length of the hospital stay. The stresses the child experiences involve fear and separation from parents, family, and friends. It also is a stressful time for the parents who, while worrying about their child's health, must often juggle time for work and for taking care of other family members. By understanding that these responsibilities weigh heavily on parents' minds and by remembering to provide reassurance and simple explanations, the radiographer can make the child's visit to the imaging department easier.

Patient Care: Physical Considerations

GENERAL MEASURES

Depending on the level of care being provided, children may arrive in the imaging department with chest tubes, IV infusions (including central venous lines), colostomies, ileostomies, or urine collection systems. Usually these children are inpatients, but in many instances outpatients (particularly in interventional cases) arrive in the department with various tubes in situ (e.g., gastrostomy or gastrojejunostomy tube placements). The radiographer must be aware of the purpose and significance of these medical adjuncts and know the ways to care for the patient with them (see p. 170).

The competent and caring radiographer takes note of the following:

1. What are the specific instructions regarding the care and management of the child during the child's stay in the department?
2. Will a nurse accompany the child?
3. Will physical limitations influence the way the examination is performed?

Many inpatients are on a 24-hour urine and stool collection routine. Therefore medical personnel who change diapers on these patients should save the old diaper for the ward/floor personnel to weigh or assess.

Hospital policy and the availability of nursing staff within the imaging department determine the amount of involvement the radiographer has with the management of IV lines. The radiographer must be able to assess the integrity of the line and must know the measures to take in the event of problems.[1]

---

[1]Torres LS: *Basic medical techniques and patient care in imaging technology,* ed 5, Philadelphia, 1997, Lippincott-Raven.

ISOLATION PROTOCOLS AND UNIVERSAL BLOOD AND BODY FLUID PRECAUTIONS

Prevention of the spread of contagious disease is of primary importance in a health care facility for children. Microorganisms are most commonly spread from one person to another by human hands. *Careful hand washing* is the single most important precaution, but unfortunately, it is often the most neglected. In addition, all equipment that comes in contact with the radiographer and patient during isolation cases must be washed with an appropriate cleanser.

The premise of universal blood and body fluid precautions is that *all blood and body fluids* are to be considered *infected*. The Centers for Disease Control and Prevention recommend that health care workers practice blood and body fluid precautions when caring for all patients. These precautions are designed to protect both patients and medical personnel from the diseases spread by infected blood and body fluids. All blood and body fluids, including secretions and excretions, must be treated as if they contain infective microorganisms. Working under this assumption, personnel can protect themselves not only from patients in whom a known infective organism is present but also from the unknown. Fig. 28-5 outlines the protective precautions the health care workers should observe while performing particular tasks.

The management of patients in isolation varies according to the type of organism or preexisting condition, the procedure itself (some can alternatively be performed with a mobile unit), and hospital/departmental policies. Decisions regarding when to bring an infectious patient to the department also often depend on the condition of other patients who may be in the vicinity. For example, patients with *multiresistant organisms* should not be close to immunocompromised patients.

The radiographer should follow all precautions outlined by the physician and nursing unit responsible for the child. Respiratory, enteric, or wound precautions for handling a patient are usually instituted to protect staff members and other patients. Isolation procedures are instituted to protect a patient from infection. Protective isolation is used, for example, with burn victims and patients with immunologic disorders. The protective clothing worn by staff members may be the same in either situation, but the method of discarding it will be different.[1]

[1]Torres LS: *Basic medical techniques and patient care in imaging technology,* ed 5, Philadelphia, 1997, Lippincott-Raven.

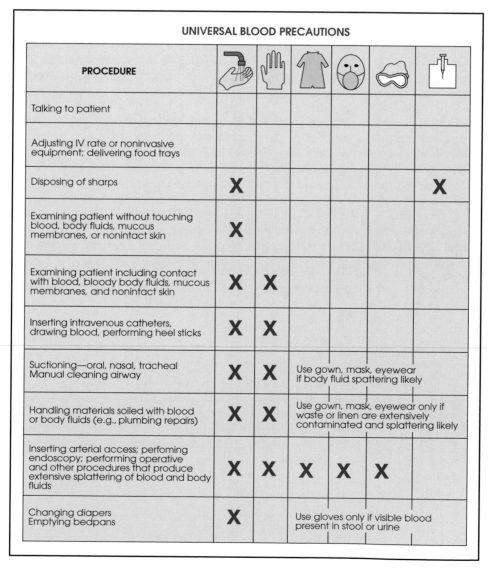

UNIVERSAL BLOOD PRECAUTIONS

PROCEDURE	🚰	🖐	👕	😷	🥽	💉
Talking to patient						
Adjusting IV rate or noninvasive equipment; delivering food trays						
Disposing of sharps	X					X
Examining patient without touching blood, body fluids, mucous membranes, or nonintact skin	X					
Examining patient including contact with blood, bloody body fluids, mucous membranes, and nonintact skin	X	X				
Inserting intravenous catheters, drawing blood, performing heel sticks	X	X				
Suctioning—oral, nasal, tracheal Manual cleaning airway	X	X	Use gown, mask, eyewear if body fluid spattering likely			
Handling materials soiled with blood or body fluids (e.g., plumbing repairs)	X	X	Use gown, mask, eyewear only if waste or linen are extensively contaminated and splattering likely			
Inserting arterial access; perfoming endoscopy; performing operative and other procedures that produce extensive splattering of blood and body fluids	X	X	X	X	X	
Changing diapers Emptying bedpans	X		Use gloves only if visible blood present in stool or urine			

Fig. 28-5 Universal blood precautions chart, designed as a quick reference guide showing the precautions that are necessary for various procedures.

(Courtesy The Hospital for Sick Children, Toronto.)

Patient Care: Special Concerns

As with most pediatric examinations, a team approach produces the best results. Cooperation among all caregivers and the child provides for a smooth examination. A few special situations that deserve individual mention are discussed in the following sections.

PREMATURE INFANT

One of the greatest dangers facing the premature and sometimes the full-term neonate is *hypothermia* (below normal body temperature). *Thermoregulation,* the balance of heat losses and gains, is crucial to the care and survival of the premature infant. The sources of heat loss—evaporation, convection, conduction, and radiation—are greater in the preterm infant. Premature babies have a greater surface area in comparison to body mass. Furthermore, they are not capable of storing the fat needed for warmth, and they have increased metabolic rates.

So that hypothermia does not occur, premature infants should be examined within the infant warmer or isolette whenever possible. Therefore general radiography must be performed with a portable or mobile unit. The radiographer should take great care to prevent the infant's skin from coming in contact with cassettes. Covering the cassette with one or two layers of a cloth diaper (or equivalent) works well; however, the material should be free of creases because these produce significant artifacts on neonatal radiographs.

When the premature infant is brought to the imaging department for gastrointestinal (GI) procedures or various types of scans, the radiographer should observe the following guidelines:

- Elevate the temperature in the room 20 to 30 minutes before the arrival of the child. The ambient temperature of the imaging room is usually cool compared with the temperature of the neonatal nursery.
- When raising the temperature is impossible, prepare the infant for the procedure while the infant is still in the isolette and remove the infant for as brief a period as possible.
- Use heating pads and radiant heaters to help maintain the infant's body temperature; however, these adjuncts are often of limited usefulness because of necessary obstructions such as the image intensifier. If heaters are used, position them at least 3 feet from the infant.
- Place large bags of IV solutions, prewarmed by soaking in a sink of warm water, beside the infant to serve as small hot water bottles.
- Monitor the infant's temperature throughout the procedure, and keep the isolette plugged in to maintain the appropriate temperature.

Because of the risk of infection to infants in the neonatal intensive care unit (NICU), most units insist on adherence to isolation protocols such as gowning and hand washing.

NOTE: *Neonatal* refers to newborn. Although premature babies comprise the highest percentage of patients in NICUs, all of the infants in these units are not necessarily premature. Full-term babies experiencing distress are also cared for in NICUs.

The radiographer must take care when positioning an infant from the NICU. Many of these infants can tolerate only minimal handling without their heart rates slowing dramatically. The conscientious radiographer is very careful when moving the infant and/or the venous or arterial lines that may be implanted in the infant.

MYELOMENINGOCELE

A *myelomeningocele* is a *congenital* defect characterized by a cystic protrusion of the meninges and the spinal cord tissue and fluid. It occurs as a result of *spina bifida,* a cleft in the neural arches of a vertebra. It can be recognized by fetal ultrasonography at the seventeenth or eighteenth week of gestation. Myelomeningoceles may cause varying degrees of paralysis and hydrocephalus. The higher the location of the myelomeningocele, the worse the neurologic symptoms.

Patients with myelomeningoceles are cared for in the prone position. Therefore, whenever possible, radiographic examinations on these patients should be performed using the prone position until the defect has been surgically repaired and the wound healed. The primary imaging modalities used in the investigation and follow-up care of myelomeningoceles include ultrasonography, computed tomography (CT), and magnetic resonance imaging (MRI).

OMPHALOCELE AND GASTROSCHISIS

An *omphalocele* is a congenital defect that resembles an enormous umbilical hernia. Omphaloceles are covered in a thin, translucent, membranous sac of peritoneum, and their contents include bowel and perhaps liver. *Gastroschisis* is a similar condition in which a portion of bowel herniates through a defect near the naval. The difference is that in gastroschisis the bowel is not included within a sac.

In both omphalocele and gastroschisis the herniated abdominal contents must be kept warm and moist. This is especially important with gastroschisis. A responsible physician or nurse should be present when patients with these conditions are examined radiographically, because they become rapidly hypothermic.

EPIGLOTTITIS

Epiglottitis is one of the most dangerous causes of acute upper airway obstruction in children and must be treated as an EMERGENCY. Its peak incidence occurs in children between the ages of 3 and 6 years. Epiglottitis is usually caused by *Haemophilus influenzae*, and the symptoms include acute respiratory obstruction, high fever, and *dysphasia* (inability to swallow or difficulty in swallowing). When epiglottitis is clinically suspected, the radiographer observes the following steps:

- **Insist** that the patient be accompanied by and transported **into** the x-ray room with the responsible physician. The patient must be supported in the upright position with an emergency physician monitoring the airway at all times.
- **Do not proceed with the necessary lateral radiograph of the nasopharynx or soft tissues of the neck without the presence of the physician.**
- Perform the single upright lateral image **without moving the patient's head or neck.**
- Take extreme care to ensure the child does not panic, cry, or become agitated.

OSTEOGENESIS IMPERFECTA

Osteogenesis imperfecta, a disease characterized by brittle bones, is often referred to by its abbreviation, OI. Because the approach and management need to be altered significantly in the imaging department to accommodate patients with OI, radiographers should be aware of this commonly used abbreviation. Children with OI are prone to spontaneous fractures or fractures that occur with minimal trauma. Although OI can vary in severity, patients with this disease need to be handled with *extreme care* by an experienced radiographer.

Children with OI are almost always accompanied by a key caregiver—usually a parent. Experience has shown that these patients are best handled with a team approach in an unhurried atmosphere. The team is comprised of the patient, parent (caregiver), and radiographer, with the radiographer observing the following guidelines:

- Constantly reassure the parent and patient that every part of the procedure will be explained before it is attempted.
- For the best results, explain the desired position to the parent in simple terms. For example, "the knee needs to point to the side" for a lateral image. Then allow the parent to do the positioning.
- Ask the older child for advice on the way the child should be moved or lifted.
- If possible, take the radiographs with the child in the bed or on the stretcher. This is often possible, given the patient's small physical stature.

Practical tip: It is wise to evaluate the technical factors by checking the first radiograph before proceeding with the rest of the series. (Generally speaking, the technical factors can be halved.) The radiographer should remember that an introduction and a few moments of explanation and reassurance that the radiograph will be done using a team approach can ensure a smooth examination in most OI patients.

SUSPECTED CHILD ABUSE

Although no *universal* agreement exists on the definition of child abuse, the radiographer should have an appreciation of the all-encompassing nature of this problem. *Child abuse* has been defined as "the involvement of physical injury, sexual abuse or deprivation of nutrition, care or affection in circumstances which indicate that injury or deprivation may not be accidental or may have occurred through neglect."[1] Although diagnostic imaging staff members are usually involved only in cases in which physical abuse is a possibility, they should realize that sexual abuse and nutritional neglect are also prevalent.

[1]Robinson MJ: *Practical pediatrics*, ed 2, New York, 1990, Churchill Livingstone.

Legal statutes in all provinces and states in North America require health care professionals to *report suspected cases* of abuse or neglect. The radiographer, while preparing or positioning the patient, may be the first person to suspect abuse or neglect. The first course of action for the radiographer should be to consult a radiologist (when available) or the attending or responsible physician. After this consultation the radiographer may no longer have cause for suspicion, because some naturally occurring skin markings mimic bruising. *If the radiographer's doubts persist, the suspicions must be reported to the proper authority, regardless of the physician's opinion.* Recognizing the complexity of child abuse issues, many hospitals have developed a multidisciplinary team of health care workers to respond to these issues. Radiographers working in hospitals have access to this team of physicians, social workers, and psychologists for the purposes of reporting their concerns; others are advised to work through their local Children's Aid Society or appropriate organization.

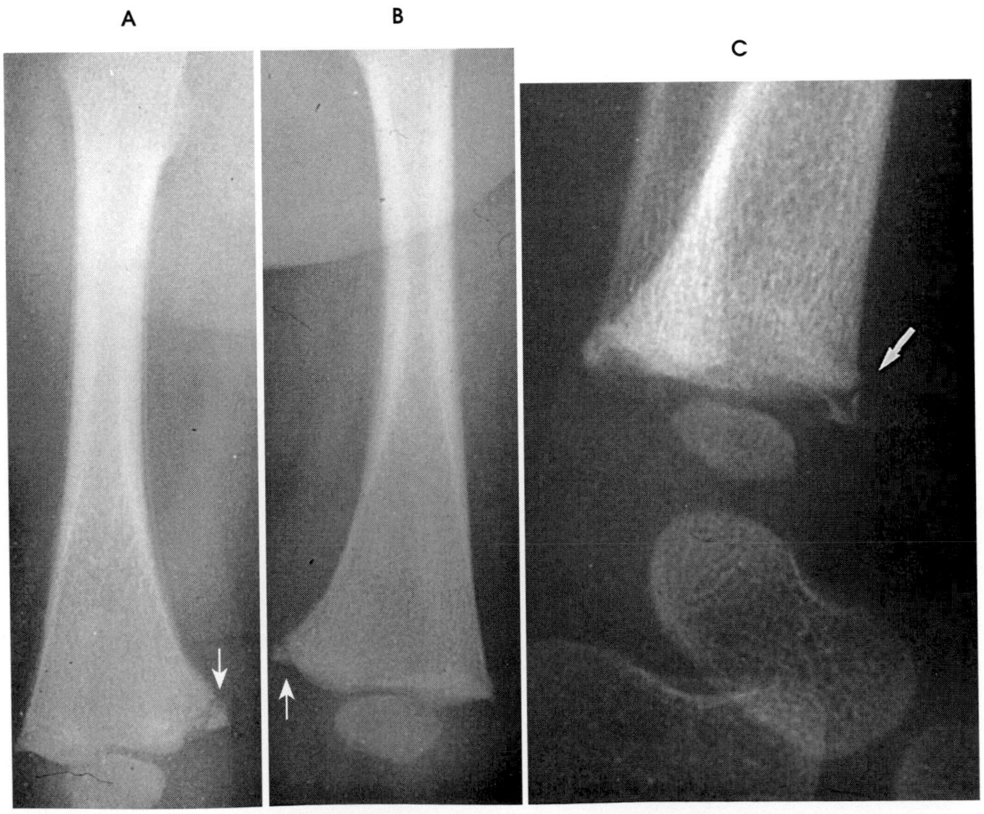

All imaging modalities can and do play a role in the investigation of suspected child abuse. Plain image radiography, often the initial imaging tool, can reveal characteristic radiologic patterns of skeletal injury. Corner fractures and "bucket-handle" fractures (or lesions) are considered *classic indicators* of physical abuse (Fig. 28-6). The presence of numerous fracture sites at varied or multiple stages of healing can also indicate long-term or ongoing abuse. These cases are often viewed by nonradiologic staff members (e.g., lawyers) as well as imaging professionals. Therefore evidence of injury must be readily apparent.

The radiographer's role is to provide physicians with diagnostic radiographs that *demonstrate bone and soft tissue equally well.* Referring physicians depend on the expertise of the diagnostic imaging service for the detection of physical abuse, and radiologists are able to estimate the date of the injury based on the degree of callous formation or the amount of healing.

The radiographer observes the following guidelines when dealing with a case of possible child abuse:

- Give careful attention to exposure factors and the recorded detail demonstrated for limb radiography. Imaging systems yielding high detail are recommended for cases of suspected child abuse because the associated skeletal injuries are often very subtle (see Fig. 28-6).
- Perform *skeletal surveys* with *multiple images of individual areas* using appropriate centering points, collimation, and technical factors. Performing a *babygram*—a 35 × 43 cm (14 × 17 inch) cassette of the entire baby—should *be avoided* because the resultant images are of reduced diagnostic quality. Distortion (because of improper centering), scatter, and underexposure and overexposure of various parts all play a part in the degradation of the image. Babygrams are no longer considered an acceptable imaging protocol for the investigation of child abuse.
- Although it may be difficult to do, give the parents of these children the same courtesy as any other parent. Remember that the parent who is present may not be responsible for the injuries. Deal with the parent in a nonjudgmental manner aimed at not jeopardizing further relations between the parent and health care providers.

Fig. 28-6 Radiographs demonstrating physical abuse. Left and right corner fractures (*arrows,* **A** and **B**) and bucket-handle fractures or lesions (*arrow,* **C**) are considered classic indicators of physical abuse in children. The bucket handle appearance is subtle and demonstrated only if the "ring" is seen on profile (*arrow*).

Protection of the Child

PROTECTION FROM INJURY

The diagnostic imaging department is responsible for ensuring that children neither injure themselves nor are injured during their stay in the department. Emphasis on quality assurance and risk management dictates that many hospitals (and, consequently, radiology departments) perform routine safety inspections to take a proactive stance in minimizing the potential for harm. These inspections are often performed by a two-person team that includes: (1) the supervising or charge radiographer and (2) a frontline worker, whose input is vital because the worker uses the equipment on a daily basis. The following guidelines are observed:

- To *avoid the possibility of injury,* supervise children while they are in the department or being transported to and from the department. Some departments clearly delineate, in their policy and procedure manuals, safety precautions to be carried out while patients are in the imaging room. Such policies relate to the use of Velcro or compression bands designed to prevent patients from rolling from the imaging table (see Figs. 28-7 and 28-13).
- Regularly inspect all immobilization tools to ensure that they are maintained in working order. Experienced radiographers should instruct all novice pediatric radiographers in proper immobilization techniques, and novice radiographers' practices should be observed by senior or supervising radiographers.
- In the event of an injury, however minor, file a report documenting the specifics of the incident and the actions taken. Some departments require that reports be filed even in the event that there was *potential* for an injury to occur.

PROTECTION FROM UNNECESSARY RADIATION

The conscientious radiographer can do much to protect children from exposure to unnecessary radiation. Radiographers should remember that bone marrow, active in the formation of blood cells, is distributed throughout the pediatric skeleton and that tissue damage is associated with ionizing radiation. Radiographers should observe the following steps:

- Direct efforts toward *proper centering and selection of exposure factors, precise collimation,* and *appropriate use of filters* (where required), which all contribute to safe practice.
- Use *strategic placement of gonadal and breast shielding* and employ *effective immobilization techniques* to reduce the need for repeat examinations.
- Instead of the AP projection, use the PA projection of the thorax and skull to reduce the amount of radiation reaching the breast tissue and lens of the eye respectively.
- During radiography of the upper limbs *protect the upper torso of all children.*
- Employ diagonal placement of small gonadal aprons along the thorax and abdomen to protect the sternum and gonads of infants and toddlers during supine radiography.
- Have older children wear child-size full lead aprons or adult aprons. (See Common Pediatric Examinations, Limb Radiography.)

Radiographers in supervisory and management positions have added responsibilities. In addition to ensuring that the previously described practices are followed, supervising radiographers should take into account the clinical needs of the radiologist and follow the ALARA (as low as reasonably achievable) principle of radiation exposure when developing technique charts or programming exposure consoles. Pediatric imaging poses conflicting demands on imaging protocols. High kilovolt (peak) (kVp) is desired to keep the milliamperes-seconds (mAs) low (thereby reducing the absorbed dose), but low mA values can present *quantum mottle* problems in the radiographic examination of small body parts, specifically pediatric limbs and neonatal chests. For acceptable diagnostic quality, relatively high resolution is needed. Practically speaking, these needs are often met by the development of a multispeed film-screen combination or *computed radiography* (CR) system. Slow-speed systems are used to demonstrate small parts (limbs and neonatal chests), and faster speeds are used for procedures involving the spine, abdomen, and GI tract. The least confusing approach is to purchase one type of film and *screens of varying speeds,* when a film-screen system is used. The cassettes are then color coded along their outer edges, and the user can be directed to a corresponding color-coded chart to select the appropriate combination.

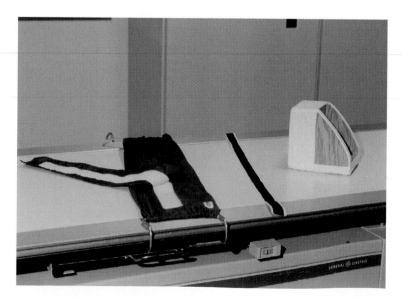

Fig. 28-7 Three tools frequently used in pediatric immobilization: *(left to right)* a Velcro band, often called a *Bucky* or *body band;* a strip of reusable Velcro; and a "bookend."

Used judiciously by experienced and knowledgeable personnel, CR can reduce the radiation dose from 33% to 50% (see Chapter 34). This technique significantly shortens the time needed to perform the procedure and optimizes or tailors the images to suit individual patient requirements. As a result of increased familiarity with the power of window level and width adjustments in CT and MRI, radiologists have developed a deeper appreciation and acceptance of the digital format. Automatic, laser-printed spot images in GI barium studies are a common general application of *image intensifier–based digital radiography.* Pulsed fluoroscopy with "last image hold" also reduces patient dose and length of examination. Furthermore, the ability to transmit the digital image directly to a laser printer to produce hard copies saves valuable radiographer time. This often allows the radiographer to spend more time with the patient or to assist the next child sooner.

A cautionary note: The fact that digitally acquired images can be "post-processed," thereby correcting some exposure errors, does not negate an important truth—*images of proper density are achieved by proper positioning.* The anatomy to be demonstrated must be in proper alignment with the photocell or ionization chamber.

Immobilization: Principles and Tools

Perhaps the two most successful tools for pediatric radiography are *effective immobilization* and *good communication skills.* Respected pediatric radiographers approach patients and parents with kindness and take care to maintain patient comfort throughout the procedure.

Naturally, a willingness to cooperate on the child's part allows for more *passive,* less aggressive immobilization techniques. *Reassurance, praise,* and conversational *distraction* are the three ingredients of successful communication. Reassurance is perhaps second only to sleep as the best passive immobilization technique. A sleeping child who is moved gently, kept comfortable and warm, and not startled by sudden or loud noises often remains asleep throughout the procedure. However, as previously noted, all chest images must be taken while the child is awake, because the rate of respiration is too shallow during sleep to provide full inspiration images.

Despite effective communication, it is often necessary to restrain children during radiography. If immobilization is not handled appropriately, difficulties can arise for the radiographer, patient, and parent. Immobilization should never become a traumatic, torturous event for the child, and no immobilization technique should cause harm to the child. Experienced radiographers should teach novice pediatric radiographers how to *carefully* restrain a child. A radiographer's lack of experience, coupled with the parent's and child's fear, can often lead to frustration on *everyone's* part. With practice, the radiographer can keep patients both comfortable and immobilized with a minimum of frustration.

The radiographer can prevent a great deal of frustration by using the communication strategies described at the beginning of this chapter and applying some *practiced* immobilization techniques. It is important to remember that the parent (presuming one is present) can do only one job. For example, a parent who assists with the radiographic examination of her 2-year-old's forearm can help only by holding the humerus and the hand; the radiographer or some other staff member has the tasks of immobilizing the other arm and both legs.

Aside from the regular sponges and sandbags, three tools frequently used in pediatric immobilization deserve mention. They are the Velcro compression band (sometimes referred to as a Bucky or body band), a strip of reusable Velcro, and a "bookend" (see Fig. 28-7). These devices are effective for the immobilization of children, although their applications are not limited to pediatric radiography.

Other tools, such as the Pigg-o-stat (Modern Way Immobilizers, Clifton, Tenn.) and the octagonal infant immobilization cradle, are described in the following sections.

Common Pediatric Examinations

CHEST RADIOGRAPHY

The most common radiographic procedure performed in hospitals and clinics is of the chest. Radiologists agree that for most diagnostic chest radiographs in pediatric patients, upright images yield a great deal more information than supine radiographs. It is, however, important to know the way to achieve diagnostic quality in both positions. Regardless of body position, accurate diagnosis depends on high-quality images made with short exposure times to reduce motion. *Expiratory images can lead to erroneous radiologic interpretations.* Therefore images acquired *on maximal inspiration* are crucially important for accurate diagnosis. Well-positioned, nonrotated radiographs are also essential for proper diagnosis because even minor degrees of rotation can significantly distort the normal anatomy.

Upright radiograph on the newborn to 3-year-old

The many challenges of obtaining upright images include preventing motion and rotation, freeing the lung fields of superimposition of humeri and scapulae, and obtaining a good inspiratory radiograph. Various methods of immobilization are used to achieve these images, often with somewhat mixed results. Fortunately these challenges are easily met with the use of a pediatric positioner and immobilization tool called the *Pigg-o-stat* (Fig. 28-8). Although the Pigg-o-stat is primarily used for chest radiography, other applications include upright abdominal images and radiography of the thoracic and lumbar spine.

The Pigg-o-stat is composed of a large support base on wheels, a small adjustable seat, and Plexiglas supports called *sleeves*. These sleeves come in two sizes. The seat, sleeves, and "turntable" base rotate as a unit to facilitate quick positioning from PA to lateral projections. Although some physicians do not favor use of the Pigg-o-stat (for aesthetic reasons and because of the possibility of sleeve artifacts), the device has been shown to be one of the safest and most versatile restraining methods available for chest and upright abdominal radiography.

Communication with parents

The Pigg-o-stat requires explanation for parents unfamiliar with its use. The radiographer should offer an explanation similar to this: "Doctors prefer chest x-rays to be performed with the child in the upright position. To help your child remain still, we have the child sit on this little seat. These plastic supports fit snugly around the child's sides and keep the arms raised. The device looks funny, and your child will probably cry, but this is usually an expression of frustration about being confined. The crying actually helps to obtain a good x-ray image because at the end of a cry your child will take a big gasp of air. At that moment the exposure will be taken."

A complete explanation is worthwhile and essential. The parent can be shown how to help place the child on the seat by guiding the feet in. Then the parent can assist by holding the arms above the child's head.

Radiographers should realize that positioning a child in a Pigg-o-stat is a *two-person job.* Radiographers can safely take children out of the Pigg-o-stat without assistance, but an extra pair of hands is needed in the initial positioning. The properly instructed parent is generally willing and able to assist.

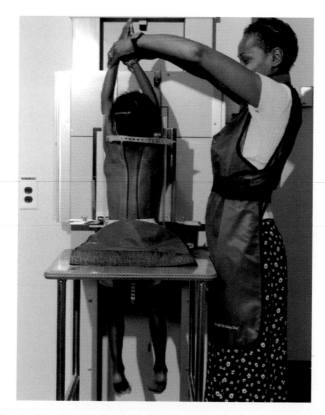

Fig. 28-8 Position for PA chest radiograph. The Pigg-o-stat (Modern Way Immobilizers, Clifton, Tenn.) is a pediatric positioner and immobilization tool. The cassette is held in the metal extension stand.

Method

The following steps are observed:

- Have the patients be undressed completely from the waist up, so that after the patient is positioned, the ribs are visible on inspiration.
- Choose the appropriate sleeve size. Sleeves should fit snugly, which often requires Velcro strips or adhesive tape wrapped around the base of the sleeves (Fig. 28-8).
- Adjust the seat height to approximately the correct level. The seat is at the correct height if, when the patient is sitting up straight, the face fits in the contours or cutout portions of the sleeves.

This one-step positioning, in which the child is sitting straight on the seat with the arms raised evenly above the head, ensures motionless and nonrotated images (Fig. 28-9). The orientation of the room (i.e., where the chest stand or cassette holder is located relative to the control panel) and the image requested determine how well the radiographer can see the child's thorax to ensure that the exposure is made during inspiration. The radiographer can detect inspiration by doing the following (listed in decreasing order of reliability):

1. Waiting for the end of a cry—the child will take a big gasp of air
2. Watching the abdomen—the child's abdomen will extend on inspiration
3. Watching the chest wall—the ribs will be outlined on inspiration
4. Watching the rise and fall of the sternum

Centering and collimation

The central ray for both PA and lateral projections is directed to the level of T6-T7, but the collimated field should extend from and include the mastoid tips to just above the iliac crests. Inclusion of the mastoid tips demonstrates the upper airway; narrowed or stenotic airways are a common source of respiratory problems in pediatric patients. By collimating just above the crests of the ilia, the radiographer can include the inferior costal margins. A significant number of children arrive in the imaging department with long lung fields resulting from hyperinflation. Noted examples include patients with cardiac disorders and asthma.

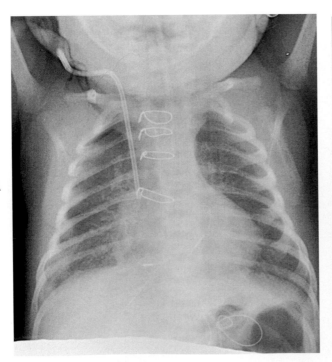 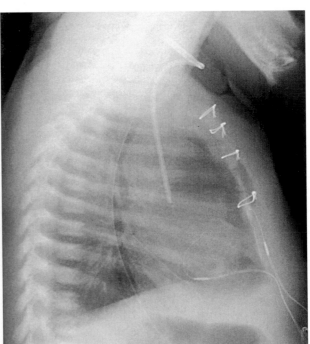

Fig. 28-9 PA **(A)** and lateral **(B)** chest images of a 10-day-old patient with a pathologic cardiac condition. The Pigg-o-stat provides motionless, nonrotated radiographs of good inspiration. Note the presence of sternal wires, cardiac pacing wires, and a central venous line. The nasogastric tube is seen well on the lateral image.

Upright radiograph on the 3- to 10-year-old

Upright radiographs on 3- to 10-years olds are easily obtained by observing the following steps:

- Help the child sit on a large wooden box, a wide-based trolley with brakes, or a stool, with the cassette supported using a metal extension stand. Children of this age are very curious and have short attention spans. By having them sit, the radiographer can prevent them from wiggling from the waist down.
- For the PA radiograph, have the child hold on to the side supports of the extension stand, with the chin on top of or next to the cassette. This prevents upper body movement.
- When positioning for the lateral radiograph, have the parent (if presence is permitted) assist by raising the child's arms above the head and holding the head between the arms (Fig. 28-10). PA and lateral chest images of a 6-year-old patient are shown in Fig. 28-11.

A

B

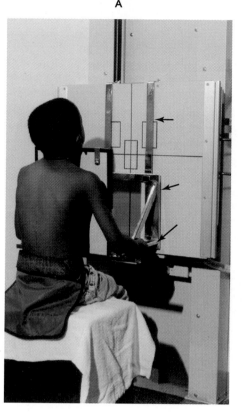
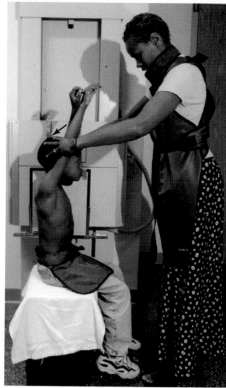

Fig. 28-10 A, PA chest radiographs should be performed on the 3- to 10-year-old with the child sitting. **B,** The parent, if present, can assist with immobilization for the lateral image by holding the child's head between the child's arms. Metal extension stands *(arrows on **A** and **B**)* are commercially available from companies that market diagnostic imaging accessories.

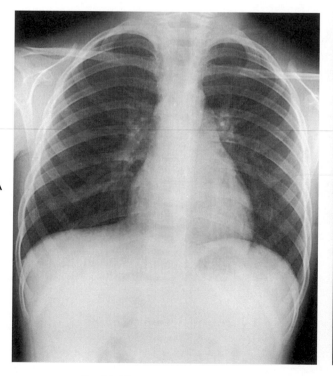
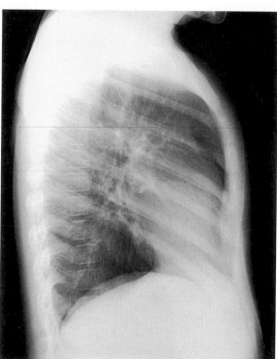

A

B

Fig. 28-11 PA **(A)** and lateral **(B)** radiographs of a seated 6-year-old boy. Large wooden boxes have the advantage of being sturdier than stools or trolleys, which often have wheels.

Supine radiograph (infant immobilizer method)

Infants needing supine and cross-table lateral radiographs can be immobilized with the immobilization device shown in Fig. 28-12. This tool is particularly useful for patients with chest tubes, delicately positioned gastrostomy tubes, or soft tissue swellings or protrusions that may be compromised by the sleeves of the Pigg-o-stat. Similar to the Pigg-o-stat, the infant immobilizer is a one-step positioning and immobilization tool.

Evaluating the image

As in adult chest radiography, the use of kVp is also desirable in pediatric chest work; however, this is relative. In adult work, high kVp generally ranges between 110 and 130 but for pediatric PA projections ranges between 80 and 90. Practically speaking, the use of a higher kVp is impossible because the corresponding mAs are too low to produce a diagnostic image. Relatively high kVp helps to provide images with long-scale contrast.

The criteria used to evaluate recorded detail include the resolution of peripheral lung markings. Evaluating any image for adequate density involves assessing the most and least dense areas of the demonstrated anatomy. In the PA chest image, the ideal technical factor is a selection that permits visualization of the intervertebral disk spaces through the heart (the most dense area) while still demonstrating the peripheral lung markings (the least dense area). Rotation should be assessed by evaluating the position of midline structures. Posterior and anterior midline structures (i.e., sternum, airway, and vertebral bodies) should be superimposed. The anatomic structures to be demonstrated include the airway (trachea) to the costophrenic angles. Similar to chest radiography in adults, the visualization of 9 to 10 posterior ribs is a reliable indicator of a radiograph taken with good inspiration (see Table 28-1).

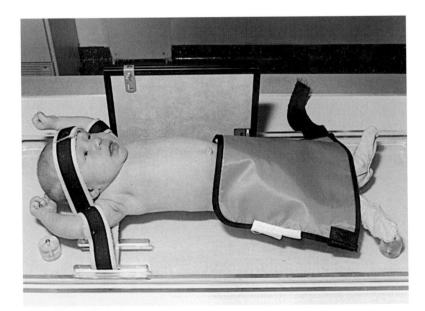

Fig. 28-12 Supine infant immobilizer, a one-step immobilization device useful when upright positioning is contraindicated. This 6-week-old baby is positioned with the arms, head, and legs immobilized with foam-lined Velcro strips. The cassette is in place for the horizontal beam lateral (cross-table lateral).

TABLE 28-1

Quick reference guide for radiograph assessment*

	Density		Recorded detail	Contrast		Anatomy	Rotation check
	Most dense	Least dense		Long scale >3 shades	Short scale <3 shades		
PA Chest	Midline; intervertebral disk spaces, heart	Peripheral lung markings	Peripheral lung markings	Airway, heart, apices, bases, mediastinum, lung markings behind diaphragm and heart		Airway to bases	Airway position, S-C joints, lung field measurement, cardiac silhouette
PA Chest	Heart	Retrocardiac space	Peripheral lung markings	Airway, heart, apices, bases		Airway to bases, spinous processes to sternum	Superimposition of ribs, spinous processes on profile
Abdomen	Lumbar spine	Peripheral edges, soft tissue above crests of the ilia	Organ silhouettes	Diaphragm, liver, kidney, spine, gas shadows		Right and left hemidiaphragm, pubic symphysis, right and left skin edges	
Limbs	Bone	Soft tissue	Bony trabecular patterns		Bone, muscle, soft tissue	Joints above and below injury, all soft tissue	AP and lateral images must not resemble obliques
Hips	Hip joints	Iliac crests	Bony trabecular pattern		Bone, soft tissue	Iliac crests, lesser trochanter	Symmetric iliac crests
Lateral Lumbar Spine	L5-S1	Spinous processes	Bony trabecular pattern		Bone	T12 to coccyx, spinous processes to vertebral bodies	Alignment of posterior surfaces of vertebral bodies

*Evaluating the radiograph to determine its diagnostic quality is a practiced skill. This chart, designed as a quick reference guide, outlines the five important technical criteria and the related anatomic indicators used in critiquing radiographs.

Common pediatric examinations

HIP RADIOGRAPHY

The hip and pelvis are commonly examined radiographically in both the pediatric and adult population. However, the clinical rationale for ordering these examinations varies tremendously. The informed radiographer who understand these differences can be of great assistance. With a basic comprehension of some of the common pediatric pathologies and disease processes, the radiographer is better able to appreciate the skills required of the radiologist to make an accurate diagnosis.

General principles

Both hips are examined, using the same projection for comparison. Hip examinations on children are most often ordered to assess for Legg-Calvé-Perthes disease and congenital dislocation of the hip and to diagnose nonspecific hip pain. Because these conditions require evaluation of the symmetry of the acetabula, joint spaces, and soft tissue, symmetric positioning is crucial.

Despite the importance of radiation protection, little written literature is available to guide radiographers on the placement of gonadal shields and when to use shielding. The radiographer should observe the following guidelines:

- *Always* use gonadal shielding on males. However, take care to prevent potential lesions of the pubic symphysis from being obscured.
- In females, use gonadal protection on all radiographs *except* the first AP projection of the *initial* examination of the hips and pelvis.
- After sacral abnormality or sacral involvement has been ruled out, use shielding on subsequent images in females.
- Before proceeding, check the girl's records or seek clarification from the parents regarding whether this is the child's first examination.
- Because the female reproductive organs are located in the mid-pelvis with their exact position varying, ensure that the shield covers the sacrum and part or all of the sacroiliac joints.

NOTE: Many children have been taught that no one should touch their "private parts." Radiographers need to be sensitive and use discretion when explaining and carrying out the procedure.

- *Never touch the pubic symphysis in a child,* regardless of whether you are positioning the patient or placing the gonadal shield.
- Remember that the superior border of the pubic symphysis is *always* at the level of the greater trochanters, and use the trochanters as a guide for both positioning and shield placement.
- In males, keep the gonadal shield from touching the scrotum by laying a 15-degree sponge or a cloth over the top of the femora. The top of the shield can be placed level with the trochanters and the bottom half of the shield can rest on top of the sponge or cloth (Fig. 28-13).
- In females, place the top, widest part of the shield in the midline, level with the anterior superior iliac spine (ASIS).

Initial images

The preliminary examination of the hips and pelvis on children includes a well-collimated AP projection and a projection in what is commonly referred to as the "frog leg" position. This position is more correctly described as a coronal image of the pelvis with the thighs in abduction and external rotation, or the frog (Lauenstein) lateral projection (see Chapter 7).

Preparation and communication

All images of the abdomen and pelvic girdle should be performed with the diaper completely removed. This is *essential* for radiography of the hips and pelvis. Diapers, especially wet diapers, produce significant artifacts on radiographs, often rendering them undiagnostic. The radiographer or imaging department staff member should place all necessary sponges, gonadal shielding, Velcro strips, and Velcro restraining bands on the table before beginning the examination.

Children are usually familiar with Kermit the Frog. Explaining that the child will pretend to be Kermit serves nicely.

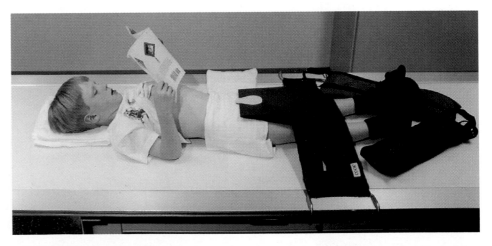

Fig. 28-13 The male gonad shield should cover the scrotum without obscuring the pubic symphysis. The greater trochanters indicate the upper border of the pubic symphysis; the top of the shield should be placed approximately $1/2$ inch below this level. The gonadal shield rests on a 15-degree sponge, which prevents the radiographer's hands from coming close to or touching the scrotal area.

Positioning and immobilization

As described previously, *symmetric positioning* is of great importance. However, as in many examinations, the hip positions that are the most uncomfortable for the patient are often the most crucial. When a child suffers from hip pain or dislocation, symmetric positioning is difficult to achieve because the patient often tries to compensate for the discomfort by rotating the pelvis. The radiographer should observe the following steps when positioning the patient:

- As with hip examinations on any patient, check that the ASISs are equidistant from the table.
- After carefully observing and communicating with the patient to discover the location of pain, the radiographer can use sponges to compensate for rotation. Sponges should routinely be used to support the thighs in the frog leg position. This can help prevent motion artifacts.
- Do not accept poorly positioned images. Expend considerable effort in attempting to achieve optimal positioning. This effort may include giving instructions, or repeating instructions to the novice pediatric radiographer.

Because *immobilization techniques* should vary according to the aggressiveness of the patient, the radiographer can follow these additional guidelines:

- Make every effort to use explanation and reassurance as part of the immobilization method. The child may require only a Velcro band placed across the legs as a safety precaution (Fig. 28-13).
- For the active (or potentially active) child, wrap a Velcro strip around the knees and place large sandbags over the arms (Fig. 28-14). The Velcro strip around the knees keep the child from wiggling one leg out from under the Velcro band. After getting one leg out, the child may get the other out and possibly roll off the table.
- If the child has enough strength to free the arms from the sandbags, ask a parent to stand on the opposite side of the table from the radiographer and hold the child's humeri. The parent's thumbs should be placed directly over the child's shoulders (Fig. 28-15). This method of immobilization is used extensively. It works well for supine abdominal images, intravenous urograms (IVUs), intravenous pyelograms (IVPs), overhead GI procedures, and spinal radiography.

Evaluating the images

Rotation or symmetry can be evaluated by ensuring that midline structures are, in fact, in the midline and that the ilia appear symmetric. Depending on the degree of skeletal maturation, visualization of the trochanters can indicate the position of the legs when the radiograph was taken. Symmetry in the skin folds is also an important evaluation criterion for the diagnostician. The anatomy to be demonstrated includes the crests of the ilia to the upper quarter of the femora. The density should be such that the bony trabecular pattern is visible in the hip joints, the thickest and most dense area within the region. The visualization of the bony trabecular pattern is used as an indicator that sufficient recorded detail has been demonstrated. This, of course, should not be at the expense of demonstrating the soft tissues—the muscles and skin folds (see Table 28-1).

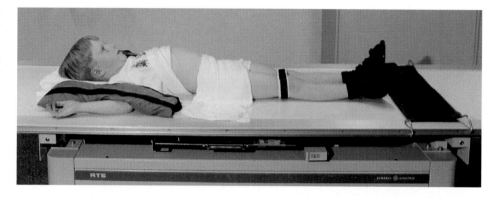

Fig. 28-14 Immobilization of the active child: sandbags over the arms, Velcro strips around the knees, and a Velcro band beside the patient's feet to be secured over the legs, as in Fig. 28-15.

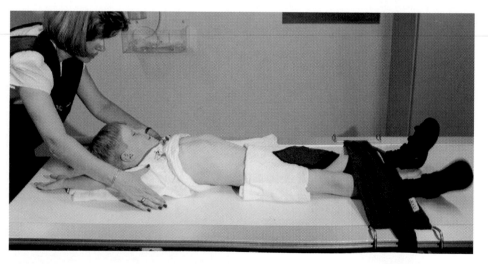

Fig. 28-15 If the child is strong enough or aggressive enough to remove the sandbags, the parent can hold the child's humeri by placing the thumbs directly over the child's shoulders.

SKULL RADIOGRAPHY

Along with radiography of the limbs, skull radiography presents some of the greatest challenges to the radiographer. Indeed, cranial radiography is usually one of the last areas students become comfortable with during their clinical education.

The reasons are twofold: (1) anatomically speaking, the skull is complex, and (2) the frequency of skull examinations has steadily decreased with the increased availability of CT and MRI. Pediatric patients such as the 3-year-old in Fig. 28-16 are an even greater challenge.

The problems associated with cranial radiography in children can be lessened by *preparing the room* before the patient and parent enter (Fig. 28-17) and avoiding *two common pitfalls:* (1) ineffective immobilization and (2) forgetting (or not taking the time) to check the first radiograph of a skull series. The first image should be treated as a *scout radiograph,* an image that permits assessment of the exposure factors and allows the radiographer to tailor the remaining images to suit the peculiarities of the individual patient. The clinical rationale for performing skull radiography differs tremendously between pediatric and adult patients. Children who arrive in the imaging department for skull examinations may have congenital abnormalities that significantly alter the bone density. Their age and consequent degree of skeletal maturation also affect bone density. These factors need to be considered as the technical factors are selected. Therefore the viewing of the initial image is very important.

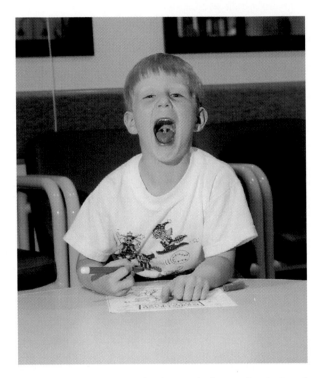

Fig. 28-16 This little boy's face indicates a challenge for skull radiography.

Immobilization

All patients 3 years old and younger should be immobilized using the "bunny" technique illustrated in Fig. 28-18. (An exception to this rule is the sleeping child.) A well-wrapped child remains that way through five to seven images. Mastering this technique is clearly one of the secrets to successful immobilization. A few words of explanation to the parent regarding the need to wrap the child, along with some instructions for ways the parent can help, are also very beneficial. Experience has shown that although children initially do not like being wrapped up using this technique, after their initial frustration and perhaps the use of a pacifier, they often settle down and occasionally fall asleep. If beneficial, the pacifier can be left in the patient's mouth for every image with the exception of the reverse PA projection. The parent must be cautioned not to unwrap the child until all radiographs have been checked for diagnostic quality.

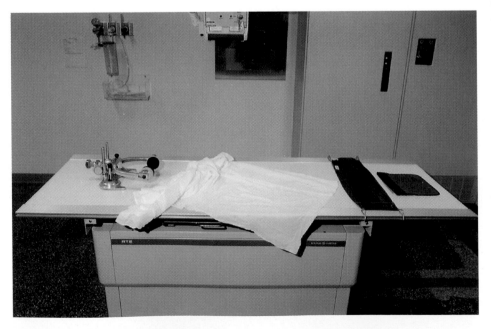

Fig. 28-17 The well-prepared radiographer can make a potentially difficult skull examination go smoothly. Note the gonadal shield, Velcro band, and head clamps in place. A standard hospital sheet has been unfolded and placed on the table to prepare for immobilization using the "bunny" technique.

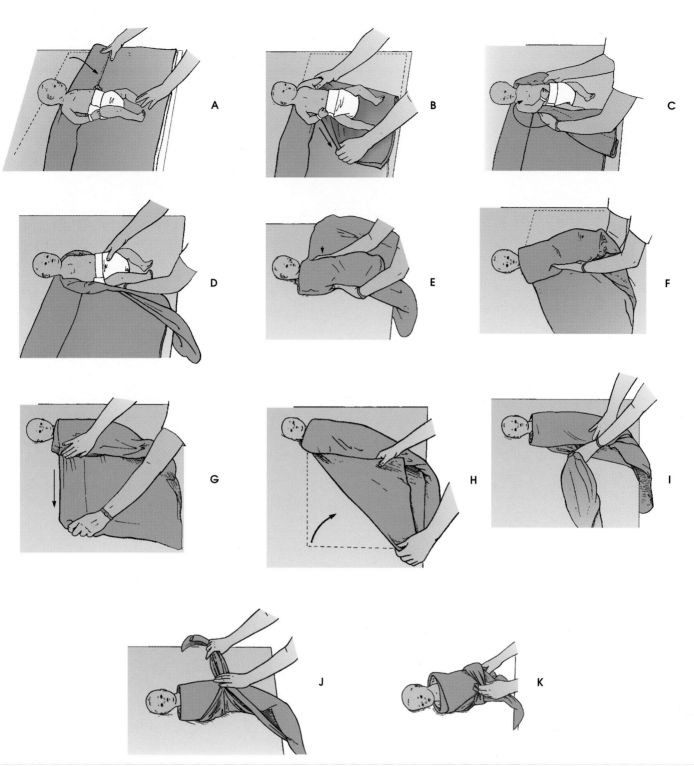

Fig. 28-18 The "bunny" method used to immobilize the patient for cranial radiography. **A** to **D** focus on immobilization of the shoulders, **E** to **G** concentrate on the humeri, and **H** to **K** illustrate the way the sheet is folded and wrapped to immobilize the legs. **A**, Begin with a standard hospital sheet folded in half lengthwise. Make a 6-inch fold at the top, and lay the child down about 2 feet from the end of the sheet. **B**, Wrap the end of the sheet over the left shoulder, and pass the sheet under the child. **C**, This step makes use of the 6-inch fold. Reach under, undo the fold, and wrap it over the right shoulder. (Steps **B** and **C** are crucial to the success of this immobilization technique because they prevent the child from wiggling the shoulders free.) **D**, After wrapping the right shoulder, pass the end of the sheet under the child. Pull it through to keep right arm snug against the body. **E**, Begin wrapping, keeping the sheet snug over the upper body to immobilize the humeri. **F**, Lift the lower body and pass the sheet underneath, keeping the child's head on the table. Repeat steps **E** and **F** if material permits. **G**, Make sure the material is evenly wrapped around the upper body. (Extra rolls around the shoulder and neck area produce artifacts on 30-degree fronto-occipital and submentovertical radiographs.) **H**, Make a diagonal fold with the remaining material (approximately 2 feet). **I**, Roll the material together. **J**, Snugly wrap this over the child's femora. (The tendency to misjudge the location of femora and thus wrap too snugly around the lower legs should be avoided.) **K**, Tuck the end of the rolled material in front. (If not enough material remains to tuck in, use a Velcro strip or tape to secure it.) (From The Michener Institute for Applied Health Sciences, Toronto.)

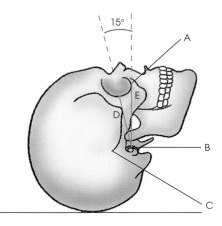

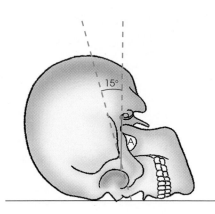

Fig. 28-19 Established tube angles and positions modified to suit the pediatric patient: *A,* Infraorbital margin; *B,* EAM; *C,* petrous ridge; *D,* OML; *E,* IOML. Note that in the young child the OML and IOML are 15 degrees apart (in contrast to older children and adults, where the difference can be 15 to 20 degrees). For simplicity, these diagrams adopt a convention of 15 degrees.

(Courtesy K. Edgell, Cook Inc., Toronto.)

Fig. 28-20 PA projection with OML perpendicular to the table. In the older child, teenager, and adult, a 15- to 20-degree caudal angulation results in the petrous ridges being projected in the lower third of the orbits. In infants and young children, a 10- to 15-degree caudal angulation achieves the same result.

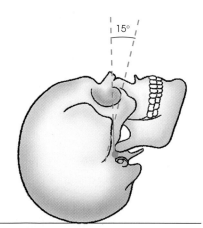

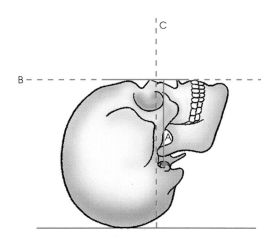

Fig. 28-21 AP projection with the OMBL perpendicular to the table. This projection requires a 15-degree cephalad angulation to project the petrous ridges in the lower third of the orbits.

Fig. 28-22 The IOML (*A*) is positioned perpendicular to the table with the patient in a *comfortable* position—one the head and neck naturally assume as the patient lies down. (A comfortable patient is more likely to remain still.) With the patient positioned this way, the tube does not have to be angled cephalad to project the petrous ridges in the lower third of the orbits (represented by dotted line *C*). With the necessary head clamps positioned, the IOML remains perpendicular to the film. With the IOML perpendicular to the cassette, the forehead and chin are parallel to the cassette (dotted line *B*).

Positioning

The skull grows rapidly in the first $2^1/_2$ years of life, approaching the 75th percentile of adult size by that age. The radiographer must understand the way this growth and the rate at which the cranium grows relative to the facial bones alter the position of the various radiographic landmarks and angles.

Practical tip: The established cranial angulations (see Chapter 20) can be adapted to suit young children by decreasing the angulation of the central ray by 5 degrees. The line diagrams in Figs. 28-19 to 28-22 put this in perspective. The PA projection is used as the basis for these diagrams because this image projects the petrous ridges in the lower one third of the orbits, which is a common baseline radiograph for many departments.

Head clamps should be used on all children, even sleeping children. Although motion may not be a factor, the sleeping child's head needs some support to maintain the required positions. (The lateral image may be an exception if the child has fallen asleep on the back with the head turned to the side.) Many radiographers believe that the use of head clamps further agitates some children.

As with any form of immobilization, acceptance of the method depends greatly on the way it is introduced to the patient and parent. If the room is prepared before the patient enters, the head clamps should already be in position. Attention need not be drawn to the head clamps until they are about to be used, and they can then be referred to as "earmuffs" (Fig. 28-23). This avoids the unnecessary anxiety that may otherwise be experienced. The degree to which the clamps are tightened depends on the situation. Some children need them only as a reminder to keep still, whereas others need to have them adjusted more tightly. Although various kinds of head clamps are available, clamps with a suction cup base are particularly effective and versatile. (The problem some users experience with the suction cups not sticking to the table is often eliminated by lightly wetting the rubber cups.)

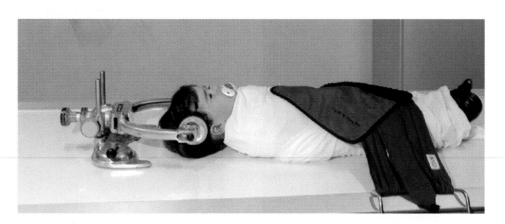

Fig. 28-23 AP projection with head clamps in place.

TABLE 28-2

Protocols for neurologic and trauma/injury radiographic routines*

Neurologic routine	Trauma/injury routine
PA or reverse PA projection (Fig. 28-23)	PA or reverse PA projection (Fig. 28-23)
30-degree frontooccipital projection	30-degree frontooccipital projection
Lateral with vertical beam (Fig. 28-24)	Lateral with horizontal beam (Fig. 23-25 A)
Submentovertical projection (Fig. 28-26)	

*The important differences between neurologic and trauma/injury routines are the inclusion of a submentovertical projection in the neurologic routine and the need for the lateral image to be performed using a horizontal beam in the trauma/injury routine. This lateral image with a horizontal beam is often referred to as a *cross-table lateral* and is performed to assess possible air/fluid levels that may occur as a result of the injury.

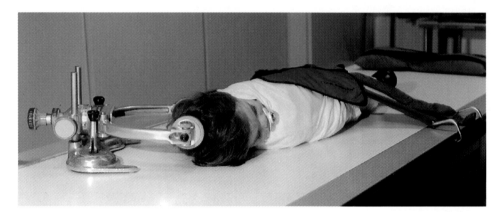

Fig. 28-24 When other methods prove unsuccessful, effective immobilization for a lateral skull radiograph with a vertical beam can be achieved with the use of a second Velcro band—*and some additional explanation to the parent.* Some radiographers question the technique because it covers the child's eyes. Turning the child's head and placing the Velcro band should be the last step (apart from a quick collimation check) before the exposure is made. Anxiousness can be alleviated if the parent bends down facing the child and talks to the child for the few seconds the radiographer needs to make the exposure.

Routines and protocols

Physicians order skull radiographs to assess neurologic problems and evaluate the extent of trauma or injury. For these reasons, many departments develop two routines: neurologic and trauma (Table 28-2; Figs. 28-24 to 28-26).

A

B

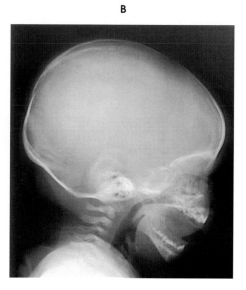

Fig. 28-25 A, Effective immobilization for lateral skull images with a horizontal beam can be achieved using the Infant Head and Neck Immobilizer. **B**, The resultant image reveals a well-positioned, nonrotated lateral skull image, including the upper cervical spine.

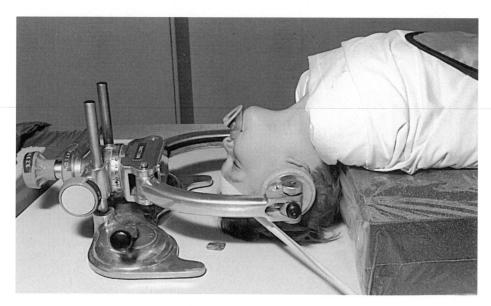

Fig. 28-26 Positioning for a submentovertical projection. Note the use of tape over the forehead to help maintain extension. (The tape is flipped over so that the nonsticky surface is in contact with the child's forehead.)

LIMB RADIOGRAPHY

Limb radiography, which accounts for a high percentage of pediatric general radiographic procedures in most clinics and hospitals, requires some explanation. The child's age and demeanor determine the method of immobilization to be employed. The immobilization methods are described here according to age group. In planning the approach, the radiographer should consider the chronologic age and psychologic outlook of the patient. For example, a very active 3 year old may be better managed using the approach for newborns to 2 year olds.

Immobilization
Newborn to 2-year-old

Limb radiography on the newborn to 2-year-old is probably the most challenging; however, it is made easier when the patient is wrapped in a towel. (A pillow case will suffice if a towel is not available.) This wrapping technique, a modification of the "bunny" method described previously, keeps the baby warm and allows the radiographer (and the parent, if assisting) to concentrate on immobilizing the injured arm. Fig. 28-27 demonstrates the method by which a piece of Plexiglas and "bookends" can be used to immobilize the hand.

Lower limbs on patients in this age group pose the greatest challenge in all pediatric limb work. In general, both arms should be wrapped in the towel and a Velcro band should be placed across the abdomen. A large sandbag is then placed over the unaffected leg (Fig. 28-28).

Preschoolers

The upper limbs of preschoolers are best examined radiographically with the child sitting on the parent's lap as shown in Fig. 28-29. If the parent is unable to participate, these children can be immobilized as described previously.

With parental participation, radiography of the lower limbs can be accomplished with the child sitting or lying on the table. Preventing the patient from falling from the table is always a primary concern with preschoolers. The parent must be instructed to remain by the child's side if the child is seated on the table. If the examination is performed with the child lying on the table, a Velcro band should be placed over the child.

School-age children

School-age children can generally be managed in the same way adult patients are for both upper and lower limb examinations.

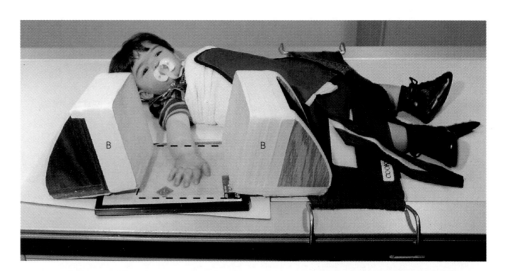

Fig. 28-27 With a simple modification of the "bunny" technique using a towel (or pillowcase), the child can be immobilized for upper limb radiography. Plexiglas *(dashed lines)* and "book-ends" *(B)* can be used to immobilize the hands of children 2 years old and younger. Note that after the child is wrapped, a Velcro band is used for safety and a small apron is placed diagonally over the body to protect the sternum and gonads. The cassette is placed on a lead mat, which prevents the image receptor from sliding on the table.

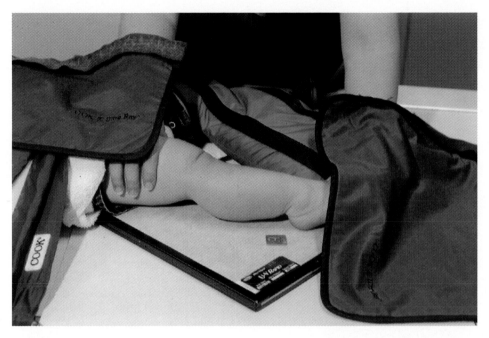

Fig. 28-28 The challenges of immobilizing lower limbs are greater than those of immobilizing upper limbs. After wrapping both of the patient's arms in a towel and placing a Velcro band over the abdomen, the radiographer can place a large sandbag over the unaffected leg. With careful collimation and proper instruction the parent can hold the limb as demonstrated. (The parent's hands shown without lead gloves and not draped in lead for illustration purposes only.)

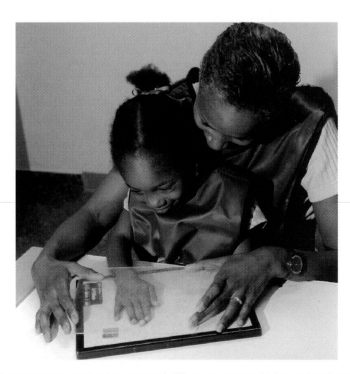

Fig. 28-29 Preschoolers are best managed sitting on a parent's lap. A lead mat is used to keep the cassette from sliding. Note use of Plexiglas to immobilize fingers.

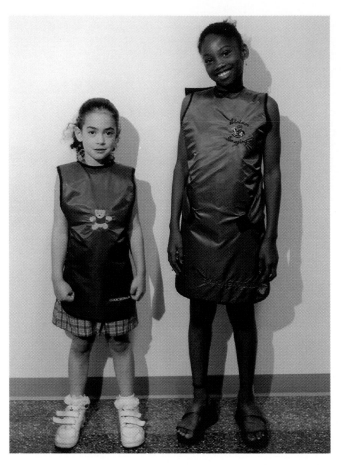

Fig. 28-30 The teddy bear on this full-length apron makes it appropriate for young children.

Radiation protection

The upper body should be protected in all examinations of the upper limbs, because of the close proximity of the thymus, sternum, and breast tissue to the scatter of the primary beam. Child-sized lead aprons with cartoon characters are both popular and practical (Fig. 28-30).

Management of fractures

As with adult patients who arrive in the imaging department with obvious fractures, the child with an obvious fracture *must* have the limb properly splinted by qualified personnel before the radiographer commences the examination. The splint protects both the patient and the radiographer, because the radiographer could cause further injury by manipulating an unsplinted limb.

Patients with fractures often arrive in the imaging department on a stretcher. The radiographer skilled at adapting routines can often obtain the necessary radiographs without moving the patient onto the table.

Ways to manage patients with OI were discussed in a previous section of this chapter (see Patient Care sections).

Evaluating the image

One of the most striking differences between adult and pediatric patients is the radiographic appearance of the limb. Radiographers develop an appreciation for these differences, which are caused by the presence of epiphyseal lines, as they gain experience in evaluating pediatric images. In departments in which the patient mix includes children and adults, preliminary limb work may require the *contralateral* side to be examined for comparison purposes. To the uneducated eye, a normally developing epiphysis may mimic a fracture. For this reason and because fractures can occur through the epiphyseal plate, physicians must learn to recognize epiphyseal lines and their appearance at various stages of ossification. Fractures that occur through the epiphysis are called *growth plate fractures*. Fig. 28-31 illustrates five types of epiphyseal fractures, referred to as *Salter-Harris type fractures*, the most widely used form of classification.

Because the growth plates are composed of cartilaginous tissue, the *density* of the radiographic image must be such that soft tissue is demonstrated in addition to bone (see Table 28-1). As previously described for radiography of the hip, the visualization of the bony trabecular pattern is used as an indicator that sufficient *recorded detail* has been demonstrated. Because of the smallness of pediatric limbs, an imaging system that provides better resolving power is usually required. As a general rule the speed of the imaging system used for limb radiography should be half that used for spines and abdomens.

A   B   C   D   E

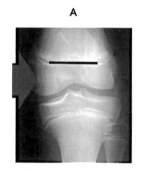 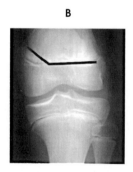 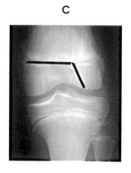 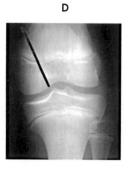 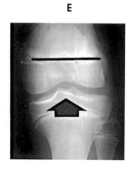

Fig. 28-31 Salter-Harris fractures. The *black lines* represent the fracture lines. **A**, A type 1 fracture occurs directly through the growth plate. **B**, A type 2 fracture extends through the growth plate and into the metaphyses. **C**, A type 3 fracture line extends through the growth plate and into the epiphyses. **D**, A type 4 fracture line extends through the metaphyses, across or sometimes along the growth plate, and through the epiphyses. **E**, A type 5 fracture involves a crushing of all or part of the growth plate. Fractures that occur through the epiphyses are significant injuries because they can affect growth if not recognized and treated properly. Proper radiographic technique is required for the demonstration of both soft tissue and bone. This is especially important with type 1 fractures, in which the growth plate is separated as a result of a lateral blow, and type 5 fractures, in which the growth plate has sustained a compression injury. Types 1 and 5 fractures do not occur through the bone.

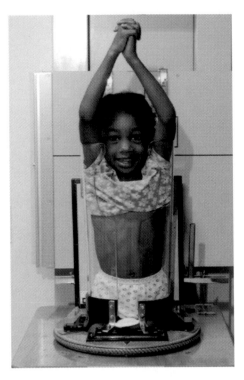

Fig. 28-32 The Pigg-o-stat, modified with the seat raised to suit upright abdominal radiography. The sleeves and seat are cleaned, and the seat is covered with a cloth diaper or thick tissue before the patient is positioned.

ABDOMINAL RADIOGRAPHY

Abdominal radiography for children is requested for different reasons than it is for adults. Consequently the initial procedure or protocol differs significantly. In addition to the supine and upright images, the assessment for acute abdomen conditions or the abdominal series in adult radiography usually includes radiographs obtained in the left lateral decubitus position. Often the series is not considered complete without a PA projection of the chest. To keep radiation exposure to a minimum, the pediatric abdominal series need only include two images: the supine abdomen and an image to demonstrate air-fluid levels. The upright image is preferred over the lateral decubitus in patients under 2 or 3 years of age because, from an immobilization and patient comfort perspective, it is much easier to perform. The upright image can be obtained with a slight modification of the Pigg-o-stat whereas the lateral decubitus position requires significant modification of the Pigg-o-stat.

Positioning and immobilization

Young children can be immobilized for supine abdomen imaging with the same methods described for radiography of the hips and pelvis (see Fig. 28-13), methods that provide basic immobilization of a patient for supine table radiography. The radiographer should observe the following guidelines for upright abdominal imaging:

- Effectively immobilize newborns and children as old as 2½ or 3 years for the upright image using the Pigg-o-stat.
- Raise the seat of the Pigg-o-stat to avoid projecting artifacts from the bases of the sleeves over the lower abdomen (Fig. 28-32).
- For the best results in the older child, have the child sit on a large box, trolley, or stool and spread the legs apart to prevent superimposition of the upper femora over the pelvis.

Lateral images of the abdomen are occasionally required in children, generally to localize something in the AP plane. Immobilization for lateral images is quite challenging; this difficulty, along with the fact that patient immobilization is the same as for lateral spine images, makes it worthy of mention here. Properly instructed, the parent can be helpful with this radiograph. The radiographer should observe the following steps:

- Remember that the *parent can do only one job.*
- Ask the parent to stand on the opposite side of the table and hold the child's head and arms.
- Immobilize the rest of the child's body using available immobilization tools. These tools include large 45-degree sponges, sandbags (large and small), a "bookend," and a Velcro band.
- Accomplish immobilization by rolling the child on the side and placing a small sponge or sandbag between the knees.
- Snugly wrap the Velcro band over the hips; to prevent backward arching, place the "bookend" against the child's back with the 45-degree sponge and sandbag positioned anteriorly (Fig. 28-33).

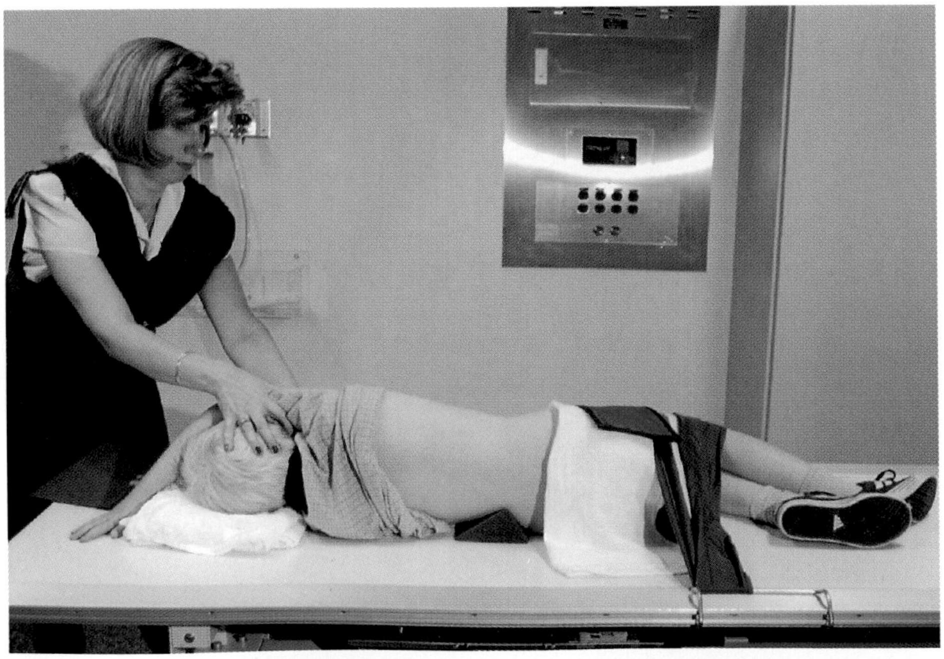

Fig. 28-33 The immobilization used for lateral abdominal imaging is also very effective for lateral thoracic and lumbosacral spine images. A 45-degree sponge and sandbag are used anteriorly.

Practical tip: It is common for pediatric clinicians to request "two views of the abdomen." The accompanying clinical information should support this request; if it does not, the radiographer should *seek clarification before proceeding*. Depending on the clinical reason for the radiographs, the two images may need to be supine and lateral. Abdominal images requested for infants in the NICU illustrate this point well. The neonatal patient with *necrotizing enterocolitis* requires supine and left lateral decubitus radiographs to rule out air-fluid levels indicative of bowel obstruction. However, the patient with an umbilical catheter needs supine and lateral images to verify the location and position of the catheter.

GASTROINTESTINAL AND GENITOURINARY PROCEDURES

In the interest of limiting radiation exposure to the GI and genitourinary systems, examinations are tailored to the individual patient. After a brief introduction, the radiographer should explain the procedure and check that the patient has undergone proper bowel preparation. The radiographer can then proceed with preparation (e.g., enema tip insertion) and immobilization of the patient.

Most procedures are performed by the radiologist. Exceptions include IVUs and in some hospitals voiding cystourethrograms (VCUGs). Notwithstanding, the radiographer has an integral role in the success of all examinations. Optimal hard-copy images require a thorough understanding of the equipment, its capabilities, and its limitations. Good patient care and organizational skills can also make the examination proceed more smoothly.

Immobilization for gastrointestinal procedures

As with other immobilization techniques, various beliefs exist regarding immobilization methods for the fluoroscopic portion of GI procedures; two methods are described. (The child may be immobilized for the "overhead" images as per the method outlined for the supine abdomen examination.)

Modified "bunny" method

The child's torso and legs are wrapped in a small blanket or towel and secured with a Velcro strip or tape. The arms are left free, raised above the head, and held by the parent (if present) (Fig. 28-34). The radiologist can then operate the carriage with one hand, holding the child's legs with the other to rotate the patient, thus obtaining the necessary coating of barium. This technique, thought by many to be more comfortable for the child, is often preferred by radiologists because small blankets are more readily available than the octagonal infant immobilization device. Success with this technique depends on someone (often a parent) assisting.

Conventional fluoroscopic suites, as contrasted to remote suites, are often preferred for GI examinations on children under 5 years old. Infants and preschoolers often require hands-on assistance to achieve desired positions and ensure their safety. In addition, the scattered dose is easier to minimize in conventional suites (see Radiation protection for GI procedures in the next section).

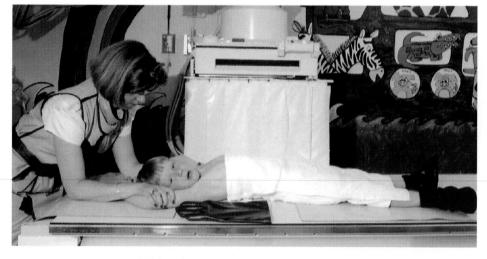

Fig. 28-34 Another modification of the "bunny" technique. The arms are left free and are raised above the head to prevent superimposition over the esophagus. In this example, tape is used to secure the blanket; however, Velcro strips are easier to use if a parent is not available to assist.

Octagonal infant immobilization method

The octagonal infant immobilization method, although effective, is less comfortable and appears more traumatic. However, with some creativity on the part of staff members, much of the child's fear can be averted by playing the "rocket ship game." The 3-year-old in Fig. 28-35 was told he would be dressed in a space suit (the hospital gown) and would go for a ride in the rocket ship.

By virtue of its construction, the octagonal immobilizer provides immobilization of the child in a variety of positions. As with the Pigg-o-stat, initial positioning of the child is a two-person process. The additional person does not have to be another radiographer; a well-instructed parent can assist. Because this technique immobilizes the head and arms, it is the method of choice when a parent is unable to provide assistance.

Radiation protection for gastrointestinal procedures

It is good practice to cover most of the tabletop of conventional fluoroscopic units with large mats of lead rubber (the equivalent of 0.5 mm of lead is recommended) (Fig. 28-35). Effective protection for operators and patients can be achieved by positioning the mats so that only the areas being examined are exposed.

Voiding cystourethrogram for genitourinary procedures

A primary purpose of the VCUG is to assess vesicoureteral reflux (reflux from the bladder to the ureters). In addition, VCUG in males can identify and evaluate urethral strictures. Radiation protection for the fluoroscopic portion should be the same as outlined above for GI examinations. The VCUG assesses bladder function and demonstrates ureteral and urethral anatomy.

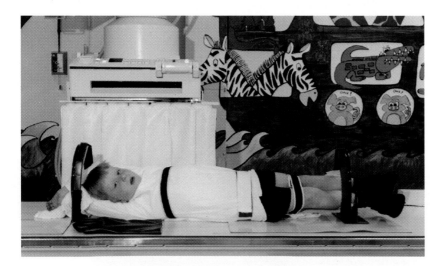

Fig. 28-35 The octagonal immobilizer (or for this child a "rocket ship") permits the child to be immobilized in a variety of positions.

Method

The patient is catheterized, a procedure that often requires two people—one to perform the catheterization and one to immobilize the legs in a frog leg position. The catheter is connected via tubing to a 500-ml bottle of contrast medium hung about 3 feet above the table. Under fluoroscopic guidance, contrast medium is dripped into the bladder until the bladder is full. Images are then taken while the patient is voiding to demonstrate reflux. This is often easier said than done! Preschoolers who have just been "toilet trained" and older children are often embarrassed. Techniques such as running tap water or pouring warm water over the genital area often encourage children to void.

Positioning

The female patient remains in the supine position, but the male patient must be placed in an oblique position during voiding to prevent the urethra from being superimposed over the pubic symphysis. After placing the male in an oblique position, the radiographer should take care to ensure the urethra is not superimposed over the femur.

Intravenous urogram for genitourinary procedures

Most pathologic conditions identified on an IVU or IVP can also be diagnosed with ultrasonography, a noninvasive, radiation-free examination. These advantages, combined with increased confidence on the part of urologists about ultrasound images and corresponding reports, are responsible for the dramatic decline in requests for IVUs. However, when IVUs are requested, most radiologists make a conscious effort to keep the number of exposures to a minimum; indeed, many examinations are completed with one preliminary radiograph and a late-stage filling radiography (between 5 and 15 minutes). Radiologists find it helpful to review previous radiographs at the time of the study so that the imaging sequence can be tailored to the patient, thereby keeping the radiation dose as low as possible.

Examinations Unique to the Pediatric Patient

BONE AGE

Children can arrive at the imaging department with either retarded skeletal development or advanced skeletal maturation. In either situation the degree of skeletal maturation is determined by the appearance, size, and differentiation of various ossification centers. The most commonly used assessment technique, developed by Greulich and Pyle,[1] compares an AP radiograph of the left hand and wrist with standards developed in the 1930s and 1940s and as later revised. Although these standards recognize the differing degrees of skeletal maturation between males and females by using separate standards for each gender, their applications are limited. Variations can also occur as a result of genetic diversity, nutritional status, and race.

Radiologists evaluate the differentiation and degree of fusion between the epiphyses and shafts of the bones of the hand and wrist by comparing the patient's radiograph with the standards printed in the atlas to determine the best match. The Greulich and Pyle method is considered extremely useful for most ages. Little change occurs in the ossification centers of the hand and wrist in the first 1 to 2 years of life, whereas the ossification of the knee and foot occurs rapidly during this time. Therefore bone age protocols for children 1 and 2 years old often include an AP radiograph of the left knee. Some department protocols specify that a knee radiograph be included for all children under the age of 2 years. In dedicated pediatric centers, others have found it more practical to specify that if, on reviewing the radiograph, the radiographer notes an apparent lack of ossification in the metacarpal epiphyses, the necessary radiograph of the left knee should then be obtained.

[1]Gruelich WW, Pyle SI: *Radiographic atlas of skeletal development of the hand and wrist,* ed 2, Stanford, Calif., 1959, Stanford University Press.

RADIOGRAPHY FOR SUSPECTED FOREIGN BODIES

Aspirated foreign body

A significant number of pediatric patients examined in emergency departments have a history that leads the physician to suspect a foreign body has been aspirated into the bronchial tree. This is a common cause of respiratory distress in children between the ages of 6 months and 3 years. In many cases the foreign body is nonopaque or radiolucent.

The foreign body, if slightly opaque and lodged in the *trachea,* may be demonstrated with filtered, high-kVp radiography of the *soft tissues of the neck.* From a radiologist's perspective, these images must be performed with the child's neck adequately extended and the shoulders lowered as much as possible. From the radiographer's perspective, this can be difficult to accomplish on the 6-month-old to 3-year-old. This challenge, however, is made easier with the use of the mc Infant Head and Neck Immobilizer (Cook [Canada], Inc., Stouffville, Ontario).

Method

The radiographer observes the following guidelines:

- Have the child be undressed from the waist up. Then position the child with the head in the contoured/cut out portion, the neck over the raised portion, and the chest on the sloped portion of the immobility device (Fig. 28-36).
- Lower and immobilize the shoulders using the provided towelette; then immobilize the head and upper thorax using the foam-lined Velcro strips. The neck extension helps to keep the trachea from appearing buckled, and the towelette and foam-lined Velcro shoulder straps keep the shoulders from being superimposed on the airway.

The Infant Head and Neck Immobilizer is specially designed for radiography of the soft tissue of the neck. However, if the device is not available, the radiographer can improvise with a 45-degree sponge and some Velcro strips.

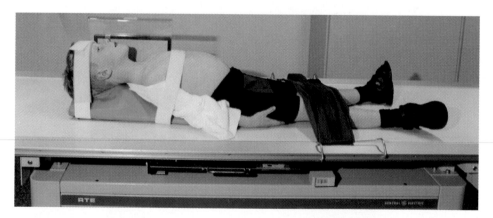

Fig. 28-36 The mc Infant Head and Neck Immobilizer provides the necessary extension of the neck for radiography of the soft tissues of the neck. The shoulders are kept low with the use of a towelette.

Aspirated foreign bodies are *more commonly lodged in the bronchial tree*, more often in the right side than the left side. Air becomes trapped on the affected side because the lodged foreign body acts as a ball valve, permitting air to enter on inspiration but preventing it from being exhaled on expiration. The result is a relatively normal-appearing inspiratory PA chest image but an abnormal appearance on the expiratory radiograph. Consequently the *routine* or *protocol* for chest examinations in patients with suspected aspirated foreign bodies should be an *inspiratory PA projection, an expiratory PA projection, and also a lateral projection.*

If satisfactory inspiration and expiration images cannot be obtained, bilateral lateral decubitus images should be obtained. (The unaffected lung will show that the heart has migrated toward the dependent lung. The affected dependent lung will remain fully inflated, preventing any downward migration of the heart.)

Ingested foreign body

Children frequently put objects in their mouths. If swallowed, these objects can cause obstruction or respiratory distress. Coins are the most commonly ingested foreign body, and, being radiopaque, they are easily identified. When ingested foreign body is known or suspected, the first imaging examination should be radiographs of the neck and chest or radiographs of the nasopharynx, chest, and abdomen.

Practical tip: In small children (approximately 1 year of age), this examination can be performed using a 35 × 43 cm (14 × 17 inch) cassette (Fig. 28-37). The radiographer needs to understand that the foreign body may be lodged anywhere between the nasopharynx and the anal canal. The presence of a foreign body cannot be ruled out if these areas are not well demonstrated. Esophageal studies are often required to demonstrate nonopaque foreign bodies.

Because of the anatomy of the esophagus and trachea, a coin identified in the coronal plane at the level of the thoracic inlet generally is lodged in the esophagus, whereas a coin found along the sagittal plane is generally lodged in the trachea.

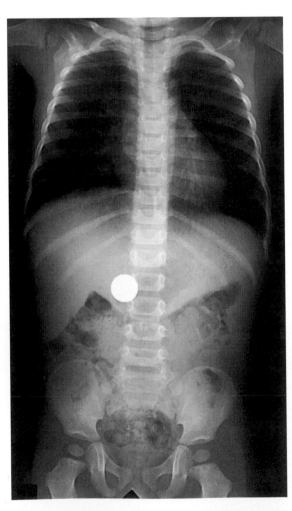

Fig. 28-37 A radiograph of the nasopharynx, chest, and abdomen is used to rule out the presence of a foreign body. If the coin this child had ingested had not been visible, a separate radiograph of the nasopharynx would have been obtained. Note that the diagonal placement of the gonadal shield over the distal pubic symphysis prevents the lower rectum from being obscured by lead.

SCOLIOSIS

Scoliosis has been defined as "the presence of one or more lateral-rotatory curvatures of the spine."[1] *Lateral* means toward the side, and *rotary* refers to the fact that the vertebral column rotates around its axis. Scoliosis can be a congenital or an acquired (e.g., posttrauma) condition. When physicians suspect scoliosis, radiographers evaluate for it using a PA or AP projection (preferably PA) on a 3-foot-long cassette of the entire spine. If the physician feels the curve has progressed to the point that further intervention is needed, a *full scoliosis series* is requested. The full scoliosis series should consist of 3-foot PA and lateral projections of the spine and probably right- and left-bending images (Fig. 28-38); (see also Figs. 8-149 and 8-150). A PA chest radiograph is included when the series is requested preoperatively. The purpose of the bending images is to assess or predict the degree of correction that can be obtained. The follow-up radiographic examination usually includes upright PA and lateral images.

[1]Silverman FN, Kuhn UP: *Caffey's pediatric x-ray diagnosis-an integrated approach,* St Louis, 1993, Mosby.

The radiographer should observe the following guidelines for obtaining the easiest and potentially most accurate method of accomplishing the bending images:

- Place the patient in the supine position on the radiographic table.
- Ask the patient to bend sideways as if reaching for the knees.
- Ensure that the ASIS remain equidistant to the table as the patient bends.
- Collimation and centering are crucial because the resultant image must include the first "normal" shaped (i.e., nonwedge-shaped) cervical or thoracic vertebra down to the crests of the ilia (see Fig. 28-38). (Experience has shown that curve progression usually stops coincident with the fusing of the epiphyses of the iliac crests.)

The geometric measurements determine the degree of curvature. The selected method of treatment is determined in part by the measurement of the angles outlined.

Radiation protection

Because scoliosis images are obtained relatively frequently to assess the progression of the curves, effective methods of radiation protection must be used:

- Obtain the 3-foot AP projection using breast shields; alternatively, position the patient for the PA projection, which makes the use of breast shields optional.
- Ensure that lead is draped over the patient's right breast tissue for the AP left-bending image, and vice versa.
- Protect gonads by placing a small lead apron at the level of the ASIS.

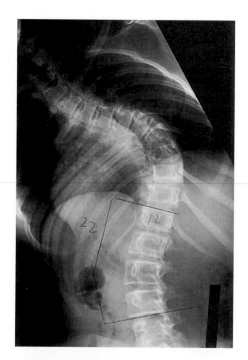

Fig. 28-38 In planning corrective surgery, orthopedic surgeons generally observe the bending images as if looking at the patient's back. The structures to be demonstrated include the uppermost non–wedge-shaped vertebrae and the iliac crests.

Overview Of Advanced Modalities

It is beyond the scope of this chapter to discuss *all* the imaging advances that have had a recent impact on pediatric imaging. The following sections highlight some advances that have had a direct impact on previously established protocols or routines in general radiography.

MAGNETIC RESONANCE IMAGING

MRI is perhaps the most dramatic and widespread technologic advancement in imaging. MRI quickly gained acceptance in the evaluation of most organ systems in the adult population. Its acceptance has been slower in pediatrics. This is somewhat ironic, considering that some of the advantages of MRI (enhanced contrast resolution, multiplanar capabilities, and lack of ionizing radiation) are crucial considerations in pediatric imaging.

The explanation for the slower acceptance of pediatric MRI lies in the length of an MRI examination. For example, a spinal MRI procedure may take from 60 to 90 minutes. During this time a child is required to remain still in an enclosed tunnel, hearing a loud and constant "hammering" noise that can be rather frightening. In a large proportion of the pediatric population, heavy sedation is often required to be able to complete an MRI examination. Conscious sedation is sometimes inadequate because the child can wake up during the scan. General anesthesia, with its risks and potential complications, is therefore needed. This being the case, MRI in young children may be a very serious and potentially risky procedure. Consequently the MRI staff need enhanced skills to care properly for these patients. It is preferable if the direct patient care team includes pediatric anesthetists and nurses. In addition, just as the successful radiologist of the twenty-first century will probably need to be proficient at MRI, the radiographer must be similarly proficient at providing high-quality diagnostic MRI studies.

MRI is documented as the method of choice for evaluating such pediatric spinal cord abnormalities as *tethered cords, lipomyelomeningoceles, neoplasms, myelination,* and *congenital anomalies.* MRI has also proved advantageous to cardiologists and cardiac surgeons. Diagnoses previously suggested on chest radiographs are now confirmed for the cardiologist. Cardiac surgeons are better able to plan corrective surgeries because MRI scans demonstrate the sites and full extent of collateral vessels necessary for grafting procedures.

As experience with pediatric limb radiography increases, the radiographer can appreciate the difficulties the physician has in diagnosing certain types of fractures of the epiphyseal plates (Salter-Harris fractures). MRI can demonstrate, through cartilaginous structures, fractures that would otherwise be missed because these areas appear lucent on the standard radiograph. Elbow surgery can be less complex for the orthopedic surgeon who can first rule out additional Salter-Harris fractures with multiplanar MRI scans. These multiplanar images include coronal, axial, and sagittal images.

MYELOGRAPHY

In imaging departments where MRI is available, the popularity of myelography has been steadily decreasing. This is especially true in the adult population but a relatively significant number of myelograms are still performed in pediatric centers. Neonatal patients, for example, sometimes develop a weakness in their upper limbs after traumatic births. If the neonate has been removed too aggressively during vaginal delivery, the nerves of the brachial plexus can be injured. If small, these tears may resolve of their own accord. Alternatively, they may worsen and require surgical repair. The diagnostic procedure of choice in this instance is a CT myelogram. After introducing a contrast medium into the subarachnoid space using a spinal needle, the radiographer performs a spinal CT scan. This scan shows any abnormal collections of contrast material where the nerve roots have been pulled. A cervical CT scan with special reconstructions in the sagittal, coronal, and oblique planes helps to visualize this condition best.

COMPUTED TOMOGRAPHY

CT has recently become a routine diagnostic tool—one that more and more general radiographers are using. Pediatric patients present unique challenges, even to the seasoned CT technologist.

In the pediatric population, CT is useful in diagnosing congenital anomalies, assessing metastases, and diagnosing bone sarcomas and sinus disease; it has virtually replaced radiographic scanography. Young children have difficulty following the instructions needed for a diagnostic scan. Suggestions regarding approach and atmosphere were presented at the beginning of this chapter. Some basic technical tips are given here. As in the care of any pediatric patient, the role of the CT technologist is important in the success of the examination. The technologist must gain the respect and confidence of the young patient and the caregiver, if present.

The CT scanner itself is a very impressive piece of equipment, one that needs careful explanation to help allay the patient's fears. One of the most significant fears is claustrophobia. Techniques to reduce claustrophobia include the use of a television/VCR and music for entertainment (Fig. 28-39). Parent participation is often encouraged for the same reasons outlined previously in the chapter.

The advent of faster scanners and the introduction of helical scanning have significantly reduced scan times, thereby lessening patient anxiety. For example, a neck, chest, abdomen, and pelvic scan can now be completed in approximately 1 minute. However, patient preparation, the injection of IV contrast material, and the computer processing of images can bring the total time of this examination to 15 to 20 minutes.

For young children, 15 or 20 minutes can be a long time, sometimes long enough to warrant the use of conscious sedation. Nursing staff then become actively involved in monitoring the sedated patient. The CT technologist should be comfortable with the use of oxygen-delivery systems, suction apparatus, and basic emergency management techniques. Generally speaking, if a reaction occurs in a pediatric patient, it will worsen significantly faster than in an adult. This underscores the need for the technologist to be well versed in the signs and symptoms of a potential reaction and the appropriate emergency response measures.

Emphasis should also be placed on mechanisms of dose reduction in CT. Examples include reducing the field of view (FOV) to allow precise collimation for the body part being examined and performing scans using preprogrammed (dose-conscious) protocols.

Technical advances in CT will bring even faster systems in the future. In fact, several manufacturers of CT scanners are currently advertising "real-time" CT. In practice this should reduce the number of patients requiring sedation, making the procedure faster, safer, and less costly. In addition to increasing scan speed, CT manufacturers have worked hard to include dose-minimizing software features and user-friendly protocol programming options. If optimized and used to their maximum potential, these features will make routine CT examinations easier, thereby opening the door of this specialty field to all technologists.

CT has largely replaced conventional radiographic examinations done to assess leg length discrepancy (LLD). *Spot scanography*, one of the relatively common conventional methods, is a technique in which three exposures of the lower limbs (centered over the hips, knees, and ankles in turn) are made on a single 35 × 43 cm (14 × 17 inch) cassette (see Chapter 11). A radiopaque rule is included for the purpose of calculating the discrepancy on the resulting image.

Studies have shown that CT digital radiography is an accurate technique for measuring LLD. It is reproducible, and positioning and centering errors are less likely to occur. More importantly, studies also report radiation dose to be less than that for conventional techniques, leading researchers to recommend that the CT scout image–type option be used particularly in young patients having serial examinations. Technical details beyond the scope of this atlas are provided in texts cited in the bibliography at the end of this chapter.

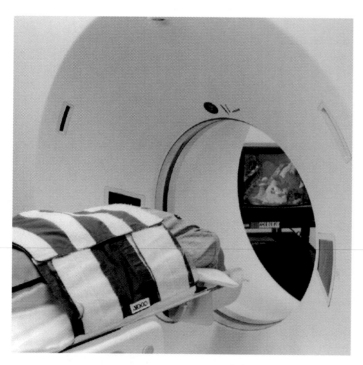

Fig. 28-39 Right coronal CT positioning is best tolerated when patient is distracted by a television positioned behind the gantry.

THREE-DIMENSIONAL IMAGING

In the pediatric population, three-dimensional images reconstructed from CT or MRI data have revolutionized surgical procedures. This new technique allows clinicians (predominantly orthopedic and plastic surgeons, but also neurosurgeons) to manipulate three-dimensional images of their patients interactively on a computer screen, rotating the image in any angle. Using this information, they can develop strategies that may change the complete treatment, management, or operative approach. Three-dimensional images are extremely useful, if not vital, in "mapping" a course of treatment for many corrective procedures for congenital malformations. Examples include craniofacial syndromes, congenital hip dysplasia, and conditions requiring plastic correction. Three-dimensional imaging also plays a major role in the management of cervical spine trauma and rotary subluxation of the spine in children.

INTERVENTIONAL RADIOLOGY

Interventional radiology has dramatically changed the role of the radiology department in both teaching and nonteaching hospitals and clinics. In the past the justifications and rationales for radiology departments were diagnostic ones. However, radiology departments with professionally instructed interventional staff can now offer hospitals therapeutic services in addition to diagnostic services. This heightened awareness has largely resulted from the nature and efficacy of the interventional procedures.

These therapeutic interventions often obviate the need for surgery. Therapeutic procedures performed in the imaging department provide an attractive alternative to surgery for the patient, parent, hospital administrator, and society. (A procedure performed in the imaging department is much less expensive than one performed in the operating room.) These procedures are minimally invasive compared with their surgical counterparts, thereby reducing recovery times. Shortened length of stay translates into economic savings for the parents of pediatric patients.

Although these interventional procedures are predominantly performed in suites previously referred to as *specials* or *angiographic suites*, many procedures, especially nonvascular procedures, are performed in digital radiography and fluoroscopy suites. These diverse locations of care and the postprocedural care involved with vascular-interventional cases provide expanded avenues for general-duty radiographers to come in contact with patients. Interventional radiology holds a privileged position in many imaging departments. Nevertheless, a detailed, descriptive explanation of this role is well beyond the scope of this text. (Detailed discussions appear in texts cited in the bibliography at the end of this chapter for further readings.)

General radiographers must be able to recognize patients who have undergone interventional procedures, particularly vascular-interventional procedures in which central venous access devices have been inserted or implanted. This heightened awareness is crucial for infection prevention. After central venous access devices are inserted, they provide a direct conduit to the heart—a conduit or route in which bacteria can readily grow.

The following paragraphs provide a brief overview of some of the most common venous access devices and indications for their use. They also illustrate the need for increased education to prevent catheter-related infections. Although estimates regarding the rate of infection vary, health care professionals involved in the management of patients with indwelling vascular access devices do not minimize the magnitude and severity of catheter-related infections. They also are among the first to admit that "intravascular devices are indispensable in modern-day medical practice."[1] Catheter-related infections can increase the length of hospital stays and put patients at risk. However, as with radiologic procedures, the benefits often outweigh the associated risks.

---

[1] Pearson, ML: *Infect Control Hosp Epidemiol* 17:439, 1996.

Interventional radiology presents an alternative to pediatric surgery for angioplasty (balloon dilation), stent placement, embolization, vascular access device insertion, and numerous other procedures. *Angioplasty* refers to the placement of a balloon-tipped catheter in the center of a narrowed vessel; the balloon is inflated and deflated several times to stretch or dilate the narrowed segment. *Embolization* refers to the occlusion of small feeder vessels with either tiny coils or specially formulated glue. This procedure is performed to cut off the blood supply to a tumor.

For simplicity, interventional radiology can be divided into vascular and nonvascular procedures. Vascular procedures are generally performed in angiographic suites. In addition to the therapy (or intervention) being provided, angiography and ultrasonography are also performed for diagnostic and guidance purposes. Angiography can be arterial or venous; pediatric vasculature is well suited to both. IV injection is favored in infants because their relatively small blood volume and rapid circulation allow for good vascular images to be obtained after the injection of contrast material into a peripheral vein. In infants, hand injections are often preferred over power injections to help avoid extravasation. Intraarterial digital subtraction angiography (DSA) (see Chapter 35) has become a valuable tool for imaging professionals. DSA is performed using diluted contrast medium, which can reduce pain, and it provides a useful "roadmapping" tool. Roadmapping, a software tool available on newer angiographic equipment, uses the intraarterial injection to provide a fluoroscopic display of arterial anatomy—a very useful tool for imaging tortuous vessels.

Vascular-interventional procedures can be neurologic, cardiac, or systemic in nature. Nonvascular procedures often involve the digestive and urinary systems. Examples include the insertion of gastrostomy and nephrostomy tubes, respectively. These tubes provide conduits from the stomach and kidneys to the skin surface.

The following paragraphs focus on the vascular side of interventional radiology, more specifically the insertion of vascular access devices. The reason for this is simple: given the number of chest radiographs ordered for pediatric patients, radiographers will far more frequently encounter patients with these devices.

Simply stated, vascular access devices are of three types: nontunneled, tunneled, and implanted. The selection of device is often determined by a combination of factors, including the purpose of the access, and proposed indwelling time. Furthermore, the physician or patient may choose a particular device in the interests of compliance or after assessing underlying clinical considerations.

Nontunneled catheters are commonly referred to as *peripherally inserted central catheters,* or *PICC lines.* They are available with single or multiple lumens. The insertion point is usually the basilic or cephalic vein, at or above the antecubital space of the nondominant arm. Multiple lumens are desirable when a variety of different medications (including total parenteral nutrition) are to be administered (Fig. 28-40). These devices must be strongly anchored to the skin because children often pull on and displace the catheters, resulting in damage to the line and potential risk to themselves. To render the catheters more secure, pediatric clinicians often tailor their insertion and anchoring techniques to help prevent the catheter from being pulled out by the patient.

As with PICC lines, tunneled catheters can have multiple lumens. However, unlike PICC lines, they are not inserted into the peripheral circulation; rather, they are inserted via a subcutaneous tunnel into the subclavian or internal jugular veins. The tunneling acts as an anchoring mechanism for the catheter to facilitate long-term placement (Fig. 28-41). Tunneled catheters are used for the administration of chemotherapy, antibiotics, and fluids; they are also used for hemodialysis. (Technologists may see or hear these referred to as *Hickman lines,* a term that has been generalized to include tunneled catheters placed in subclavian or internal jugular veins.)

A

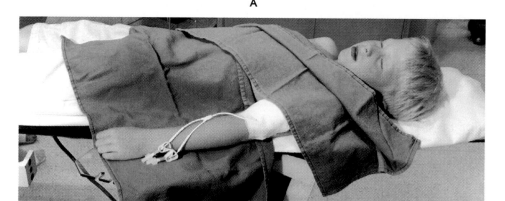

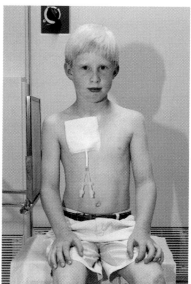

Fig. 28-41 External appearance of tunneled, double-lumen central venous access device. These catheters are used for long-term therapy. Their short track to the heart can increase the risk of infection, necessitating proper care for maintenance.

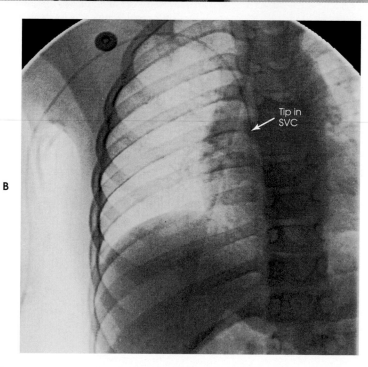

Tip in SVC

B

Fig. 28-40 A, Postinsertion image of a double-lumen peripherally inserted central catheter (PICC) line in a 7-year-old boy (shown in the interventional suite). Conscious sedation was used for this procedure. **B,** Digital image of PICC line demonstrating the distal tip of the catheter positioned in the superior vena cava.

Implanted devices are often referred to as *ports*. These are titanium or polysulfone devices with silicone centers, and they are attached to catheters. The whole device is implanted subcutaneously with the distal end of the catheter tip further implanted, often into the superior vena cava or right atrium. A port is the device of choice for noncompliant children or adults who, for aesthetic purposes, would rather not have the limb of a catheter protruding from their chest (Fig. 28-42).

In summary, vascular access devices have dramatically changed the course of treatment for many patients in a very positive way. Patients who would have previously been hospitalized for antibiotic therapy can now go home with the device in place. This is good news. The increased prevalence of these devices means that patients with vascular access devices are in the community and visiting radiology departments everywhere. Therefore the need has grown for increased education for patients and those who come in contact with them. PICC lines have a smaller likelihood of introducing catheter-related infections; tunneled lines present a greater risk.

Radiographers must recognize vascular access devices and treat them with utmost care. They should report dislodged bandages and sites showing signs of infection (i.e., redness, exudate) *immediately*. Catheter-related infections compound recovery courses, sometimes in life-threatening ways. They cost hospitals many thousands of dollars each year.

Postprocedural care currently represents a very significant and ongoing challenge for all personnel who treat, manage, and come in contact with patients who have vascular access devices. To date, this challenge has not been adequately addressed. *To whom does the responsibility of postprocedural care rest?* It is the responsibility of all these personnel.

NUCLEAR MEDICINE

If bladder function is the *only* concern for the physician who requests a VCUG, a nuclear medicine *direct radionuclide cystogram (DRC)* can be performed. The DRC emphasizes the assessment of bladder function. Radiographers should recognize that *nuclear medicine studies assess function rather than demonstrate anatomy*. The DRC permits observation of reflux during imaging over a longer period. In addition, it allows for accurate quantification of postvoiding residual volume. The radiation dose to the patient is less with this procedure than with the VCUG, making it an attractive option for the pediatric patient. (Technical details on nuclear medicine are presented in texts cited in the selected bibliography at the end of this chapter.)

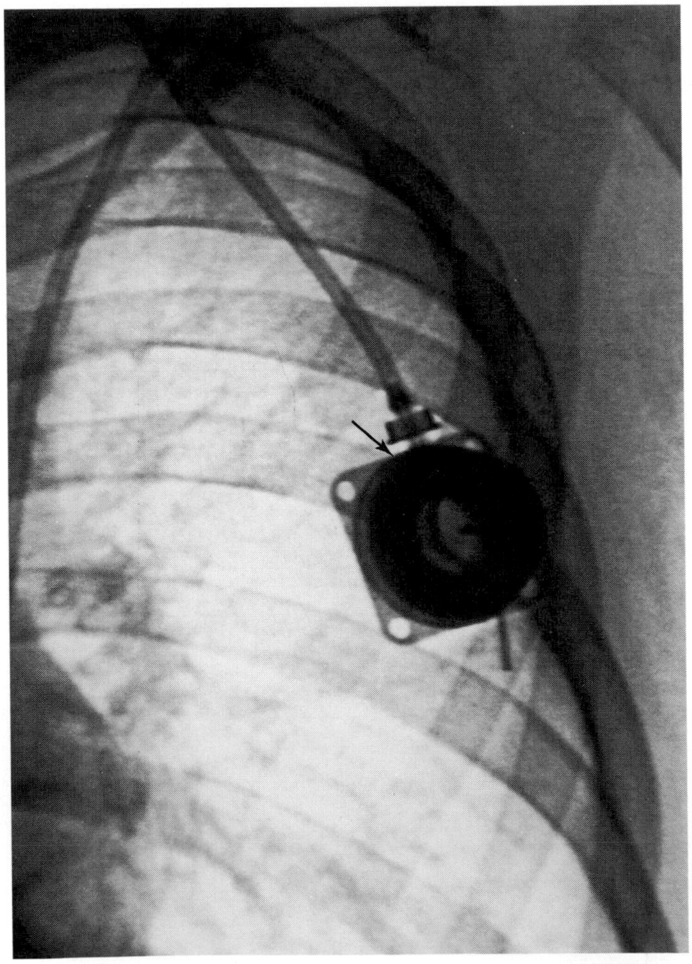

Fig. 28-42 Digital image of port *(arrow)*. Ports are vascular devices that must be accessed subcutaneously. They are preferred for active children and for aesthetic reasons.

Conclusion

Although no one can prevent a child from experiencing the fear engendered by a visit to the hospital, much can be done to allay that fear. Questions from children such as "Am I going to have a needle?" require a truthful response. However, the manner in which the response is delivered can make a tremendous difference. Children are impressionable and dependent on their caregivers, but they are also often the best teachers radiographers can have. Radiographers should watch and listen to these small patients, observe their body language and facial expressions, and note their questions and reactions for cues regarding ways to respond to them. The rewards—a child's smile and trust—are given more frequently than might be expected.

ACKNOWLEDGMENT

The authors wish to acknowledge the contributions of GE Medical Systems Canada, Mississauga, Ontario, and Cook (Canada), Inc., Stouffville, Ontario, which made the color illustration program for this chapter possible.

DEDICATION

To Alyssa, Alexander, Aaron, Andrew, Erik, Keisha, Richard, and the many other children who depend on us. They are our best teachers—and our future.

Selected bibliography

Aitken AGF et al: Leg length determination by CT digital radiography, *AJR* 144:613, 1985.

Campbell WE et al: Radiologic insertion of long term venous access devices, *Semin Intervent Radiol* 2:1994. {AU: Please provide beginning page number.}

Dietrich RB: *The Raven MRI teaching file, pediatric MRI*, New York, 1991, Raven Press.

Duck S: Neonatal intravenous therapy, *J Intravenous Nurs,* 20(3):366, 1997.

Godderidge C: *Pediatric imaging,* Philadelphia, 1995, WB Saunders.

Green M: Tech-tips, *Can J Med Rad Tech* 22:119, 1991.

Green RE, Oestman JW: *Computed digital radiography in clinical practice*, New York, 1992, Thieme.

Gruelich WW, Pyle SI: *Radiographic atlas of skeletal development of the hand and wrist*, ed 2, Stanford, Calif., 1959, Stanford University Press.

Jester JR, Scanlan BE: Fast, informative, low in dose: the digital instant image. Initial clinical experience. *Electromedica* 56:134, 1988.

Jones D, Gleason CA, Lipstein SU: *Hospital care of the recovering NICU infant*, Baltimore, 1991, Williams & Wilkins.

Kleinman PK: *Diagnostic imaging of child abuse*, Baltimore, 1987, Williams & Wilkins.

Laudicina P: *Applied pathology for radiographers*, Philadelphia, 1989, WB Saunders.

Maynar M et al: Vascular interventional procedures in the pediatric age group. In Casteneda-Zunigo WR, editor: *Interventional radiology*, Baltimore, 1992, Williams & Wilkins.

McBride KD et al: A comparative analysis of radiological and surgical placement of central venous catheters, *Cardiovasc Intervent Radiol* 20:17, 1997.

Miller KD, Christine DL: Experience with PICC at a university medical center, *J Intravenous Nurs* 20:141, 1997.

Milne DA et al: *Hospital for Sick Children diagnostic imaging—procedure manual*, Toronto, 1993, Hospital for Sick Children.

Nelson WE, Behrman RE, Vaughan VC, III: *Textbook of pediatrics*, ed 12, Philadelphia, 1983, WB Saunders.

Ozonoff MB: *Pediatric orthopedic radiology*, Philadelphia, 1992, WB Saunders.

Pearson ML: Guideline for prevention of intravascular-device–related infections, *Infect Control Hosp Epidemiol* 7:439, 1996.

PQ CT imaging systems, notes, Cleveland, Ohio, 1996, Picker International Inc.

Reed ME: *Pediatric skeletal radiology*, Baltimore, 1992, Williams & Wilkins.

Robinson MJ: *Practical pediatrics*, ed 2, New York, 1990, Churchill Livingstone.

Silverman FN, Kuhn UP: *Essentials of Caffey's pediatric x-ray diagnosis—an integrated approach*, St Louis, 1990, Mosby.

Silverman FN, Kuhn UP: *Caffey's pediatric x-ray diagnosis—an integrated imaging approach*, St Louis, 1993, Mosby.

Torres LS: *Basic medical techniques and patient care for radiologic technologists*, ed 5, Philadelphia, 1997, Lippincott.

Toshiba Corporation Medical Systems: *Kid CT, product brochure*, Tokyo, 1997.

Medical review, special edition, Tokyo, 1996, Toshiba Corporation Medical Systems.

Wilmot DM, Sharko GA: *Pediatric imaging for the technologist*, New York, 1987, Springer-Verlag.

Woodward et al: *MRI for technologists*, New York, 1995, McGraw-Hill.

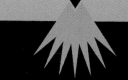

TOMOGRAPHY

JEFFREY A. BOOKS

RIGHT: Early planigraphic (tomographic) device designed by Ziedses des Plantes. The x-ray tub *(top)* is attached with a bar to the Bucky tray. The continuous metal bar extends downward to the front side of the Bucky tray assembly. Mounted on the floor is a peg with a string attached. One operator turned the lower bar while a colleague made the exposure. As the bar turned, the string wrapped itself around the peg with a spiral movement. The result was a tomographic image.

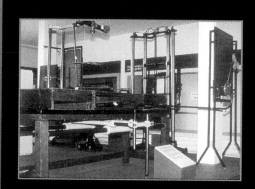

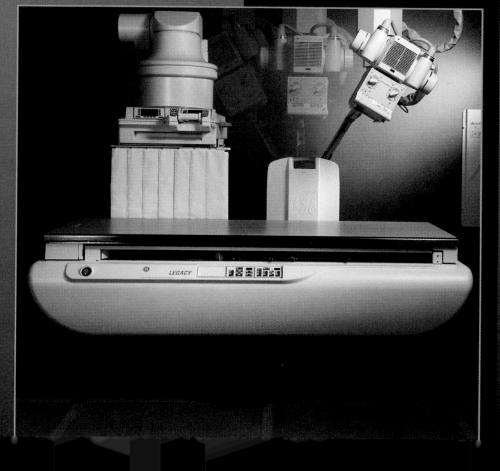

Tomographic unit with image intensifier in park position, 1999.

(Courtesy General Electric Medical Systems.)

Historical Development

Since its inception in the 1890s, radiography has faced the problem of trying to record three-dimensional body structures accurately as two-dimensional images. This unavoidably results in the superimposition of structures, which often obscures important diagnostic information. One attempt to overcome this problem is the use of right-angle images. Over the years many other techniques have been developed that partially circumvent the problem of superimposition, such as multiple radiographs, stereoscopic images, and subtraction techniques in angiography.

The partial or complete elimination of obscuring shadows by the effect of motion on shadow formation is a common technique used in radiography. This effect is frequently used with conventional projections. For example, in conjunction with a long exposure time, breathing motion is used to reduce rib and pulmonary shadows to a background blur on frontal images of the sternum and lateral radiographs of the thoracic spine.

Body-section radiography (or more appropriately, *tomography*) is a term used to designate a radiographic technique by which most of the problems of superimposed images are overcome. *Tomography** is the term used to designate the technique whereby a predetermined plane of the body is demonstrated in focus on the radiograph. Other body structures above or below the plane of interest are eliminated from the image or are rendered as a low-density blur caused by motion.

---

*Almost all italicized words are defined at the end of this chapter.

The origin of tomography cannot be attributed to any one person; in fact, tomography was developed by several different gifted individuals experimenting in different countries at about the same time without any knowledge of each other's work. In 1921, Dr. André-Edmund-Marie Bocage, a French dermatologist, described in an application for a patent many of the principles used in modern tomographic equipment. Many other early investigators made significant contributions to the field of tomography. Each of these pioneers applied a different name to a particular device or process of body-section radiography. Bocage (1922) termed the result of his process *moving film roentgenograms;* the Italian Vallebona (1930) chose the term *stratigraphy;* the Dutch physician Ziedses des Plantes (1932), who made several significant contributions, called his process *planigraphy.* The term *tomography* came from the German investigator Grossman, as does the *Grossman principle,* which is discussed later in this section.

Tomography was invented in the United States in 1928 by Jean Kieffer, a radiographer who developed the special radiographic technique to demonstrate a form of tuberculosis that he had. His process was termed *laminagraphy* by another American, J. Robert Andrews, who assisted Kieffer in the construction of his first tomographic device, the laminagraph.[1]

A great deal of confusion arose over the many different names given to the general process of body-section radiography. To eliminate this confusion, the International Commission of Radiological Units and Standards appointed a committee in 1962 to select a single term to represent all of the processes. *Tomography* is the term the committee chose, and this term is now recognized throughout the medical community as the single appropriate term for all forms of *body-section radiography.*[2]

---

[1]Littleton JT: *Tomography: physical principles and clinical application,* Baltimore, 1976, Williams & Wilkins.

[2]Vallebona A, Bistolfi F: *Modern thin-section tomography,* Springfield, Ill, 1973, Charles C Thomas.

Physical Principles

As with conventional radiography, tomography has three basic requirements: an x-ray source, an object, and a recording medium (generally film). However, to create an image of a single plane of tissue in tomography, a fourth requirement must be met-synchronous movement of two of the three essential elements during the x-ray exposure. This is achieved by moving the x-ray source and cassette in opposing directions about the stationary patient. Because of the end effects, tomography may be thought of as a process of controlled blurring.

The basic tomographic blurring principle is demonstrated in Fig. 29-1. At the beginning of the exposure, the tube and cassette are at positions T_1 and F_1, respectively (with T indicating the x-ray tube and F indicating the cassette). During the exposure the tube and cassette travel in opposite directions, and their movements are terminated at the end of the exposure at positions T_2 and F_2. The *focal plane* is at the level of the axis of rotation, or *fulcrum,* and is considered parallel with the tabletop. Structures at the same level of the focal plane remain in focus, whereas structures in other planes above and below this level are blurred across the image. The star located above the level of the fulcrum is projected to the right side of the image receptor at the beginning of the exposure. At the end of the exposure the relative position of the star has now moved to the left of the receptor. Because this is not a static image but a dynamic one, the structure is now nothing more than a blurred density image. The round structure located at the level of the focal plane, however, is projected at the same place on the receptor throughout the entire exposure; therefore it is not blurred but remains in focus.

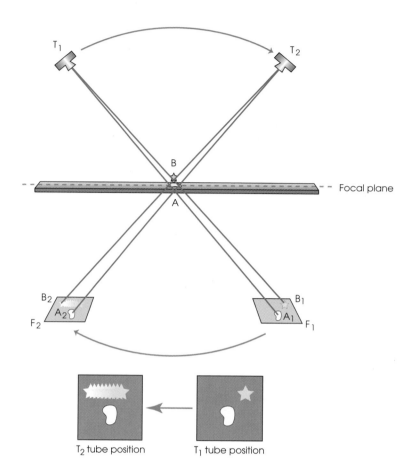

Fig. 29-1 Fundamental tomographic blurring principle depicting x-ray tube (*T*), focal plane (patient), and x-ray image receptor (*F*).

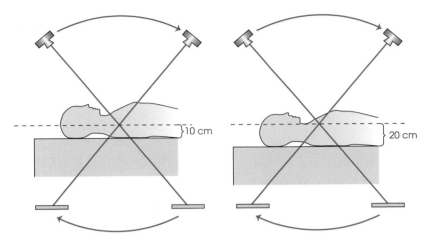

Fig. 29-2 Grossman principle (fixed fulcrum). Tabletop height is changed to alter fulcrum level.

Tomographic sections at different fulcrum heights may be obtained by altering the level of the focal plane. This may be accomplished by one of two methods, depending on the principle used in the design of the tomographic device. These two principles, the *planigraphic principle* and the *Grossman principle,* are the basis of all modern tomographic equipment. The Grossman principle uses a *fixed fulcrum* system in which the axis of rotation remains at a fixed height (Fig. 29-2). The focal plane level is changed by raising and lowering the tabletop and patient through this fixed point to the desired height. In contrast the planigraphic principle uses an *adjustable fulcrum* system (Fig. 29-3). The actual fulcrum or pivot point is raised or lowered to the height of the desired focal plane level, whereas the tabletop and patient remain stationary at a fixed height.

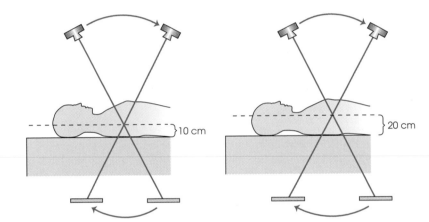

Fig. 29-3 Planigraphic principle (adjustable fulcrum). Pivot point height is changed to alter fulcrum level.

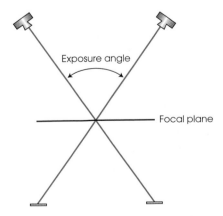

Fig. 29-4 Tomographic exposure angle.

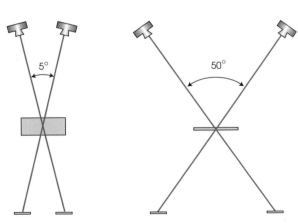

Fig. 29-5 Narrow exposure angles yield thick tomographic sections *(left);* wide exposure angles yield thin tomographic sections *(right).*

The *exposure angle* (*tomographic angle*) is the angle of arc described by the movement of the tube and image receptor during the tomographic exposure (Fig. 29-4). The width of the focal plane or the plane of tissue that is in maximum focus is called the *section thickness* (Fig. 29-5). The thickness of the tomographic section may be changed by altering the exposure angle. Because no blurring would occur in a tomogram employing a stationary x-ray tube (an exposure angle of 0 degrees), the resulting image would yield a conventional radiograph demonstrating all planes of tissue contained within the part being imaged (an infinite section thickness). In tomography, as the exposure angle increases from 0 degrees, the section thickness decreases. Tomograms using wide exposure angles demonstrate thin sections; conversely, smaller exposure angles demonstrate comparatively thicker sections.

The range of section thickness produced by wide-angle tomography is approximately 1 to 5 mm, and that produced by narrow-angle tomography, or *zonography*, ranges from slightly less than ⅜ inch (1 cm) to about 1 inch (2.5 cm). Zonography, the tomographic technique used to demonstrate relatively thick sections, or zones, of tissue, was first described by des Plantes, who recommended it for examining sections of the cranium and spinal column.

Zonography is now used in a number of other regions of the body. Its blurring characteristics make it ideally suited to demonstrate structures that are low in contrast relative to adjacent structures. Zonography is frequently employed in the abdomen, where the structures that make up the soft tissue organs are extremely low in contrast relative to each other and therefore are difficult to differentiate on conventional radiographs.

The degree to which definition decreases with distance from the focal plane depends on the width of the angle described by the tube motion. Wide angles of tube movement provide excellent blurring of structures both close to and remote from the focal plane. Narrow angles of tube movement provide excellent blurring of structures remote from the focal plane but only moderate to slight blurring of structures close to the focal zone.

Although visibility of the objective area is greatly enhanced by the partial or complete elimination of obscuring shadows, the appearance of the tomogram is quite different from that of a conventional radiograph. The customary sharp definition and clear contrast are diminished, and the contours of all but the thinnest structures are absent. The contrast is reduced because of the way the blurring action diffuses elements in other planes over the focal plane image. This creates an overall increase in the density on the tomogram, which, in turn, results in an overall decrease in contrast for the structures demonstrated.

The formation of the tomographic image is a cumulative process. The shadows of structures in the plane of focus accumulate on the image receptor as the area traversed by the beam of radiation swings over the arc. The images are not sharp because the radiation traverses structures from many angles, outlining clearly only those boundaries to which the beam is momentarily tangential in its passage.

Zonograms are comparable in appearance with conventional radiographs for the following reasons:

1. The cuts are thick enough to show structural contours.
2. The narrow arc described by the tube directs the radiation at only slightly oblique angles so that it projects structural contours more nearly true to shape.
3. With the reduced effects of less blurring, the contrast and detail produced are superior to those possible in wide-angle tomography. However, a zonogram does not necessarily provide more diagnostic information than a wide-angle tomogram; instead, each has its place in tomography. The choice between using a wide or narrow *exposure angle* depends primarily on the thickness of the structure or structures in the tomogram and their proximity to other structures outside the focal plane.

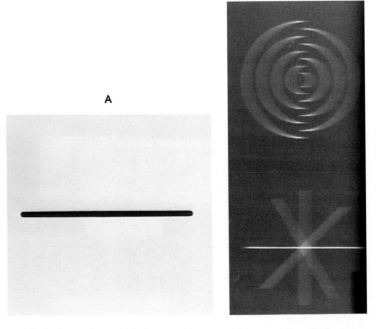

Blurring Motions

Modern tomographic equipment offers a variety of different blurring patterns. These blurring motions fall under two categories: (1) *unidirectional (linear)* and (2) *pluridirectional (complex) tomographic motions,* which include circular, elliptic, hypocycloidal, and spiral motions. A basic understanding of the characteristics of these blurring patterns is necessary to understanding their advantages and limitations.

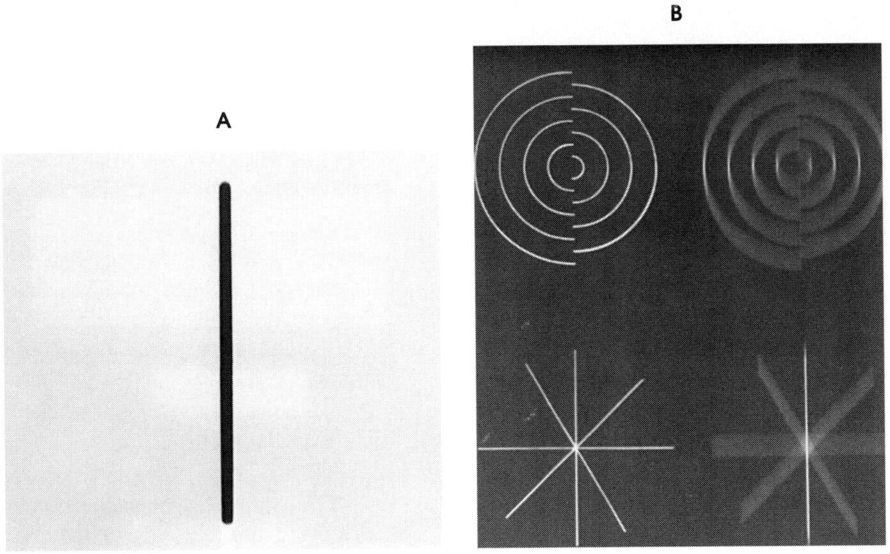

UNIDIRECTIONAL MOTION

The basic tomographic blurring pattern is the *unidirectional,* or linear, motion. The blurring action of linear motion is provided by elongation of structures outside the focal plane so that they become indistinguishable linear streaks or blurs over the focal plane image. Maximum blurring occurs to those elements of structures outside the focal plane that are oriented perpendicular to the relative motion of the tube (Figs. 29-6 through 29-8). In linear tomography, therefore, elements of structures oriented parallel to the motion of the tube are incompletely blurred and can form false shadows, or *phantom images,* over the focal plane image. This results in an inaccurate representation of the focal plane because of the summation of the focal plane image and the images of some structures outside the plane of focus. This characteristic is demonstrated in the tomogram of a test object. The test object consists of two wire patterns: pattern 1 is located at the level of the focal plane (*left-hand image* in Fig. 29-6, *B*); pattern 2 (*right-hand image*) is 5 mm away from the level of the focal plane and therefore exhibits the effects of the blurring motion used.

Fig. 29-6 A, Pinhole tracing of 45-degree longitudinal linear motion. **B,** Tomogram of test object at 45-degree longitudinal linear motion. *(Left)* The pattern is at level of focal plane. *(Right)* The pattern is 5 mm above level of focal plane. With linear motion the most blurring occurs to elements of the test object oriented perpendicular to the movement of the tube; the least blurring occurs to elements oriented parallel to the tube.

Fig. 29-7 A, Pinhole tracing of 45-degree transverse linear motion. **B,** Tomogram of test object at 45-degree transverse linear motion.

The most blurring occurs to elements of the patterns that are perpendicular to the tube movement, and the least occurs to those parallel. In linear tomography, structures to be blurred must be oriented at right angles to the tube movement. For example, in tomography of the chest the tube movement is oriented perpendicularly to the ribs for maximum blurring of those structures.

PLURIDIRECTIONAL MOTION

A more efficient blurring motion is one in which all elements of an object are perpendicular to the movement of the tube at some time during the exposure. This is the principle of the second type of blurring motion—the pluridirectional, or complex, motion.

Circular motion

The basic *pluridirectional* motion is the circular pattern (Fig. 29-9). The circular motion does not blur by mere elongation (as in linear motion) but by evenly diffusing the densities of structures outside the focal plane over the focal plane image. Tomograms using a circular or other complex motion therefore exhibit more even contrast, but they show less contrast than linear tomograms with their characteristic linear streaking. All elements of the test pattern are equally blurred, regardless of their orientation. The circular motion maintains a constant radius and angle throughout the exposure, which results in a sharp cutoff margin of the blurred structures. This in turn may result in the formation of phantom images superimposed over the focal plane image.

The phenomenon of phantom images occurs more often in circular tomography using small angles, such as circular zonography. The phantom images are created by fusion of the margins of the blurred shadows of structures slightly outside the focal plane or by annular (circular) shadows of dense structures, again slightly outside the focal plane.

These phantom images are usually less dense and less distinct than the actual focal plane images. They can be identified as such on successive tomograms as the real structure(s) or come(s) into focus.

The characteristics of wide-angle circular tomography are identical to those of small-angle circular tomography, with one exception. The wider angle results in greater displacement of the blurred shadows, thereby reducing the possibility of phantom image formation.

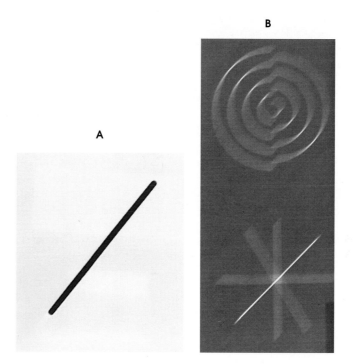

Fig. 29-8 A, Pinhole tracing of 45-degree oblique linear motion. **B,** Tomogram of test object at 45-degree oblique linear motion.

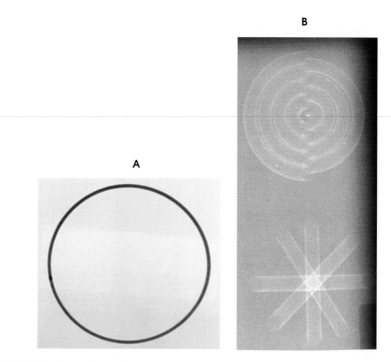

Fig. 29-9 Circular motion of 45 degrees. **A,** Pinhole tracing. **B,** Tomogram of test object demonstrating annular shadow formation and fusion of marginal blur pattern, which are characteristics of circular motion.

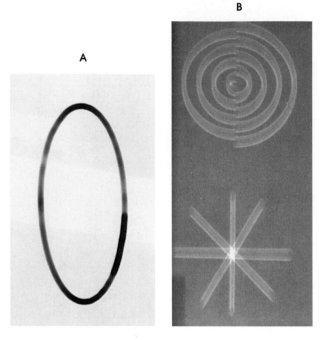

Fig. 29-10 Elliptic motion. **A,** Pinhole tracing. **B,** Tomogram of test object demonstrating characteristics of both linear and circular motions.

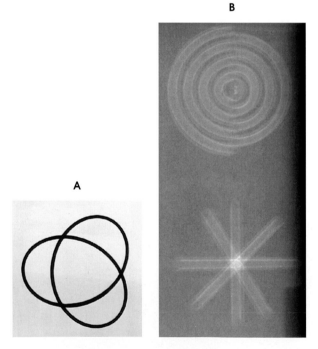

Fig. 29-11 Hypocycloidal motion. **A,** Pinhole tracing. **B,** Tomogram of test object demonstrating excellent blurring characteristics.

Elliptic motion

Because elliptic motion has both linear and circular aspects to its pattern, it exhibits the blurring characteristics of both (Fig. 29-10). It requires the same perpendicular orientation as linear motion and exhibits phantom shadow characteristics similar to both linear and circular motions. Although it is a more efficient blurring motion than the simple linear motion, the quality of blur is much less than in the circular motion or the more complex motions, hypocycloidal and spiral motion.

Hypocycloidal motion

Hypocycloidal motion (i.e., a compound type of continuous egg-shaped motion) offers excellent displacement of the marginal blur pattern, nearly eliminating the possibility of phantom image formation (Fig. 29-11). It provides excellent blurring of structures both close to and remote from the focal plane and has a focal plane thickness of slightly less than 1 mm.

Spiral motion

Tomographic equipment capable of producing a spiral motion is usually designed for a three-spired (trispiral) or five-spired motion (Fig. 29-12). The spiral motion, although different in pattern from the hypocycloidal motion, also offers excellent displacement of the marginal blur pattern, exceptional resolving power, and a section thickness of less than 1 mm.

These excellent blurring characteristics make both the hypocycloidal and spiral motion useful in tomographic examinations of any area of the body. They are especially useful in examinations of the skull, where structures are very small and compact and require greater separation of tissue planes (Fig. 29-13).

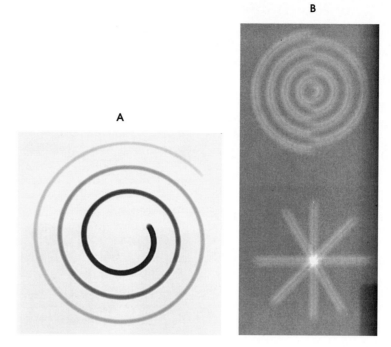

Fig. 29-12 Trispiral motion. **A,** Pinhole tracing. **B,** Tomogram of test object demonstrating excellent blurring characteristics.

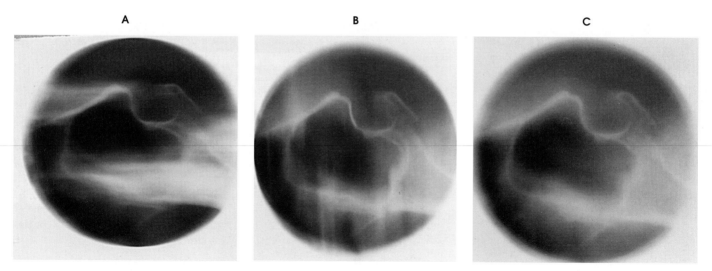

Fig. 29-13 Tomograms of sella turcica in lateral position through midplane. **A,** Transverse linear motion. **B,** Longitudinal linear motion. **C,** Trispiral motion demonstrating the sella turcica much more clearly and without the parasitic linear streaking found in **A** and **B**.

Factors Affecting the Tomographic Image

In 1976 Littleton[1] noted the following: "The difference between a high quality tomogram and a poor one is very slight; hence, it is extremely important that attention be given to all the parameters which contribute to the focal plane image." The factors that affect the tomographic image can be divided into two categories: (1) patient variables and (2) equipment variables.

PATIENT VARIABLES

As in conventional radiography, proper positioning of the patient and proper centering of the central ray are crucial. An equally important factor that must be considered in tomography is selection of the proper focal plane level. The part must be adequately immobilized because any motion adds unwanted blur to the focal plane image. Object size and the relative density of structures affect density and contrast of the image.

---

[1]Littleton JT: *Tomography: physical principles and clinical application,* Baltimore, 1976, Williams & Wilkins.

EQUIPMENT VARIABLES

The tomographic principle used affects several properties of the image, with magnification the factor most affected. Tomographic machines using the *fixed fulcrum,* or Grossman, principle maintain a constant magnification factor at any focal plane level, because the distance between the focal plane and cassette remains the same at any level. Conversely, with the *adjustable fulcrum,* or planigraphic, system, the focal plane-image receptor distance changes as the fulcrum height is varied, resulting in different magnification of the focal plane image at different fulcrum heights. However, at most working levels this magnification is less than the fixed rate of magnification of the fixed fulcrum machines.

The degree to which structures outside the focal plane are blurred is a function of the geometry of the blurring pattern and the angle of the tomographic arc. The more complex the blurring pattern, the greater the effacement of structures outside the focal plane. Wide exposure angles provide greater blurring of structures both close to and remote from the focal plane. The exposure angle also determines the thickness of the focal plane image. As previously mentioned, the wider the exposure angle, the thinner the section thickness, and, conversely, the narrower the exposure angle, the thicker the section thickness.

Each blurring pattern requires a specific amount of time to complete its motion. Therefore the exposure time must be sufficient to allow completion of the motion before termination of the exposure. Linear motions generally take less time to complete than do more complex pluridirectional movements. Exposure time is one half of the milliampere-second (mAs) formula, but because each pattern has different restrictions for certain exposure times, the mAs and kilovolt (peak) (kVp) must be altered to change the density. Because contrast levels are inherently low in tomography, high milliamperes and relatively low kVp techniques are used in most examinations to enhance the contrast between structures. Collimating to the smallest possible field size also improves the contrast of the image.

The focal spot size affects the recorded detail of the focal plane image. In areas in which great recorded detail is required, such as the skull, cervical spine, and limbs, the smallest available focal spot should be used. In other areas, fine recorded detail may not be required; therefore, to prolong the life of the x-ray tube, the large focal spot may be used when possible. The radiographer must take extreme care not to exceed the recommended tube limits or cooling rate.

Tomographic machines must provide synchronous, vibration-free movement of the tube and image receptor because any mechanical instability may transmit unwanted motion and create additional blur to the focal plane image. For this reason, most manufacturers have designed tomographic equipment to begin the exposure after the motion has begun, allowing enough time for any unwanted motion and vibration that may have been caused by the rapid acceleration of the tube and cassette to be stabilized. The exposure is then terminated just before the end of the movement to avoid any motion that may occur during the rapid deceleration of the tube and image receptor.

Because the thicknesses of image receptors vary with each manufacturer, one type of cassette should be used throughout the entire examination. Otherwise, the focal plane images will not be successively consistent from level to level because the height of the image receptor and therefore the focal plane image will vary with each image receptor.

The image receptor-speed combination greatly affects the tomographic image. Very low speed combinations produce images with very good recorded detail, but they require a greater amount of radiation. A faster combination produces images with good recorded detail and contrast with much less radiation. Other combinations using rare-earth intensifying screens produce radiographs with excellent detail but slightly lower contrast.

Equipment

Tomography machines may be varied in appearance and function, but all have certain common requirements. Aside from the usual features of any radiographic machine, such as an x-ray source, timer, and mAs and kVp selector, any x-ray machine capable of producing a tomographic image must have three additional features:

1. Some type of linkage connecting the x-ray source and image receptor carriage to provide synchronous, vibration-free movement of the tube and receptor in opposite directions during the tomographic exposure.
2. A means of imparting motion to the tube and receptor carriage for each different tomographic movement.
3. A means of adjusting the fulcrum height for tomograms at different levels.

As the x-ray tube moves in one direction, the image receptor carriage always moves in the opposite direction (Fig. 29-1). The receptor moves synchronously with the movement of the tube, maintaining a constant relationship with it. This mechanical type of linkage is the basic type of linkage that most tomographic machines use, from the simplest machines to highly sophisticated pluridirectional units. The major difference between the two is that in the pluridirectional machines, the simple metal rod is replaced by a heavier metal beam or a parallelogram of thick rods that attach at either end to the x-ray tube and image receptor carriage. The heavier material used for the linkage is required to withstand the great centrifugal force created by the tube and receptor carriage as it swings rapidly through the complex motions.

Advances in computer technology have made possible another type of linkage. Current manufacturers have developed a radiographic machine capable of linear tomography with no direct mechanical linkage between the tube and receptor carriage. The x-ray tube is mounted on the ceiling and is electronically linked to the image receptor carriage through a microcomputer. The microcomputer controls separate drive motors that maintain the tube and image receptor in alignment throughout the linear motion. This design allows for greater mobility of the x-ray tube for radiographic examinations because it is free floating when not in the tomographic mode, making it much more versatile than the standard radiographic/tomographic unit.

The second requirement is a means of imparting motion to the tube and image receptor carriage for each tomographic motion. Modern machines employ motors that drive the tube and receptor for the blurring movement. The motor drive and linkage mechanism must provide stable, vibration-free movement of the tube and image receptor. Any unwanted motion may cause additional blurring of the focal plane image.

All tomographic machines must also have some means of adjusting the height of the fulcrum. In machines using the adjustable or planigraphic principle, the motor drive alters the actual pivot point of the tube-image receptor carriage assembly by raising and lowering the axis of rotation. Tomographic machines using the fixed fulcrum, or Grossman, principle have a tabletop that is raised or lowered by a motor to the desired height.

Tomographic equipment has changed considerably since the early days of Vallebona and des Plantes. Their first machines were crude although ingeniously designed contrivances operated with ropes, pulleys, and hand cranks. Present-day equipment is motor driven and ranges from simple radiographic tables that can change into linear tomography devices to highly sophisticated machines designed primarily for pluridirectional tomography. The more elaborate tomographic machines offer several automatic functions such as automatic fulcrum height adjustment and motorized cassette shift for multiple exposures on one cassette. The pluridirectional machines are capable of several complex motions as well as simple linear movement.

TESTING OF TOMOGRAPHIC EQUIPMENT

Tomographic equipment is carefully checked and calibrated by the manufacturer's service representative when it is installed. The tube-image receptor tray movement must be stable and exactly balanced, and the travel time and exposure time at each of the exposure angles and tomographic movements must be synchronized. These are checked with a pinhole test device, a lead plate with a very small beveled hole in the middle. The device is positioned on the tabletop directly in line with the central ray; the pinholes must be placed either above or below the focal plane. The tomographic exposure is made, tracing on the image receptor the actual pattern of the tomographic motion used. Any mechanical instability or aberration in the correct exposure time can be noted on the pinhole tracing. (For examples of pinhole tracings, see Figs. 29-6 to 26-12.)

Another test device is the *tomographic test phantom.* This device is used to determine the accuracy of the fulcrum height indicator and the section thickness of the different exposure angles and blurring motions. The blurring characteristics of the different motions may also be determined with the phantom (see Figs. 29-6 and 29-13). Different phantoms are available, but most manufacturers of tomographic equipment recommend the test phantom developed by Dr. J. T. Littleton. This is the type of device used in Figs. 29-6 to 29-12.

Clinical Applications

Tomography is a proven diagnostic tool that can be of significant value when a definitive diagnosis cannot be made from conventional radiographs. This is because tomography can remove confusing shadows from the point of interest. Tomography may be used in any part of the body but is most effective in areas of high contrast such as bone and lung. Body-section radiography is used to demonstrate and evaluate a number of different pathologic processes, traumatic injuries, and congenital abnormalities. A basic familiarization with the clinical applications of tomography helps the tomographer to be more effective. Some of the major clinical applications of tomography are described in the following sections. However this versatile technique has other applications as well.

PATHOLOGIC PROCESSES IN SOFT TISSUES

Tomography is frequently used to demonstrate and evaluate benign processes and malignant neoplasms in the lungs. Benign lesions and malignancies cannot always be differentiated with conventional chest radiography. However, tomography is capable of defining the location, size, shape, and marginal contours of a lesion.

Benign lesions characteristically have smooth, well-marginated contours and frequently contain bits of calcium. The presence of calcium in a chest lesion usually confirms it as being benign. The benign lesions most commonly found in the lungs are granulomas, which form as a tissue reaction to a chronic infectious process that has healed.

Conversely, carcinogenic neoplasms characteristically have ill-defined margins that feather or streak into the surrounding tissue and rarely contain calcium (Figs. 29-14 and 29-15). Lung cancers may originate in the lung, in which case the neoplasm is termed a *primary malignancy*. Bronchogenic carcinoma is an example of a primary malignancy that may develop in the chest. Lung cancers may develop as the result of the spread of cancer from another area of the body to the lungs. These malignancies are termed *secondary,* or *metastatic, tumors*. Breast cancer, testicular cancer, and other malignancies may metastasize to the lungs.

When an apparent solitary nodule is noted on a conventional chest radiograph, the presence or exclusion of other lesions may be determined with general tomographic surveys of both lungs. These "whole-lung" or "full-lung" tomograms are used to exclude the possibility of metastatic disease from other organs. Frequently these lesions cannot be visualized by conventional radiographic techniques, and tomography is one means to identify these occult nodules. Demonstration of the number of tumors and their location, size, and relationship to other pulmonary structures is crucial to the physician's plan of treatment and the prognosis for the patient. Reexamination by tomography may be performed at a later date to check on the progress of the disease and the effectiveness of the therapy.

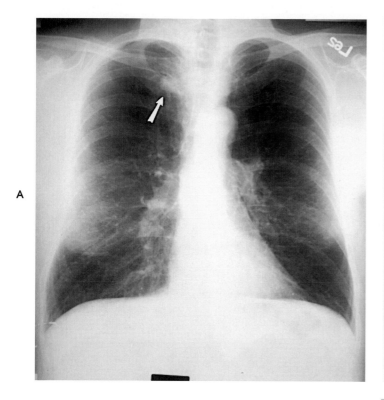

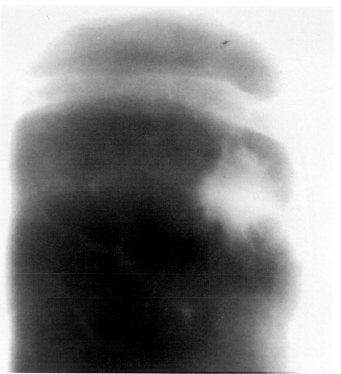

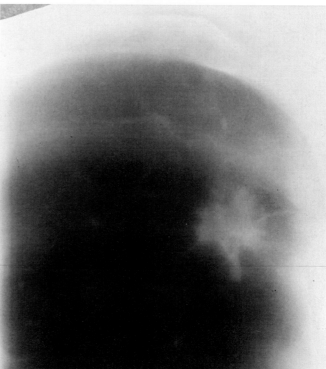

Fig. 29-14 A, PA chest radiograph demonstrating ill-defined density *(arrow)* in right upper chest. **B** and **C,** Collimated AP tomograms of patient in **A,** demonstrating lesion in posterior chest plane with ill-defined margins that feather or streak into surrounding lung tissue, characteristic of a malignant chest lesion.

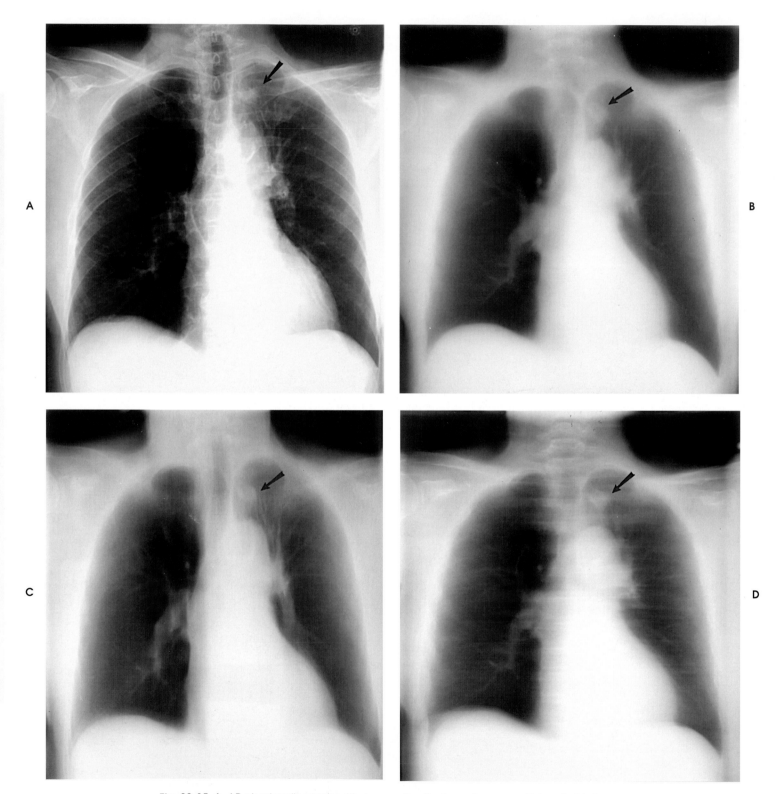

Fig. 29-15 A, AP chest radiograph with vague density *(arrow)* over medial end of left clavicle. **B** to **D,** AP full-lung tomograms of patient in **A,** taken to exclude the possibility of other occult lesions. **B,** Trispiral tomogram ³/₈ inch (1 cm) anterior to hilar plane at level of tumor. Radiographic appearance of lesion *(arrow)* is consistent with malignant chest neoplasm. **C,** Longitudinal linear tomogram of 40 degrees at same fulcrum level as **B.** Visualization of lesion *(arrow)* is decreased because of linear streaking and incomplete blurring of other structures outside the focal plane. **D,** A 40-degree transverse linear tomogram at the same level as **B** and **C,** again demonstrating poor visualization of lesion *(arrow)* because of linear blurring characteristics. Blurring of anterior ribs is incomplete.

PULMONARY HILA

Neoplasms involving the pulmonary hila are effectively evaluated by tomography, which can determine if and to what degree the individual bronchi are patent or obstructed. This partial or complete obstruction may occur when a neoplasm develops within the bronchus and bulges into the bronchial airspace when a tumor grows adjacent to the bronchus. As the lesion grows, it may press against the bronchus, reducing the size of the lumen and thus restricting or obstructing airflow to that part of the lung. Pneumonia, atelectasis, and other inflammatory or reactive changes that may occur with the obstruction may further hinder conventional imaging of this area. Demonstration of bronchial patency through a density is strong evidence that the lesion is inflammatory and not malignant (Fig. 29-16).

SOFT TISSUE LESIONS AFFECTING BONY STRUCTURES

Tomography is also used to demonstrate and evaluate soft tissue neoplasms in the presence of bony structures. Because of the high density of bone and the relatively low density of soft tissue neoplasms, the actual lesion usually cannot be demonstrated, but the bony destruction caused by the tumor may be demonstrated with great clarity.

For example, neoplasms involving the pituitary gland (e.g., pituitary adenoma) usually cause bony changes or destruction of the floor of the sella turcica, which indicates the presence of a pituitary adenoma. In addition to showing destruction caused by the tumor, tomography can demonstrate bony septations in the sphenoidal sinus, which aids the surgeon in removal of the tumor (Fig. 29-17).

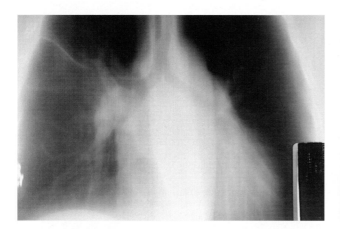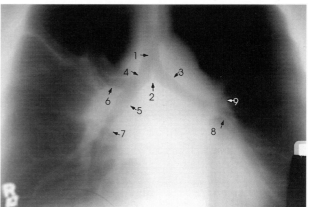

Fig. 29-16 Normal branchotomogram through midplane of hilum. **A,** Linear tomogram. **B,** Trispiral tomogram demonstrating the hilar structures more clearly: *1,* trachea; *2,* carina; *3,* left main bronchus; *4,* right main bronchus; *5,* intermediate bronchus; *6,* right upper lobe bronchus; *7,* right lower lobe bronchus; *8,* left lower lobe bronchus; *9,* left upper lobe bronchus.

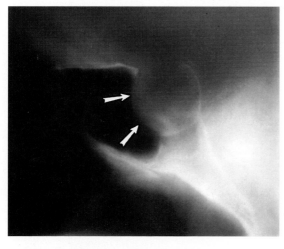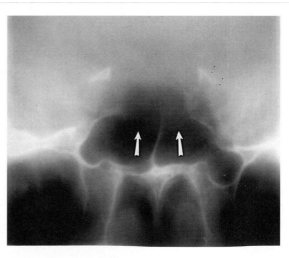

Fig. 29-17 Tomograms through midplane of sella turcica demonstrating destruction of floor *(arrows)* caused by a pituitary adenoma. **A,** Lateral tomogram. **B,** AP tomogram.

LESIONS IN BONE

Subtle changes that may occur as a result of a pathologic process in bone tissue may be noted on conventional radiographs, but in many instances only tomography can determine the true nature and extent of the involvement (Fig. 29-18). Pathologic processes involving bony structures are normally characterized by bone destruction and changes in bone tissue or surface margins. More specifically, in tomography an attempt is made to identify the extent of bone destruction; the status of the cortex of the bone (i.e., whether destruction extends through the cortical bone); the presence of any periosteal reaction to the lesion, changes in the bone matrix, new bone formation; and the status of the zone between diseased and normal bone.

Destruction or other alterations of bone may result from a multitude of benign or malignant processes that manifest themselves in different ways. Some benign processes such as osteomyelitis are characterized by areas of bone destruction, whereas others such as osteomas appear as abnormal growths of bone from bone tissue. Some processes may exhibit a combination of bone destruction and new growth, as occurs in Paget's disease and rheumatoid arthritis.

Malignant neoplasms in bone tissue may occur in the form of primary lesions or secondary lesions resulting from the metastatic spread of cancer from another area of the body. Some forms of cancer occurring in bone exhibit areas of both destruction and new growth, whereas others exhibit only areas of extensive destruction.

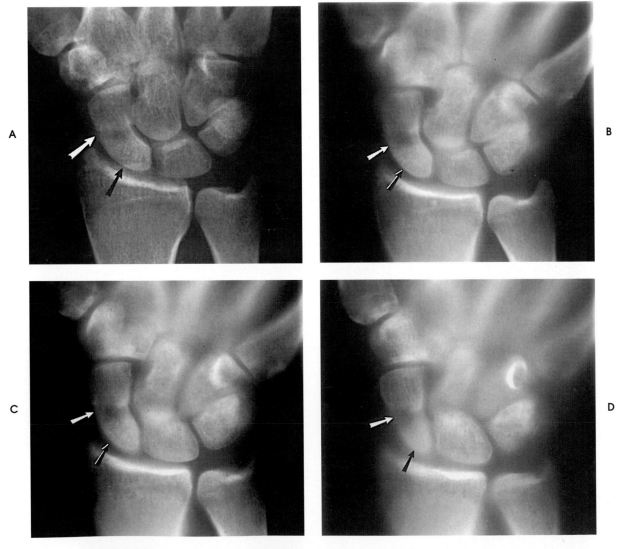

Fig. 29-18 A, PA wrist radiograph demonstrating healing fracture *(white arrow)* of scaphoid bone and increased density *(black arrow)* of proximal end. **B** through **D,** Tomograms at 3-mm intervals demonstrating fracture site *(white arrows)* with dense area *(black arrows)* of sclerotic bone at proximal end of scaphoid bone, consistent with aseptic necrosis.

FRACTURES

The three major clinical applications for tomography when dealing with known and suspected fractures are (1) identification and evaluation of occult fractures, (2) better evaluation of known fractures, and (3) evaluation of the healing process of fractures.

Occult fractures

If a fracture is suspected clinically but cannot be ruled out or identified by conventional imaging techniques, tomography may be indicated. Tomography is often used when fractures are suspected in areas of complex bone structures such as the cervical spine. The cervical spine projects a myriad of confusing shadows, often hiding fracture lines and making an accurate diagnosis impossible. Tomography can identify and evaluate these occult fractures (Fig. 29-19). Knowledge of these fractures can be crucial to the plan of treatment and the prognosis for the patient.

The skull is another area that frequently requires tomographic evaluation for occult fractures. The skull has many complicated bone structures that often make identification and evaluation of fractures extremely difficult without the use of tomography. The facial nerve canal that courses through the temporal bone is just one of many areas that are difficult to evaluate for fractures without tomography. Blowout fractures of the orbital floor also frequently require tomographic evaluation because of the difficulty in identifying and evaluating fractures and fragments of the thin bones composing the floor and medial wall of the orbit (Fig. 29-20).

Known fractures

Tomography may also be used to evaluate known fractures with greater efficiency than is possible with conventional radiography. In some instances a fracture may be visualized on a conventional radiograph, but because of the complex nature of the fracture or superimposition of shadows from adjacent structures, the fracture site cannot be adequately evaluated without the use of tomography. This is often the case in hip fractures involving the acetabulum. In acetabular fractures, portions of the acetabulum are often broken into many fragments that may be difficult to identify. With tomography the fragments and any possible femoral fracture can be evaluated before an attempt is made to reduce the fracture.

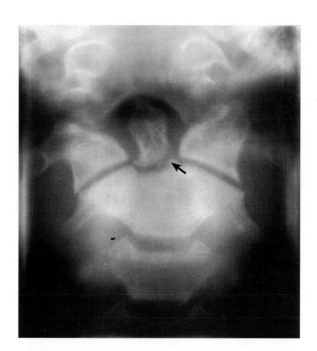

Fig. 29-19 AP tomogram of C1-C3 demonstrating complete fracture at base of dens *(arrow)*.

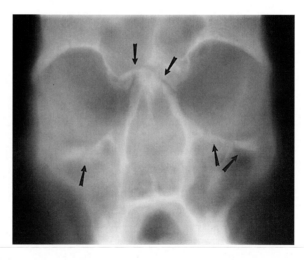

Fig. 29-20 Frontal tomogram using reverse Caldwell method, demonstrating multiple facial fractures *(arrows)*.

Healing fractures

Tomography may also be used to evaluate the healing process of fractures when conventional imaging techniques prove inadequate because of overlying shadows of fixation devices, adjacent structures, or bone callus. In these situations, tomography may be essential to assess whether the bone is healing properly throughout the fracture site. Tomography also can identify areas of incomplete healing in the fracture (Fig. 29-21).

ABDOMINAL STRUCTURES

Because of the relatively homogeneous densities of abdominal structures, both radiographic and tomographic imaging of this area are most effectively performed in conjunction with the use of contrast materials. Zonography is usually preferred for tomographic evaluation of these organs. As previously stated, zonography produces focal plane images of greater contrast than is possible with thin-section tomography. This increased level of contrast aids in visualization of the relatively low-density organs of the abdomen. The extensive blurring of remote structures that occurs with wide-angle tomography is not necessary in the abdomen because relatively few high-density structures exist in this area to compromise the zonographic imaging of the abdominal structures. Thick sections of organs are depicted with each zonogram, and entire organs can be demonstrated in a small number of tomographic sections.

A circular motion with an exposure angle of 8 or 10 degrees is recommended for use in the abdomen. Occasionally, an angle of 15 degrees may be necessary to eliminate bowel-gas shadows if the smaller angle does not provide adequate effacement (blurring) of the bowel.

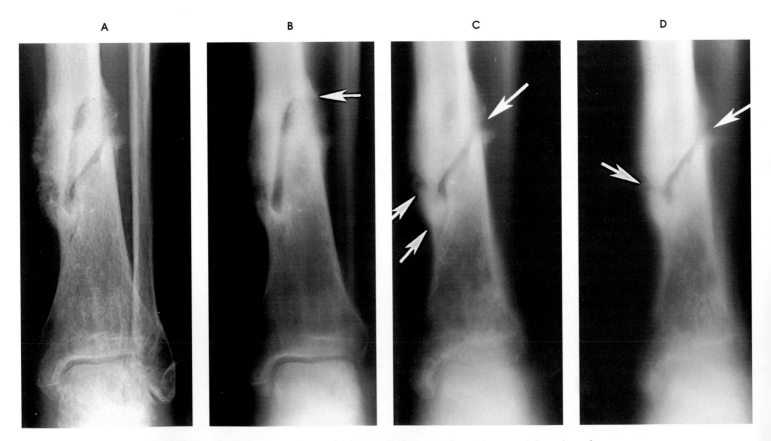

Fig. 29-21 A, AP distal tibia radiograph demonstrating questionable complete union of fractures. **B,** AP tomogram of same patient as in **A,** demonstrating incomplete union of longitudinal fracture *(arrow).* **C** and **D,** Tomograms demonstrating incomplete union of oblique fractures *(arrows)* through shaft of tibia of same patient as in **A** and **B. C,** Tomogram obtained 0.5 cm to **B. D,** Tomogram obtained ³/₈ inch (1 cm) posterior to **B.**

Zonography using a linear movement is not recommended because it does not provide adequate blurring of structures outside the focal plane. If a linear movement is employed, an exposure angle of 15 degrees should be used to provide adequate blurring. Linear tomography does not produce accurate focal plane images because of the incomplete blurring effect of structures oriented parallel to the tube movement. Although the possibility of false image formation exists with circular tomography, the image of the focal plane is far more accurate than with linear tomography. Linear tomograms are higher in contrast than circular tomograms, but this is actually a result of the linear streaking caused by the incomplete blurring characteristics of linear motion. Circular motion, on the other hand, produces an accurate focal plane image with slightly less but even contrast.

The most common tomographic examinations of the abdomen are of the kidneys and biliary tract. These examinations are normally performed with contrast material.

Renal tomography

Many institutions include tomography of the kidneys as part of the intravenous urography (IVU) procedure (Fig. 29-22). The tomograms are usually taken immediately after bolus injection of the contrast material. At this time the kidney is entering the nephrogram phase of the IVU, in which the nephrons of the kidney begin to absorb the contrast material, causing the parenchyma of the kidney to become somewhat radiopaque. Zonography may then be used to demonstrate lesions in the kidney that may have been overlooked with conventional radiography.

Another typical renal tomographic examination is the nephrotomogram. The major difference between this and the IVU is the method of introduction of the contrast material. In nephrotomography the contrast material is drip-infused throughout the examination instead of introduced in a single bolus injection. This method allows for a considerably longer nephrographic effect because the nephrons opacify the kidney as they continuously absorb and excrete the contrast material.

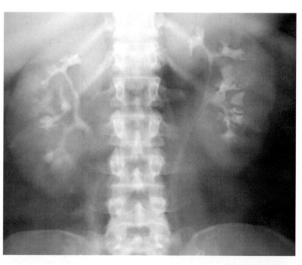

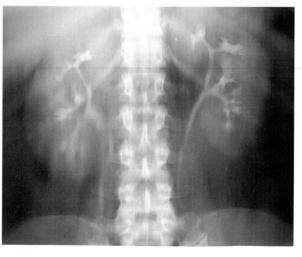

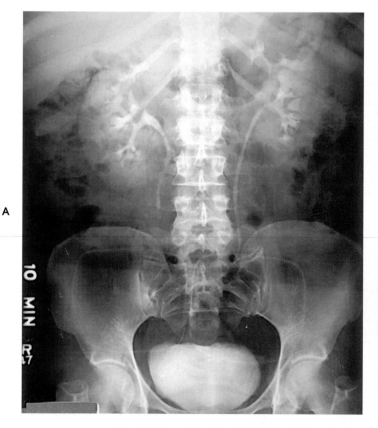

Fig. 29-22 A, IVU, AP abdomen radiograph. Bowel shadows obscure kidneys.
B, AP tomogram of same patient as in **A,** obtained through midplane of kidneys using 8-degree circular motion. Bowel shadows are absent, and compared with **C,** visualization of kidneys is improved. **C,** AP tomogram of same patients as in **A** and **B** and at same levels as in **B,** but employing 20-degree linear motion. Note linear streaking and loss of detail of collecting systems and kidney borders.

Intravenous cholangiograms

The biliary tract is another organ system that may require tomography for adequate evaluation. If an oral cholecystogram does not yield sufficient information for a diagnosis or if biliary ductal disease is suspected in a patient after cholecystectomy, an intravenous cholangiogram (IVC) may be indicated. The IVC is performed by infusing a solution of the contrast material Cholografin into the bloodstream, where it is first absorbed into and then excreted by the liver into the biliary ducts. The drip infusion should be administered slowly over approximately 20 to 30 minutes to reduce the possibility of anaphylactic shock.

Opacification of the ducts is generally not great enough for adequate evaluation with conventional radiography alone. The ducts may also be partially or completely obscured by the superimposition of structures in the abdomen. Even if the ducts may be well opacified on conventional radiographs, tomography should be performed to obtain information not provided by conventional radiography (Fig. 29-23).

Zonography is normally used for IVCs. Sometimes, however, more blurring or a thinner tomographic section is desired. For those instances a trispiral or hypocycloidal motion may be preferred. If a linear motion is to be employed, an exposure angle of 15 to 20 degrees should be used.

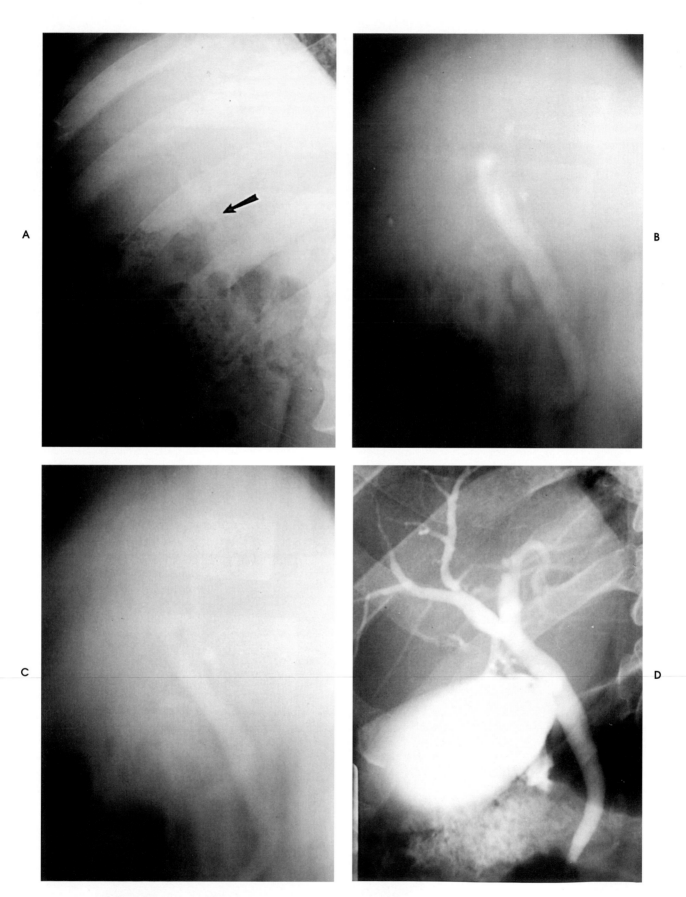

Fig. 29-23 A, IVC, AP oblique projection, RPO body position. Faintly opacified common bile duct *(arrow)* is obscured by bowel gas and liver. **B** and **C,** RPO tomograms of same patients as in **A** through level of common bile duct. Visualization of duct is improved over the plain image study in **A. D,** Transhepatic cholangiogram of same patient as in **A** to **C.**

Basic Principles of Positioning

Rarely in conventional radiography does one single radiographic image contain all the diagnostic information necessary to make an accurate diagnosis. This is also true in tomography; one series of tomograms in a single plane usually does not contain enough information to make an accurate diagnosis. As in radiography, two or more image planes are usually required for most tomographic examinations. For bilateral structures such as the internal acoustic canals, only one radiograph may be used. In such cases, tomograms of the contralateral side are obtained for comparison.

Many fundamental radiographic body positions are used in tomography. The AP and lateral projections are basic to most tomographic examinations. Occasionally a special oblique projection may be necessary for optimal visualization of the part under investigation. The radiographer should observe the following positioning guidelines:

- In tomography, orient the structures either parallel or perpendicular to the tomographic plane. For example, when evaluating structures in the base of the skull, position the patient's head for a basal projection so that the base of the skull is oriented parallel to the section plane. This parallel position not only produces images that are more anatomically correct but also reduces the total number of tomograms necessary to cover the area of interest. If the base of the skull is not parallel but is slightly oblique, more tomograms are required to evaluate the area of interest adequately. This also pertains to other areas of the body in which large, relatively flat surfaces occur, such as in long bones.
- When producing tomograms of long bones such as the femur, adjust the long axis of the bone to be parallel to the tomographic plane.
- For some structures such as the sella turcica, use a perpendicular orientation for tomography. Because the presence of a pituitary adenoma usually affects the floor of the sella, orient the floor perpendicular to the section plane. AP and lateral radiographs are routinely used; for both images, the floor remains perpendicular to the tomographic plane.

Very few areas in radiology place greater demand on the knowledge and ability of the radiographer than the field of tomography. The tomographer must possess a strong background and understanding of anatomy and the spatial relationships of the structures of the body (see Chapter 27). The tomographic radiographer must know where certain structures of the general body parts are located, the best way to position those structures for tomographic examination, the depth at which particular structures are located, and the way the tomographic image should look. On many occasions, even experienced tomographers must rely heavily on the knowledge and instruction of the radiologist monitoring the examination. The radiographer and radiologist should work together closely because no two tomographic examinations are exactly alike and each patient must be considered individually. The radiographer should observe the following guidelines when assisting with the tomographic examination:

- Provide the radiologist with an adequate clinical history of the patient. If this information is not provided on the examination requisition, obtain it by studying the patient's medical records or interviewing the patient.
- Review and discuss this clinical information and any pertinent radiographs with the radiologist before beginning the examination. After reviewing the information, the radiologist and radiographer can then decide on the area of interest, the optimum position, the size of the field of exposure, the type of blurring motion and exposure angle to be used, the separation intervals between tomographic sections, and the parameters for the fulcrum height. The most complex motion available should be used whenever possible.
- Complete all equipment preparation before positioning the patient. This reduces the amount of time that the patient is required to maintain an often uncomfortable position.

- Briefly and simply explain the procedure to the patient, and offer a rough estimate of the expected length of the examination. Many patients are under the mistaken impression that the procedure consists of a few radiographs taken in a matter of minutes and that they will then be permitted to leave. They are not aware that they will be required to maintain a certain position throughout the procedure. The patient who knows what to expect will be better able to cooperate throughout the lengthy examination.
- Ensure the patient's comfort, which is extremely important. The use of a suitable table pad is recommended for tomographic examinations. A table pad that is $1\frac{1}{2}$ inches (3.8 cm) thick adds an insignificant amount to the overall patient thickness and greatly increases the patient's comfort. If uncomfortable, even the most cooperative patient will be unable to hold still for the examination.
- When needed, use angle sponges and foam blocks to help the patient maintain the correct position. Do not, however, use foam sponges in tomographic examinations of the head. Section intervals of 1 or 2 mm are often employed in this area, and foam sponges do not give firm enough support to the head. With little change in pressure the head may move, drastically altering the desired focal plane levels. Use folded towels to support the head if needed; they offer greater resistance to any downward pressure.

Immobilization Techniques

The most effective immobilization technique is the radiographer's instructions to the patient. No amount of physical restraint can keep patients from moving if they do not fully understand the importance of holding still from the first preliminary image to the end of the tomographic series. The radiographer should observe the following guidelines:

- Because suspension of respiration is mandatory in examinations of the chest and abdomen, give explicit breathing instructions to the patient for examinations of these areas.
- In chest tomography, instruct the patient to take a consistent, uniform deep breath for each tomogram. Caution the patient not to strain to take in the maximum breath because the patient may have difficulty in holding the breath during the exposure. Tell the patient to take a moderately deep breath that can be comfortably held for the duration of the tomographic exposure. This not only allows for optimum inflation of the lungs but also provides consistency between the focal plane levels throughout the tomographic series. Consistency in inspirations is vitally important if the area of interest is located near the diaphragm. Slight variations in the amount of air taken in may result in obscuring of the area of interest by the elevated diaphragm. Suspension of respiration is also necessary to prevent blurring of structures by the breathing motion.
- Have the patient suspend respiration in the expiratory phase in examinations of the abdomen to elevate the diaphragm and visualize more of the abdomen. As in chest tomography, the suspension of respiration assists in maintaining consistency in tissue planes and reduces motion artifacts.

- Use suspended respiration techniques in tomographic examinations of the head if needed. Unwanted motion of the head may occur when obese patients or patients with large breasts are positioned in the right anterior oblique (RAO) body position for lateral skull tomography. This problem may be resolved by having the patient suspend respiration during the exposure or by turning the patient over into a left posterior oblique (LPO) body position.
- Mark the entrance point of the central ray on the patient's skin. If the patient moves, this mark can be used as a reference point for repositioning, eliminating the need to take another scout image to recheck the position. If the mark is made with a grease pencil, it can easily be removed after the examination.
- When performing tomographic examination of the skull in the lateral position, place a small midline mark on the patient's nasion to facilitate measuring for the midline tomogram and to recheck the position between the scout image and the actual tomographic series. By ensuring that this mark is still at the same level from the tabletop, the interpupillary line is still perpendicular to the tabletop, and the central ray is still entering at the reference mark, the correct position can be maintained throughout the examination.

Scout Tomograms

Three preliminary tomograms are usually taken to locate the correct levels for the tomographic series. One tomogram is taken at the level presumed to be at the middle of the structure or area to be examined. The other two scout tomograms are taken at levels higher and lower than this midline tomogram. The separation interval between these tomograms depends on the thickness of the structure. Tomograms of small structures such as those found in the skull may be made at 5-mm or 1-cm intervals for the preliminary images. After the correct planes have been determined, the tomographic series is taken at smaller intervals. When the total depth of the area of interest is several centimeters thick, the separation interval for these scout tomograms is increased to 3/4 inch (1.9 cm) or more. Table 29-1 includes separation intervals for the preliminary tomograms and tomographic series. The following guidelines are observed:

Use external landmarks as reference points to assist in determining the proper fulcrum level.

- In some cases, such as chest lesions that can be identified on PA and lateral chest radiographs, take measurements from these radiographs to aid in the selection of the scout tomogram levels. For example, to determine the proper level for AP tomography of a chest lesion, measure the distance on the conventional lateral chest radiograph from the posterior chest wall to the middle of the lesion. Add this distance to the thickness of the table pad. Ensure that a scout tomogram taken at this fulcrum height is in the middle of the lesion.
- Use a similar process for tomography in the lateral position, taking the measurements from the AP chest radiograph.
- If the area of interest is not localized on the scout images, take a plain radiograph using the same centering as for the preliminary tomograms. This confirms that the area of interest is actually in the collimated field of interest and recentering is not required.

TABLE 29-1

Positioning for tomography

Examination part	Projection	Central ray position	Preliminary tomographic levels	Separation intervals	Comments
Sella turcica	AP	Glabella	1.5, 2.5, and 3.5 cm anterior to tragus	2 mm	Shield eyes
	Lateral	2.5 cm anterior and superior to tragus	−1, 0, and +1 cm to midline of skull	2 mm	Place water bag under patient's chin for support
Middle ear (internal acoustic canal, facial nerve canal)	AP	Midpoint between inner and outer canthi	−0.5, 0, and +0.5 mm to tip of tragus	1 or 2 mm	Shield eyes
	Lateral	5 mm posterior and superior to external acoustic canal	At level of outer canthus and 1 and 2 cm medial	1 or 2 mm	Place water bag under patient's chin for support
Paranasal sinuses (general survey) and orbital floors	Reverse Caldwell	Intersection of midsagittal plane and infra-orbital rims	−2, 0, and +2 cm to level of outer canthus	3 to 5 mm	Infraorbitomeatal line should be perpendicular to tabletop
	Lateral	2 cm posterior to outer canthus	−3 and +3 cm to midline of skull	3 to 5 mm	Place water bag under patient's chin for support
Base of skull	Submentovertex	Midpoint between angles of mandible	−1, 0, and +1 cm	2 or 3 mm	Orbitomeatal line should be parallel to tabletop
Cervical spine	AP	To vertebral body/bodies of interest	0, −2, and −4 cm to external acoustic meatus	3 or 5 mm	
	Lateral	To vertebral body/bodies of interest	−2, 0, and +2 cm from midline of back	3 or 5 mm	Place water bag under patient's chin for support and two or more on neck to equalize density for entire cervical spine
Thoracic spine	AP	To vertebral body/bodies of interest	3, 5, and 7 cm from tabletop	5 mm	Flex knees slightly to straighten spine
	Lateral	To vertebral body(ies) of interest	−2 and +2 cm from midline of back	5 mm	Flex knees, and place sponge against patient's back for support

TABLE 29-1

Positioning for tomography—cont'd

Examination part	Projection	Central ray position	Preliminary tomographic levels	Separation intervals	Comments
Lumbar spine	AP	To vertebral body/bodies of interest	4, 7, and 10 cm from tabletop	5 mm	Flex knees slightly to straighten spine
	Lateral	To vertebral body/bodies of interest	−2, 0, and +2 cm from midline of back	5 mm	Flex knees and place sponge against patient's back for support
Hip	AP	Head of femur	−2, 0, and +2 cm for greater trochanter	5 mm	Place water bag over area of greater trochanter to equalize density to hip
	Lateral (frog leg)	Head femur	5, 7, and 9 cm from tabletop	5 mm	Place water bag over area of femoral neck to equalize density
Limbs	AP and lateral	At area of interest	5 mm to 1.5 cm, depending on size of limb	2 to 5 mm	Adjust limb to be parallel to tabletop
Chest (whole lung and hila)	AP	9 to 12 cm below sternal notch	10, 11, and 12 cm above tabletop	1 cm	Use through filter (80 to 90 kVp)
	Lateral	Midchest at level of pulmonary hila	−5, 0, and +5 cm from midline of back	1 cm	Place sponge against patient's back for support
Chest (localized lesion)	AP and lateral	Measure distance to lesion from chest wall on plain radiographs, and center at this point on patient	Measure distance to lesion on lateral chest image and thickness of table pad; −2, 0, and +2 cm from measurement	2, 3, or 5 cm	Use low kVp (50 to 65) for high contrast
Nephrotomogram	AP	Midpoint between xiphoid process and top of iliac crests	7 cm for small patient; 9 cm for average patient; 11 cm for large patient	1 cm	Use 8 to 10 degrees of circular movement or 15 to 20 degrees of linear movement
Intravenous cholangiogram	AP oblique, 20 degree right posterior oblique (RPO)	10 cm lateral to lumbar spine	10, 12, and 14 cm for small patient; 12, 14, and 16 cm for average patient; 13, 16, and 19 cm for large patient	5 mm to 1 cm	Use 8 to 10 degrees of circular movement or 15 to 20 degrees of linear movement

General Rules for Tomography

The following rules are essential:
- Know the anatomy involved.
- Position the patient as precisely as possible.
- Use proper immobilization techniques.
- Use a small focal spot for tomography of the head and neck and limbs.
- Use a large focal spot for other areas of the body where fine recorded detail is not crucial.
- Use low kVp when high contrast is desired.
- Use high kVp when contrast differences between structures must be reduced; for example, whole-lung tomography requires a high kVp-80 to 90 kVp-in conjunction with a trough filter.
- When necessary, use water or flour bags to absorb primary or secondary radiation. For example, in lateral cervical spine tomography, place the bags on the upper cervical spine area to reduce the density difference between the spine and dense shoulders. Collimate the beam as tightly as possible to reduce patient exposure and improve contrast.
- Shield the patient, especially the eyes, in examinations of the skull and upper cervical spine.
- Use the proper blurring motion. In general, use the most complex blurring motion available. If zonography is required, use a circular motion. If only linear motion is available, take care to orient the part correctly to the direction of the tube.
- Mark each tomogram with the correct layer height. This may be done by directly exposing lead numbers on each tomogram or by marking each tomogram after it is processed. Another technique is to shift vertically the right or left marker used on each successive image. If the level of the first image is known, the correct level for each successive image can be determined. If multiple tomograms are taken on one image receptor, follow the same shift sequence to avoid confusion in marking the layer heights.

TOMOGRAPHY OF THE SKULL

Strict immobilization techniques must be used for any tomographic examination of the skull. Reference points should be marked on the patient for rechecking of the position.

The basic skull positions are outlined in the following sections and are to be used in conjunction with Table 29-1.

AP projection
- Adjust the patient's head to align the orbitomeatal line (OML) and the midsagittal plane perpendicular to the tabletop.
- Ensure that the distances from the tabletop to each tragus (the tonguelike projection of the ear just in front of the external acoustic meatus) are equal; this indicates that the head is positioned perfectly.

AP projection: reverse Caldwell method
- Position the infraorbitomeatal line (IOML) and the midsagittal plane perpendicular to the tabletop.
- Ensure that the tragi are equidistant from the tabletop.

Lateral projection
- Position the midsagittal plane parallel to the tabletop.
- Ensure that the interpupillary line is perpendicular to the tabletop.
- Check that the OML is approximately parallel to the lower border of the image receptor.

TOMOGRAPHY OF OTHER BODY PARTS

Standard radiographic projections (AP, lateral, and oblique) are used for most areas of the body. The same general rules of tomography apply to all areas. In general the projection that best demonstrates the area of interest in a conventional radiograph is usually the best for tomography. Selected tomograms are shown in Figs. 29-24 to 29-29.

Information on panoramic tomography, which is used to demonstrate the entire mandible and temporomandibular joint using one tomographic type of exposure, is provided in Chapter 21 of this atlas.

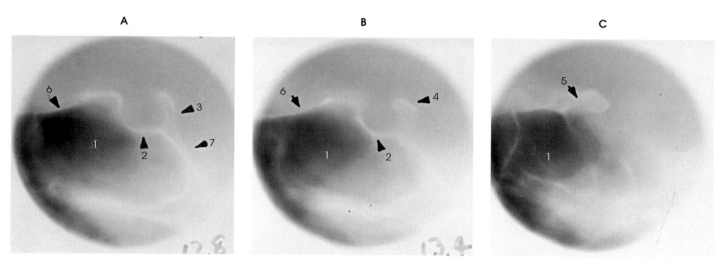

Fig. 29-24 Lateral sella turcica. **A,** Tomogram through midplane of sella. **B,** Tomogram 5 mm lateral to **A**. **C,** Tomogram ⅜ inch (1 cm) lateral to **A**. *1,* Sphenoidal sinus; *2,* floor of sella; *3,* dorsum sellae; *4,* posterior clinoid process; *5,* anterior clinoid process; *6,* planum sphenoidale; *7,* clivus.

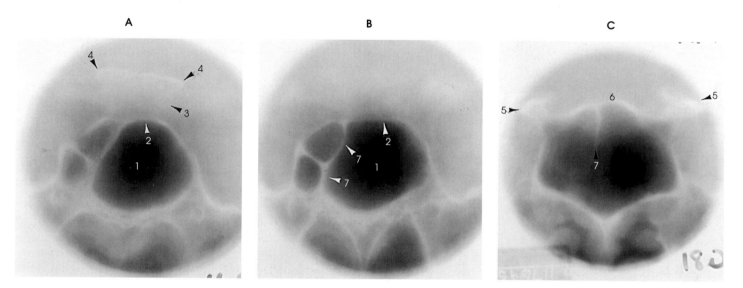

Fig. 29-25 AP tomograms of sella turcica. **A,** Tomogram in posterior plane of sella turcica. **B,** Tomogram 3/8 inch (1 cm) anterior to **A**, demonstrating floor of sella. **C,** Tomogram 2 cm anterior to **A**, demonstrating anterior clinoid processes. *1,* Sphenoidal sinus; *2,* floor of sella; *3,* dorsum sellae; *4,* posterior clinoid processes; *5,* anterior clinoid processes; *6,* planum sphenoidale; *7,* septations of sphenoidal sinus.

A   B   C

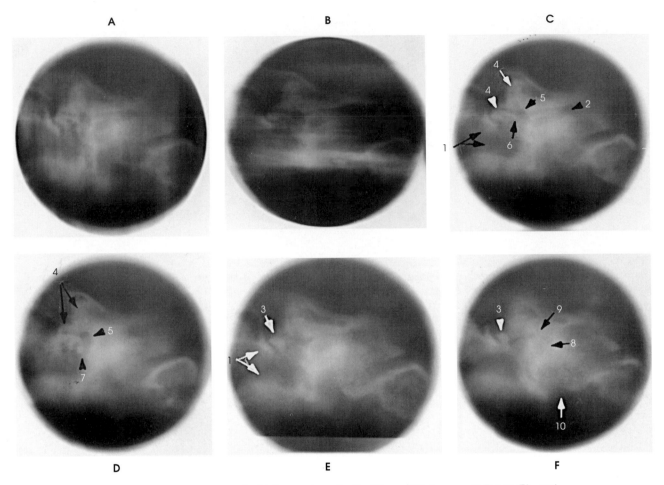

D   E   F

Fig. 29-26 AP tomograms of middle ear. Longitudinal linear (**A**), transverse linear (**B**), and trispiral (**C**) motion are at same posterior level of middle ear. Note improved visualization of structures with trispiral motion. AP tomograms anterior to level of **C** by 2 mm (**D**), 4 mm (**E**), and 6 mm (**F**). *1*, External acoustic canal; *2*, internal acoustic canal; *3*, ossicular mass, including malleus, incus, and lateral and superior semicircular canals; *4*, acoustic ossicles; *5*, vestibule; *6*, fenestra vestibuli; *7*, fenestra cochlea; *8*, cochlea; *9*, cochlea portion of facial nerve canal; *10*, carotid canal.

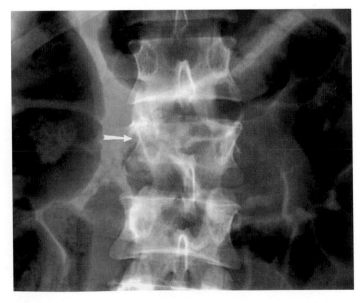

Fig. 29-27 AP lumbar spine showing suspected fracture (*arrow*) of L2 (see Fig. 29-28).

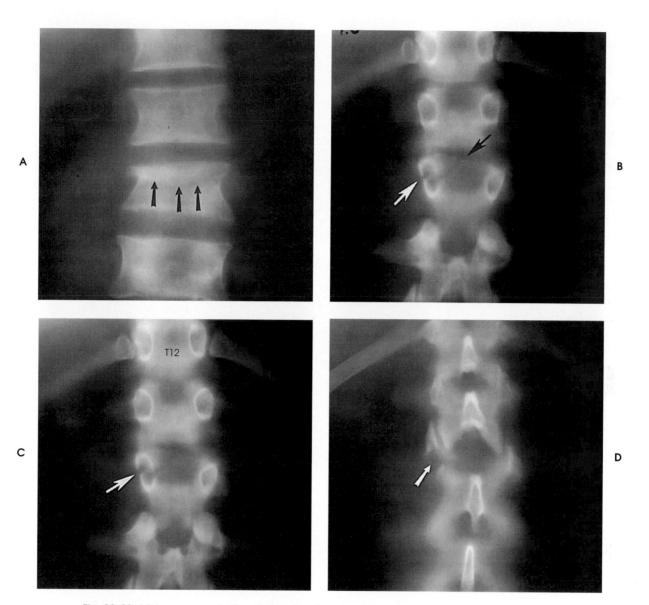

Fig. 29-28 AP tomograms further delineating fracture site shown in AP radiograph in Fig. 29-27. **A,** Tomogram through anterior plane of vertebral body, demonstrating wedging of vertebral body of L2 (*arrows*). **B,** AP tomogram 2 cm posterior to **A** through lane of pedicles. Fracture line extends through right pedicle *(white arrow)* and vertebral body *(black arrow)*. **C,** AP tomogram 3 cm posterior to **A**, demonstrating displacement of fracture *(arrow)*. **D,** AP tomogram 4 cm posterior to **A**, demonstrating displaced fracture *(arrow)* of superior articular process of L3.

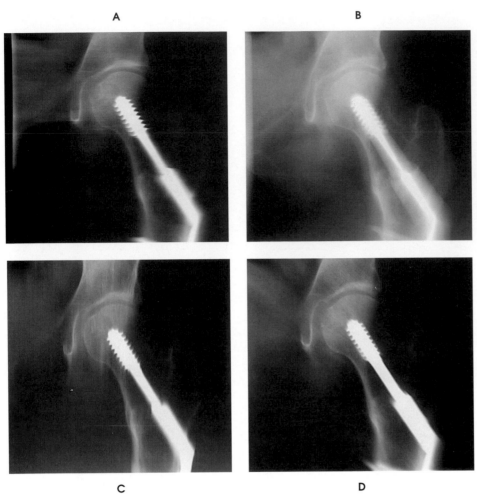

A

B

C

D

Fig. 29-29 AP tomograms of hip with fixation device at same level, comparing different blurring motions: **A,** Trispiral; **B,** circular; **C,** longitudinal linear; **D,** oblique linear.

Conclusion

Tomography has changed dramatically since the early days of Bocage and des Plantes. Their crude devices bear little resemblance to today's modern tomographic machines. Tomography has been widely accepted as an extremely useful diagnostic tool. Linear tomographic machines can now usually be found in even the smallest hospitals. Many large hospitals have one or more linear units in addition to a pluridirectional machine.

Computed tomography (CT) and magnetic resonance imaging (MRI) have certainly proved themselves as extremely valuable diagnostic tools, and in most cases their images are far superior to those of conventional tomography. However, in many instances tomography can provide sufficient information for an accurate diagnosis at a cost far less than that of the more sophisticated imaging modalities. Furthermore, most MRI and CT scanners are extremely busy, and many cannot handle the high workload. Conventional tomography can often answer diagnostic questions satisfactorily or at least screen patients for further evaluation by the other, more sophisticated imaging modalities.

Although many equipment manufacturers still market a variety of x-ray machines capable of performing linear tomography, the more expensive, complex motion tomography units have been dropped from their product lines. In this era of cost containment, most health care facilities can ill afford to dedicate a piece of radiographic equipment solely for conventional tomography. Equipment manufacturers have taken note of this and have responded accordingly. Most equipment companies now offer a variety of tomographic options to their line of radiographic and fluoroscopic and fixed radiographic units.

"Add-on" tomography devices of the twenty-first century look nothing like their crude predecessors, with their long metal bar attachments with sliding sleeves and thumbscrews to adjust fulcrum heights. The new units are simple to connect and usually provide push-button control for adjusting amplitude and layer height. Some of these devices do not even have a mechanical linkage but rather use microprocessor-controlled motorized drive units for the tube and Bucky, or other image receptor, trays to impart their motion. Although the linear tomographic images produced by these units do not quite compare with those produced by pluridirectional units, they are often considered quite acceptable. In this cost-conscious era, tomography will likely remain for many years a valuable diagnostic imaging tool for both small and large hospitals.

Definition of Terms

adjustable fulcrum Tomographic fulcrum that is either raised or lowered to achieve the desired fulcrum height (see planigraphic principle).

body-section radiography See *tomography*.

complex tomographic motion See *pluridirectional tomographic motion*.

exposure angle Degree of arc angulation described by the movement of the x-ray tube and cassette during a tomographic motion.

fixed fulcrum Tomographic fulcrum remains at a fixed height (see *Grossman principle*).

focal plane Plane of tissue that is in focus on a tomogram.

fulcrum Point of axis of rotation for a tomographic motion.

Grossman principle Tomographic principle in which the fulcrum or axis of rotation remains at a fixed height; the focal plane level is changed by raising or lowering the tabletop through this fixed point to the desired height.

laminagraphy See *tomography*.

linear tomographic motion Basic tomographic movement that occurs when x-ray tube and cassette movement occurs with the longitudinal axis of the tomographic table.

moving film roentgenogram See *tomography*.

phantom images False tomographic images that appear but do not represent an actual object or structure within the focal plane; these images are created by the incomplete blurring or the fusion of the blurred margins of some structures characteristic to the type of tomographic motion used.

planigraphic principle Tomographic principle in which the fulcrum, or axis of rotation, is raised or lowered to alter the level of the focal plane; the tabletop height remains constant.

planigraphy Synonymous with *tomography*.

pluridirectional tomographic motion Tomographic motion in many different directions.

section thickness Tomographic plane that is in maximum focus.

stratigraphy Synonym for *tomography*.

tomographic angle See *exposure angle*.

tomography Radiographic technique that depicts a single plane of tissue by blurring images of structures above and below the plane of interest.

unidirectional tomographic motion Tomographic motion in only a linear direction.

zonography Tomography that uses exposure angles of 10 degrees or less to depict thick sections or zones of tissue.

Selected bibliography

Andrews JR: Planigraphy. I. Introduction and history, *AJR* 36:575, 1936.

Berrett A: *Modern thin-section tomography*, Springfield, Ill, 1973, Charles C Thomas.

Bocage AEM: French patent no. 536464, 1922.

Bosniak MA: Nephrotomography: a relatively unappreciated but extremely valuable diagnostic tool, *Radiology* 113:313, 1974.

Chasen MH et al: Tomography of the pulmonary hila: anatomical reassessment of the conventional 55 posterior oblique view, *Radiology* 149:365, 1983.

Durizch ML: *Technical aspects of tomography*, Baltimore, 1978, Williams & Wilkins.

Ho C, Sartoris DJ, Resnick D: Conventional tomography in musculoskeletal trauma, *Radiol Clin North Am* 27:929, 1989.

Holder JC et al: Metrizamide myelography with complex motion tomography, *Radiology* 145:201, 1982.

Kieffer J: United States patent, 1934.

Littleton JT: *Tomography: physical principles and clinical applications*, Baltimore, 1976, Williams & Wilkins.

Littleton JT et al: Adjustable versus fixed-fulcrum tomographic systems, *AJR* 117:910, 1973.

Littleton JT et al: Linear vs. pluridirectional tomography of the chest: correlative radiographic anatomic study, *AJR* 134:241, 1980.

Maravilla KR et al: Digital tomosynthesis: technique for electronic reconstructive tomography, *AJR* 141:497, 1983.

Older RA et al: Importance of routine vascular nephrotomography in excretory urography, *Radiology* 136:282, 1980.

Potter GD et al: Tomography of the optic canal, *AJR* 106:530, 1969.

Sone S et al: Digital image processing to remove blur from linear tomography of the lung, *Acta Radiol* 32:421, 1991.

Stanson AW et al: Routine tomography of the temporomandibular joint, *Radiol Clin North Am* 14:105, 1976.

Valvasori GE: Laminagraphy of the ear: normal roentgenographic anatomy, *AJR* 89:1155, 1963.

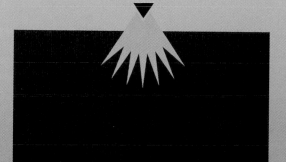

MOBILE RADIOGRAPHY

KARI J. WETTERLIN

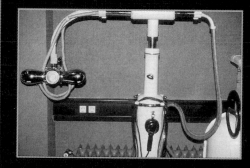

RIGHT: Portable radiographic unit, early 1940s. Note the exposed glass ends of the x-ray tube. A spring-wound mechanical timer is hanging on the vertical support.

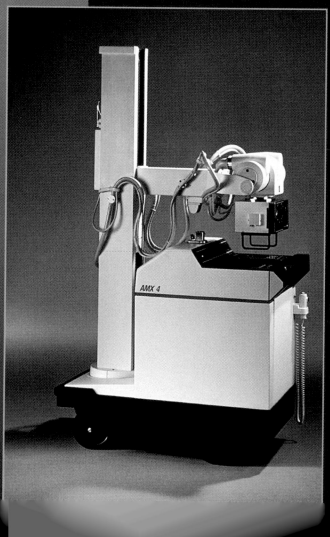

Battery-operated mobile radiographic unit, 1999.

(Courtesy General Electric Medical Systems.)

Principles of Mobile Radiography

Mobile radiography using transportable radiographic equipment allows imaging services to be brought to the patient. In contrast to the large stationary machines found in radiographic rooms, compact mobile radiography units can produce diagnostic images in virtually any location (Fig. 30-1). Mobile radiography is commonly performed in patient rooms, emergency rooms, intensive care units, surgery and recovery rooms, and nursery and neonatal units. Some machines are designed for transport by automobile or van to nursing homes, extended care facilities, or other off-site locations requiring radiographic imaging services.

Mobile radiography was first used by the military for treating battlefield injuries during World War I. Small portable units were designed to be carried by soldiers and set up in field locations. Although mobile equipment is no longer "carried" to the patient, the term *portable* has persisted and is often used in reference to mobile procedures.

This chapter focuses on the most common projections performed with mobile radiography machines. The basic principles of mobile radiography are detailed, and helpful hints are provided for successful completion of the examinations. An understanding of common projections enables the radiographer to perform most mobile examinations ordered by the physician.

Mobile X-Ray Machines

Mobile x-ray machines are not as sophisticated as the larger stationary machines in the radiology department. Although mobile units are capable of producing images of most body parts, they vary in their exposure controls and power sources (or generators).

A typical mobile x-ray machine has controls for setting kilovolt (peak) (kVp) and milliampere-seconds (mAs). The mAs control automatically adjusts milliamperage (mA) and time to preset values. Maximum settings differ among manufacturers, but mAs typically range from 0.04 to 320 and kVp from 40 to 130. The total power of the unit varies between 15 and 25 kilowatts (kW), which is adequate for most mobile projections. By comparison, the power of a stationary radiography unit can reach 150 kW (150 kVp, 1000 mA) or more.

Some mobile x-ray machines have anatomic programming similar to stationary units. The anatomic programmer automatically sets all exposure factors to preset values based on the selected examination. The radiographer can adjust these settings as needed to compensate for differences in the size or condition of a patient. Automatic exposure control (AEC) may be available for some mobile machines. A paddle containing an ionization chamber is placed behind the cassette and is used to determine the exposure time. However, with the increasing use of computed radiography (CR), anatomic programming and AEC may not be as useful. The much wider dynamic range available with CR and the ability to manipulate the final image with the computer result in images of proper density without the use of automatic systems.

Mobile x-ray machines are classified into two categories—*battery operated* and *capacitor discharge*—depending on the power source.

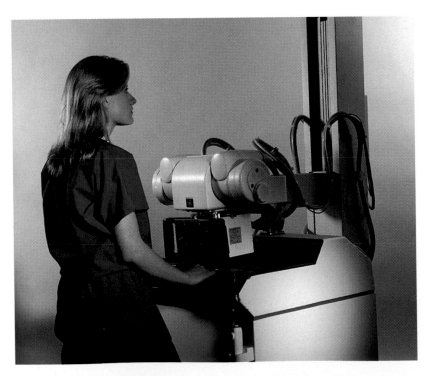

Fig. 30-1 Radiographer driving a battery-operated mobile radiography machine to a patient's room.

BATTERY-OPERATED MOBILE UNITS

Battery-operated machines use two different sets of batteries. One set, consisting of as many as 10 12-V lead acid batteries, controls the x-ray power output; the other set provides the power for the self-propelled driving ability. When the batteries are fully charged, these machines can be used for as many as 10 to 15 x-ray exposures and can be driven reasonable distances around the institution. Recharging after heavy use may be necessary to ensure maximum consistency in radiation output. The driving mechanisms include forward and reverse speeds; because of the power drive, a strong "deadman" type of brake is standard. A deadman brake stops the machine instantly when the push-handle is released. The advantages of these machines are that they are cordless and they provide constant kVp and mAs.

CAPACITOR-DISCHARGE MOBILE UNITS

Capacitor-discharge mobile machines contain a capacitor-discharge unit and do not operate on batteries. A capacitor is a device that stores electrical energy. The radiation is generated when an electrical discharge is sent across the x-ray tube electrodes from a bank of high-voltage capacitors. The capacitor must be charged briefly before each exposure, with the power coming from a standard 110-V outlet. Larger capacitor-discharge machines may require a 220-V outlet. These machines are not self-propelling, and they are typically much lighter as a result of not having batteries. They are moved around the institution manually.

In a capacitor-discharge system, the kVp drops constantly during the length of the exposure. For example, the kVp may start at 100 and may drop to 80 by the end of an exposure. This may result in inadequate penetration of thick body areas. Consequently, special attention must be given to creating a technique chart that uses higher kVp and lower mAs than would normally be used with a conventional generator. If the desired technique normally requires 90 kVp at 20 mAs on noncapacitor discharge machines, using a technique of 100 kVp on a capacitor-discharge unit is preferred because the average kVp during the exposure is about 92. The advantages of capacitor-discharge machines are their smaller size and ease in movement. They also do not require long capacitor charging times before the exposure.

Technical Considerations

Mobile radiography presents the radiographer with challenges different from those experienced in performing examinations with stationary equipment in the radiology department. Although the positioning of the patient and placement of the central ray are essentially the same, three important technical matters must be clearly understood to perform optimum mobile examinations: the *grid,* the *anode heel effect,* and the *source-to-image receptor distance (SID).* In addition, exposure technique charts must be available (see Fig. 30-4).

GRID

For optimum imaging, a *grid* must be level, centered to the central ray, and correctly used at the recommended focal distance, or radius. When a grid is placed on an unstable surface such as the mattress of a bed, the weight of the patient can cause the grid to tilt "off-level." If the grid tilts transversely, the central ray forms an angle across the long axis. Image density is lost as a result of grid "cutoff" (Fig. 30-2). If the grid tilts longitudinally, the central ray angles through the long axis. In this case, grid cutoff is avoided, but the image may be distorted or elongated.

A grid positioned under a patient can be difficult to center. If the central ray is directed to a point transversely off the midline of a grid more than 1 to $1\frac{1}{2}$ inches (2.5 to 3.8 cm), a cutoff effect similar to that produced by an off-level grid results. The central ray can be centered longitudinally to any point along the midline of a grid without cutoff. Depending on the procedure, beam-restriction problems may occur. If this happens, a portion of the image is "collimated off," or patient exposure is excessive because of an oversized exposure field.

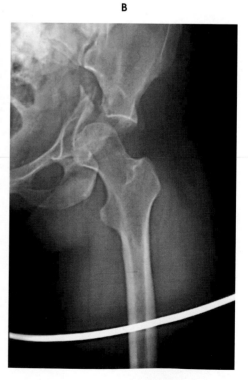

A **B**

Fig. 30-2 Mobile radiograph of a proximal femur and hip, demonstrating comminuted fracture of the left acetabulum. **A,** Poor-quality radiograph resulted when the grid was transversely tilted far enough to produce significant grid cutoff. **B,** Excellent- quality repeat radiograph on the same patient, performed with the grid accurately positioned perpendicular to the central ray.

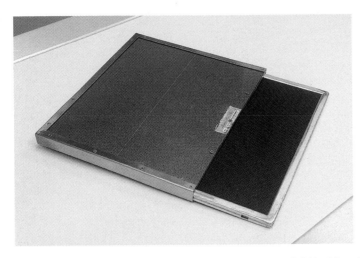

Fig. 30-3 Grid mounted on a rigid frame device and protected. Grid holder allows easy insertion of a cassette for mobile radiography uses.

TABLE 30-1

Cathode placement for mobile projections*

Part	Projection	Cathode placement
Chest	AP	Diaphragm
	AP—decubitus	Down side of chest
Abdomen	AP	Diaphragm
	AP—decubitus	Down side of abdomen
Pelvis	AP	Upper pelvis
Femur	AP	Proximal femur
	Lateral	Proximal femur
Cervical spine	Lateral	Over lower vertebrae (40-inch (102-cm) SID only)
Chest and abdomen in neonate	All	No designation†

AP, anteroposterior; SID, source-to-image receptor distance.
*The cathode side of the beam has the greatest intensity.
†Not necessary because of small field size of the collimator.

Grids used for mobile radiography are often of the focused type. Many radiology departments, however, continue to use the older, parallel-type grids for some or all mobile examinations. All focused grids have a recommended focal range, or radius, that varies with the grid ratio. Projections taken at distances greater or less than the recommended focal range can produce cutoff in which image density is reduced on lateral margins. Grids with a lower ratio have a greater focal range, but they are less efficient for cleaning up scatter radiation. The radiographer must be aware of the *exact* focal range for the grid used. Most focused grids used for mobile radiography have a ratio of 6:1 or 8:1, and they have a focal range of about 36 to 44 inches (91 to 112 cm). This focal range allows mobile examinations to be performed efficiently. Inverting a focused grid causes a pronounced cutoff effect similar to that produced by improper distance.

Today most grids are mounted on a protective frame, and the cassette is easily inserted behind the grid (Fig. 30-3). A final concern regarding grids relates to the use of "tape-on" grids. If a grid is not mounted on a cassette holder frame but instead is manually fastened to the surface of the cassette with tape, care must be taken to ensure that the tube side of the grid faces the x-ray tube. The examinations described in this chapter present methods of ensuring proper grid cassette placement for projections that require a grid.

ANODE HEEL EFFECT

Another consideration in mobile radiography is the *anode heel effect*. The heel effect causes a decrease of image density under the anode side of the x-ray tube. The heel effect is more pronounced with the following:
- Short SID
- Larger field sizes
- Small anode angles

Short SIDs and large field sizes are common in mobile radiography. Furthermore, in mobile radiography, the radiographer has control of the anode-cathode axis of the x-ray tube relative to the body part. Therefore correct placement of the anode-cathode axis with regard to the anatomy is essential. When performing a mobile examination, the radiographer may not always be able to orient the anode-cathode axis of the tube to the desired position because of limited space and maneuverability in the room. For optimum mobile radiography, the anode and cathode sides of the x-ray tube should be clearly marked to indicate where the high-tension cables enter the x-ray tube, and the radiographer should use the heel effect maximally (Table 30-1).

SOURCE-TO-IMAGE RECEPTOR DISTANCE

The *SID* should be maintained at 40 inches (102 cm) for most mobile examinations. A standardized distance for all patients and projections helps to ensure consistency in imaging. Longer SIDs—40 to 48 inches (102 to 122 cm)—require increased mAs to compensate for the additional distance. The mA limitations of a mobile unit necessitate longer exposure times when the SID exceeds 40 inches (102 cm). Despite the longer exposure time, a radiograph with motion artifacts may result if the SID is greater than 40 inches (102 cm). In addition, motion artifacts may occur in the radiographs of critically ill adult patients and infants or small children who require chest and abdominal examinations but may not be able to hold their breath.

RADIOGRAPHIC TECHNIQUE CHARTS

A radiographic technique chart should be available for use with every mobile machine. The chart should display, in an organized manner, the standardized technical factors for all the radiographic projections done with the machine (Fig. 30-4). A caliper should also be available; this device, is used to measure the thickness of body parts to ensure that accurate and consistent exposure factors are used. Measuring the patient also allows the radiographer to determine the optimum kVp level for all exposures (Fig. 30-5).

MOBILE RADIOGRAPHIC TECHNIQUE CHART					
AMX—4 40-inch SID Lanex medium screens/TML 8:1 grid					
Part	**Projection**	**Position**	**cm—kVp**	**mAs**	**Grid**
Chest	AP	Supine/upright	21—85	1.25	No
	AP	Lateral decubitus	21—85	6.25	Yes
Abdomen	AP	Supine	23—74	25	Yes
	AP	Lateral decubitus	23—74	32	Yes
Pelvis	AP	Supine	23—74	32	Yes
Femur (distal)	AP	Supine	15—70	10	Yes
	Lateral	Dorsal decubitus	15—70	10	Yes
C-spine	Lateral	Dorsal decubitus	10—62	20	Yes
NEONATAL					
Chest/abdomen	AP	Supine	7—64	0.8	No
	Lateral	Dorsal decubitus	10—72	1	No

Fig. 30-4 Sample radiographic technique chart showing the manual technical factors used for the 10 common mobile projections described in this chapter. The kVp and mAs factors are for the specific centimeter measurements indicated. Factors vary depending on the actual centimeter measurement.

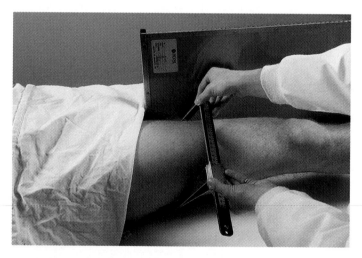

Fig. 30-5 Radiographer measuring the thickest portion of the femur to determine exact technical factors needed for the examination.

Radiation Safety

Radiation protection for the radiographer, others in the immediate area, and the patient is of paramount importance when mobile examinations are performed. *Mobile radiography produces some of the highest occupational radiation exposures for radiographers.* The radiographer should wear a lead apron and should stand as far away from the patient, x-ray tube, and useful beam as the room and the exposure cable allow (Fig. 30-6). The recommended *minimal* distance is 6 feet (2 m). When possible, the radiographer should stand at a right angle (90 degrees) to the primary beam and the object being radiographed. The least amount of scatter radiation occurs at this position. However, shielding and distance have a greater effect on exposure reduction and therefore should always be considered first.

The single most effective means of radiation protection is *distance*. The radiographer should inform all persons in the immediate area that an x-ray exposure is about to occur so that they may leave to avoid exposure. Lead protection should be provided for any individuals who are unable to leave the room and for those who may have to hold a patient or cassette.

The patient's gonads should be shielded with appropriate radiation protection devices for any of the following situations:

- X-ray examinations performed on children
- X-ray examinations performed on patients of reproductive age
- Any examination for which the patient requests protection
- Examinations in which the gonads lie in or near the useful beam
- Examinations in which shielding will not interfere with imaging of the anatomy that must be demonstrated (Fig. 30-7)

In addition, the source-to-skin distance (SSD) cannot be less than 12 inches (30 cm), in accordance with federal safety regulations.[1]

---

[1]National Council on Radiation Protection: Report 102: *Medical x-ray, electron beam and gamma ray protection for energies up to 50 MeV,* Bethesda, Md, 1989.

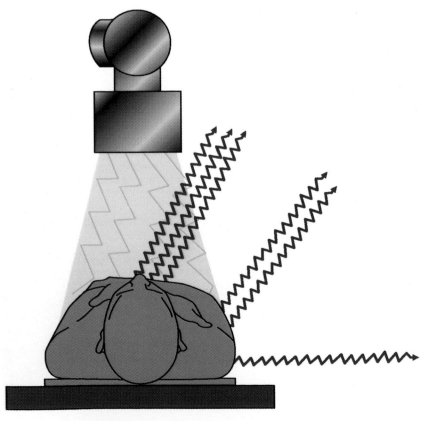

Fig. 30-6 Whenever possible, the radiographer should stand at least 6 feet (2 m) from the patient and useful beam. The lowest amount of scatter radiation occurs at a right angle (90 degrees) from the primary x-ray beam.

Isolation Considerations

Two types of patients are often cared for in isolation units: (1) patients who have infectious microorganisms that could be spread to health care workers and visitors and (2) patients who need protection from potentially lethal microorganisms that may be carried by health care workers and visitors. Optimally, a radiographer entering an isolation room should have a full knowledge of the patient's disease, the way it is transmitted, and the proper way to clean and disinfect equipment before and after use in the isolation unit. However, because of the confidentiality of patient records, the radiographer may not be able to obtain information about a patient's specific disease. Therefore all patients must be treated with universal precautions. If isolation is used to protect the patient from receiving microorganisms (reverse isolation), a different protocol may be required. Institutional policy regarding isolation procedures should be available and strictly followed.

When performing mobile procedures in an isolation unit, the radiographer should wear the required protective apparel for the specific situation—gown, cap, mask, shoe covers, and gloves. All of this apparel is not needed for every isolation patient. For example, a mask, a gown, and gloves are worn by all persons entering a strict isolation unit, but only gloves are worn for drainage secretion precautions. The radiographer should always wash the hands with warm, soapy water before putting on gloves. The x-ray machine is taken into the room and manipulated into position. The cassette is placed into a clean, protective cover. Pillowcases will not protect the cassette or the patient if bodily fluids soak through them. A clean, impermeable cover should be used in situations in which bodily fluids may come into contact with the cassette. For examinations of patients in strict isolation, two radiographers may be required to maintain a safe barrier (see Chapter 1).

After finishing the examination, the radiographer should remove and dispose of the mask, cap, gown, shoe covers, and the gloves according to institutional policies. All equipment that touched the patient or the patient's bed must be wiped with a disinfectant according to appropriate aseptic technique. The radiographer should wear new gloves, if necessary, while cleaning equipment. Hand washing is repeated before the radiographer leaves the room.

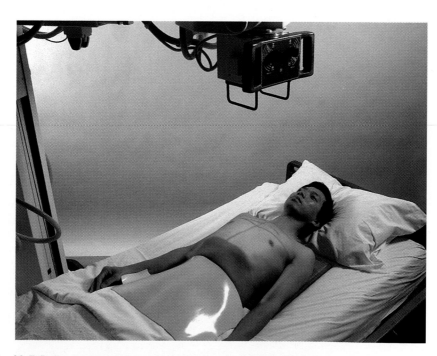

Fig. 30-7 Patient ready for a mobile chest examination. Note lead shield placed over the patient's pelvis. This shield does not interfere with the examination.

Performing Mobile Examinations

INITIAL PROCEDURES

The radiographer should plan for the trip out of the radiology department. Ensuring that all of the necessary devices (cassette, grid, tape, measuring caliper, markers, blocks) are transported with the mobile x-ray machine provides greater efficiency in performing examinations. Many mobile x-ray machines are equipped with a storage area for transporting cassettes and supplies. If a battery-operated machine is used, the radiographer should check the machine to ensure that it is charged properly. An inadequately charged machine can interfere with performance and affect the quality of the radiograph.

Before entering the patient's room with the machine, the radiographer should follow several important steps (Box 30-1). The radiographer begins by checking that the correct patient is going to be examined. After confirming the identity of the patient, the radiographer enters, makes an introduction as a radiographer, and informs the patient about the x-ray examinations to be performed. While in the room, the radiographer observes any medical appliances, such as chest tube boxes, catheter bags, and IV poles, that may be positioned next to or hanging on the sides of the patient's bed. The radiographer should ask family members or visitors to step out of the room until the examination is finished. If necessary, the nursing staff should be alerted that assistance is required.

Communication and cooperation between the radiographer and nursing staff members are essential for proper patient care during mobile radiography. In addition, communication with the patient is *imperative,* even if the patient is or appears to be unconscious or unresponsive.

THE EXAMINATION

Chairs, stands, IV poles, wastebaskets, and other obstacles should be moved from the path of the mobile machine. Lighting should be adjusted if necessary. If the patient is to be examined in the supine position, the base of the mobile machine should be positioned toward the middle of the bed. If a seated patient position is used, the base of the machine should be toward the foot of the bed.

For lateral and decubitus radiographs, positioning the base of the mobile machine parallel to or directly perpendicular to the bed allows the greatest ease in positioning the x-ray tube. Room size can also influence the base position used.

At times, the radiographer may have difficulty accurately aligning the x-ray tube parallel to the cassette while standing at the side of the bed. When positioning the tube above the patient, the radiographer may need to check the x-ray tube and cassette alignment from the foot of the bed to ensure that the tube is not tilted.

For all projections, the primary x-ray beam must be collimated no larger than the size of the cassette. When the central ray is correctly centered to the cassette, the light field coincides with or fits within the borders of the cassette.

A routine and consistent system for labeling and separating exposed and unexposed cassettes should be developed and maintained. It is easy to "double expose" cassettes during mobile radiography, particularly if many examinations are performed at one time. Most institutions require additional identification markers for mobile examinations. Typically the time of examination (especially for chest radiographs) and technical notes such as the position of the patient are indicated. A log may be maintained for each patient and kept in the patient's room. The log should contain the exposure factors used for the projections and other notes regarding the performance of the examination.

PATIENT CONSIDERATIONS

Patients requiring mobile radiography often are in extended care facilities or are immobile and among the most sick. They may be awake and lying in bed in traction because of a broken limb, or they may be critically ill and unconscious. A brief but total assessment of the patient must be conducted both before and during the examination. Some specific considerations to keep in mind are described in the following sections.

Assessment of the patient's condition

A thorough assessment of the patient's condition and room allows the radiographer to make necessary adaptations to ensure the best possible patient care and imaging outcome. The radiographer assesses the patient's level of alertness and respiration and then determines the extent to which the patient is able to cooperate and the limitations that may affect the procedure. Some patients may have varying degrees of drowsiness because of their medications or medical condition. Many mobile examinations are performed in patient's rooms immediately after surgery; these patients may be under the influence of various anesthetics.

Box 30-1

Preliminary steps for the radiographer before mobile radiography is performed

- Announce your presence to the nursing staff, and ask for assistance if needed.
- Determine that the correct patient is in the room.
- Introduce yourself to patient and family as a radiographer and explain the examination.
- Observe the medical equipment in the room as well, as other apparatus and IV poles with fluids. Move the equipment if necessary.
- Ask family members and visitors to leave.*

---

* A family member may need to be present for the examination of a small child.

Patient mobility

The radiographer must never move a patient or part of the patient's body without assessing the patient's ability to move or tolerate movement. At all times, *gentleness* and *caution* must prevail. If unsure, the radiographer should always check with the nursing staff or physician. For example, many patients who undergo total joint replacement may not be able to move the affected joint for a number of days or weeks. However, this may not be evident to the radiographer. Some patients may be able to indicate verbally their ability to move or their tolerance for movement. *The radiographer should never move a limb that has been operated on or is broken unless the nurse, the physician, or sometimes the patient grants permission.* Inappropriate movement of the patient by the radiographer during the examination may harm the patient.

Fractures

Patients can have a variety of fractures and fracture types, ranging from one simple fracture to multiple fractures of many bones. A patient lying awake in a traction bed with a simple femur fracture may be able to assist with a radiographic examination. However, another patient may be unconscious and have multiple broken ribs, spinal fractures, or a severe closed head injury.

Few patients with multiple fractures are able to move or tolerate movement. The radiographer must be cautious, resourceful, and work in accordance with the patient's condition and pain tolerance. If a patient's trunk or limb must be raised into position for a projection, the radiographer should have ample assistance so that the part can be raised safely without causing harm or intense pain.

Interfering devices

Patients who are in intensive care units or orthopedic beds because of fractures may be attached to a variety of devices, wires, and tubing. These objects may be in the direct path of the x-ray beam and consequently produce artifacts on the image. Experienced radiographers know which of these objects can be moved out of the x-ray beam. When devices such as fracture frames cannot be moved, it may be necessary to angle the central ray or adjust the cassette to obtain the best radiograph possible. In many instances the objects have to be radiographed along with the body part (Fig. 30-8). The radiographer must exercise caution when handling any of these devices and should never remove traction devices without the assistance of a physician.

Positioning and asepsis

During positioning, the cassette (with or without a grid) often is perceived by the patient as cold, hard, and uncomfortable. Therefore before the cassette is put in place, the patient should be warned of possible discomfort and assured that the examination will be for as short a time as possible. The patient will appreciate the radiographer's concern and efficiency in completing the examination as quickly as possible.

If the surface of the cassette touches bare skin, it can stick, making positioning adjustments difficult. *The skin of older patients may be thin and dry and can be torn by manipulation of the cassette if care is not taken.* A cloth or paper cover over the cassette can protect the patient's skin and alleviate some of the discomfort by making it feel less cold. The cover also helps to keep the cassette clean. Cassettes that contact the patient directly should be wiped off with a disinfectant for asepsis and infection control.

The cassette must be enclosed in an appropriate, impermeable barrier in any situation in which it may come in contact with blood, body fluids, and other potentially infectious material. A contaminated cassette can be difficult and sometimes impossible to clean. Approved procedures for disposing of used barrier must be followed.

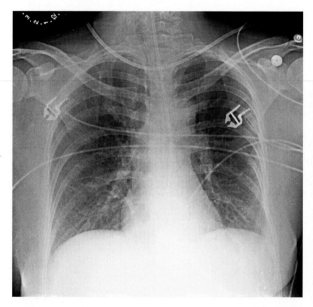 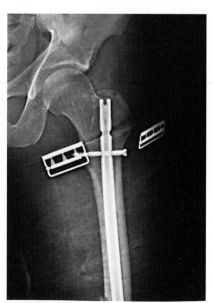

Fig. 30-8 A, Mobile radiograph of the chest. Note the variety of objects in the image that could not be removed for the exposure. **B,** Mobile radiograph of proximal femur and hip. Metal buckles could not be removed for the exposure.

🦅 AP PROJECTION*
Upright or supine

Image receptor: 35 × 43 cm (14 × 17 inch) lengthwise or crosswise, depending on body habitus; a nongrid or grid cassette can be used, depending on patient size or institutional policy

Position of patient
Depending on the condition of the patient, elevate the head of the bed to a semierect or sitting position. The projection should be performed with the patient in the upright position or to the greatest angle tolerated by the patient whenever possible. Use the supine position for critically ill or injured patients.

---

*The nonmobile projection is described in Chapter 10.

Position of part
Center the midsagittal plane to the cassette.
- To include the entire chest, position the cassette under the patient with the top about 2 inches (5 cm) above the *relaxed* shoulders. The exact distance depends on the size of the patient. When the patient is supine, the shoulders may move to a higher position relative to the lungs. Adjust accordingly.
- Be certain that the patient's shoulders are relaxed; then internally rotate the patient's arms to prevent scapular superimposition of the lung field, if not contraindicated.
- Ensure that the patient's upper torso is not rotated or leaning toward one side (Fig. 30-9).
- *Shield gonads.*
- *Respiration:* Inspiration, unless otherwise requested. If the patient is receiving respiratory assistance, carefully watch the patient's chest to determine the inspiratory phase for the exposure.

Central ray
- Perpendicular to the long axis of the sternum and the center of the cassette. The central ray should enter about 3 inches (7.6 cm) below the jugular notch at the level of T7)

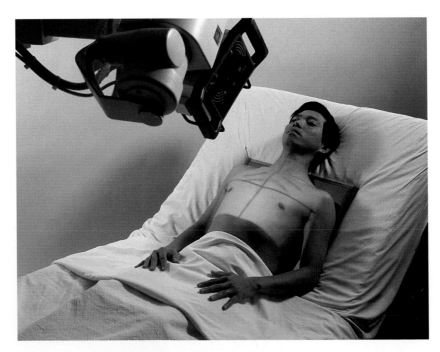

Fig. 30-9 Mobile AP chest: partially upright.

COMPUTED RADIOGRAPHY

A grid must be used for all mobile computed radiography chest examinations if the exposure technique is more than 90 kVp. (Review the manufacturer's protocol for the exact kVp levels for the unit that is used.) When a crosswise-positioned grid is used, the central ray must be perpendicular to the grid to prevent grid cutoff.

Structures shown

This projection demonstrates the anatomy of the thorax, including the heart, trachea, diaphragmatic domes, and most importantly the entire lung fields, including vascular markings (Fig. 30-10).

EVALUATION CRITERIA

The following should be clearly demonstrated:

- No motion. Well defined (not blurred) diaphragmatic domes and lung fields
- Lung fields in their entirety, including costophrenic angles
- Pleural markings
- Ribs and thoracic intervertebral disk spaces faintly visible through heart shadow
- No rotation with medial portion of clavicles and lateral border of ribs equidistant from vertebral column

NOTE: To ensure the proper angle from the x-ray tube to the cassette, the radiographer can double-check the shadow of the shoulders from the field light projected onto the cassette. If the shadow of the shoulders is thrown far above the upper edge of the cassette, the angle of the tube must be corrected.

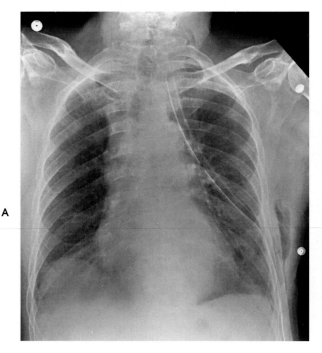

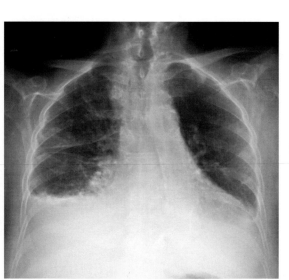

Fig. 30-10 Mobile AP chest radiographs in critically ill patients. **A,** Patient with postoperative left thoracotomy and chest tube, infiltrate or atelectasis in the left base, segmental elevation of the right hemidiaphragm, and soft tissue emphysema on the left. **B,** Patient with small left pleural effusion and moderate right effusion, cardiomegaly, mild pulmonary vascular congestion, and calcification and torsion of the aorta.

AP OR PA PROJECTION*
Right or left lateral decubitus position

Image receptor: 35 × 43 cm (14 × 17 inch) lengthwise; a nongrid or grid cassette can be used, depending on patient size

Position of patient
- Place the patient in the lateral recumbent position.
- Flex the patient's knees to provide stabilization, if possible.
- Place a firm support under the patient to elevate the body 2 to 3 inches (5 to 8 cm) and prevent the patient from sinking into the mattress.
- Raise both of the patient's arms up and away from the chest region, preferably above the head. An arm lying on the patient's side can imitate a region of free air.
- Ensure that the patient cannot roll out of bed.

*The nonmobile projection is described in Chapter 10.

Position of part
- Position the patient for the AP projection whenever possible. It is much easier to position an ill patient (particularly the arms) for an AP.
- Adjust the patient to ensure a lateral position. The coronal plane passing through the shoulders and hips should be vertical.
- Place the cassette behind the patient and below the support so that the lower margin of the chest will be visualized.
- Adjust the grid so that it extends approximately 2 inches (5 cm) above the shoulders. The cassette should be supported in position and not leaning against the patient to avoid distortion (Fig. 30-11).
- *Shield gonads.*
- *Respiration:* Inspiration unless otherwise requested.

Central ray
- Horizontal and perpendicular to the center of the cassette, entering the patient at a level of 3 inches (7.6 cm) below the jugular notch

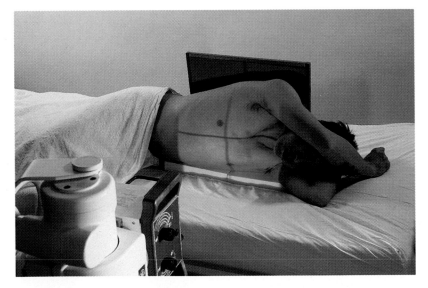

Fig. 30-11 Mobile AP chest: left lateral decubitus position. Note yellow block placed under the chest to elevate it. The block is necessary to ensure that the left side of the chest is included on the image.

Structures shown

This projection demonstrates the anatomy of the thorax, including the entire lung fields and any air or fluid levels that may be present (Fig. 30-12).

The following should be clearly demonstrated:

- No motion
- No rotation
- Affected side in its entirety (upper lung for free air and lower lung for fluid)
- Patient's arms out of region of interest
- Proper identification to indicate that decubitus position was used

NOTE: Fluid levels in the pleural cavity are best visualized with the affected side down, which also prevents mediastinal overlapping. Air levels are best visualized with the unaffected side down. The patient should be in position for at least 5 minutes before the exposure is made to allow air to rise and fluid levels to settle.

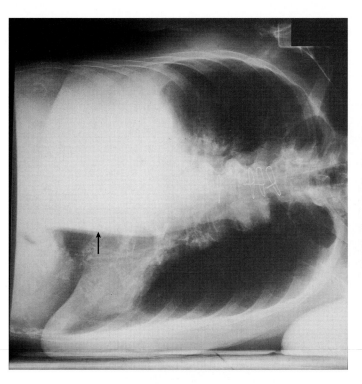

A

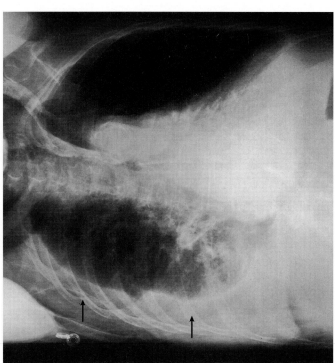

B

Fig. 30-12 Mobile AP chest radiographs performed in lateral decubitus positions in critically ill patients. **A**, Left lateral decubitus position. The patient has a large right pleural effusion *(arrow)* and no left effusion. Note that the complete left side of thorax is visualized because of elevation on a block. **B**, Right lateral decubitus position. The patient has right pleural effusion *(arrows)*, cardiomegaly, and mild pulmonary vascular congestion. Note that the complete right side of thorax is visualized because of elevation on a block.

AP PROJECTION*

Image receptor: 35 × 43 cm (14 × 17 inch) lengthwise grid

Position of patient

- If necessary, adjust the patient's bed to achieve a horizontal bed position.
- Place the patient in a supine position.

---

*The nonmobile projection is described in Chapter 16.

Position of part

- Position the grid under the patient to demonstrate the abdominal anatomy from the pubic symphysis to the upper abdominal region.
- Keep the grid from tipping side to side by placing it in the center of the bed and stabilizing it with blankets or towels if necessary.
- Use the patient's draw sheet to roll the patient; this makes it easier to shift the patient from side to side during positioning of the cassette, and it provides a barrier between the patient's skin and the grid.
- Center the midsagittal plane of the patient to the midline of the grid.

- Center the grid to the level of the iliac crests. If the emphasis is on the upper abdomen, center the grid 2 inches (5 cm) above the iliac crests or high enough to include the diaphragm.
- Adjust the patient's shoulders and pelvis to lie in the same plane (Fig. 30-13).
- Move the patient's arms out of the region of the abdomen.
- *Shield gonads.* Note that this may not be possible in a female patient.
- *Respiration:* Expiration.

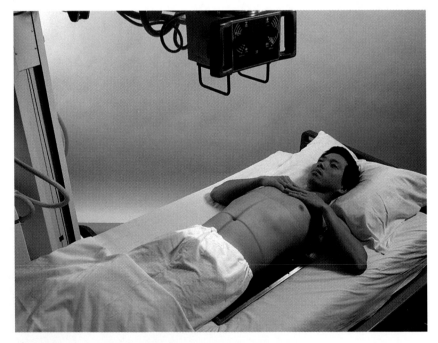

Fig. 30-13 Mobile AP abdomen.

Central ray

- Perpendicular to the center of the grid along the midsagittal plane and at the level of the iliac crests or the tenth rib laterally

Structures shown

This projection demonstrates the following: the inferior margin of the liver; the spleen, kidneys, and psoas muscles; calcifications; and evidence of tumor masses. If the image includes the upper abdomen and diaphragm, the size and shape of the liver may be seen (Fig. 30-14).

The following should be clearly demonstrated:

- No motion
- Outlines of the abdominal viscera
- Abdominal region, including pubic symphysis or diaphragm (both may be seen on some patients)
- Vertebral column in center of image
- Psoas muscles, lower margin of liver, and kidney margins
- No rotation
- Symmetric appearance of vertebral column and iliac wings

NOTE: Hypersthenic patients may require two separate projections using a crosswise grid. One grid is positioned for the upper abdomen and the other for the lower abdomen.

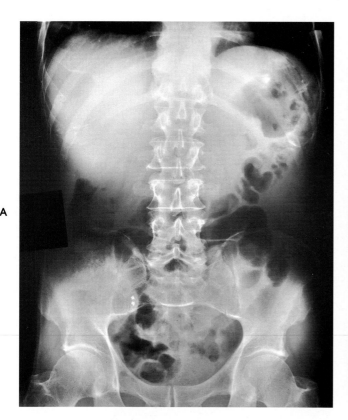 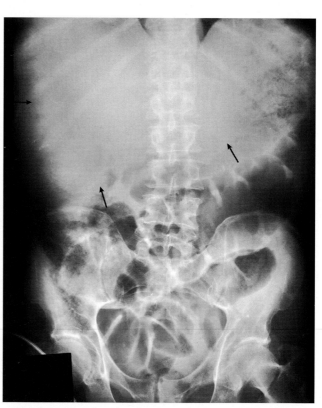

Fig. 30-14 Mobile AP abdomen radiographs. **A**, Abdomen without pathology. Note that the entire abdomen is seen in this patient. **B**, Patient with hepatomegaly encompassing the entire upper abdomen (*arrows*). Note that the diaphragm cannot be seen in this patient, who has a longer abdomen than the patient in **A**.

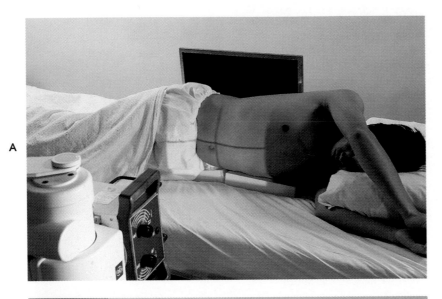

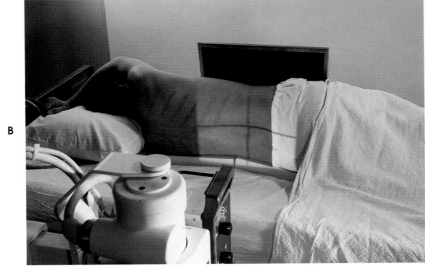

Fig. 30-15 Mobile AP abdomen radiograph: left lateral decubitus position. **A,** AP projection. **B,** PA projection. Note yellow blocks placed under the abdomen to level the abdomen and keep the patient from sinking into the mattress.

AP OR PA PROJECTION*
Left lateral decubitus position

Image receptor: 35 × 43 cm (14 × 17 inch) lengthwise grid.

Position of patient
- Place the patient in the left lateral recumbent position unless requested otherwise.
- Flex the patient's knees slightly to provide stabilization.
- If necessary, place a firm support under the patient to elevate the body and keep the patient from sinking into the mattress.
- Raise both of the patient's arms away from the abdominal region, if possible. The right arm lying on the side of the abdomen may imitate a region of free air.
- Ensure that the patient cannot fall out of bed.

Position of part
- Use the PA or AP projection, depending on the room layout.
- Adjust the patient to ensure a true lateral position. The coronal plane passing through the shoulders and hips should be vertical.
- Place the grid vertically in front of the patient for a PA projection and behind the patient for an AP projection. The grid should be supported in position and not leaned against the patient; this position prevents grid cutoff.
- Position the grid so that its center is 2 inches (5 cm) above the iliac crests to ensure that the diaphragm is included. The pubic symphysis and lower abdomen do not have to be visualized (Fig. 30-15).
- Before making the exposure, be certain that the patient has been in the lateral recumbent position for at least 5 minutes to allow air to rise and fluid levels to settle.
- *Shield gonads.*
- *Respiration:* Expiration.

*The nonmobile projection is described in Chapter 16.

Abdomen

Central ray

- Horizontal and perpendicular to the center of the grid, entering the patient along the midsagittal plane

Structures shown

Air or fluid levels within the abdominal cavity are demonstrated. These projections are especially helpful in assessing free air in the abdomen. The right border of the abdominal region must be visualized (Figs. 30-16).

EVALUATION CRITERIA

The following should be clearly demonstrated:

- No motion
- Well-defined diaphragm and abdominal viscera
- Air or fluid levels, if present
- Right and left abdominal wall and flank structures
- No rotation
- Symmetric appearance of vertebral column and iliac wings

NOTE: Hypersthenic patients may require two projections with the 35 × 43 cm (14× 17 inch) grid positioned crosswise to visualize the entire abdominal area. A patient with a long torso may require two projections with the grid lengthwise to visualize the entire abdominal region.

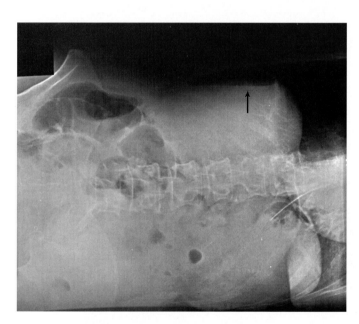

Fig. 30-16 Mobile AP abdomen radiograph: left lateral decubitus position. Free intraperitoneal air is seen on the upper or right side of the abdomen *(arrow).* The radiograph is slightly underexposed to demonstrate the free air more easily.

▲ AP PROJECTION*

Image receptor: 35 × 43 cm (14 × 17 inch) grid crosswise

Position of patient
- Adjust the patient's bed horizontally so that the patient is in a supine patient position.
- Move the patient's arms out of the region of the pelvis.

---

*The nonmobile projection is described in Chapter 7.

Position of part
- Position the grid under the pelvis so that the center is midway between the anterior superior iliac spine (ASIS) and the pubic symphysis. This is about 2 inches (5 cm) inferior to the ASIS and 2 inches (5 cm) superior to the pubic symphysis.
- Center the midsagittal plane of the patient to the midline of the grid. The pelvis should not be rotated.
- Rotate the patient's legs medially approximately 15 degrees when not contraindicated (Fig. 30-17).
- *Shield gonads:* Note that this may not be possible in female patients.
- *Respiration:* Suspend.

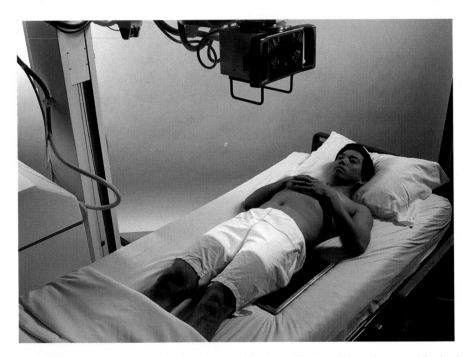

Fig. 30-17 Mobile AP pelvis. Note that the grid is placed horizontal and perpendicular to the central ray.

Central ray

- Perpendicular to the midpoint of the grid, entering the midsagittal plane. The central ray should enter the patient 2 inches (5 cm) above the pubic symphysis and 2 inches (5 cm) below the ASIS.

Structures shown

This projection demonstrates the pelvis, including the following: both hip bones; the sacrum and coccyx; and the head, neck, trochanters, and proximal portion of the femurs (Fig. 30-18).

The following should be clearly demonstrated:

- Entire pelvis, including proximal femurs and both hip bones
- No rotation
- Symmetric appearance of iliac wings and obturator foramina
- Both greater trochanters and ilia equidistant from edge of radiograph
- Femoral necks not foreshortened and greater trochanters in profile

NOTE: It is not uncommon for the weight of the patient to cause the bottom edge of the grid to tilt upward. The x-ray tube may need to be angled caudally to compensate and maintain proper grid alignment, thereby preventing grid cutoff. However, the exact angle needed is not always known or easy to determine. The radiographer may want to lower the foot of the bed slightly (Fowler's position), thereby shifting the patient's weight more evenly on the grid and allowing it to be flat. A rolled-up towel or blanket placed under the grid also may be useful to prevent lateral tilting. If the bed is equipped with an inflatable air mattress, the maximum inflate mode is recommended. Tilting the bottom edge of the grid downward is another possibility. Check the level of the grid carefully and compensate accordingly.

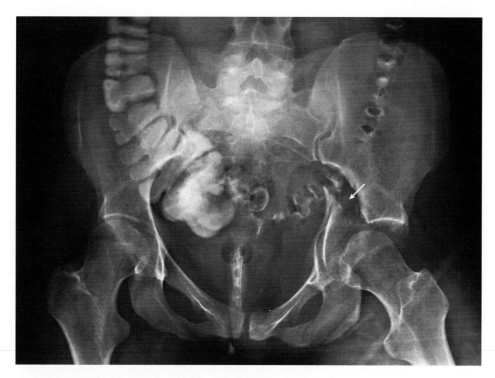

Fig. 30-18 Mobile AP pelvis radiograph. This patient has a comminuted fracture of the left acetabulum with medial displacement of the medial acetabular wall *(arrow)*. Residual barium is seen in the colon, sigmoid, and rectum.

🦅 AP PROJECTION*

Most mobile AP and lateral projections of the femur may be radiographs of the middle and distal femur taken while the patient is in traction. The femur cannot be moved, which presents a challenge to the radiographer.

Image receptor: 35 × 43 cm (14 × 17 inch) grid lengthwise

Position of patient

- The patient is in the supine position.

___

*The nonmobile projection is described in Chapter 6.

Position of part

- *Cautiously* place the grid lengthwise under the patient's femur with the distal edge of the grid low enough to include the fracture site, pathologic region, and knee joint.
- Elevate the grid with towels, blankets, or blocks under each side, if necessary, to ensure proper grid alignment with the x-ray tube.
- Center the grid to the midline of the affected femur.
- Ensure that the grid is placed parallel to the plane of the femoral condyles (Fig. 30-19).
- *Shield gonads.*
- *Respiration:* Suspend.

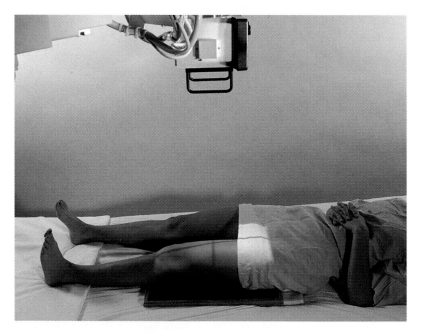

Fig. 30-19 Mobile AP femur.

Central ray

- Perpendicular to the long axis of the femur and centered to the grid.
- Be certain that the central ray and grid are aligned to prevent grid cutoff.

COMPUTED RADIOGRAPHY

The thickest portion of the femur (proximal area) must be carefully measured and an appropriate kVp must be selected to penetrate this area. The computer cannot form an image of the anatomy in this area if penetration does not occur. A light area of the entire proximal femur will result. Positioning the cathode over the proximal femur will improve CR image quality.

Structures shown

The distal two thirds of the femur, including the knee joint, are demonstrated (Fig. 30-20).

EVALUATION CRITERIA

The following should be clearly demonstrated:

- Majority of femur, including knee joint
- No knee rotation
- Adequate penetration of proximal portion of femur
- Any orthopedic appliance, such as plate and screw fixation.

NOTE: If the entire length of the femur needs to be visualized, an AP projection of the proximal femur can be performed by placing a 35 × 43 cm (14 × 17 inch) grid lengthwise under the proximal femur and hip. The top of the grid is placed at the level of the ASIS to ensure that the hip joint is included. The central ray is directed to the center of the grid and long axis of the femur (see Fig. 30-2).

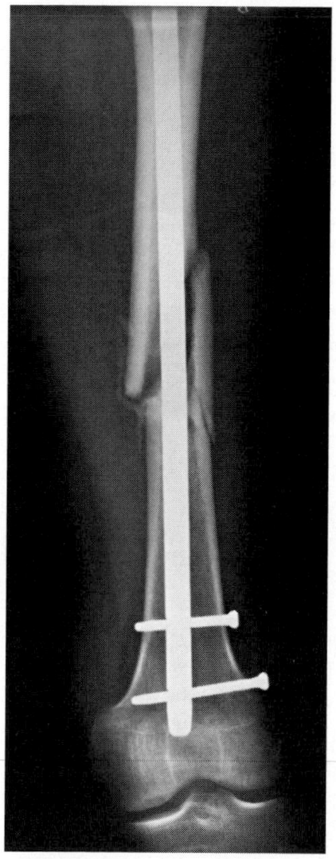

Fig. 30-20 Mobile AP femur radiograph showing a fracture of the midshaft with femoral rod placement. Note that the knee joint is included on the image.

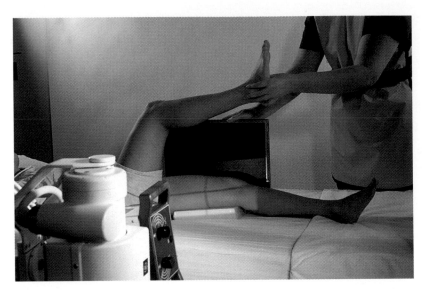

Fig. 30-21 Mobile *mediolateral* left femur. An assistant wearing a lead apron is holding and positioning the right leg and femur and steadying the grid.

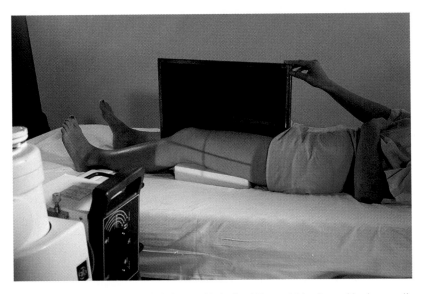

Fig. 30-22 Mobile *lateromedial* left femur. Note that the grid is placed between the legs and steadied by the patient.

 LATERAL PROJECTION*
Mediolateral or lateromedial
Dorsal decubitus position

The femur may not be able to be moved, which presents a challenge to the radiographer. The *mediolateral* projection is generally preferred because more of the proximal femur is demonstrated.

Image receptor: 35 × 43 cm (14 × 17 inch) grid lengthwise

Position of patient

- The patient is in the supine position.

Position of part

- Determine whether a mediolateral or lateromedial projection will be performed.

Mediolateral projection

- Visualize the optimum length of the patient's femur by placing the grid in a vertical position next to the lateral aspect of the femur.
- Place the distal edge of the grid low enough to include the patient's knee joint.
- Have the patient, if able, hold the upper corner of the grid for stabilization; otherwise, support the grid firmly in position.
- Support the unaffected leg by using the patient's support (a trapeze bar if present) or a support block.
- Elevate the *unaffected* leg until the femur is nearly vertical. An assistant may need to elevate and hold the leg of a critically ill patient. The assistant may also steady the grid and must wear a lead apron for protection (Fig. 30-21).

Lateromedial projection

- Place the grid next to the medial aspect of the affected femur (between the patient's legs), and ensure that the knee joint is included (Fig. 30-22).
- Ensure that the grid is placed *perpendicular* to the epicondylar plane.
- *Shield gonads.*
- *Respiration:* Suspend.

---

*The nonmobile projection is described in Chapter 6.

Central ray

- Perpendicular to the long axis of the femur, entering at its midpoint.
- Ensure that the central ray and grid are aligned to prevent grid cutoff; the central ray is centered to the femur and not to the center of the grid.

COMPUTED RADIOGRAPHY

The thickest portion of the femur (proximal area) must be measured carefully, and an appropriate kVp must be selected to penetrate this area. The computer cannot form an image of any anatomy in this area if penetration does not occur. A light area of the entire proximal femur will result. Positioning the cathode over the proximal femur will improve CR image quality.

Structures shown

This projection demonstrates the distal two thirds of the femur, including the knee joint, without superimposition of the opposite thigh (Fig. 30-23).

EVALUATION CRITERIA

The following should be clearly demonstrated:

- Majority of femur, including knee joint
- Patella in profile
- Superimposition of femoral condyles
- Opposite femur and soft tissue out of area of interest
- Adequate penetration of proximal portion of femur
- Orthopedic appliance, if present

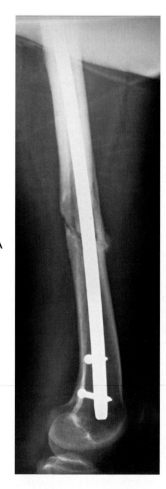

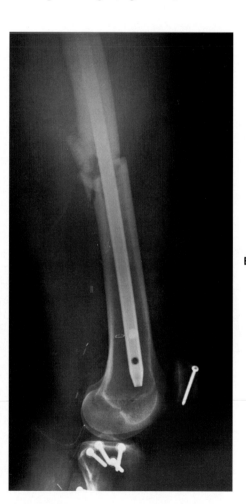

Fig. 30-23 Mobile lateral femur radiographs demonstrating midshaft fractures and femoral rod placement. Note that the knee joints are included on the image. **A**, Mediolateral. **B**, Lateromedial.

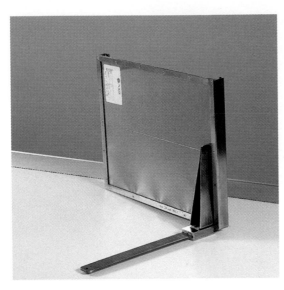

Fig. 30-24 Measuring caliper used to hold a 24 × 30 cm (10 × 12 inch) grid in place for mobile lateral cervical spine radiography.

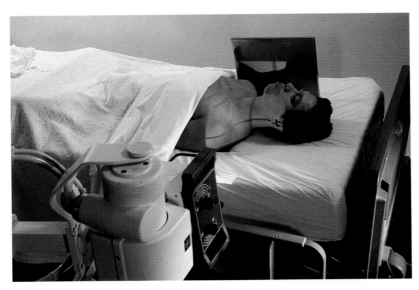

Fig. 30-25 Mobile lateral cervical spine.

LATERAL PROJECTION*
Right or left dorsal decubitus position

Image receptor: 24 × 30 cm (10 × 12 inch) grid lengthwise; may be performed with a nongrid cassette in smaller patients

Position of patient
- Position the patient in the supine position with arms extended down along the sides of the body.
- Observe whether a cervical collar or another immobilization device is being used. *Do not remove the device without the consent of the nurse or physician.*

Position of part
- Ensure that the upper torso, cervical spine, and head are not rotated.
- Place the grid lengthwise on the right or left side, parallel to the neck.
- Place the top of the grid approximately 1 to 2 inches (2.5 to 5 cm) above the external acoustic meatus (EAM) so that the grid is centered to C4 (upper thyroid cartilage).
- Raise the chin slightly. *In the patient with new trauma, suspected fracture, or known fracture of the cervical region, check with the physician before elevating the chin. Improper movement of a patient's head can disrupt a fractured cervical spine.*
- Immobilize the grid in a vertical position. The grid can be immobilized in multiple ways if a holding device is not available. The best method is to use the measuring caliper. Slide the long portion of the caliper under the shoulders of the patient, with the short end of the caliper pointing toward the ceiling and the grid held between the ends of the caliper (Fig. 30-24). Another method is to place pillows or a cushion between the side rail of the bed and the cassette, thereby holding the cassette next to the patient. Tape also works well in many instances (Fig. 30-25).
- Have the patient relax the shoulders and reach for the feet, if possible.
- *Shield gonads.*
- *Respiration*: Full expiration to obtain maximum depression of the shoulders.

---

*The nonmobile projection is described in Chapter 8.

Central ray

- Horizontal and perpendicular to the center of the grid. This should place the central ray at the level of C4 (upper thyroid cartilage).
- Ensure that proper alignment of the central ray and grid is maintained to prevent grid cutoff.
- Because of the great object-to-image distance (OID), a SID of 60 to 72 inches (158 to 183 cm) is recommended. This also helps to demonstrate C7.

COMPUTED RADIOGRAPHY

To ensure that the lower cervical vertebrae are fully penetrated, the kVp must be set to penetrate the C7 area.

Structures shown

This projection demonstrates the seven cervical vertebrae, including the base of the skull and the soft tissues surrounding the neck (Fig. 30-26).

EVALUATION CRITERIA

The following should be clearly demonstrated:

- All seven cervical vertebrae, including interspaces and spinous processes
- Neck extended when possible so that rami of mandible are not overlapping C1 or C2
- C4 in center of grid
- Superimposed posterior margins of each vertebral body

NOTE: It is essential that C6 and C7 be included on the image. To accomplish this, the radiographer should instruct the patient to relax the shoulders toward the feet as much as possible. If the examination involves pulling down on the patient's arms, the radiographer should exercise extreme caution and evaluate the patient's condition carefully to determine whether pulling of the arms can be tolerated. Fractures or injuries of the upper limbs, including the clavicles, must be considered. Furthermore, applying a strong pull to the arms of a patient in a hurried or jerking manner can disrupt a fractured cervical spine. If the lateral projection does not adequately visualize the lower cervical region, the Twining method, sometimes referred to as the "swimmers" position, which eliminates pulling of the arms, may be recommended for individuals who have experienced trauma or have a known cervical fracture. One arm must be placed above the patient's head (see Twining method, Chapter 8).

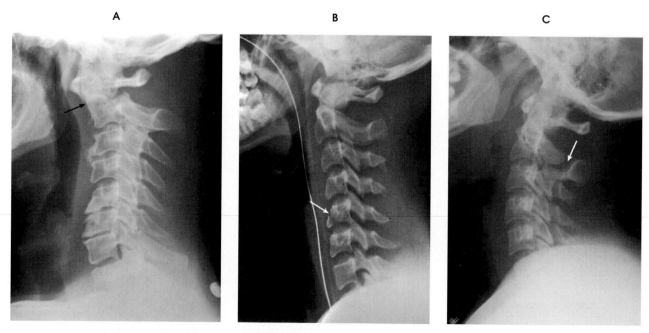

Fig. 30-26 Mobile lateral cervical spine radiographs performed at the patient's bedside several weeks after trauma. **A**, Entire cervical spine shows slight anterior subluxation of the dens on the body of C2 *(arrow)*. **B**, Entire cervical spine shows a nearly vertical fracture through the body of C5 with slight displacement *(arrow)*. **C**, The first five cervical vertebrae show vertical fractures through posterior aspects of C2 laminae *(arrow)* with 4-mm displacement of the fragments. Earlier radiographs demonstrated that C6 and C7 were unaffected and did not need to be included in this follow-up radiograph.

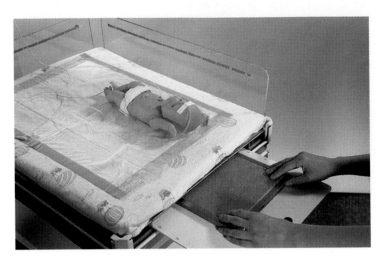

Fig. 30-27 Cassette being placed on a special tray for placement below the infant. Numbers along the side of tray correspond with numbers along the side of the bed railing to allow accurate positioning of the cassette.

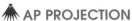

AP PROJECTION

The chest and abdomen combination described here is typically ordered for neonatal premature infants who are in the neonatal intensive care unit. If a chest or abdomen projection is ordered separately, the radiographer should adjust the central ray and collimator accordingly.

Image receptor: 8 × 10 inch (20 × 24 cm) lengthwise

Position of patient

Position the infant supine in the center of the cassette. Some bassinets have a special tray to hold the cassette. Positioning numbers along the tray permits accurate placement of the cassette (Fig. 30-27). If the cassette is directly under the infant, cover it with a soft, warm blanket.

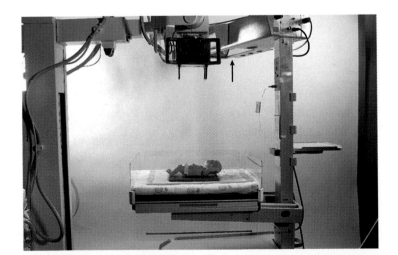

Fig. 30-28 Neonatal intensive care unit bassinet with premature infant. Overhead heating unit *(arrow)* is moved out of the way to accommodate the mobile x-ray machine tube head.

Position of part

- *Carefully* position the x-ray tube over the infant (Fig. 30-28).
- Ensure that the chest and abdomen are not rotated.
- Move the infant's arms away from the body or over the head and bring the legs down and away from the abdomen. The arms and legs may have to be held by a nurse, who should wear a lead apron.
- Leave the head of the infant rotated. (See note at end of this section.)
- Adjust the collimators closely to the chest and abdomen (Fig. 30-29).
- *Shield gonads.*
- *Respiration:* Inspiration. The neonatal infant has an extremely fast respiratory rate and cannot hold the breath. Make the best attempt possible to perform the exposure on full inspiration (Fig. 30-30).

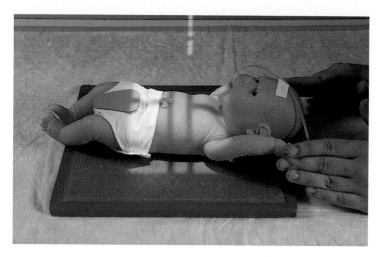

Fig. 30-29 Mobile chest and abdomen radiograph of neonate. Note the male gonad shield. (In actual practice the cassette is covered with a soft, warm blanket.)

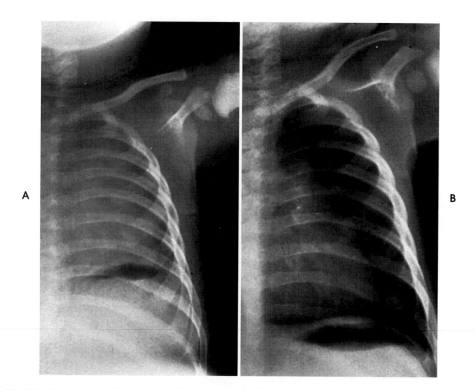

Fig. 30-30 Radiographs on inspiration and expiration in a neonatal infant. **A,** Left side of chest is shown at full *expiration*. Note the lack of normal lung markings and the illusion of massive pulmonary disease. The diaphragm is not seen, and the heart appears enlarged. **B,** Repeat radiograph of the same patient performed correctly at full *inspiration*. The diaphragm may be seen correctly at the level of the tenth posterior rib. The same technical factors were used for both exposures.

(Courtesy Department of Radiology, Rochester General Hospital, Rochester, NY; from Cullinan AM, Cullinan JE: *Producing quality radiographs,* ed 2, Philadelphia, 1994, Lippincott.)

Central ray

- Perpendicular to the midpoint of the chest and abdomen along the midsagittal plane

Structures shown

The anatomy of the entire chest and abdomen is demonstrated (Fig. 30-31).

EVALUATION CRITERIA

The following should be clearly demonstrated:

- Anatomy from apices to pubic symphysis in the thoracic and abdominal regions
- No motion
- No blurring of lungs, diaphragm, and abdominal structures
- No rotation of patient

NOTE: When performing an AP or lateral projection of the chest, the radiographer should keep the head and neck of the infant straight so that the anatomy in the upper chest and airway is accurately visualized. However, straightening the head of a neonatal infant in the supine position can inadvertently advance an endotracheal tube too far into the trachea. Therefore it is sometimes more important to leave the head of an intubated neonatal patient rotated in the position in which the infant routinely lies to obtain accurate representation of the position of the endotracheal tube on the radiograph.

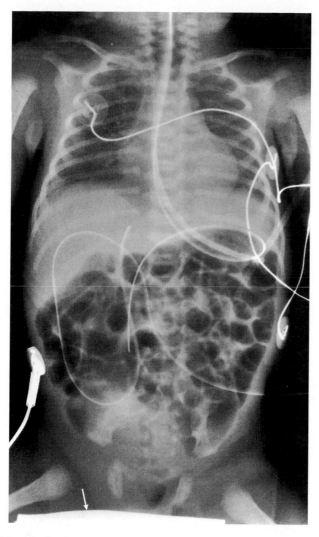

Fig. 30-31 Mobile AP chest and abdomen radiograph of a neonate. The exposure technique demonstrates the anatomy of the entire chest and abdomen. Note the gonad shield accurately positioned on this male infant *(arrow)*.

LATERAL PROJECTION
Right or left dorsal decubitus position

Image receptor: 8 × 10 inch (20 × 24 cm) lengthwise

Most neonatal premature infants cannot be turned on their sides or placed upright for a lateral projection.

Position of patient
- *Carefully* place the x-ray tube to the side of the bassinet.
- Position the infant supine on a radiolucent block covered with a soft, warm blanket. If a radiolucent block is not readily available, an inverted box of tissues works well.

Position of part
- Ensure that the infant's chest and abdomen are centered to the cassette and not rotated.
- Move the infant's arms above the head. The arms will have to be held up by a nurse, who should wear a lead apron.
- Place the cassette lengthwise and vertical beside the patient and then immobilize it.
- Leave the head of the infant rotated. (See note on p. 234).
- Adjust the collimators closely to the chest and abdomen (Fig. 30-32).
- *Shield gonads.*
- *Respiration:* Inspiration. The neonatal infant has an extremely fast respiratory rate and cannot hold the breath. Make the best attempt possible to perform the exposure on full inspiration.

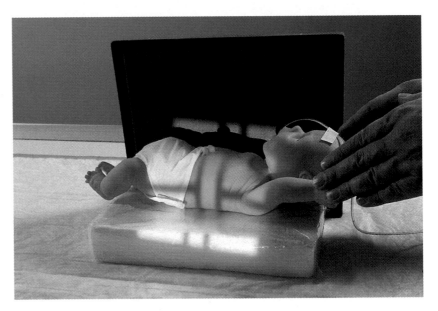

Fig. 30-32 Mobile lateral chest and abdomen of a neonate in the dorsal decubitus position. The infant is positioned on a raised block with the cassette below the block.

Chest and Abdomen: Neonate

Central ray

- Horizontal and perpendicular to the midpoint of the chest and abdomen along the midcoronal plane

Structures shown

This projection demonstrates the anatomy of the entire chest and abdomen, with special attention to the costophrenic angles in the posterior chest. If present, air and fluid levels are visualized (Fig. 30-33).

Selected bibliography

Adler AM, Carlton RR: *Introduction to radiography and patient care*, Philadelphia, 1994, WB Saunders.

Bontrager KL: *Textbook of radiographic positioning*, ed 4, St Louis, 1997, Mosby.

Bushong SC: *Radiologic science for technologists*, ed 6, St Louis, 1997, Mosby.

Carlton RR, Adler AM: *Principles of radiographic imaging: an art and a science*, ed 2, Albany, NY, 1996, Delmar.

Cullinan AM, Cullinan JE: *Producing quality radiographs*, ed 2, Philadelphia, 1994, Lippincott.

Drafke MW: *Trauma and mobile radiography*, Philadelphia, 1990, FA Davis.

Ehrlich RA, McClosky ED: *Patient care in radiography*, ed 4, St Louis, 1997, Mosby.

Gray JE et al: *Quality control in diagnostic imaging*, Rockville, Md, 1983, Aspen.

Kowalczyk N, Donnet K: *Introductory patient care for the imaging professional*, ed 2, St Louis, 1998, Mosby.

Statkiewicz-Sherer MA, Visconti PJ, Ritenour ER: *Radiation protection in medical radiography*, St Louis, 1998, Mosby.

Thompson MA et al: *Principles of imaging science and protection*, Philadelphia, 1994, WB Saunders.

Torres LS: *Basic medical techniques and patient care in imaging technology*, Philadelphia, 1997, Lippincott.

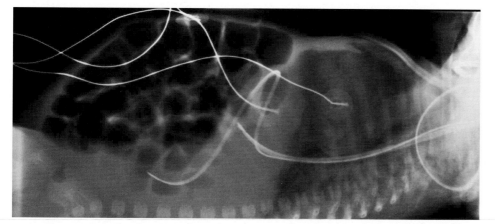

Fig. 30-33 Mobile lateral chest and abdomen radiograph of a neonate in the dorsal decubitus position. The exposure technique demonstrates the anatomy of the entire chest and abdomen.

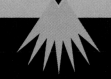

CARDIAC CATHETERIZATION

JEFFREY A. HUFF

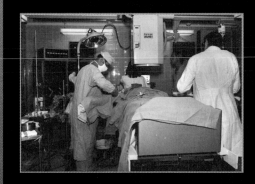

RIGHT: Catheterization laboratory from the 1970s.

(Courtesy Sedgewick Archives, College of Medicine, The Ohio State University, Columbus, Ohio.)

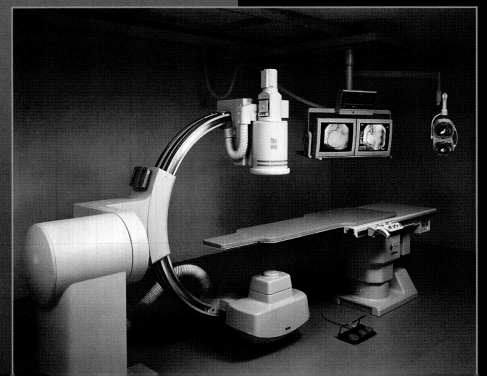

LEFT: Modern single-plane digital catheterization with "smart handle" technology.

(Courtesy Toshiba America Medical Systems.)

Cardiac catheterization is a comprehensive term used to describe a minor surgical procedure involving the introduction of specialized catheters into the heart and surrounding vasculature for the purpose of diagnostic evaluation and therapy (*intervention**) associated with a variety of cardiovascular-related disorders in both children and adults. Thus cardiac catheterization can be classified as either a diagnostic study or an interventional procedure. The primary purpose of diagnostic studies is to collect data necessary to evaluate the patient's condition. Cardiac interventional procedures involve the application of therapeutic measures through catheter-based systems to treat disorders of the vascular and conduction systems within the heart mechanically or pharmaceutically.

---

*Almost all italicized terms are defined at the end of this chapter.

Historical Development

As early as 1844, experimental placement of catheters into the hearts of animals led to the successful catheterization of both the right and left ventricles of a horse by Claude Bernard, a French physiologist. The first human cardiac catheterization was reported in 1929 by Forssman, a 25-year-old surgical resident who placed a catheter into his own heart and then walked to the radiology department where a chest radiograph was produced to document his medical achievement. Catheterization of the heart soon became a valuable tool used primarily for diagnostic purposes. Through the 1940s the basic catheterization study remained relatively uncomplicated and easy for physicians to perform; however, the risk to the patient was significant.

In the years that followed, catheterization methods and techniques increased in number and complexity and were refined. The refinements included the development of the Seldinger technique (see Chapter 26) and the introduction of the transseptal left-heart catheter. Selective coronary *angiography* was first reported by Sones in 1959, when he inadvertently injected contrast medium into the right coronary artery of a patient who was undergoing routine aortography. By the early 1960s, coronary angiography was an accepted selective procedure. In 1962, Ricketts and Abrams described the first percutaneous method for selective coronary angiography. This method was further perfected in the late 1960s with the introduction of preformed catheters designed to seek out the ostium of both the right and left coronary arteries.

The 1960s and 1970s brought tremendous advances in radiologic and cardiovascular medicine and technology. Radiographic imaging and recording equipment, physiologic monitoring equipment, and cardiovascular pharmaceuticals and supplies became increasingly reliable. Since the 1970s major efforts have been made to increase the dependability, applicability, and diversity of cardiac catheterization interventional techniques. The use of computers in the catheterization laboratory has facilitated the development of this rapidly growing subspecialty of the cardiovascular medical and surgical sciences. These advances and trends have enabled cardiac catheterization to evolve from a simple diagnostic investigation to its current state as a sophisticated diagnostic study and interventional procedure.

Principles of Cardiac Catheterization

General indications, contraindications, and risks are associated with diagnostic and interventional cardiac catheterizations. The physician must consider these factors when attempting to determine the appropriateness of any type of catheterization.

GENERAL INDICATIONS

Cardiac catheterization is performed to identify the anatomic and physiologic condition of the heart. The data gathered during catheterization provide the physician with information to develop management strategies for patients who have cardiovascular disorders. Coronary *angiography* is currently the most definitive procedure for visualizing the coronary anatomy. The anatomic information gained from this procedure may include the presence and extent of obstructive coronary artery disease, thrombus formation, coronary artery collateral flow, coronary anomalies, aneurysms, and spasm. Coronary artery size can also be determined.

Coronary artery disease is the most common disorder necessitating catheterization of the adult heart. This disease is caused primarily by the accumulation of fatty intracoronary *atheromatous* plaque, which leads to *stenosis* and *occlusion* of the coronary arteries. Coronary artery disease is symptomatically characterized by chest pain *(angina pectoris)* or a heart attack *(myocardial infarction [MI])*. Treatment of coronary artery disease includes both medical and surgical intervention.

Diagnostic cardiac catheterization of the adult patient with coronary artery disease is conducted to assess the appropriateness and feasibility of various therapeutic options. For example, cardiac catheterization is performed before open-heart surgery to provide *hemodynamic* and angiographic data to document the presence and severity of disease. In selected circumstances, postoperative catheterization is performed to assess the results of surgery. An interventional procedure (such as *percutaneous transluminal coronary angioplasty [PTCA]*, *intracoronary stent*, or *atherectomy*) may be indicated for the relief of *arteriosclerotic* coronary artery stenosis.

Diagnostic studies of the adult heart also aid in evaluating the patient who has confusing or obscure symptoms (such as chest pain of undetermined cause). These studies are also used to assess diseases of the heart not requiring surgical intervention, such as certain *cardiomyopathies*.

In children, diagnostic heart catheterization is employed in the evaluation of congenital and valvular disease, disorders of the cardiac conduction system, and selected cardiomyopathies. Interventional techniques are also performed in children, primarily to alleviate the symptoms associated with certain congenital heart defects.

With the complexity of cardiovascular disease and the numerous catheterization procedures that are available, establishing a comprehensive list of the indications for cardiac catheterization is difficult. Instead, because coronary angiography is the procedure most frequently performed in the catheterization laboratory, the indications for this procedure as established by the American College of Cardiology and the American Heart Association (ACC/AHA) are discussed in this chapter (see selected bibliography). The indications include the following disease states:

- Known or suspected coronary heart disease, both symptomatic and asymptomatic
- Atypical chest pain of uncertain origin
- Acute *myocardial infarction (MI)* (evolving, completed, and convalescent)
- Valvular heart disease
- Known or suspected congenital heart disease
- Conditions such as dilated cardiomyopathy and disease affecting the aorta

The ACC/AHA guidelines also indicate the risks, benefits, and uses of the procedure by placing the previously discussed disease categories into three classifications:

Class 1—conditions for which general agreement exists that coronary angiography is justified

Class 2—Conditions for which coronary angiography is frequently performed, but for which a divergence of opinion exists with respect to its justification in terms of value and appropriateness

Class 3—conditions for which coronary angiography ordinarily is not justified

CONTRAINDICATIONS AND ASSOCIATED RISKS

Cardiac catheterization has associated inherent risk factors. However, many physicians agree that the only absolute contraindication to this procedure is refusal of the procedure by a mentally competent person.

Contraindications for coronary angiography are relatively few when the appropriateness of the procedure is based on the benefit-risk ratio. Relative contraindications may include the following:

- Active gastrointestinal bleeding
- Renal insufficiency
- Recent stroke
- Fever from infection or the presence of an active infection
- Severe electrolyte imbalance
- Severe anemia
- Short life expectancy because of other illness
- Digitalis intoxication
- Patient refusal of therapeutic treatment such as PTCA or bypass surgery
- Severe uncontrolled hypertension
- *Coagulopathy* and bleeding disorders
- Pulmonary edema
- Uncontrolled ventricular *arrhythmias*

Some of these conditions may be temporary, or they may be treated and reversed before cardiac catheterization is attempted.

The risks of cardiac catheterization vary according to the type of procedure and the status of the patient undergoing the procedure. Variables include the anatomy to be studied; type of catheter and approach used; history of drug allergy; presence of basic cardiovascular disease or noncardiac disease such as asthma or diabetes; *hemodynamic* status; and age and other patient characteristics.

As with any invasive procedure, complications can be expected during cardiac catheterization. The Society for Cardiac Angiography and Interventions (SCA&I) reviewed the catheterizations for 53,581 patients performed in 66 member laboratories from October 1979 to December 1980 and found the major complication rate for the entire group was 1.82%. Major complications included death, MI, cerebrovascular accident (CVA, or stroke), major arrhythmias, vascular injury, and other miscellaneous complications. More recently the SCA&I reviewed the catheterizations of an additional 222,553 patients performed over a 3-year period from 1984 through 1987 and found that the major complication rate for the entire group was 1.74%.

The risks associated with cardiac catheterization have decreased in recent years. However, as the severity of the patient's disease increases, so do the risks associated with the procedure. Therefore the benefits expected to be derived from cardiac catheterization must be weighed against the associated risks of the procedure.

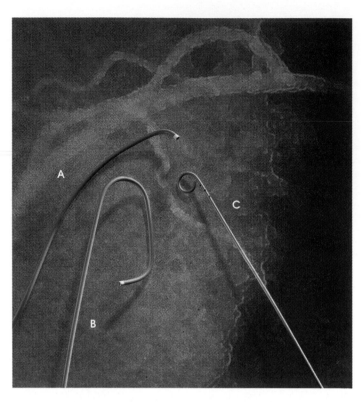

Fig. 31-1 Catheters used during cardiac catheterization: *A,* Judkins right; *B,* Judkins left; *C,* pigtail.

(Courtesy Cordis Corp., Miami.)

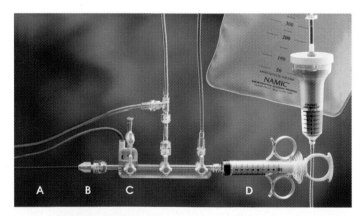

Fig. 31-2 Disposable 3 valve Compensator Morse manifold, with a Selector catheter *(A),* rotating adapter *(B),* pressure transducer *(C),* and angiographic control syringe *(D).*

(Courtesy SCHNEIDER/NAMIC, Glens Falls, New York.)

Specialized Equipment

Cardiac catheterization has developed into a highly complex, sophisticated procedure requiring specialized equipment and supplies. Unlike earlier radiographic examinations of the intracardiac structures, modern cardiac catheterization requires more than a simple fluoroscope and a recording modality such as that used in overhead radiography.

Equipment required for cardiac catheterization can be categorized in five groups: (1) cardiovascular, (2) fluoroscopic, (3) cineangiographic, (4) digital imaging, and (5) ancillary equipment and supplies. The following are examples of equipment typically contained in each group.

CARDIOVASCULAR EQUIPMENT
Catheters

Catheters are long, thin tubes placed in the human vasculature (Fig. 31-1). They are available in various lengths, shapes, and diameters, and they also have varying numbers of side holes. The physician decides which catheter to use in a particular circumstance. Cardiac catheters are radiopaque, presterilized, preshaped, and disposable.

The catheter (or catheters) placed in a patient's vasculature can function as a fluid-filled column for hemodynamic data or as a conduit for contrast media, *thrombolytic* agents, and mechanical devices. Blood samples can be drawn directly from selected cardiac chambers for the purpose of *oximetry* or other laboratory analysis. So that these and other tasks can be performed, three or four valves (stopcocks) are combined to form a *manifold* attached to the proximal end of the coronary catheter (Fig. 31-2). Using a manifold allows such functions as drawing blood samples, administering medications, and recording blood pressures to be performed without disconnecting the catheter.

Physiologic monitoring equipment

The physiologic recorder is integral to cardiac catheterization procedures. It is used to monitor and record vital patient functions, including electrical activity within the heart and certain hemodynamic parameters such as the pressures within various intracardiac chambers (Fig. 31-3). Patients are monitored during the entire catheterization procedure (regardless of the type performed) with periodic electrocardiographic (ECG or EKG) and pressure recordings.

For the collecting of hemodynamic data during catheterization, the physiologic recorder (receiving information in electrical form) must be connected to the catheter (carrying information as physical fluid pressure). Devices called *transducers* are interfaced between the manifold and the physiologic recorder to convert fluid (blood) pressure into an electrical signal (see Fig. 31-2).

For a standard cardiac catheterization, physiologic recorders usually have four channels: two for ECG recordings and two for pressure recordings. However, a physiological recorder can have as many as 16 channels. A channel, or module, is an electrical component of the physiologic recorder that is capable of measuring an individual parameter such as a specific type of ECG or intravascular pressure. The number of channels required for a particular catheterization increases as the amount of detailed information required increases. Increasingly these systems are produced with detailed information and procedural databases for the collection and maintenance of patient clinical data as well as the concurrent generation of a report at the time of catheterization.

Pressure injector

The pressure injector for the administration of radiographic contrast medium (Fig. 31-4) is used not only during cardiac catheterization but also in general angiography (see Chapter 26). In the catheterization laboratory the pressure injector is generally used to inject a large amount (25 to 50 ml) of contrast material into the left ventricle (the main pumping chamber of the heart) or to visualize the aortic root and pulmonary vessels. Administration of contrast medium into the coronary arteries generally does not require a high-pressure injector.

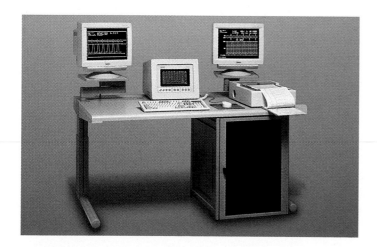

Fig. 31-3 Computer-based physiologic monitor used to monitor patient ECG and hemodynamic pressures during cardiac catheterization.

(Courtesy Quinton Instrument Co., Bothell, Wash.)

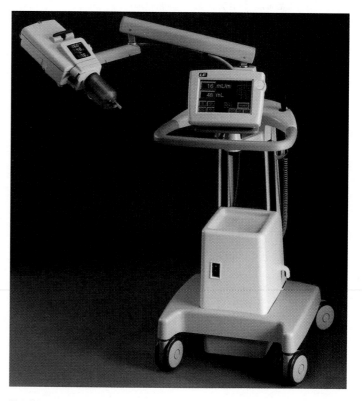

Fig. 31-4 The Angiomat (ILLUMENA) high-pressure injector for radiographic contrast medium.

(Courtesy Liebel-Flarsheim, a product of Mallinckrodt, Inc., Cincinnati.)

FLUOROSCOPIC IMAGING

The fluoroscopic imaging equipment found in the cardiac catheterization laboratory is essentially the same as that found in the vascular angiography suite. The catheterization laboratory requires an electrooptical system capable of producing fluoroscopic images with the greatest amount of recorded detail available. Maximum resolution from the optical system is crucial because of the small size of the cardiac anatomy.

Fluoroscopic tubes must be capable of producing ionizing radiation for the long periods of time necessary for fluoroscopy and therefore must be designed to withstand greater heat loading. For most catheterization imaging, multifocal-spot, high-speed rotating fluoroscopic tubes are desirable. Extremely short exposure times are required to accommodate the rapid-exposure sequencing of the various recording systems.

A high-resolution imaging and recording system requires several pieces of equipment, including an image intensification tube. This tube should produce the maximum recorded detail necessary for cardiac catheterization. The image intensification tube used in the cardiac catheterization laboratory generally comes with a choice of two, three, or four magnification modes to allow for enhanced visualization of small anatomic structures. For viewing "live" fluoroscopic images, a television camera is coupled to the output phosphor of the image intensifier, and its signal is fed to television monitors placed so that the images can be easily observed during the procedure.

CINEANGIOGRAPHIC AND VIDEOTAPE IMAGE RECORDING

Cineangiography ("cine" meaning *film*) and videotape systems permanently record images on film and at the same time allow for immediate playback and review during the procedure. Permanent recording of the cineangiographic image is made on 35-mm black-and-white movie film. For this purpose, a high-resolution motion picture camera is attached to the image intensifier to record the image at 30 or 60 frames per second. Cineangiographic recording and videotape recording occur simultaneously.

DIGITAL ANGIOGRAPHIC IMAGE RECORDING

Digital angiography has gained universal acceptance in the catheterization laboratory. Digital imaging now produces resolution comparable with that of the 35-mm cineangiographic film image. The resolution possible with early digital equipment was a drawback to the use of digital imaging in the catheterization laboratory. Larger matrix size, the obvious solution to this problem, allowed for acceptable resolution but also created another problem: how to acquire and store large volumes of digital information.

In the late 1970s and early 1980s the high-speed parallel transfer disk was introduced to solve the acquisition and short-term storage problem. This new disk acquired and stored an entire coronary angiogram and made real-time digital playback during the procedure possible.

Permanent storage of the digital images remained a problem. Floppy disk and computer tape storage were not adequate solutions because they required significant amounts of time and supplies.

Long-term storage of large amounts of digital images has benefited from advances in computer technology. Larger hard drives, digital tape storage, magnetooptical disks, compact discs, and digital video disks (DVD) are a few of the new storage media. These storage devices provide a high-speed, large-capacity method of storage, capable of acquiring large amounts of data (32 gigabytes [GB]) with very high resolution.

A committee composed of industry representatives was established to set standards for digital imaging. The Digital Communications Committee (DICOM) has set guidelines for a universal exchange standard in digital imaging. The committee determined that the compact disc recordable (CD-R) would be the preferred storage medium for single-patient study transfer between institutions. The CD-R, which is the same size as the compact disc read-only memory (CD-ROM), is a one-time recording medium capable of storing 650 megabytes (MB) of information. Because the CD-R can store such a large amount of information, it is quickly becoming the equivalent of a cineangiography film. Applications involving DVD are still evolving. Eventually it will be possible to store up to 14 GB of information on one DVD. (Definitions and other information on computer fundamentals are presented in Chapter 32.)

The speculation that digital imaging systems will someday replace cineangiography film as the standard for cardiac catheterization imaging is now nearly a reality. Problems regarding ways to transport and view digital images easily have been addressed by the DICOM standard. To conform to this standard, equipment manufacturers will continue to produce digital products that can be accessed by any other manufacturer's product line.

One disadvantage of the CD-R is the need to purchase the equipment to download and play back the images. Currently all catheterization laboratories have a cineangiographic projector to view 35-mm film angiograms, but not every catheterization laboratory has the equipment necessary to view the CD-R. Until all laboratories have the equipment to meet the DICOM standard, cineangiographic imaging will continue to be used.

Today the cineangiography versus digital question is solved through the use of *simultaneous acquisition* technology, which means that cineangiographic film and digital images are acquired at the same time. This technology combines the practicality of 35-mm cineangiographic film with the image manipulation and analysis capabilities (e.g., left ventricular ejection fraction calculations, coronary artery stenosis sizing) of digital angiograms.

ANCILLARY EQUIPMENT AND SUPPLIES

Because of the nature of the patient's condition and the inherent risks of cardiac catheterization, each catheterization room requires a fully equipped emergency cart. The cart typically contains emergency medications, cardiopulmonary resuscitation equipment, defibrillators, intubation equipment, and other related supplies. Oxygen and suction must also be readily available. Oximeters are used to determine the oxygen saturation of the blood samples obtained during adult and pediatric catheterizations (Fig. 31-5).

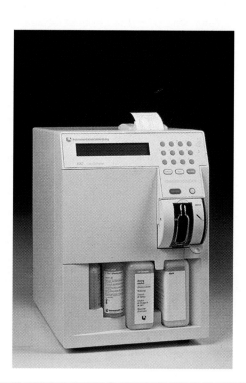

Fig. 31-5 Oximeter used to measure oxygen saturation in blood.

(Courtesy Instrumentation Laboratories, Lexington, Mass.)

Several iodinated radiographic contrast media are approved for intravascular, intracardiac, and intracoronary use in both adults and children. Transient (temporary) ECG changes during and immediately after the injection of contrast medium are common. Because of their properties, nonionic contrast media and ionic low-osmolar contrast media have gained acceptance and are now used in many cardiac catheterization laboratories. Unfortunately, the newer contrast media are considerably more expensive. Nonionic contrast media have some definite advantages over ionic high-osmolar contrast media. For example, they are associated with a reduced incidence of cardiovascular reactions and side effects as a result of their lower osmotic pressure. Most catheterization laboratories now use the newer contrast media.

Patient Positioning for Cardiac Catheterization

Procedures such as selective coronary arteriography and certain pediatric catheterizations require imaging equipment to be positioned to reduce the superimposition created by the cardiac vasculature. Moving the patient during the catheterization is not desirable, particularly when catheters have been carefully positioned to demonstrate specific anatomic structures or to record certain data.

In most catheterization laboratories the image intensifier and fluoroscopic tube are mechanically suspended in a C-arm configuration to allow for equipment rotation around the patient and to provide cranial or caudal angulation. In this configuration the image intensifier is above the plane of the table, and the fluoroscopic tube is beneath the table. During catheterization procedures the patient is placed on the examination table in a supine position. For optimal images, the imaging equipment should be rotated around the patient. In some interventional procedures, biplane C-arms are advantageous because they allow simultaneous imaging of cardiac structures in two different planes (Fig. 31-6).

Adult and pediatric coronary anatomy has both normal and pathologic variations. Therefore projections for each type of catheterization procedure cannot be specified. Instead, each patient's anatomy must be fluoroscopically evaluated to ascertain the optimum degree of rotation and cranial or caudal angulation necessary to visualize each structure of interest.

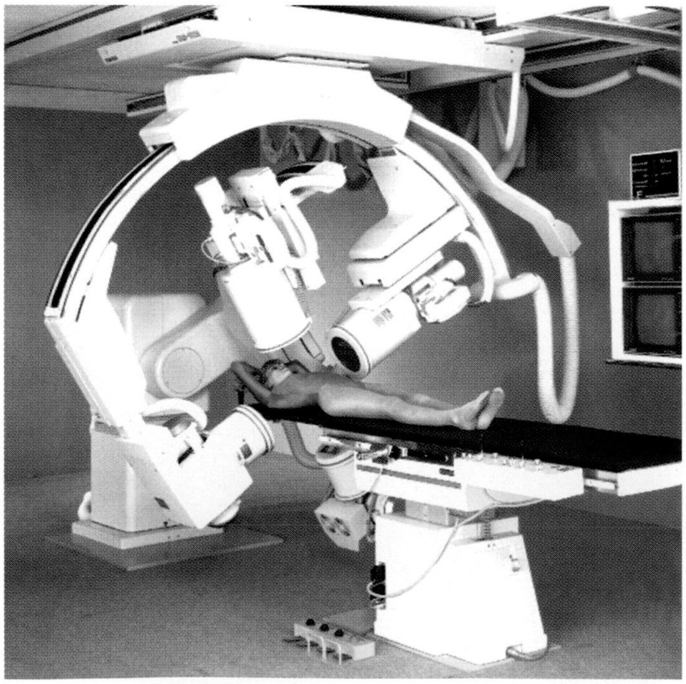

Catheterization Methods and Techniques

Different cardiac catheterizations require various combinations of methods and techniques to allow for precise data acquisition and the application of therapeutic interventions. Some methods and techniques common to most cardiac catheterizations are discussed in the following sections.

PRECATHETERIZATION CARE

Before the catheterization is performed, the procedure is explained and informed consent is obtained. Testing before catheterization normally includes the following:
- Patient history
- Physical examination
- Chest x-ray examination
- Blood work
- ECG
- Echocardiogram
- Exercise stress test

Various medications are frequently administered for sedation and control of nausea.

Patients brought to the catheterization laboratory typically are not allowed anything to eat or drink for 4 to 6 hours before the procedure. During all catheterizations a protocol, or detailed record, of the procedure is maintained. The record includes hemodynamic data, fluoroscopy time, medications administered, supplies used, and other pertinent information.

Fig. 31-6 Biplane radiology equipment used in the cardiac catheterization laboratory.

(Courtesy Toshiba America Medical Systems.)

CATHETER INTRODUCTION

After the patient has been transported to the catheterization laboratory, ECG and blood pressure monitoring are initiated. The appropriate site for catheter introduction must be prepared using aseptic technique to minimize the risk of subsequent infection. The area of the body to be entered is shaved, and an antiseptic solution is applied. Numerous sites can be used for catheter introduction. The specific sites vary according to the age and body habitus of the patient, the preference of the physician, and the procedure attempted.

For catheterization of the femoral artery or vein, the percutaneous approach is employed. (See the Seldinger technique, which is detailed in Chapter 26, Fig. 26-11.) In the Seldinger technique the skin is aseptically prepared and infiltrated with a local anesthetic. The skin is punctured with a special angiography needle that is then placed in the desired vessel. A guide wire is advanced through the needle into the artery or vein; the needle is removed, leaving the guide wire in the vessel. An introducer, essentially a one-way valve, is placed over the guide wire and advanced into the vessel. This creates a controlled access into which catheters may be introduced with very little loss of blood. The catheter is placed over the guide wire and advanced toward the heart. The guide wire may be removed or temporarily left in place to facilitate further placement of the catheter. When the catheter is in the proper position, the guide wire is removed, the catheter is connected to the manifold, and the coronary angiogram may begin.

If the percutaneous approach cannot be used, a cut-down technique is employed. This technique requires that a small incision be made in the skin to allow for direct visualization of the artery or vein the physician wants to catheterize. The skin is aseptically prepared and infiltrated with local anesthetic, and the vessel or vessels are bluntly dissected and exposed. After an opening is created in the desired vessel (*arteriotomy* or *venotomy*), the catheter is introduced and advanced toward the heart. Cut-down procedures are frequently performed in the right antecubital fossa to access the basilic vein or brachial artery.

DATA COLLECTION

The acquisition of certain data is essential, regardless of the type of catheterization performed. Physiologic data typically collected include hemodynamic parameters and ECG and oximetry readings.

Hemodynamic parameters include blood pressure and *cardiac output.* The monitoring and recording of both intracardiac (within the heart) and extracardiac (outside the heart) vascular pressures require the use of the catheter-manifold-transducer-physiologic apparatus system described previously in this chapter. *Cardiac output,* an important indicator of the overall ability of the heart to pump blood, can be measured in the catheterization laboratory. Several methods are used to obtain estimates of cardiac output. The ECG is continuously monitored during catheterization and can be simultaneously recorded with intracardiac or extracardiac pressures (Fig. 31-7). Blood samples are obtained from the various chambers of the heart to determine *oxygen saturation* levels.

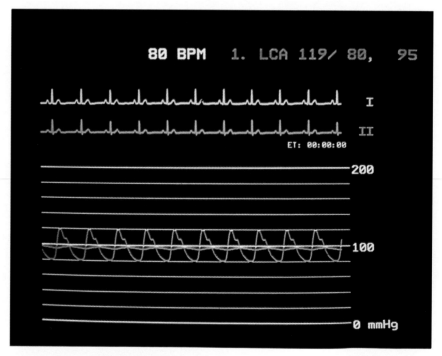

Fig. 31-7 Simulated electrocardiogram *(top)* and aortic pressure *(bottom).*

(Courtesy Quinton Instrument Co., Bothell, Wash.)

Catheterization Studies and Procedures

The primary purpose of the diagnostic cardiac catheterization is data collection, and the primary purpose of the interventional procedure is therapy. The following sections briefly describe some of the more commonly performed diagnostic and interventional heart catheterizations.

BASIC DIAGNOSTIC STUDIES OF THE VASCULAR SYSTEM

Adults

Catheterization of the left side of the heart is a widely performed, basic diagnostic cardiac study. The catheter may be introduced through the brachial or femoral artery, advanced to the ascending aorta, and passed through the aortic valve into the left ventricle. Arterial oximetry is performed, and pressures are taken in the left ventricle; these measurements are repeated as the catheter is withdrawn across the aortic valve. Selective angiography of the right coronary artery and left coronary artery is performed, with different projections used for each coronary artery to prevent superimposition with overlapping structures. Coronary angiography allows the extent of intracoronary stenosis to be evaluated (Figs. 31-8 and 31-9).

Because of the complexity of the anatomy involved, the variations in patient body habitus, and the presence of anomalies, a comprehensive guide for angiographic projections is difficult to establish. Instead, projections commonly used during coronary angiography are included in Table 31-1. The physician determines the projections that best demonstrate the artery of interest. Coronary arteriograms are obtained in nearly all catheterizations of the left side of the heart.

Angiography of the left ventricle is performed in nearly all catheterization studies of the left side of the heart (Fig. 31-10). Left ventriculography provides information about *valvular competence, interventricular septal integrity,* and the efficiency of the pumping action of the left ventricle (ejection fraction).

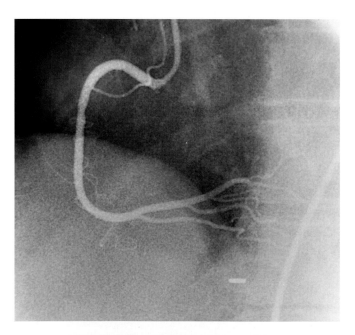

Fig. 31-8 Normal right coronary artery.

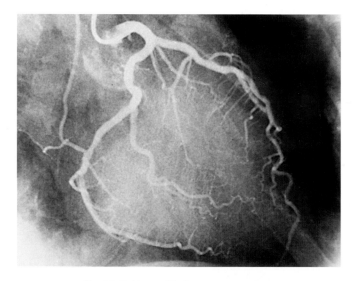

Fig. 31-9 Normal left coronary artery.

Catheterization of the right side of the heart is another commonly performed procedure. During right heart catheterization, a catheter is inserted into a vein in the groin or antecubital fossa and advanced to the vena cava, into the right atrium, across the tricuspid valve, to the right ventricle, and through the pulmonary valve to the pulmonary artery, until it is wedged distally in the pulmonary artery. Pressure measurements and oximetry are performed in each of the heart chambers as the catheter is advanced. The pressure measurements are used to determine the presence of such disorders as valvular heart disease, congestive heart failure, and certain cardiomyopathies. The oximetry data are used to determine the presence of an intracardiac shunt. Cineangiography is performed as appropriate.

Exercise *hemodynamics* are often required in the evaluation of valvular heart disease when symptoms of fatigue and *dyspnea* are present. In such cases, simultaneous catheterization and pressure measurements of the right and left heart are performed at rest and during peak exercise. Exercise often consists of pedaling a stationary bicycle, exercycle-type device—an *ergometer*—which is placed on top of the examination table. During simultaneous catheterization a catheter is placed in a vein (femoral or basilic) and an artery (femoral or brachial).

TABLE 31-1

Common angiographic angles for specific coronary arteries

Coronary artery	Vessel segment	Projection*
Left coronary artery	Left main	PA or RAO 5 to 15 degrees
	Left anterior descending	LAO 30 to 40 degrees, cranial 20 to 40 degrees
		RAO 5 to 15 degrees, cranial 15 to 45 degrees
		RAO 20 to 40 degrees, caudal 15 to 30 degrees
		RAO 30 to 50 degrees
		Lateral
	Circumflex	RAO 20 to 40 degrees, caudal 15 to 30 degrees
		LAO 40 to 55 degrees, caudal 15 to 30 degrees
		LAO 40 to 60 degrees
Right coronary artery	Middle right	LAO 20 to 40 degrees
		RAO 20 to 40 degrees
	Posterior descending	LAO 5 to 30 degrees, cranial 15 to 30 degrees

*PA, Posteroanterior; *RAO*, right anterior oblique; *LAO*, left anterior oblique.

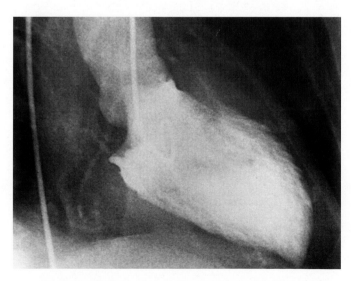

Fig. 31-10 Normal left ventriculogram during diastole.

Children

A primary indication for diagnostic catheterization studies in children is the evaluation and documentation of specific anatomy, hemodynamic data, and selected aspects of cardiac function associated with congenital heart defects. Methods and techniques used for catheterization of the pediatric heart vary depending on age, heart size, type and extent of defect, and other coincident pathophysiologic conditions.

Pediatric cardiac catheters are often introduced *percutaneously* into the femoral vein and in older children sometimes into the femoral artery. In very young patients, it may be possible to pass a catheter from the right atrium to the left atrium (thereby allowing access to the left side of the heart) through either a *patent foramen ovale* or a preexisting atrial septal defect. If the atrial septum is intact, temporary access to the left atrium may be obtained using a transseptal catheter system. With the transseptal catheter system, a long introducer and needle are used to puncture the right atrial septum of the heart to gain access to the left atrium if access cannot be attained as previously described.

ADVANCED DIAGNOSTIC STUDIES OF THE VASCULAR SYSTEM: ADULTS AND CHILDREN

An example of an advanced diagnostic study of the vascular system is *endomyocardial biopsy*, which is performed to provide a tissue sample for direct pathologic evaluation of cardiac muscle. A special biopsy catheter with a bioptome tip (Fig. 31-11) is advanced under fluoroscopic control from either the jugular or femoral vein to the right ventricle (Fig. 31-12). After the bioptome is advanced into the ventricle, the jaws of the device are opened and the catheter is advanced to the ventricular septum. After the bioptome is in contact with the septum, its jaws are closed and a gentle tugging motion is applied to retrieve the tissue sample. Several biopsy specimens are acquired in this manner. The specimens are immediately fixed in either glutaraldehyde or buffered formalin before being sent for pathologic evaluation. Endomyocardial biopsy is frequently used to monitor cardiac transplantation patients for early signs of tissue rejection and to differentiate between various types of cardiomyopathies.

A
B

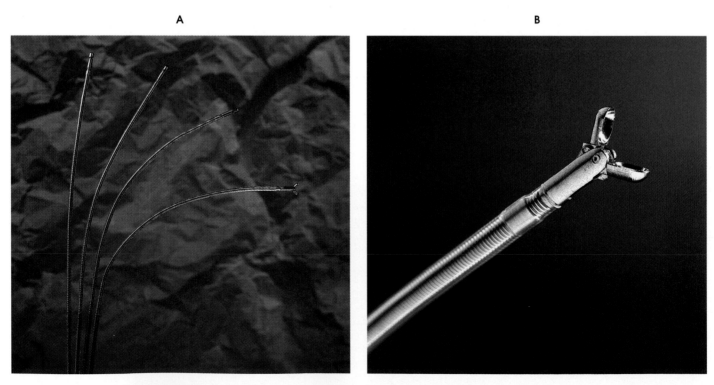

Fig. 31-11 A, Standard biopsy catheters. **B,** Bioptome catheter tip used for myocardial biopsy. The jaws on the tip close and take a "bite" from the inside of the heart muscle.

(Courtesy Cordis Corp., Miami.)

ADVANCED DIAGNOSTIC STUDIES OF THE CONDUCTION SYSTEM: ADULTS AND CHILDREN

Electrophysiology studies involve the collection of sophisticated data to facilitate detailed mapping of the electrical conduction system within the heart. The procedures involve the placement of numerous multipolar catheters within the heart (Fig. 31-13). Electrophysiology studies are used to analyze the conduction system, induce and evaluate arrhythmias, and determine the effects of therapeutic measures in treating arrhythmias.

Electrode catheters are introduced into the femoral vein, internal jugular vein, or subclavian vein. Because several catheters are used, multiple access sites are needed. It is not uncommon to have three introducer sheaths placed within the same vein. The catheters consist of several insulated wires, each of which is attached to an electrode on the catheter tip that serves as an interface with the intracardiac surface. The arrangements of the electrodes on the catheter allow its dual function of recording the electrical signals of the heart (intracardiac electrograms) and pacing the heart. The pacemaker function is performed to introduce premature electrical impulses to determine possible arrhythmias. After characterization of the precise defect occurs, an appropriate course of therapy can be undertaken.

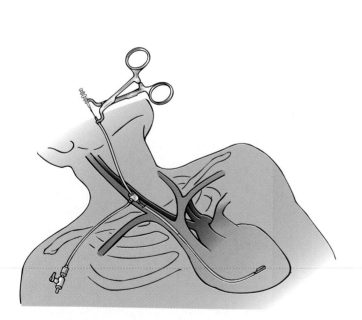

Fig. 31-12 The bioptome tip in the right ventricular apex, pointing toward the ventricular septum.

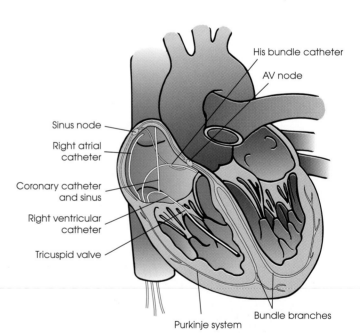

Fig. 31-13 Catheter positions for routine electrophysiologic study. Multipolar catheters are positioned in the high right atrium near the sinus node, in the area of the atrioventricular apex, and in the coronary sinus.

INTERVENTIONAL PROCEDURES OF THE VASCULAR SYSTEM
Adults

Interventional cardiac catheterization techniques requiring special-purpose catheters have expanded significantly since the late 1970s. Percutaneous transluminal cardiac angioplasty is a technique that employs balloon dilation of a coronary artery stenosis to increase blood flow to the heart muscle. The first successful PTCA was performed in 1977 by Gruentzig.

During PTCA, a specially designed guiding catheter is placed into the orifice of the stenotic coronary artery as determined by coronary angiography (Fig. 31-14). A steerable guide wire is inserted into the balloon catheter and advanced within the guiding catheter (Fig. 31-15). The guide wire is advanced across the stenotic area; it serves as a support platform so that the balloon catheter can be advanced and centered across the stenosis. Controlled and precise inflation of the balloon fractures and compresses the fatty deposits into the muscular wall of the artery. This compression, in conjunction with the stretching of the external vessel diameter, is necessary for successful angioplasty. The balloon is deflated to allow rapid *reperfusion* of blood to the heart muscle. The inflation procedure, followed by arteriography, may be repeated several times until a satisfactory degree of patency is observed (Fig. 31-16). The limiting factor of PTCA is *restenosis,* which occurs in approximately 30% to 50% of the patients who undergo the procedure.

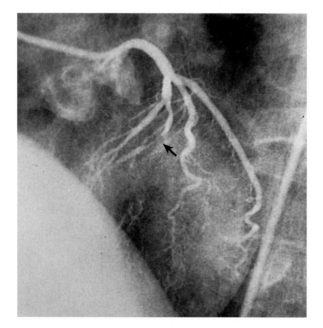

Fig. 31-14 Stenotic coronary artery before PTCA. The arrow indicates the stenotic area, estimated at 95%, with minimum blood flow distal to the lesion.

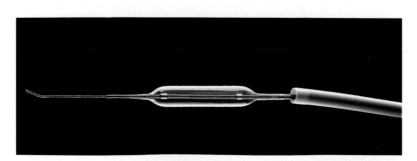

Fig. 31-15 Catheter system for PTCA. The three sections of the system are the outer guiding catheter *(right)*, central balloon catheter *(middle)*, and internal steerable guide wire *(left)*.

(Courtesy Codis Corp., Miami.)

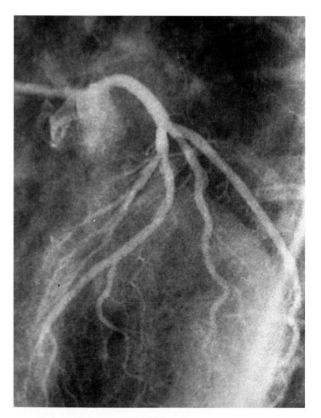

Fig. 31-16 Coronary arteriogram after PTCA in the same patient as in Fig. 31-14. The blood flow is estimated to be 100%.

Another interventional procedure being performed more frequently on adult patients with coronary artery stenosis is the placement of an expandable *intracoronary stent.* The procedure is similar to PTCA and is performed in the same manner, except that a metallic stent is mounted on the PTCA balloon (Fig. 31-17). For optimum stent deployment, the stent is centered across the entire length of the stenosis. Deployment of the stent is achieved with the inflation and deflation of the PTCA balloon. After the stent is deployed, the angioplasty balloon is removed and a high-pressure balloon is advanced within the stent. Inflation of the high-pressure balloon is performed to embed the metallic struts of the stent in the walls of the blood vessel. Restenosis rates are lower in patients receiving intracoronary stents than in those who undergo conventional angioplasty.

Atherectomy devices have also been used in the treatment of coronary artery disease. Unlike PTCA balloons, atherectomy devices remove the fatty deposit or thrombus material from within the artery (Fig. 31-18). The *directional coronary atherectomy (DCA)* procedure uses a specially designed cutting device to shave the plaque out of the lumen of the artery. As the cutting blade is advanced, the excised atheroma is pushed forward into the distal nose-cone collection chamber. The *rotational burr atherectomy* procedure uses an elliptic brass burr coated with fine diamond chips as the cutting mechanism. The burr, which operates at an extremely high speed of rotation, preferentially ablates and pulverizes atheromatous tissue into microparticles as it is advanced through the stenosis. The microparticles are removed by the reticuloendothelial system. The *transluminal extraction atherectomy* procedure uses a cutting device that consists of a pair of stainless-steel cutting blades arranged in a conical configuration. The central lumen of the cutting device is attached to a vacuum bottle that aspirates thrombus and atheromatous tissue as the cutting blade is advanced through the lesion. Atherectomy procedures generally require adjunctive PTCA or intracoronary stent placement to achieve an optimum angiographic result.

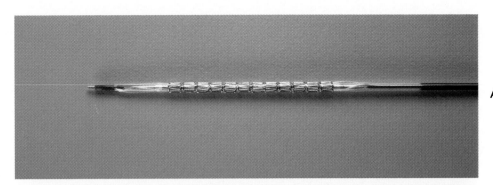

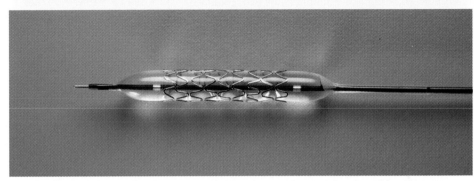

Fig. 31-17 Balloon expandable intracoronary stent: **A,** Before stent balloon inflation; **B,** After stent balloon inflation.

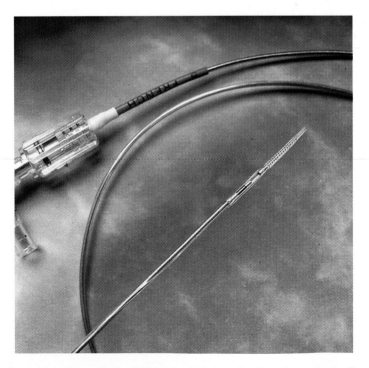

Fig. 31-18 Coronary atherectomy device used during directional coronary atherectomy. The balloon on the inferior aspect of the cutting device is inflated inside the coronary artery; plaque is forced into the opening, then shaved off and collected in the tip.

(Courtesy Guidant Vascular Intervention, Santa Clara, Calif.)

Because of the risks associated with mechanical interventions of the vascular system, open-heart surgical facilities must be immediately available. Coronary occlusion, for example, is a major complication requiring emergency surgery in patients undergoing catheter-based mechanical interventions.

Interventional pharmacologic procedures in adults consist of the therapeutic administration of medications during cardiac catheterization. An example is the intracoronary infusion of urokinase, which is a *thrombolytic* agent used in the early hours of an acute MI in an effort to modify its course. Estimates indicate that thrombotic coronary artery occlusion is present in 75% to 85% of patients with acute MI. If reperfusion of the *ischemic* myocardium is effective, scarring is reduced. Reperfusion in the early stages of MI offers greater potential for heart muscle salvage.

Children

A number of congenital cardiac defects in children are amenable to interventional procedures performed in the catheterization laboratory. As with PTCA procedures, cardiovascular surgical support services must be readily available.

When successful, certain pediatric interventional procedures negate the need for surgical correction of defects. Some procedures, however, are performed for palliative purposes to allow the child to grow to a size and weight at which subsequent open-heart surgery is feasible.

One such technique, *balloon atrial septostomy,* may be used to enlarge a patent foramen ovale or preexisting atrial septal defect. Enlargement of the opening enhances the mixing of right and left atrial blood, resulting in an improved level of systemic arterial oxygenation. *Transposition of the great arteries* is a condition for which atrial septostomy is performed.

Balloon septostomy requires a catheter similar to the type used in PTCA. The balloon is passed through the atrial septal opening into the left atrium, inflated with contrast medium, and then snapped back through the septal orifice. This causes the septum to tear. Often the technique must be repeated until the septal opening is sufficiently enlarged to allow the desired level of blood mixing as documented by oximetry, intracardiac pressures, and angiography.

If the atrial septum does not contain a preexisting opening, an artificial defect can be created. A transseptal system approach is employed, and a special catheter containing an internal folding knifelike blade is advanced into the left atrium (Fig. 31-19). After the catheter is inside the left atrium, the blade is advanced out of its protective outer housing and pulled back to the right atrium, creating an incision in the septal wall. This technique may be repeated. A balloon septostomy is then performed to widen the new opening, and the condition of the patient is monitored by oximetry, blood pressures, and angiography.

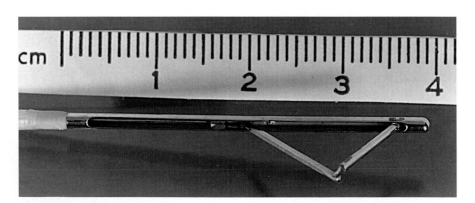

Fig. 31-19 Blade on catheter tip used to incise septal walls in pediatric interventional procedures.

A patent ductus arteriosus is sometimes evident in the newborn. In utero the pulmonary artery shunts its blood flow into the aorta through the ductus arteriosus, which normally closes after birth. Patent ductus arteriosus occurs when this channel fails to close spontaneously. In some instances, closure can be induced with medication. If this measure is unsuccessful and the residual shunt is deemed significant, surgical closure (ligation) of the vessel is appropriate.

For some patients, occlusion of a patent ductus arteriosus can be accomplished in the catheterization laboratory. A catheter containing an occlusion device, such as an *umbrella*, is advanced to the ductus. After the position of the lesion is confirmed by angiography, the occluder is released. Subsequent clotting and fibrous infiltration permanently stop the flow and subsequent mixing of blood.

INTERVENTIONAL PROCEDURES OF THE CONDUCTION SYSTEM: ADULTS AND CHILDREN

Permanent implantation of an antiarrhythmic device is a manipulative procedure that is being performed with greater frequency in cardiac catheterization laboratories, rather than in operating rooms (Fig. 31-20). Antiarrhythmic devices include *pacemakers* for patients with *bradyarrhythmias* and/or disease of the electrical conduction system of the heart and *implantable cardioverter defibrillators (ICDs)* for patients with lethal ventricular *tachyarrhythmias* originating from the bottom of the heart.

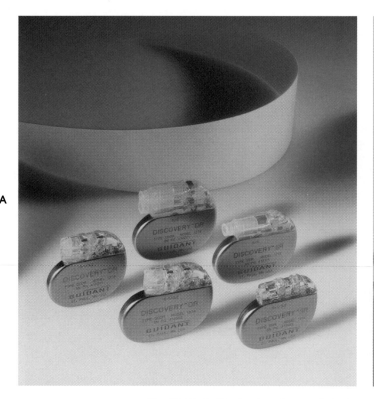
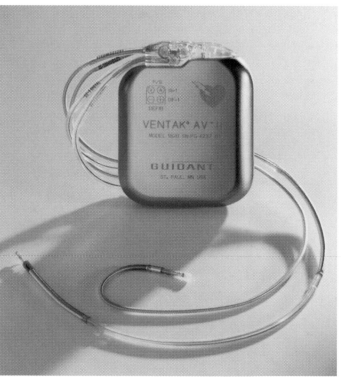

A

B

Fig. 31-20 A, Single-chamber and dual-chamber pacemakers. **B,** Implantable cardioverter defibrillator.

(Courtesy Guidant Corp., Cardiac Pacemakers, Inc., St. Paul, Minn.)

Pacemaker implantation can be successfully performed under local anesthesia in selected adult and pediatric patients. ICD implantation requires conscious sedation or general anesthesia because of the type of testing required at the time of implantation. Insertion of either a pacemaker or an ICD involves puncturing the subclavian or cephalic vein and introducing leads (electrically insulated wires with distal electrodes). The leads are manipulated so that their tips are in direct contact with the right ventricular or right atrial endocardium, or both. The leads are then tested for stimulation and sensing properties to ascertain proper functioning before they are attached to the pulse generator. During ICD implantation, defibrillation threshold testing is performed to determine the amount of energy required to defibrillate a patient from ventricular *tachycardia* or *fibrillation*. After testing is completed, the proximal end of the lead(s) is then attached to a battery pack (pacemaker or ICD) and implanted in a subcutaneous or subpectoral pocket created in the thorax (Fig. 31-21). Current pacemakers have a longevity of 5 to 10 years, and ICDs have a longevity of 6 to 8 years.

Another interventional procedure being performed to treat disorders of the conduction system in the cardiac catheterization laboratory is *radiofrequency (RF) ablation.* Several different arrhythmias previously treated with ICD implantation or drug therapy can now be treated with RF ablation. The procedure is normally performed at the time of the diagnostic electrophysiology study if an underlying mechanism or *arrhythmogenic* focus is identified.

RF ablation is achieved by delivering a low-voltage, high-frequency alternating current directly to the endocardial tissue through a specially designed ablation catheter. The current desiccates the underlying abnormal myocardial conduction tissue and creates a small, discrete burn lesion. Localized RF lesions create areas of tissue necrosis and scar, subsequently destroying the arrhythmogenic focus. Several RF lesions may be necessary to eliminate the abnormal conduction circuit.

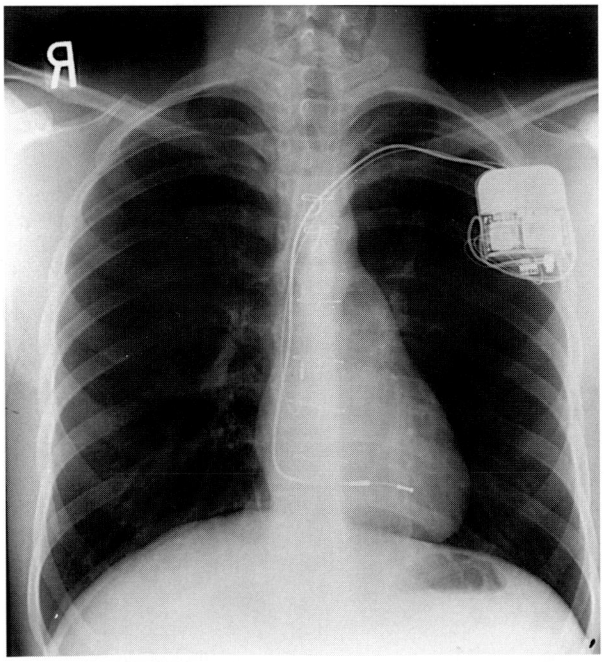

Follow-up electrophysiologic testing is performed to document the resolution of the arrhythmia. RF ablation of the atrioventricular (AV) node and pacemaker insertion are fast becoming the preferred treatment for chronic atrial fibrillation with rapid irregular responses. The AV junction is destroyed intentionally; consequently the rapid irregular electrical impulses from the atrium are not conducted into the ventricle. A pacemaker is then implanted, and a more consistent, regular heart rate is achieved.

POSTCATHETERIZATION CARE

When the catheterization procedure is completed, all catheters are removed. If a cut-down approach was used, the arteriotomy or venotomy is repaired as appropriate. If a percutaneous approach was used, pressure is placed on the puncture site until the bleeding is controlled. Wound sites are cleaned and dressed to minimize the risk of infection. Elastic dressings are often used to encourage *hemostasis.*

Postcatheterization medications are prescribed by the physician. The puncture site must be observed for hemorrhage or *hematoma,* and the status of the distal pulse is recorded on the protocol record before the patient leaves the catheterization laboratory. Vital signs should be monitored regularly for at least 24 hours after the catheterization. The ingestion of fluids should be encouraged, and pain medication may be indicated.

Cardiac catheterization may also be performed on an outpatient or same-day treatment basis. The patient is monitored for 4 to 8 hours in a recovery area and then allowed to go home. Instructions for home-care recovery procedures are usually given to the patient or a family member before the patient leaves the recovery area.

Fig. 31-21 Chest radiograph of a patient with a permanent pacemaker implanted. Note the pacemaker location in the superior and anterior chest wall, with the distal leads located in both the right ventricle and right atrium of the heart.

Cardiac Catheterization Trends

Techniques and methods for cardiac catheterization continue to be developed and refined. Angiographic imaging and recording devices are becoming even more sophisticated and therefore yielding ever-greater resolution and detail. Magnetic resonance imaging of the cardiovascular system is now a well-recognized investigational technique. Magnetic resonance coronary arteriography is now able to reliably assess anomalous coronary artery anatomy and to identify the presence of calcification in the coronary arteries and bypass grafts. The clinical use of intravascular ultrasound imaging and other improved computerized image enhancements should allow for more precise data collection and more tailored methods of determining the interventional method to use in treating coronary artery disease.

Many experts feel that the greatest area for growth in the field of cardiac catheterization is in interventional procedures. Despite the use of such techniques as PTCA, intracoronary stenting, and atherectomy in coronary artery disease, restenosis continues to be prevalent and of major concern. The majority of the research in interventional procedures is geared toward finding a technique to prevent or greatly limit restenosis after an intervention. Newly designed devices and techniques using beta irradiation are currently being investigated to determine their efficacy in treating restenosis. Procedures classified as experimental or investigational in the late 1980s are now being performed regularly. Existing and new interventional procedures should continue to provide patients with viable, relatively low-risk, financially reasonable alternatives to open-heart surgery.

Current trends indicate that the number and variety of outpatient cardiac catheterizations will continue to increase. The equipment used and procedures performed in the cardiac catheterization laboratories of the future are likely to be significantly different from those associated with existing facilities. However, despite changes in cardiovascular technology and medical techniques, cardiac catheterization laboratories will continue to provide essential patient care services necessary for the diagnosis and treatment of a vast number of cardiovascular-related diseases.

Definition of Terms

angina pectoris Severe form of chest pain and constriction near the heart; usually caused by a decrease in the blood supply to cardiac tissue; most often associated with stenosis of a coronary artery as a result of atherosclerotic accumulations or spasm. The pain generally lasts for a few minutes and is more likely to occur after stress, exercise, or other activity resulting in increased heart rate.

angiography Radiographic demonstration of blood vessels after the introduction of a contrast medium.

arrhythmia Variation from normal heart rhythm.

arrhythmogenic Producing an arrhythmia.

arteriosclerotic Indicative of a general pathologic condition characterized by thickening and hardening of arterial walls, leading to general loss of elasticity.

arteriotomy Surgical opening of an artery.

atherectomy Excision of atherosclerotic plaque.

atheromatous Characteristic of degenerative change in the inner lining of arteries caused by the deposition of fatty tissue and subsequent thickening of arterial walls that occurs in atherosclerosis.

bradyarrhythmia Irregular heart rhythm in conjunction with bradycardia.

bradycardia Any heart rhythm with an average heart rate of less than 60 beats per minute.

cardiac output Amount of blood pumped from the heart per given unit of time; can be calculated by multiplying stroke volume (amount of blood in milliliters ejected from the left ventricle during each heartbeat) by heart rate (number of heart beats per minute). A normal, resting adult with a stroke volume of 70 ml and a heart rate of 72 beats per minute has a cardiac output of approximately 5.0 L per minute.

cardiomyopathies Relatively serious group of heart diseases typically characterized by enlargement of the myocardial layer of the left ventricle and resulting in decreased cardiac output; hypertrophic cardiomyopathy is a condition often studied in the catheterization laboratory.

cineangiography High-speed, 35-mm motion picture film recording of a fluoroscopic image of structures containing radiographic contrast medium.

coagulopathy Any disorder that affects the blood-clotting mechanism.

directional coronary atherectomy (DCA) Excision of atheroma through a percutaneous transcatheter approach using a rotating cutting device supported by a balloon positioned on the back of the catheter.

dyspnea Labored breathing.

ejection fraction Measurements of ventricular contractility expressed as the percentage of blood pumped out of the left ventricle during contraction; can be estimated by evaluating the left ventriculogram; normal range is between 57% and 73%, with an average of 65%. A low ejection fraction indicates failure of the left ventricle to pump effectively.

ergometer Device used to imitate the muscular, metabolic, and respiratory effects of exercise.

fibrillation Involuntary, chaotic muscular contractions resulting from spontaneous activation of single muscle cells or muscle fibers.

hematoma Collection of extravasated blood in an organ or a tissue space.

hemodynamics Study of factors involved in circulation of blood. Hemodynamic data typically collected during heart catheterization are cardiac output and intracardiac pressures.

hemostasis Arrest of blood flow in a hemorrhage.

intervention Therapeutic modality—mechanical or pharmacologic—used to modify the course of a disease process.

interventricular septal integrity Continuity of the membranous partition that separates the right and left ventricles of the heart.

intracoronary stent Metallic device placed within a coronary artery across a region of stenosis.

ischemic Indicative of a local decrease of blood supply to myocardial tissue associated with temporary obstruction of a coronary vessel, typically as a result of thrombus (blood clot).

myocardial infarction (MI) Acute ischemic episode resulting in myocardial damage and pain; commonly referred to as a *heart attack.*

occlusion Obstruction or closure of a vessel, such as a coronary vessel, as a result of foreign material, thrombus, or spasm.

oximetry Measurement of oxygen saturation in blood.

oxygen saturation Amount of oxygen bound to hemoglobin in blood, expressed as a percentage.

patent foramen ovale Opening between the right atrium and left atrium that normally exists in fetal life to allow for the essential mixing of blood. The opening normally closes shortly after birth.

percutaneous transluminal coronary angioplasty (PTCA) Manipulative interventional procedure involving the placement and inflation of a balloon catheter in the lumen of a stenosed coronary artery for the purpose of compressing and fracturing the diseased material, thereby allowing subsequent increased distal blood flow to the myocardium.

percutaneously Performed through the skin.

reperfusion Reestablishment of blood flow to the heart muscle through a previously occluded artery.

restenosis Narrowing or constriction of a vessel, orifice, or other type of passageway after interventional correction of primary condition.

rotational burr atherectomy Ablation of atheroma through a percutaneous transcatheter approach using a high-speed rotational burr.

stenosis Narrowing or constriction of a vessel, an orifice, or other type of passageway.

tachyarrhythmia Irregular heart rhythm in conjunction with tachycardia.

tachycardia Any heart rhythm having an average heart rate in excess of 100 beats per minute.

thrombolytic Capable of causing the breakup of a thrombus.

transducer Device used to convert one form of energy into another. Transducers used in cardiac catheterization convert fluid (blood) pressure into an electrical signal displayed on a physiologic monitor.

transluminal extraction atherectomy Excision and aspiration of atheroma and thrombus through a percutaneous transcatheter approach using a low-speed cutting and suction device.

transposition of the great arteries Congenital heart defect requiring interventional therapy. In this defect the aorta arises from the right side of the heart and the pulmonary artery arises from the left side of the heart.

umbrella Prosthetic interventional device consisting of two opposing polyurethane disks connected by a central loop mounted on a spring-loaded assembly to provide opposing tension.

valvular competence Ability of the valve to prevent backward flow while not inhibiting forward flow.

venotomy Surgical opening of a vein.

Selected bibliography

ACC/AHA Task Force on Assessment of Diagnostic and Therapeutic Cardiovascular Procedures: guidelines for coronary angiography, *J Am Coll Cardiol* 10:935, 1987.

Amplatz K et al: Mechanics of selective coronary artery catheterization via femoral approach, *Radiology* 89:1040, 1967.

Baim D et al: Adjunctive angioplasty before and after directional atherectomy, *J Am Coll Cardiol* 19:351A, 1992.

Beatt K et al: Restenosis after coronary angioplasty: the paradox of increased lumen diameter and restenosis, *J Am Coll Cardiol* 19:258, 1992.

Bernard Claude: *Des substances toxiques,* Paris, 1857, JB Baillière et fils.

Berné R, Levy ML: *Cardiovascular physiology,* ed 5, St Louis, 1986, Mosby.

Bertrand M et al: Percutaneous transluminal coronary rotary ablation with Rotablator (European experience), *Am J Cardiol* 69:470, 1992.

Braunwald E: *Heart disease: a textbook of cardiovascular medicine,* vols 1 and 2, Philadelphia, 1980, WB Saunders.

Calkins H et al: Diagnosis and cure of the Wolff-Parkinson-White syndrome or paroxysmal supraventricular tachycardias during a single electrophysiologic test, *N Engl J Med* 324:1612, 1991.

Ciuffo AA et al: Benefits of nonionic contrast in coronary arteriography: preliminary results of a randomized double-blind trial comparing iopamidol and Renografin-76, *Invest Radiol* 19:S197, 1984.

Clanville AR et al: The role of right ventricular endomyocardial biopsy in the long term management of heart-lung transplant recipients, *J Heart Lung Transplant* 6:375, 1987.

Daily E, Schroeder J: *Hemodynamic waveforms—exercises in identification and analysis,* St Louis, 1983, Mosby.

de Feyter PJ et al: Emergency PTCA in unstable angina pectoris refractory to optimal medical treatment, *N Engl J Med* 313:342, 1985.

DeWood MA et al: Prevalence of total coronary occlusion during the early hours of transmural myocardial infarction, *N Engl J Med* 303:897, 1980.

Ellenbogen KA: *Cardiac pacing,* Boston, 1992, Blackwell.

Fischman DL et al: A randomized comparison of coronary stent placement and balloon angioplasty in the treatment of coronary artery disease, *N Engl J Med* 331:496, 1994.

Ford RD: *Cardiovascular disorders,* ed 4, Philadelphia, 1984, Springhouse.

Fowles RE, Mason JW: Role of cardiac biopsy in the diagnosis and management of cardiac disease, *Prog Cardiovasc Dis* 27:153, 1984.

Freed M, Grines C: *Manual of interventional cardiology,* Birmingham, Ala.,1992, Physicians Press.

Gertz EW et al: Clinical superiority of a new nonionic contrast agent (iopamidol) for cardiac angiography, *J Am Coll Cardiol* 5:250, 1985.

Grines CL et al: Comparison of immediate angioplasty with thrombolytic therapy for acute myocardial infarction, *N Engl J Med* 328:673, 1993.

Grossman W: *Cardiac catheterization and angiography,* ed 3, Philadelphia, 1986, Lea & Febiger.

Gruentzig A, Senning A, Siegenthaler WE: Nonoperative dilatation of coronary artery stenosis: percutaneous transluminal coronary angioplasty, *N Engl J Med* 301:61, 1979.

Hess DS et al: Permanent pacemaker implantation in the cardiac catheterization laboratory: the subclavian approach, *Cathet Cardiovasc Diagn* 8:453, 1982.

Hirshfield JW Jr: Cardiovascular effects of iodinated contrast agents, *Am J Cardiol* 66:9F, 1990.

Hurst JW: *The heart,* ed 5, vols 1 and 2, New York, 1976, McGraw-Hill.

Jackman WM et al: AV node reentry tachycardia, *N Engl J Med* 327:313, 1992.

Jackman WM et al: Catheter ablation of atrioventricular junction using radiofrequency current in 17 patients. Comparison of standard and large-tip catheter electrodes, *Circulation* 83:1562, 1991.

Johnson LW et al: Coronary arteriography 1984-1987: a report of the Registry of the Society for Cardiac Angiography and Interventions. Part 1: results and complications, *Cathet Cardiovasc Diagn,* 17:5, 1989.

Judkins MP: Selective coronary arteriography. Part 1. A percutaneous transfemoral technic, *Radiology* 89:815, 1967.

Kennedy JW: Registry Committee of the Society for Cardiac Angiography. Complications associated with cardiac catheterization and angiography, *Cathet Cardiovasc Diagn* 8:5, 1982.

Kern MJ: *The cardiac catheterization handbook,* St Louis, 1995, Mosby.

Koller PT et al: Success, complications and restenosis following rotational atherectomy of coronary ostial stenoses, *J Am Coll Cardiol* 19:333A, 1992.

Kramer B et al: Coronary atherectomy in acute ischemic syndromes: implications of thrombus on treatment outcome, *J Am Coll Cardiol* 17:385A, 1991.

Leimgruber PP et al: Restenosis after successful coronary angioplasty in patients with single-vessel disease, *Circulation* 73:710, 1986.

Leon MB et al: Strategies for coronary revascularization using different atherectomy devices: a NACI registry report, *J Am Coll Cardiol* 19:92A, 1992.

Lozner EC et al: Coronary arteriography 1984-1987: a report of the Registry of the Society for Cardiac Angiography and Interventions. Part 2: an analysis of 218 deaths related to coronary arteriography, *Cathet Cardiovasc Diagn* 17:11, 1989.

Mabin TA, Holmes DR, Smith HC: Intracoronary thrombus: role in coronary occlusion complicating PTCA, *J Am Coll Cardiol* 5:198, 1985.

Macaya C et al: Continued benefit of coronary stenting versus balloon angioplasty: one-year clinical follow-up of Benestent trial, *J Am Coll Cardiol* 27:255, 1996.

Mancini GBJ et al: Hemodynamic and electrocardiographic effects in man of a new nonionic contrast agent (iohexol): advantages over standard ionic agents, *Am J Cardiol* 51:1218, 1983.

Mason JW: Techniques for right and left ventricular endomyocardial biopsy, *Am J Cardiol* 41:887, 1978.

Mason JW, O'Connell JB: Clinical method of endomyocardial biopsy, *Circulation* 79:971, 1989.

Nobuyoshi M et al: Restenosis after successful percutaneous transluminal coronary angioplasty: serial angiographic follow-up of 229 patients, *J Am Coll Cardiol* 12:616, 1988.

Pavlides GS et al: Safety and efficacy of urokinase during elective coronary angioplasty, *Am Heart J* 121:731, 1991.

Pepine CJ, Hill JA, Lambert CR: *Diagnostic and therapeutic cardiac catheterization,* Baltimore, 1989, Williams & Wilkins.

Peterson KL, Nicod P: *Cardiac catheterization: methods, diagnosis, and therapy,* ed 1, Philadelphia, 1997, WB Saunders.

Rapaport E: Thrombolytic agents in acute myocardial infarction, *N Engl J Med* 320:861, 1989.

Ricketts HJ, Abrams HL: Percutaneous selective coronary cine arteriography, *JAMA* 181:620, 1962.

Salem DN et al: Comparison of the electrocardiographic and hemodynamic responses to ionic and nonionic radiocontrast media during left ventriculography: a randomized double blind study, *Am Heart J* 111:533, 1986.

Schatz RA et al: Clinical experience with the Palmaz-Schatz coronary stent: initial results of a multicenter study, *Circulation* 83:148, 1991.

Serruys PW et al: A comparison of balloon-expandable stent implantation with balloon angioplasty in patients with coronary artery disease, *N Engl J Med* 331:489, 1994.

Sones FM et al: Cine-coronary arteriography, *Circulation* 20:773, 1959.

Sones FM Jr, Shirey EK: Cine-coronary arteriography, *Mod Concepts Cardiovasc Dis* 31:735, 1962.

Swan HJC: Acute myocardial infarction: a failure of timely, spontaneous thrombolysis, *J Am Coll Cardiol* 13:1435, 1989.

Taylor AM, Pennell DJ: Recent advances in cardiac magnetic resonance imaging, *Curr Opin Cardiol* 6:635, 1996.

Tilkian AG, Daily EK: *Cardiovascular procedures: diagnostic techniques and therapeutic procedures,* St Louis, 1986, Mosby.

Topol E: *Textbook of interventional cardiology,* ed 1, Philadelphia, 1990, WB Saunders.

Tuzcu EM et al: The dilemma of diagnosing coronary calcification: angiography versus intravascular ultrasound, *J Am Coll Cardiol* 27:832, 1996.

Verel D, Grainger RD: *Cardiac catheterization and angiography,* ed 3, New York, 1978, Churchill Livingstone.

Verin V et al: Feasibility of intracoronary beta-irradiation to reduce restenosis after balloon angioplasty. A clinical pilot study, *Circulation* 95:1095, 1997.

Willerson JT: Selection of patients for coronary angiography, *Circulation* 72:V3, 1985.

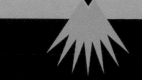

COMPUTER FUNDAMENTALS AND APPLICATIONS IN RADIOLOGY

JANE A. VAN VALKENBURG

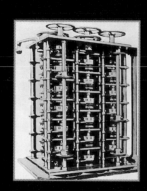

RIGHT: First mechanical forerunner of the computer, the "difference machine," introduced in 1812. This machine was used for mathematical calculations such as logarithms.

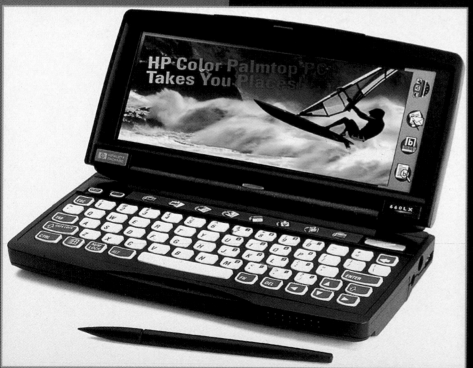

LEFT: State-of-the-art 1999 660LX Color Palmtop PC with 32MB RAM, 10MB ROM, and 56.6 Kbps external modem.

(Courtesy Hewlett-Packard Company, Santa Clara, Calif.)

Principles of Computer Applications in Radiology

The progressive and evolutionary growth in medicine would not be possible without the aid of computers. As a result of computer applications in the storage, analysis, and manipulation of data, pathologic conditions can be diagnosed more accurately and earlier in the disease process, resulting in an increased patient cure rate. With the increasing use of computers in medical science, there is clearly a need for qualified personnel who can understand and operate computerized equipment. This chapter introduces the fundamental concepts and principles of computer technology and briefly discusses the application of computers in diagnostic imaging, management, utilization, and education.

DEFINITIONS

The *computer** is a fast, computational, electronic machine that receives input data, processes the data by performing arithmetic/logic operations using a program stored in its memory, and then generates output data that are displayed on the appropriate equipment.

As a machine, the computer is limited to performing arithmetic/logic operations and cannot make rational diagnostic judgments. However, with the development of medical artificial intelligence-based expert computer systems, such as ICON (see following paragraph), the observations of the radiologist can be compared with clinical information about the case, and the case can then be compared with similar cases. As a result, the radiologist and/or physician can make more informed judgments.

*Almost all italicized terms are defined at the end of this chapter.

Artificial intelligence may be described as comparing computer function with human judgment. In medicine the concentration has been on developing computer systems that contain detailed data about specific medical subjects. In contrast, *expert computer systems* contain vast amounts of data used for making decisions about a specific problem. Expert systems are designed to duplicate the human reasoning process, thereby providing a differential diagnosis or critique of the diagnosis. When the artificial intelligence system and the expert system are integrated, the information generated aids in analytic reasoning and decision making. The artificial intelligence-based expert system used in radiology is known as the *IMAGE/ICON system.*

Historical Development

The abacus, known as the first "digital" calculator, was used as early as the sixth century BC. The abacus is a device with beads strung on parallel wires or sticks, which are attached to a frame.

In 1642 a young Frenchman, Blaise Pascal, built a small mechanical adding device to aid him in his work as an accountant. The device consisted of cogwheels in a box; each cogwheel had 10 teeth, and each tooth represented one digit from 0 through 9. As one of the wheels passed from the position of 9 to 0, a small sprocket on the wheel interdigitated with the next wheel and provided an automatic carryover. This first mechanical adding machine was known as the "arithmetic machine." The operation of the mechanical paper-tape adding machines is based on the same technique, which was also used in the development of the clock industry.

In 1694 Gottfried Wilhelm von Leibnitz, using Pascal's arithmetic machine concept, developed a mechanism that used step-cylinders instead of cogwheels. The machine could add, multiply, and divide and was known as a "calculating machine." The machines developed by Pascal and Leibnitz, are the predecessors of modern keyboard adding machines.

A French inventor, Joseph Jacquard, displayed an automatic weaving loom at the Paris Industrial Exhibition in 1801. The sequence of the loom's operations was based on coded information punched into thick paper cards. The pattern of the tapestry woven on this loom was produced by the holes in the punched cards. The positioning of the threads was determined by the presence and position of the holes on the card. Approximately 24,000 punched cards were used to produce a single tapestry.

In 1812 Charles Babbage, considered the originator of the modern computer, presented an outline for a machine that could calculate celestial tables used in the navigation of ships. Errors in calculating these tables had caused ships to go off course, often resulting in shipwrecks. The machine's calculations were based on the constant variation, or difference, in a series of multiplications, additions, divisions, or squares, and the instrument could tabulate up to 20 decimals with seven differences. Because this "difference machine," as it was called, required accurate precision in the positioning of the cogs, wheels, shafts, and sprockets, the engineering technology was not available to accurately construct it, although the design was sound (Fig. 32-1). Babbage spent 20 years attempting to build this machine, but he was never able to complete it.

Meanwhile, Babbage had been presented with one of Jacquard's tapestries and was intrigued by Jacquard's idea of a punched card and its application to constructing a machine to perform calculations. In 1834, Babbage presented the principle of what he called an "analytic engine," from which today's computer was developed. Babbage divided the construction of this machine into two main components: the "store," which is comparable to the *memory,* and the "mill," which is similar to the *central processing unit (CPU)* in modern computers. The mill performed the calculations and was controlled by a punched card. The store held the numbers for use as the calculation proceeded. Babbage devoted years to the development of this analytic engine, but unfortunately he never finished it. After his death the analytic machine was constructed using his complete and detailed drawings.

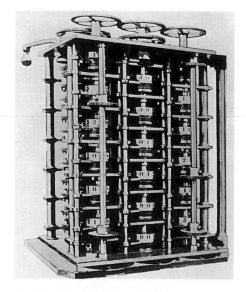

Fig. 32-1 The idea for a "difference machine" that would compute mathematical tables, such as logarithms, was first conceived by Babbage in 1812. After 20 years of labor, financial difficulties compelled him to stop work, and the machine was never completed.

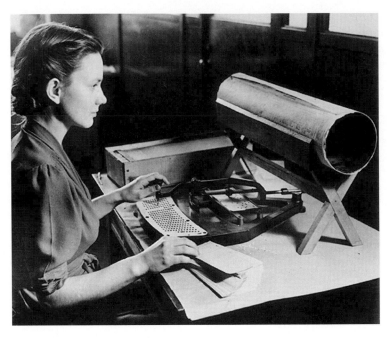

Fig. 32-2 Dial cabinet used by Hollerith to count the holes in the punched cards. The properly punched cards were then filed for future use.

(Courtesy IBM Corp., Atlanta)

During the 1880s Herman Hollerith and James Powers, who worked with the U.S. Bureau of the Census, were concerned about tabulating the census for the growing American population and decided that an automatic process must be developed. Working independently, they constructed versions of punched-card tabulating machines, and the 1890 census was tabulated using these machines. Hollerith obtained a patent on his machine and founded a company to further develop his ideas (Figs. 32-2 and 32-3). In 1911 this company merged with two other companies to form the Computer Tabulating Recording Company. In 1924 this company became International Business Machine Corporation (IBM), a leader in the development of computer technology.

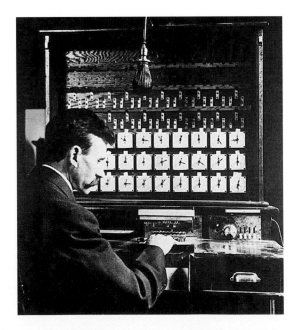

Fig. 32-3 Device used by Hollerith to punch programs, singly and manually, in cards.

(Courtesy IBM Corp., Atlanta.)

After 1920 computer development progressed at a rapid rate. A summary of important events in the advancement of computer development is provided in Table 32-1.

The significant changes in the development of computers are referred to as *generations* (Table 32-2). Since 1973 computers have become faster in performing computations as a result of miniaturization of the circuits embedded on silicon chips.

As circuits become the size of molecules, the possibility of using biologic material, such as amino acid protein chains, is being investigated for the transmission of data. Predictions are that biologic material will be used in the fifth generation of computers, which will be known as *quantum computers.*

TABLE 32-1

Important events in computer development

Date	Developer	Event
1937-1944	Howard Aiken, Harvard University	Using Babbage's mechanical design, IBM joined Aiken in the development of Mark 1, an electromechanical, automatic, sequenced-controlled calculator; program sequencing was done with paper tape
1943-1946	John Mauchley and J. Presper Eckert, University of Pennsylvania	A high-speed electronic calculator, the Electronic Numeric Integrator and Calculator (ENIAC); first machine to use vacuum tubes, which allowed faster switching functions
1946-1952	John Von Neumann, University of Pennsylvania	Designed a machine with a stored memory, Electronic Discrete Variable Automatic Computer (EDVAC); capable of reading instructions from memory and executing them in proper sequence, which allowed programming
1951	Eckert-Mauchley	The first commercially available computer, Universal Automatic Computer I (UNIVAC), using a stored memory; used by the U.S. Census Bureau; company later bought by Sperry-Rand Corporation
1954	Bell Telephone Laboratories	First computer to use solid-state transistors and diodes, Transistor Digital Computer (TRADIC); allowed development of much smaller machines
1963-1964	Numerous researchers	Integrated circuits and semiconductors; development based on principles presented by Wilhelm Schottky
1973	Numerous researchers	Miniaturization of electronic circuits or microchips; marketing of the minicomputer to general public

TABLE 32-2

Evolution of computer development

Generation	Development	Date
First	Vacuum tubes	1943–1946
Second	Solid-state transistors	1954
Third	Integrated circuits and semi-conductors	1963–1964
Fourth	Silicon chips or microchips	1973

Types of Computers

Computers can be divided into three categories: the microcomputer, the minicomputer, and the mainframe computer. The smallest computer, the *microcomputer,* usually contains the circuitry or CPU on a single integrated-circuit chip. The main limitation of this system is that it is typically a one-person or one-function system.

Minicomputers usually have faster responding CPUs and more memory and storage. Unlike most microcomputers, minicomputers are multiuser or *multitasking* systems in that a number of people (2 to 30) may use the system at one time. Minicomputers are also capable of more tasks, and they can use various programs because they contain several chips or one or more printed circuit boards filled with many integrated circuits. Minicomputers are also known as *PCs, desktop,* or *laptop computers.*

Mainframe computers are used when the need for data storage, processing speed, and memory requirements increases and when the number of users also increases. The distinction between the mainframe computer and the minicomputer is becoming less distinct as a result of innovative technology and miniaturization of computer components. Tasks that were once performed only by mainframe computers are now being handled by minicomputers. The advantage of the large mainframe system is its ability to process large amounts of data efficiently. Mainframe computers are used by the U.S. Census Bureau, the Internal Revenue Service, large corporations, research libraries, universities, and other organizations requiring the processing, acquisition, and storage of large amounts of information.

The *supercomputer* is a type of mainframe computer developed to process mathematically intense operations, such as rapid processing of deep-space images for the National Aeronautics and Space Administration (NASA), astronomic projections, and real-time national weather forecasting. This type of computer is currently used by the U.S. Census Bureau. Supercomputers, also known as *maxicomputers,* have computing speeds approaching ten billion *floating point operations* per second, have one billion bytes of memory, and can switch from one transmission state to another in one thousandth of a billionth second, or 1 picosecond. The future promises revolutionary changes in the development of computer circuitry, resulting in minicomputers that have the capabilities of maxicomputers and making obsolete the supercomputers presently being used.

The computers used in radiology departments are *microcomputers* and *minicomputers*. The applications of these computers are divided into two categories: *control* and *data management*. Microcomputers perform a specific, or specialized, function and are typically used to control operations in radiographic/fluoroscopic rooms, regulate automatic processing, and control rapid film changers. Minicomputers are found in computed tomography (CT) units and equipment used for image reconstruction. Minicomputers are also used for word processing, billing, and inventory management. Special-purpose hardware interfaced with a minicomputer is necessary for *real-time imaging,* which is used in ultrasound and digital radiography where immediate data manipulation is important.

Functional Components of the Computer

The term *hardware* is used to describe the functional equipment components of a computer and includes the parts of the computer that are visible. The term *software* designates the parts of the computer system that are invisible, such as the *machine language* and *programs*. A computer program is a clearly defined set of *instructions* that gives the computer specific tasks to perform. Programs are written in *high-level languages* that are intelligible to the user and translated into machine languages that are then intelligible to the computer.

The computer hardware consists of four functionally independent components:

1. *Input devices*
2. CPU, which houses the *control unit* and the *arithmetic/logic unit (ALU)* (Fig. 32-4)
3. *Primary memory*
4. *Output devices.*

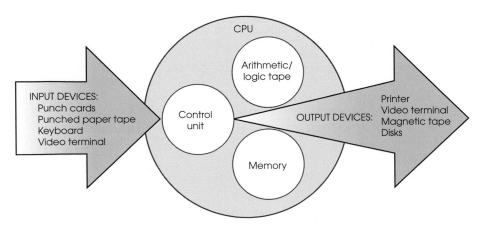

Fig. 32-4 Fundamentals of a computer: central processing unit (CPU), or operating system.

INPUT DEVICES

Input devices are the units that "read" the instructions represented on the input medium such as a keyboard. They then transform this information into *binary* digits and feed it to the CPU for processing.

Input media used in the past were punched cards and punched paper tape. Today the *keyboard* (similar to a typewriter) and *video terminal* are common devices used to give instructions to the CPU. The input device reads the coded instructions represented by the holes punched in the cards or paper tape, commands typed on a keyboard, or data drawn directly on a video terminal by means of a light pen attachment. The coded instructions enable the input device to translate the external data into binary representations that can then be handled by the CPU.

Other forms of input devices are *magnetic ink readers, optical scanners,* and *magnetic disks* or tapes. Magnetic ink, made from iron oxide particles, is used to provide direct instructions to the input device. Optical scanners are frequently employed by testing agencies to score examinations by using a light or lens system to scan a sheet of paper for information that is then converted to digital information by the input device. Magnetic disks and tapes may contain information or data to be screened and changed to binary representations by the input device (Fig. 32-5).

CONTROL UNIT

The sequence of events or tasks performed by the computer is regulated and coordinated by the control unit housed within the CPU. The control unit retrieves information from the memory and sends it to the arithmetic/logic unit (ALU) to be processed. After this processing, the control unit sends the data to the storage memory or the appropriate output device. Like a police officer stationed at a busy intersection, the control unit prevents mass confusion by directing "traffic" into the proper lanes in an orderly fashion.

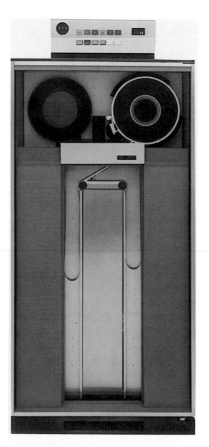

Fig. 32-5 Magnetic tape memory system. The tape loops in the lower center area and is suspended in a vacuum compartment to facilitate the tape's passage at high speeds.

(Courtesy IBM Corp., Atlanta.)

When the operator initiates a specified program, the control unit retrieves the information from the memory and sends it to the ALU for processing. On completion of the tasks by the ALU, the control unit transmits the processed information or data back to the memory or to an output device, as instructed by the operator. These functions occur in microseconds, milliseconds, and nanoseconds, depending on the circuitry of the machine, which determines the speed of the functions.

ARITHMETIC/LOGIC UNIT

The ALU does all of the computations, comparisons, and logical operations using binary numbers for additions, subtractions, multiplications, and/or divisions. The control unit determines the numbers to be acted on and the operation to be performed. After completion of the calculations, the information can be displayed immediately or placed in the memory for future use.

The calculations take place within the ALU in areas known as *registers* or *accumulators.* For example, if the task is to combine two numbers, the numbers are called from the memory by the control unit and are placed in two separate registers. The control unit passes control to the ALU to perform the computation. When the operation is completed, the result is displayed on an output device or sent back to the memory for future use.

MEMORY

Memory storage may be divided into two types: *primary* and *secondary*. The primary memory is an integral part of the circuitry and can store data for immediate retrieval when needed. Data contained in the primary memory can be transferred back and forth to the CPU for further calculations. The primary memory is described according to the *storage capacity* and is quantified by the letter *K,* which is derived from the metric system and denotes the quantity of 1000. However, because 1024 rather than an even 1000 is a mathematic integral power of 2, *K* stands for 1024 when applied to computer technology. For example, a 256K memory means that approximately 256,000 locations exist within the primary memory for data storage; however, the more accurate figure is 262,144 locations. The memory is divided into small sections called locations, with each location having a storage *address*. The address is usually represented by a number or numbers that the CPU uses to find the information for further processing or display.

The primary memory of a computer, has two types of addressable memory: the *random access memory (RAM)* and the *read-only memory (ROM)*. It is possible to read, change, delete, and store on the RAM with immediate access to data. However, if the voltage to the computer suddenly drops or fluctuates, the information is lost unless it has been stored in secondary or auxiliary storage areas such as magnetic tapes or disks. The ROM was developed to correct this deficiency in the primary memory and to prevent the loss of important instructions that are needed to operate the computer without reprogramming for each usage. The contents of the ROM are generally imprinted at the factory. Instructions and information within the ROM are nonvolatile (i.e., whether the computer is on or off does not affect the ROM). Although the CPU can retrieve the information on the ROM, the information or instructions cannot be changed or deleted and new instructions cannot be stored. The ROM is used primarily to secure frequently used programs that need to be accessible as soon as the computer is turned on.

In computers with a smaller capacity, the ROM may be removed by the operator and changed (e.g., the cartridges and disks used for video games). In the computers used in radiology departments the ROM is an integral part of the circuitry that is "burned in" at the factory. When diagnostic imaging studies are performed, data must be transmitted very quickly between the CPU and the ROM; therefore, in these computers the ROM is often located within the CPU. The ROM is a program and is usually considered software. When the ROM is part of the circuitry and is purchased as an integral part of the computer, it is referred to as *firmware*. The ROM can be changed in these special types of computers, but a person skilled in computer circuitry is needed to do the task.

The primary memory, consisting of the RAM and the ROM, is limited in storage capacity. It is relatively expensive to add circuitry for storage purposes. Use of less expensive, mass-capacity storage areas is necessary to keep records for long periods of time. The *secondary* memory storage areas, such as magnetic tapes, disks, and magnetic drums, fill this need. These secondary or auxiliary storage mediums can be removed from the computer and stored separately. When needed, they can then be inserted into a device that is interfaced with the computer, and information can be retrieved from them by use of the storage address.

OPERATING SYSTEM

An *operating system (OS)* is a set of programs to help other programs use the computer and its peripheral devices, such as printers and video terminals. These sets of programs serve four basic functions:

1. They request programs and cause the computer to execute the instructions in the program.
2. They manage the input and output and the use of peripheral devices.
3. They manage the information within the *files* and the priority of processing.
4. They manage the information stored in the RAM.

The control unit within the CPU directs the functions of the operating system and sees that the correct programs are performed. The CPU responds to the request for a program, locates the program in the operating system, copies it into a work space in the primary memory, and begins execution of the program's instructions. An operating system eliminates the need to *write* instructions into every program the operator wishes to perform.

Contained within each operating system are three management systems for instructions, sometimes called *managers*. The *input/output (I/O) manager* coordinates all transfers of information between devices connected to the computer. This manager also knows which peripheral device is connected to what other devices in the computer. Consequently each peripheral device is able to send and receive information in different ways from different locations. The file manager handles all the information that is to be stored in auxiliary storage areas by packing the information into indexed groups. The file manager also keeps track of where individual files are located by recording the file name and location with the indexed information groups. As a result, information can be retrieved when needed. When a storage disk or magnetic tape is inserted into the computer, the file manager reads where the file is stored, locates it, and loads (copies) it into a waiting area called a *buffer*. The third manager handles all of the computer's immediate records stored in the RAM.

In an operating system, when a program is requested from an input device such as a video terminal, the CPU monitors the terminal, interprets the request for a program, and then requests the file manager to retrieve the data from the files, unless this program is stored in the RAM, where it can be immediately found.

The file manager searches its directory for the file needed and loads the file onto a buffer. The file manager reports the file's status to the CPU. If the file is not found, the file manager reports that the file is "not found." If the file is found, the manager informs the CPU that the file is in the buffer. The CPU then requests that the memory manager reserve a portion of the primary memory for the program. The program moves from the buffer to the designated space, and the CPU starts operation of the program.

If the program needs additional memory or needs to use a peripheral device, a request is transmitted to the CPU, which then refers this request to the memory manager, I/O manager, or file manager. When the program is completed, the CPU gains control of the system and waits for additional *commands.*

OUTPUT DEVICES

Output devices display the results of the computations or tasks the computer has been instructed to complete. The most common devices are the video terminal and/or *cathode ray tube (CRT),* the high-speed printer, and magnetic tapes or *disk drives.* Other output devices include the modem, multiformat camera, and *servers.* These devices respond only when directed by the control unit of the CPU.

The copies made by high-speed printers and the information recorded on magnetic tapes or disks provide permanent records of the tasks completed. The printers are usually used when visual data are required, whereas magnetic tape drives and disk drives are used when data need to be stored for records or possible further computations and usage. The data stored on magnetic tapes or disks can be retrieved and displayed on a video screen (CRT) when desired, and further data can be added or deleted. Output devices are also used as input devices if the data are being retrieved from storage or are being transmitted from another location.

Mass information is usually stored on magnetic tapes, which are inexpensive and can store millions of pieces of information. Reel-to-reel magnetic tape drives are rather large, and their initial cost is quite high. Therefore this output device is used only when large amounts of information are to be stored.

Magnetic disk drives are the most popular output devices and are called either *hard disk drives* or *floppy disk drives.* The hard disks are rigid and larger, can store *megabytes (MB)* or *gigabytes (GB)* of information, and range in size from a long-playing phonograph record to a compact disc. In 1972, when IBM introduced these hard disks, they were called *30-30 disks,* or *Winchester disk drives,* because each disk would hold 30 MB of information, now considered a small storage capacity.

Disk drives range in size from 3½ to 8 inches (9 to 20 cm) in diameter and are made of a flexible plastic material. These disks or diskettes are lightweight and relatively inexpensive. They are used primarily in minicomputers. They have a slower access time and lower storage capacity than other recording media.

Computer Operations
ANALOG COMPUTERS

Unaltered electricity, demonstrated in the form of a continuous sine wave, can be used to run a computer. A computer designed to operate directly from unaltered or continuous electricity is called an *analog computer.* The tasks performed by this type of computer depend on the ability to measure distinctions in the various voltages and the precision of the circuitry. Because the electricity is in an unbroken or continuous sine wave, discrete values are difficult to measure. Therefore, if a new or different function needed to be performed, the circuit would have to be rewired.

DIGITAL COMPUTERS

Digital computers were developed to overcome the inherent problems with analog computers. Digital computers break up the electricity sine wave into distinct, measurable values (Fig. 32-6). A familiar example of this is the digital electronic timing system used in sporting events, which breaks the time or sine wave into hundredths of a second. A computer is capable of breaking the sine wave into millionths of a second. With this finer digitization the sine wave would approach an almost smooth-looking curve.

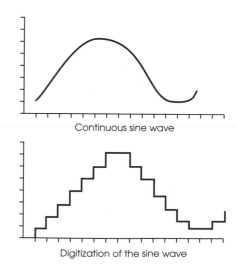

Continuous sine wave

Digitization of the sine wave

Fig. 32-6 A continuous sine wave is used in analog computers. Digital computers use a sine wave broken into distinct time increments.

Because digital computers are faster and more accurate, most computers are now digital. Much of the information from examinations performed in a radiology department is initially in the form of raw or unaltered electricity. Therefore, for the purpose of obtaining more uniform and consistent results, the computers contain an *analog-to-digital converter (ADC)*, which changes the sine wave into digital form with discrete values that can be transmitted. Digitization of the sine wave also allows the transfer of data from one location to another.

BINARY SYSTEM

A digital computer operates on a binary system that is similar to the Morse code. However, instead of dots and dashes, two digits are used—1 and 0. The American Standard Code for Information Interchange (ASCII) established a standard code consisting of a string of eight zeros and ones, referred to as a *byte,* and a string of sixteen zeros and ones, known as a *word.* Each individual digit is called a *bit (bi*nary digi*t).* The coded instructions contained in the first four bits tell the computer if the information is a number, letter, or symbol. For example, a prefix of 1011 signifies a number, and 1100 or 1101 a letter, depending on its placement within the alphabet. A different set of instructions represents a method of encoding four bits of memory into a binary representation of one decimal digit or number and is known as a *binary coded decimal (BCD).* An example of a BCD method is 0 = 0000; 1 = 0001; 2 = 0010; 3 = 0011; 4 = 0100; 5 = 0101; 6 = 0110; 7 = 0111; 8 = 1000; 9 = 1001.

The binary system forms the basis for digital electronics by allowing only two voltage levels. Information is stored by activating electronic switches or logic gates to an "off" position, represented by 0, and to the "on" position, represented by 1. By stringing these zeros and ones together, the coded instructions are received by the computer as to which function or task to perform. When the operator executes a command using the computer, the program places the zeros and ones in proper sequence. The resulting instruction to the computer is then accepted as a letter/word (such as in word processing), numerical calculations, or medical image production.

Integrated microscopic circuits are etched onto wafer-thin layers of silicon. Each of these silicon layers, or *chips,* contains a circuit that has a carefully and specifically designed maze of logic gates or switches. The integrated circuits on each of the silicon chips are then assembled into a larger circuit on a board, with the output of one circuit interfacing with the input of another. The circuit boards are designed to enable the computer to perform specialized functions and operate at higher speeds.

Although the complexity of a computer can become enormous as a result of the number of circuit boards involved, the basic circuitry or electronics using the binary system and logic gates remains the same.

PROGRAMMING

A computer program is a series of simple arithmetic steps in the binary system that occurs in a millionth of a second in the circuitry of the computer. The construction of the circuit boards within a computer determines the machine language that must be used to operate a specific computer; therefore, a certain type or brand of computer, such as the Macintosh computer, operates only on the machine language designed for it.

Computer programs stored within the primary memory or inserted in the secondary memory are known as *computer software.* When coded instructions are received by the control unit, data are retrieved from the memory and transferred to the ALU in the order of their memory location for computations. An example of a control program is Windows 98.

Because the development of computer programs is time-consuming, tedious, and prone to programming errors that can become costly, the computer industry devised what are known as *high-level languages.* These languages can be translated into a specific machine language by special programs called *compilers* or interpreters. Some of the high-level languages developed to perform specific types of tasks that are relevant to a certain field or discipline are listed in Table 32-3.

The use of high-level languages such as FORTRAN (which is used in imaging processing) has allowed the formation of sophisticated computer systems that can process the large amounts of data generated by the equipment used in a radiology department. The explosive growth of digital imaging modalities has resulted in the development of an integrated medical image management system known as the *picture archiving and communication system (PACS).* The group of computer programs that constitutes the PACS system allows a radiology department to electronically acquire images on a terminal or CRT, transmit them to various places, store the images, and catalog them on magnetic tapes or optical disks.

TABLE 32-3

High-level computer languages

Language	Uses
BASIC	Beginner's all-purpose symbolic instruction code; the standard language provided with most personal computers
COBOL	Common business-oriented language; used for financial applications; sometimes used for medical information systems
ALGOL or PASCAL	Algorithmic language; language used by mathematicians
FORTRAN	Formula translation; language for scientific programs that performs calculations based on complex formulas
PL/1	Programming language, version 1; developed by IBM to replace COBOL, FORTRAN, and ALGOL; used as a literary searcher for filer
MUMPS	Massachusetts General Hospital Utility Multiprogramming System; originally developed for medical information-processing applications; most radiology information management systems have been developed from this language
VISUAL ++ VISUAL BASIC	Visual programming language; designed for creating Windows applications

Applications in Radiology

Although the CPU of a computer system defines the processing of data, the *interfaces* with the *peripheral* input/output devices are important in radiology. The various imaging modalities depend on specific peripheral imaging devices that interface with a computer. Therefore, in the purchase of a computer system, an important consideration is the ability to upgrade the system to accommodate the newer peripherals.

BASICS OF INTERFACING PERIPHERAL DEVICES

The transfer of data among the CPU, memory, and input/output devices must occur rapidly when an examination is performed in the radiology department. To enable computers to process this rapid influx of data, a "bus" structure was developed to provide standardization and flexibility in the operating system. The bus consists of parallel conductors on a circuit board, known as a *mother board*. The circuit boards that contain the CPU, the memory, and the interface to the peripheral input/output devices are plugged into the mother board and communicate with each other by way of the bus.

The parallel conductors on the bus serve in three definite capacities: (1) as address lines that select a memory location or a specific input/output interface; (2) as data lines that carry a specified number of data bits; and (3) as control lines that carry the timing, status, and initiation of signals from one device to another. Because the bus communicates the data to and from the CPU by means of these parallel circuits instead of a string of serial bits, the processing is many times faster (Fig. 32-7).

ANALOG-TO-DIGITAL CONVERTERS AND VIDEO IMAGE PROCESSORS

Devices that produce images of real objects, such as patients, produce an analog rather than a digital signal. The electrical signal being emitted from the output phosphor of an image intensifier on a fluoroscopic unit, the scintillation crystal of a nuclear medicine detector, the ionization chamber or scintillation detector of a CT unit, or the piezoelectric crystal of an ultrasound machine is in analog form with a variance in voltage. For the signals to be read as data by the computer, they must be digitized and converted into the binary number system. The peripheral device that performs this task is the ADC, which transforms the sine wave into discrete increments with binary numbers assigned to each increment. The assignment of the binary numbers depends on the output voltage, which in turn represents the degree of attenuation of the various tissue densities within the patient.

The basic component of an ADC is the *comparator,* which outputs a 1 when the voltage equals or exceeds a precise analog voltage and outputs a 0 if the voltage does not equal or exceed this predetermined level. The most significant parameters of an ADC are (1) *digitization depth,* which is the number of bits in the resultant binary number; (2) *dynamic range,* which is the range of voltage or input signals that result in a digital output; and (3) *digitization rate,* which is the rate at which digitization takes place. Achieving the optimum digitization depth is necessary for resolution quality and flexibility in image manipulation. Digitization depth and dynamic range are analogous to producing optimum contrast and latitude in a radiograph.

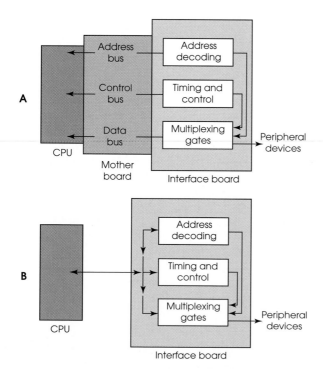

Fig. 32-7 A, Simplified diagram of the bus system, which allows rapid data transfer of up to 32 bits at a time. **B,** Data transferred to CPU in a serial or single string of bits; a longer time is required for transmission.

For production of a video image, the field size of the image is divided into many cubes or a matrix, with each cube assigned a binary number value proportional to the degree of the attenuation of the x-ray beam or intensity of the incoming signal. The individual three-dimensional cubes with length, width, and depth are called *voxels* (*vo*lume *el*ements), with the degree of attenuation or intensity of the incoming voltage determining their composition and thickness (Fig. 32-8). For example, as a result of attenuation of the x-ray beam, the contrast medium used in a CT or digital fluoroscopy examination would produce voxels with less digitization depth than the surrounding tissues. Digitization depth allows flexibility in the manipulation of the image.

The technology for displaying three-dimensional objects is continually being expanded; however, a two-dimensional square or *pixel* (*pic*ture *el*ement) represents the voxel on the television display monitor or cathode ray tube. The matrix is an array of pixels arranged in two dimensions, length and width, or rows and columns. The more pixels contained in an image, the larger the matrix becomes, with the resolution quality of the image improving. For instance, a matrix containing 256 × 256 pixels has a total of 65,536 pixels, or pieces of data, whereas a matrix of 512 × 512 pixels contains 262,144 pieces of data.

Field size should not be confused with matrix size. It is possible to combine a small field size and a large matrix size, or vice versa, depending on the equipment. The larger matrix also allows for more manipulation of the data or the image displayed on the television monitor. A larger matrix is also very beneficial and useful in imaging modalities such as digital subtraction fluoroscopy, CT, nuclear medicine, and ultrasonography.

After the image has been produced on the video display unit, *hard copies* are then printed on a single-emulsion image receptor using a multiformat camera or a laser camera that directs a laser beam onto the receptor. The laser camera also permits the images to be reproduced on paper. In addition, the images may be stored on magnetic tape or a disk for future reference. A computer system that has one or more peripherals included in the system is called a *multiprogramming system* (Fig. 32-9).

ARRAY PROCESSORS AND OTHER SPECIAL-PURPOSE PROCESSORS

To acquire a 512 × 512 pixel matrix at 30 television frames per second, an ADC must be able to process 107 digitizations per second, with each pixel being 8 to 16 digits deep to allow for satisfactory image manipulation. The hardware developed to handle this mass amount of data is the *array processor*, or special-purpose processor. The array processor, initially designed to calculate arithmetic operations at speeds 10 to 1000 times faster than the CPU, has since progressed to the point that it has become a specialized small computer. However, it is still considered peripheral to the host computer. Its function is to speed the processing of the matrices and other array of numbers by means of highly repetitive arithmetic operations.

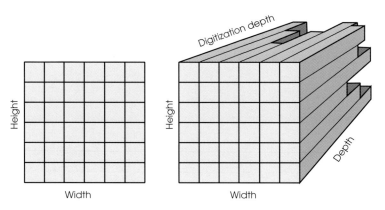

Fig. 32-8 Comparison between pixel *(left)* and voxel *(right)*.

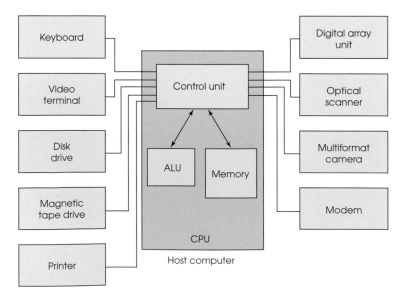

Fig. 32-9 Host computer with various input/output devices.

The arithmetic operations performed within the array processor are aided by *fast Fourier transforms,* which reduce the amplitude and increase the frequency of the sine wave through mathematic manipulation to allow faster processing. Because sine waves are not of equal intensity, the Fourier transform is a complex mathematical summation and/or multiplication of the sine waves that depict a spatial location within the body to provide a more accurate analysis and manipulation of the data. Other methods that speed up the processing are matrix multiplication, inversion, and convolution. Because of the special design of the array processor, many different operations are performed simultaneously. One definition given of an array processor is this:

It has at least one adder and one multiplier that can run simultaneously and do floating-point arithmetic; it can be programmed; and it achieves high performance through parallel processing, or pipelining.[1]

The alternatives to the array processor for arithmetic operations are the *dedicated single-component microprocessor* and the *bit-slice microprocessor.* These two special processors are less expensive but have considerably slower *response time* than the array processor.

[1]Burdett A et al: *A glossary of computing terms,* ed 6, Essex, England, 1995, Longman Group Informatics Society, British Informatics Society.

Array processors are designed to handle massive amounts of data. Therefore their use is justified in medical imaging procedures in which vast amounts of photons or signals are being emitted, such as from the output phosphor of an image intensifier, an ionization chamber, the scintillation detector of a CT unit, or the antenna of a magnetic resonance imaging (MRI) unit. All these units require an array processor to "crunch the numbers" so that they may be handled by the host computer (Fig. 32-10). For a 512×512 matrix image, the reconstruction process can take several minutes without the use of an array processor; with an array processor the task can be completed in less than 5 seconds (some in less than 1 second), with each rotation of an image requiring at least 5 million operations.

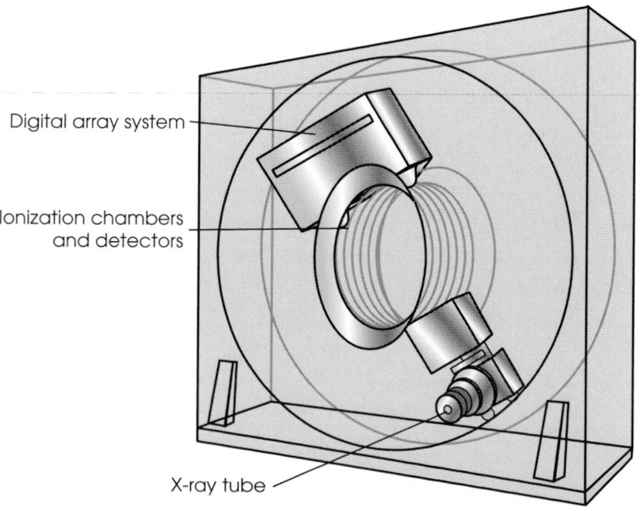

Fig. 32-10 Gantry of a third-generation CT unit. The digital array system contains the ionization chambers and detectors, an analog-to-digital converter, and a digital array unit. The attenuated x-rays are converted to an electrical signal, digitized, and transmitted to the array processor for image reconstruction.

Labels: Digital array system; Ionization chambers and detectors; X-ray tube

GRAPHIC DISPLAY DEVICES

Although many graphic display systems are available, they have not been used extensively in the medical imaging field. True graphic display is used extensively in the designing-type industries (e.g., automobiles and architecture). Gray-level mapping is used in CT, MRI, sonography, and nuclear medicine and is referred to as *graphs.* However, radiation therapy departments have used graphic display devices to demonstrate two-dimensional representations of tumors or even three-dimensional representations of tumors with shading within the graphic.

A graphic display system houses a display processing unit (DPU) and a dedicated computer with its own set of commands, data formats, and memory. The DPU creates an image on a display monitor and then regenerates this image 30 to 60 times a second to avoid a flicker in the image. For image display and regeneration of the image, the raster-scan or television-type system is used, dividing the picture into horizontal lines. Regeneration of the image takes place one line at a time. Similar equipment is used to display *virtual images,* also termed *virtual reality.* With virtual reality, moving images are displayed, and the operator is able to control their movement. This equipment has been used extensively by the motion picture industry.

A display list processor, which is housed in the host computer, transmits instructions to the DPU to create a graphic picture. The DPU then executes these instructions from 30 to 60 times per second to maintain the image on the television screen. Increased use of virtual reality in medicine will make graphic display devices obsolete.

Many graphic display systems use the "frame buffer" display technology, in which the digitization depth of each voxel is written into the DPU's memory. Manipulation of the image is less flexible with this system, but selective erasure of background intensity levels or anatomic structures can be performed. Another advantage of this system is that the host computer can perform contrast stretching, windowing, and other functions without disturbing the image data stored in the DPU's memory.

Gray-level mapping may be thought of as a graph of the gray levels within an image, and it is sometimes referred to as *histogram stretching, windowing,* or *contrast enhancement.* A histogram of the image is produced using gray-level mapping and represents a bar chart of the number of pixels versus gray levels (Fig. 32-11). The production of a gray-scale histogram or graph is made possible by a scan conversion memory tube within the computer system that uses a logarithmic transformation of the image into relative exposure values. The histogram is then easily changed into a graph representing the gray levels within an image. A low-contrast histogram representing an image has a wide histogram or a long scale of contrast (Fig. 32-13, *A*), whereas a high-contrast histogram has a narrower histogram or a short scale of contrast (Fig. 32-13, *B*).

In medical imaging equipment, *window width* refers to the width of the steep part of the curve, or the contrast within the image; *window level* refers to the location of the steep part of the curve within the gray levels and is analogous to image brightness or darkness (Fig. 32-14). The gray-level map or graph can be thought of as analogous to the density scale of a radiographic film, an H&D curve, or a characteristic curve. A windowing operation involves the selection of a certain range of the gray scale displayed as an image and the use of the full brightness scale of the television equipment to display only a specific preselected range of gray levels. The remainder of the gray scale outside of the window is subtracted from the gray-scale map, leaving only the desired portion of the image displayed (see Fig. 32-12).

Machine language is coded in binary numbers (0 and 1; on or off), and the shortest possible *word* is a bit. Each voxel depicts an individual depth level of grayness and is represented by a bit, or two *characters,* 0 and 1. The number of shades of gray in an image, representing depth, that can be present is determined by a formula, 2 raised to the power of the number of bits, or 2^n. A gray scale with discrete values is assigned to the bits of voxel depth. For example, 2^2 equals 4 gray levels; 2^8 equals 256 gray levels; 2^{10} equals 1024 gray levels; and 2^{16} equals 65,536 gray levels.

Bytes, or longer words, are necessary in digital imaging for faster processing. An 8-bit word is known as a byte; however, by convention, the computer system is referred to as an 8-bit system, a 10-bit system, or a 16-bit system. Gray levels are conceptualized as being parallel to contrast latitude: the more levels or shades of gray, the more contrast latitude. Discrete values assigned to the brightness of the levels of gray are known as *Hounsfield units* in CT; however, this concept is used by computer systems in digital radiography, nuclear medicine, MRI, and sonography.

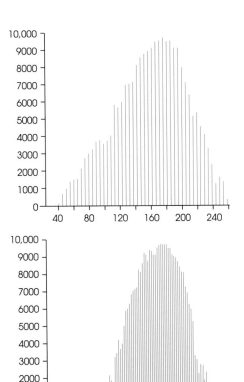

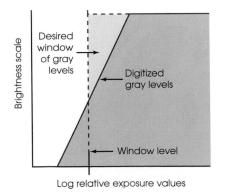

Fig. 32-11 A, Histogram demonstrating low (long-scale) contrast in an image. **B,** Histogram demonstrating high (short-scale) contrast in an image.

Fig. 32-12 Gray level windowing.

Digital Imaging Processing

Within the computer system, digital images are represented as groups of numbers. These numbers can be changed by applying mathematic operations; as a result the image is altered. This important concept has provided extraordinary control in contrast enhancement, image enhancement, subtraction techniques, and magnification without losing the original image data.

CONTRAST ENHANCEMENT

Contrast enhancement is accomplished by windowing, which was explained in the previous section of this chapter. Window width encompasses the range of densities within an image. A narrow window is comparable to the use of a high-contrast radiographic film. As a result, image contrast is increased. Increasing the width of the window allows more of the gray scale to be visualized or more latitude in the densities of the image visualized (Fig. 32-13). A narrow window is valuable when subtle differences in subject density need to be better visualized. However, the use of a narrow window increases image noise, and the densities outside of the narrow window are not visualized.

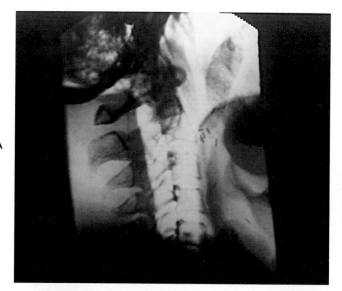

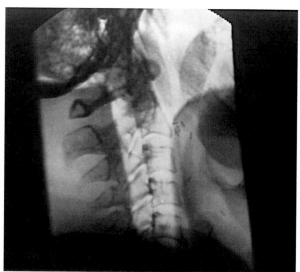

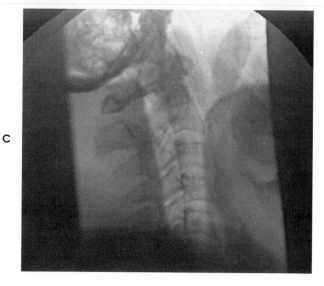

Fig. 32-13 Lateral cervical spine image using different window settings. Window widths as follows: **A,** 381; **B,** 658; and **C,** 2544. Notice that as the window width increases in numeric value, the scale of contrast increases (more long scale).

IMAGE ENHANCEMENT OR RECONSTRUCTION

Image enhancement or reconstruction is accomplished by *digital processing* or *filtering,* which can be defined as the accenting or attenuating of selected frequencies in the image. The filtration methods used in medical imaging are classified as convolution, low-pass filtering (smoothing), band-pass filtering, and high-pass filtering (edge enhancement). The background intensities within a medical image consist mainly of low spatial frequencies, whereas an edge, typifying a sudden change in intensities, is composed of mainly high spatial frequencies. (An example of an edge is the bone-to-air interface on the skull when CT is used.) Spatial noise originating from within the computer system is usually high spatial frequencies. Filtration reduces the amount of high spatial frequencies inherent in the object. The percentage of transmission versus spatial frequency, if plotted on a graph, is called *modulation transfer function (MTF).* One effort of continuing research in medical imaging is to develop systems with higher MTF.

Convolution

Convolution is accomplished automatically with computer systems that are equipped with fast Fourier transforms. In these systems the convolution process is implemented by placing a filter mask array (or matrix) over the image array (or matrix) in the memory. A filter mask is a square array or section with numbers, usually consisting of an area of 3×3 elements. The size of the filter mask is determined by the manufacturer of the equipment, although larger masks are seldom used because they take longer to process. The convolution filtering process can be conceptualized as placing the filter mask over an area of the image matrix, multiplying each element value of the filter mask by the image value directly beneath it, obtaining a sum of these values, and then placing that sum within the output image in the exact location as it was in the original image (Fig. 32-14). Convolution filtering is performed primarily to attenuate the higher frequencies within the image. The result of the convolution process is a blurring of the higher frequencies or intensities within the image.

Smoothing

Smoothing, or low-pass filtering, can also be used to remove the high-frequency noise within an image. Smoothing is accomplished by replacing the individual pixel values in the output image by gaining an average of the pixel values around each pixel. Each pixel's value in the output image is replaced by gaining the simple average of the eight neighboring pixels (Fig. 32-15). The averaging of the pixels is completed for each pixel within the matrix. The smoothing process attenuates the sudden differences in intensities or densities in the image by removing the higher frequencies within the image matrix (Fig. 32-16).

Band-pass filtration

Band-pass filtration removes or attenuates all frequencies or intensities within the image, except those in a preselected range. Band-pass filtering corresponds to the windowing process previously discussed.

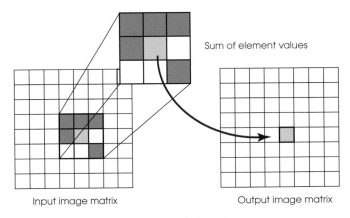

Sum of element values

Input image matrix

Output image matrix

Fig. 32-14 Convolution filtering.

9	8	7	9
7	6	3	7
8	9	9	8
9	6	7	6

9	8	7	9
7	7.3	7.3	7
8	7.1	6.7	8
9	6	7	6

Fig. 32-15 Smoothing, or low-pass filtering.

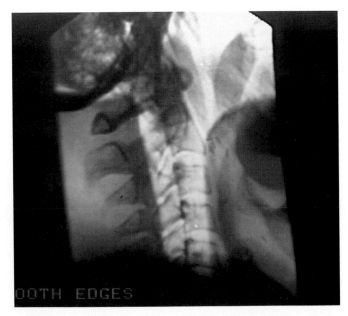

Fig. 32-16 Smoothing technique.

High-pass filtration

High-pass filtration, or *edge enhancement,* uses a special edge filter to produce an edge-sharpening effect. If a standard high-pass filter were to be used in medical imaging, a remarkably high-contrast image would be produced. An edge filter provides a more diagnostic image by averaging the gray levels similarly to the convolution process and then establishing a threshold within the gray-level scale. Thresholding allows saturation to black of all the gray levels below the threshold value and saturation to white of all the levels above the threshold. The thresholding process generates a higher contrast image of the anatomic area of interest and is particularly useful in demonstrating small structures. Research is being conducted with mammography equipment using high-pass filtration to accentuate the fine structural details within the breast and to minimize the background of the breast tissue. Digital subtraction angiography is well known for using high-pass filtration or edge enhancement to accentuate smaller vessels filled with contrast media (Fig. 32-17).

SUBTRACTION TECHNIQUES

The advantages of using *digital subtraction* include the ability to visualize small anatomic structures and the ability to perform an examination using venous injection of contrast media. The most common digital subtraction techniques are temporal subtraction and dual-energy subtraction. Hybrid subtraction is a combination of these two methods.

Temporal subtraction may be defined as a digital imaging process based on time intervals or limited by time. In its simplest form, temporal subtraction is produced by obtaining a mask (similar to a scout radiograph) and subtracting the pixel values of the mask from the pixel values of a postinjection image (see Chapter 35). The images should not change except for the contrast media-filled vasculature, and the subtracted image should primarily demonstrate the opacified blood vessels.

A serious problem with temporal subtraction is the probability of patient motion between exposures. For digital processing, a *time interval difference (TID)* mode is used to correct the motion problem. The TID technique involves obtaining a series of mask images and storing the images in adjacent memory locations. When the contrast medium is injected, a series of exposures is made at a very rapid rate, such as 15 images per second for 4 seconds. The postinjection images are identified as frame numbers and stored in adjacent memory locations. The frames, or postinjection data, are then subtracted from the masks, or original data, by allowing the computer to follow a set, programmed procedure. Examples of this set procedure are subtracting mask 1 from frame 2, mask 2 from frame 4, and so on.

Dual-energy subtraction does not require the acquisition of images before the injection of contrast media. After an iodinated contrast medium is injected, a series of rapid exposures is made at a high kilovolt (peak) (kVp) setting above the K-edge of iodine, 35 keV, and another series of exposures is made at a low kVp setting, below the 35 keV attenuation coefficient of iodine. The high kVp setting will diminish the bone contrast in the image, whereas the low kVp setting will enhance the less dense anatomic structures (e.g., the small vessels). A subtraction process of the two sets of images is then performed, with the outcome being increased contrast of the opacified vessels. For digital performance of the dual-energy subtraction technique after the images have been acquired, the densities of the straight-line portion of the film's H&D curve are correlated to the desired window level to produce the image. Advantages of dual subtraction are (1) patient motion is less of a problem than in the temporal subtraction method and (2) the high and low kVp images allow the display of bone only, soft tissue only, or a combination of the tissues.

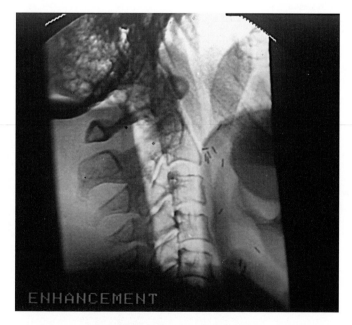

Fig. 32-17 Edge enhancement.

Hybrid subtraction is a combination of the temporal subtraction, TID, and dual-energy subtraction methods. When the hybrid subtraction method is used, a set of masks is obtained for the high kVp setting and for the low kVp setting. Therefore, two sets of masks and two sets of frames with iodinated contrast media are acquired. The low kVp masks are subtracted from the frames with contrast media, and the high kVp masks are subtracted from the high kVp frames. The hybrid subtraction procedure eliminates bone, leaving only the contrast-filled vessels.

Mask registration is a procedure that is useful when patient motion occurs between the time of the mask exposures and the time of the contrast media frames. For correction of the motion problem, the absolute density value of each pixel within the matrix of each mask and each frame is calculated and portrayed as a reregistration of the image. Calculation of the absolute values of the pixels is similar to the smoothing filtration method described previously.

MAGNIFICATION

Magnification, sometimes called *zooming,* is a process of selecting an area of interest and copying each pixel within the area an integer number of times. Large magnifications may give the image an appearance of being constructed of blocks. To provide a more diagnostic image, a smoothing or low-pass filter operation can be done to smooth out the distinct intensities between the blocks.

THREE-DIMENSIONAL IMAGING

When three-dimensional imaging was first introduced, the images were less than optimal because the resolution was too low to adequately visualize anatomic structures deeper within the body. The images often adequately displayed only the more dense structures closer to the body surface, or surface boundaries that appeared blocky and jagged. Consequently the soft tissue or less dense structures were not visualized. With the use of three-dimensional fast Fourier transforms, new *algorithms* for mathematic calculations, and computers with fast processing time, three-dimensional images have become smooth, sharply focused, and realistically shaded to demonstrate soft tissue. The ability to demonstrate soft tissue in three-dimensional imaging is referred to as a *volumetric rendering technique.*

Volumetric rendering is a computer program whereby "stacks" of sequential images are processed as a volume, with the gray-scale intensity information in each pixel being interpolated in the z axis (perpendicular to the x and y axes). Interpolation is necessary in that the field of view of the scan (the x and y axes) is not the same as the z axis because of interscan spacing. Following this computer process, new data are generated by interpolation, resulting in each new voxel having all the same dimensions. The volumetric rendering technique enables definition of the object's thickness, a crucial factor in three-dimensional imaging and in visualizing subtle densities.

Generation of three-dimensional images typically requires a stack of 50 scans with a resolution of 256×256, for a total of 6 MB of information and the processing capability of 5 million instructions per second. An average examination takes approximately 25 to 40 minutes of scan time to complete. The entire examination generally requires more than 1 hour, figured from the time the patient enters the department to the time the patient exits the department.

OPTICAL STORAGE AND RETRIEVAL SYSTEMS

Optical storage technology was developed to cope with the storage and retrieval problems within a radiology department. Optical storage technology embraces the concept of using some form of optical device to record and retrieve information from a light-sensitive medium. The optical devices currently in use are either gas or diode lasers. The media used for recording are compact discs, which resemble long-playing phonograph records.

Manufacturers of optical disk systems use minute holes made in the disk by the laser beam for the recording of information. The pits made in the media surface range in size from 1 to 2 micromillimeters (μmm), with the spacing between the rows 1.5 to 2 μmm. Using a matrix of $1024 \times 1024 \times 8$ bits per image, a laser optical disk can store approximately 3000 images; a matrix of $2048 \times 2048 \times 12$ bits per image allows approximately 400 images to be stored. Research currently being conducted should significantly increase the storage capability of compact discs in the near future.

Digital computer imaging systems using the binary system can send instructions to the optical laser system to encode the disk. The length of the pits and the distance between them made by the laser beam on the disk represent a digital coding scheme that can be retrieved. The advantages of this system are that, unlike radiographs, a disk does not deteriorate and requires very little storage space.

Information on the disk is retrieved using a reading laser that produces a light source directed at the surface of the disk. If no information is on the portion of the disk where the laser is focused, the light is reflected back. When the reading laser is focused on an area that has been encoded, or where there is a pit, the light is partially refracted according to the length and depth of the pit. The refraction of the light is then transmitted to the surface, where a photodetector is excited, produces a lower voltage, and is processed through digitization of the sine wave.

Digital optical systems can be used throughout the radiology department for the processing, transmission, storage, and retrieval of data. They can be used not only in the area of image processing but also for management services. As the technology develops, the radiology department of the future will use less film-screen technology. Instead the radiologist will be able to correlate, integrate, and evaluate images within the medical records of a single patient by use of a digital optical system.

Another form of image processing, developed primarily by NASA, is the use of a digitizing camera for the analysis of data. This type of image processing should have an impact of the field of radiography. A radiograph exposed and processed using current methods can be digitized by placing the film in a micro-densitometer on a lightbox in front of a digitizing camera that operates in a fashion similar to optical laser devices. The image is then digitized and processed by the computer system, which allows the image to be manipulated. Such a system would obviate repeat radiographs.

An innovative application of the digitizing camera and special image processors, called *teleradiography,* uses the digitizing camera to digitize the radiographic images of examinations for transmission by means of a *modem (Modulator/demodulator)* over conventional telephone lines or by satellite to a remote facility. The images are then processed by a special image processor and displayed on video terminals for diagnosis by physicians in prominent medical centers. This system enables small, rural hospitals and off-site facilities to provide improved medical care without the great expense of obtaining sophisticated computer equipment. Networks connecting large medical research centers and smaller hospitals and clinics through the use of teleradiography will thus provide more accurate diagnosis in pathologic conditions and trauma situations.

NETWORKS AND DATA TRANSMISSION

Transmission of images involves a large amount of data. A technique called *image compression* is used to reduce the number of bits per image. The compression technique uses an algorithm to change the original array of pixels to an intermediate set of data, much like the filtering process described previously in this chapter. Adjacent pixels within the image area that have the same density values are represented by a single intensity level, with a description of the area occupied by the pixels. The process of reducing the number of pixels representing an image is known as *encoding.* When the encoding process has been completed, the compressed image may be either stored or transmitted more quickly to another locality.

A *network* is a system of interconnected computer stations that can be controlled by a single mainframe or a central computer connected to and used by multiple computers in a time-sharing fashion. This type of network allows information to be transferred from one station to another or to the mainframe computer. Another type of network used in diagnostic imaging is a system of interconnected independent stations that consists of image acquisition stations, remote image acquisition and transmission stations, storage devices, departmental mainframes, and a hospital mainframe. Each point of input or output, or computer station, is called a *node* within the network. The nodes are interconnected and allow data to be transferred within the institution or to remote sites.

The methods of data transmission from one locality to another include dual-conductor telephone lines, coaxial cables, microwave radio signals, and communication satellites. The choice of transmission data depends on the speed of transmission needed, the distance from one location to another, and the cost.

Dual-conductor telephone lines are inexpensive and may already be in place. Their main disadvantages are the slow speed of data transmission and the reduced clarity of images on the receiving end. With telephone lines, it is difficult to transmit more than 1 million bits of data per second.

Coaxial cable, which uses fiberoptic light conductors, is more expensive than telephone lines but is often used in local area networks (LANs) for the transmission of data between a central health care facility and remote clinics or hospitals, within a single institution (Hospital Information System [HIS]), or within a radiology department (Radiology Information System [RIS]). The coaxial cable lines are similar to cable television lines and are called integrated services digital network (ISDN) lines. Through the use of a micro-densitometer, the image is digitized, with each pixel representing discrete density values within the sine waves; the sine waves are changed to light waves using the optical laser system. The fiberoptic system uses very fine glass fibers that confine the light and are immune to electrical interference. The light waves, representing the image, are pulsed by a light-emitting diode connected to the interface circuitry. On the receiving end of the LAN, a light-sensitive transducer converts the light pulses into digitized electrical signals, allowing the image to be reconstructed. ISDN lines transmit a high *baud rate,* or tens of millions of bits per second, with very good image clarity.

Digitized data are also transmitted using *radio microwave signals* and *communication satellites* when the image must be transmitted great distances. Long distance transmission uses a wide area network (WAN). The most familiar WAN is the World Wide Web, or Internet. A radio microwave system is a closed system and requires special sending and receiving equipment and is frequently used for teleconferencing. Telephone companies primarily control the communication satellites; however, the U.S. Department of Defense provides satellite transmission of images from sites all over the world to medical centers within the United States. The baud rate of data transmission using radio microwaves and satellites is in the hundreds of millions of bits per second, with image clarity equivalent to the original image.

INFORMATION AND MANAGEMENT SYSTEMS

Most of the information and management computer systems used in radiology have been developed from the MUMPS programming languages (see Table 32-3). The modules contained in the majority of information management systems are registration, scheduling, process control, image file management, and reporting. The use of these modules also contributes to the quality control of the department.

The function of the *registration module* is to record the dates and types of examinations a patient has had. Use of a computer file provides more accurate recording of information and much faster retrieval of the file.

Combined with the registration program is the *scheduling module* that makes the patient's appointment. This program aids in smoothing out the department's workload, thus making better use of equipment and personnel. Another function of this program is to check the patient's file for previous examinations and to sequence the examinations in the proper order. This module can also check to see what rooms are available for the study, calculate the average time it takes to complete the examination, print workloads for the entire department or a particular room, and produce schedules for the nursing stations, outpatient clinics, and physicians.

The *process module* tracks the process of performing and interpreting the examination. This process starts with the arrival of the patient in the department and includes the examinations performed, the rooms used, the radiographer who performed the examination, the number of radiographs per examination, whether retakes were required and the reason for the retakes, and whether any medications or contrast media were used. Before the patient leaves, a computer check is done to determine whether the patient needs to be scheduled for further examinations or whether all examinations have been completed. The program also records the time the report was dictated, transcribed, and signed by the radiologist. Use of this module or program can provide a very detailed repeat analysis that can be used to justify repair of equipment, new equipment purchases, or inservice education or further education of the radiographers.

Computer management of the image file provides a library system that records the files within the department, location of the files, and individual radiographs loaned to outside departments, doctors, clinics, and medical facilities. The system can provide lists of files or radiographs that are overdue, which helps in the recovery of these medical records before they are permanently lost. Used with a scheduling module, the image file module can produce a list of patients and the previous examinations completed on each patient; this information may then be retrieved from the file archives the day before the scheduled examinations. Lastly, this program also prints adhesive labels that can be attached to the file jacket to record the date and type of examination performed.

A *reporting program* assists in the preparation and interpretation of the examinations. This module usually includes a word processing program used by the transcriptionist. The use of Certified Record Techniques (CRTs) in transcription and proofreading can save clerical time and improve the accuracy of reports. Some systems even allow the radiologist to electronically sign the reports. A teaching file can also be developed with this system by having the radiologist dictate a code to be included with the transcription. The code enables the computer to identify the more interesting cases to be used for educational purposes.

All of these modules can be used on a time-sharing basis. *Time sharing* is a computer system in which each person using the system is given, for a small fraction of time, the total use or resources of the larger, multiprogram computer. The use of the large computer is rotated among the users under the direction of the operating programs and is determined by priorities. A time-sharing computer system makes a computerized information management system cost effective, even for small hospitals and clinics.

The other modules that can be included in an information management system contain *administrative* and *financial* programs. The most common of these is a *billing system* that can provide accurate and detailed itemized lists of expenses.

An overall benefit of the modules and the data or information generated is the potential to enhance quality control throughout the entire department and hospital. Management decisions based on the statistics provided by such a system promote efficiency and improve operations, thereby providing quality patient care.

Applications in Education

Computers have been used to facilitate learning for several decades. The development of miniaturized transistors and semiconductors has led to the mass distribution of microcomputers and minicomputers. As a result, computer-assisted instruction is now used at all educational levels.

It is important to distinguish between computer-assisted instruction (CAI) and computer-managed instruction (CMI). CAI programs involve learning of new information and actually assist in the teaching process. Methods incorporated in CAI are the presentation of new material with reinforcement through immediate feedback, questioning, and graphics. Learning can be ensured by testing the students' knowledge and repeating the training if necessary. Educational institutions are using CAI in distance-learning courses conducted through the Internet. CMI uses testing procedures and then directs the student to reference material for further information or help; no initial instruction is performed by the computer. Many CMI programs serve as electronic bookkeepers because their function is to grade tests, provide test scores, and provide statistical data on the tests. Certification agencies are adopting this technology.

Instruction using a CAI system is concentrated on the presentation and learning of concepts, principles, and rules, or what is known as the *cognitive domain* of learning. Its effectiveness is limited in the teaching of psychomotor skills, such as radiographic positioning, and in the *affective domain,* the learning of professional attitudes and empathy. Learning in the latter domain may be enhanced by adding a compact or video disc system to the computer system.

Although CAI has a high potential for the enhancement of learning, it will not replace the instructor in the classroom or clinical setting, just as the computer will not replace human judgment in making a diagnosis. A distinct advantage of CAI is that students exposed to this method of instruction will have the opportunity to become familiar with computers and their operation and therefore will more readily adapt to the computerized equipment in the clinical setting.

Conclusion

Radiology departments in the future will become more reliant on the computer for imaging, therapeutic purposes, file management, billing, quality assurance, patient monitoring, education, and research. Radiologists will find their time absorbed and divided among the various imaging and therapeutic procedures. As this occurs, radiologic technologists will assume additional responsibility and will be required to possess the knowledge and skills necessary to understand and operate computerized equipment, just as they must know how radiation is produced.

Definition of Terms

address Label, name, or number identifying a register, location, or unit where data are stored. In most cases, the address refers to the location in the computer memory.

algorithm Defined set of instructions that will lead to the logical conclusion of a task.

analog computer Computer that performs operations on continuous signals.

analog-to-digital converter (ADC) Input device for changing continuous (analog) signals into digital form (i.e., discrete numbers).

arithmetic/logic unit (ALU) That part of the computer that performs computations, comparisons, and logical operations.

array processor Central processor designed to allow any machine instruction to operate simultaneously on a number of data locations (data arrays). This design enables problems involving the same calculations on a range of data to be solved very quickly.

assembler Computer program used to assemble machine code from symbolic code.

assembly language Computer programming language that is machine oriented and can be translated directly into machine instructions.

baud rate Rate at which information is transmitted serially from a computer; expressed in bits per second.

binary Numbering system based on 2's rather than 10's (decimals); the individual element can have a value of 0 or 1 and in computer memory is known as a *bit.*

bit Constructed from *bi*nary digi*t.* The term refers to a single digit of a binary number; for example, the binary number 101 is composed of three bits.

boot Process of initializing a computer operating system, also referred to as *booting up.*

buffer Auxiliary storage area for data input to match the speed differences between machines.

bug Common term used to describe an error in operation or in a program.

byte Term used to define a group of bits, usually eight, being treated as a unit by the computer to store one character.

cathode ray tube (CRT) Electronic tube (like the familiar television tube) that makes the computer output visible; sometimes called a *visual display unit (VDU).*

central processing unit (CPU) Brain of the computer. It is the circuitry that actually processes the information and controls the storage, movement, and manipulation of data.

character Any letter, digit, or punctuation mark. Characters are usually represented by a binary code composed of 8 bits, or 1 byte.

command Portion of code that represents an instruction for the computer.

compiler Set of programs that compiles or converts a program into the machine language instructions for a particular computer.

console Usually the front panel of the CPU by which the operator supervises and controls the machine.

control unit That part of the CPU that directs the sequence of operations, such as which instruction is to be executed next.

cursor A character, usually an underline or a graphics block, that indicates position on a display screen.

data acquisition unit Peripheral device that acquires signals from equipment and transmits them to the computer.

data base Large file of organized information that is produced, updated, and manipulated by one or more programs.

digital computer Computer in which discrete numbers are used to express data and instructions.

digitization depth Dimension of depth within a matrix; represented by a number of pixels, which in turn signify the levels or shades of gray available within an image.

digitization rate Amount of time needed to change data from analog form to digital form.

direct access Access to data independent of the previously obtained data; it may also be called *random access.*

disk Circular plate coated with magnetic material and used to store data.

disk drive Device used to read data from and to write data onto disks.

downtime Time a computer system is out of operation, usually for repairs and/or maintenance; often expressed as a percentage of the normal operating hours.

dynamic range Range of voltage or input signals that result in a digital output.

encode To place a message into; to convert into a machine language.

file Collection of related data or information kept as a unit.

floating point operation A number in which the decimal point may be in any position.

generation Group of computers produced within the same period, based on the model of an earlier product.

gigabyte (GB) Storage capacity of one billion bytes (see *byte*).

hard copy Any readable output from a computer; usually on paper. In radiology the output of images is usually on radiographic film or other laser-printed medium.

hardware Physical devices and/or equipment of a computer system.

high-level language Computer language in which each user instruction corresponds to multiple instructions when converted to machine code; examples: FORTRAN, FOCAL, COBOL, and ALGOL.

image compression Process whereby adjacent pixels with the same values are consolidated to store data as one value, thus saving computer storage space.

input Information the computer receives via media such as magnetic tape, disks, punched cards, or keyboards.

input/output terminal (I/O terminal) Machine or device capable of both feeding information into and retrieving information from the computer.

instruction Program step that tells the computer exactly what to do for a single operation in a program.

interface Device that serves as a common boundary between two other devices; a connection between two pieces of computer hardware.

K Symbol for 1000; in computer language, it means 210 or 1024 and denotes the number of units a computer can store in its memory; example: $32 \times 1024 = 32,768$ or 32K.

language Defined set of characters that, when used alone or in combination, form a meaningful set of words and symbols; used to write instructions for a computer; examples: ALGOL, COBOL, BASIC, and FORTRAN.

machine language Programming language consisting only of numbers or symbols that the computer can understand without translation.

magnetic memory Memory device that uses magnetic fields as a means of storing data; example: magnetic tape or disks.

megabyte (MB) 1,048,576 bytes (see *byte*).

memory Storage of information and data by the computer.

modem (*modulator/demodulator*) Device that allows data to be transmitted long distances, usually over telephone lines, by impressing digital pulses onto an analog carrier wave.

multiprogramming Ability of a computer system to permit execution of more than one separate task at a time; used in time-sharing and/or multiuser systems.

multitasking Computer system or a single machine that can process several programs.

network Interconnected system of computers used to share information; also called a *net*.

node Individual computer, or sometimes another type of unit, within the same computer network; also a connection point in the data structure system.

off-line Portions of the computer that are not under the direct control of the CPU or the operator.

on-line Portions of the computer that are directly under the control of the CPU and the operator.

optical scanner Device that scans the light either reflected or transmitted through a surface and then converts the signal into a machine-readable input.

output Results generated when the computer has performed the requested combinations of tasks.

peripheral Device that is separate but connected to the computer for the purpose of supplying input and/or output capability.

pixel (*picture element*) One individual cell surface within an image matrix used for CRT image display.

primary memory Portion of a computer that is used to store information, either data or programs. The size of a computer may be referred to by the amount of user memory; usually measured in kilobytes.

random access Ability to access locations of data without regard to sequential data. Access may be accomplished by going directly to the location.

random access memory (RAM) Pertaining to a storage device in which access time is effectively independent of the location of the data.

read-only memory (ROM) Memory similar to RAM except that data cannot be written into it but is capable of being read.

real time Computer operations that occur fast enough to be analyzed and used immediately for decision making.

register Device in the CPU that stores information for future use.

response time Time between the input of information into a computer and the response or output.

serial processing Digital computer processing in which programs are run sequentially, rather than simultaneously or together.

server Host computer containing software programs that communicate with users of the World Wide Web.

software Applies to any program or set of instructions that can be loaded into a computer.

storage capacity Amount of data that can be stored in the computer memory; usually expressed in terms of kilobytes.

terminal Input/output device, usually consisting of a keyboard and display screen.

time sharing Process of accomplishing two or more tasks at (apparently) the same time. The computer will process one task at a time, but only a small portion, before switching to the next. Because the computer can process a large amount of data in a short period of time, the switching between tasks is not noticed by human observation.

voxel (*volume element*) Individual pixel with the associated volume of tissue based on the slice thickness.

Winchester disk drive Smaller, less-expensive hard disk drive capable of transferring data at an increased rate with sophisticated error detection and correction procedures.

window Arbitrary numbers used for image display based on various shades of gray. Window *width* controls the overall gray level and affects image contrast; window *center* (level) controls subtle gray images within a certain width range and ultimately affects the brightness and overall density of an image.

word Number of bits processed as a single unit in an arithmetic operation.

write To record data on a memory device.

Selected bibliography

Brice J: Execs diagnose impact of reform on radiology, *Diagn Imaging* 17:67, 1995.

Burdett A et al: *A glossary of computing terms,* ed 6, Essex, England, 1995, Longman Group Informatics Society, British Informatics Society.

Bushong SC: *Radiologic science for technologists—physics, biology, and protection,* ed 6, St Louis, 1997, Mosby.

Chandler R: PACS: applications in the modern radiology department, *Admin Radiol,* June 1987.

Convey HD et al: *Computers in the practice of medicine, introduction to computer concepts,* vol 1, Reading, Mass, 1980, Addison-Wesley.

Cook LT et al: Image processing: shape analysis, texture analysis, and three-dimensional display, *Appl Radiol* 13:123, 1984.

Choyke PL et al: Morphing radiographic images: applications on a desktop computer, *Am J Radiol* 166:527, 1996.

Curry T et al: *Christensen's introduction to the physics of diagnostic radiology,* ed 4, Philadelphia, 1990, Lea & Febiger.

Dwyer SJ III et al: Computer applications and digital imaging, Proceedings of the RSNA meeting, Chicago, Nov 1992, 78th Scientific Meeting.

Edwards M et al: Computers in radiology—interfacing with peripheral devices, *Appl Radiol* 2:37, 1984.

Enlander D: *Computers in medicine—an introduction,* St Louis, 1980, Mosby.

Fishman EK et al: Volumetric rendering techniques applications for three-dimensional imaging of the hip, *Radiology* 163:737, 1987.

Folger, T: The best computer in all possible worlds, *Discover,* October, p. 91, 1995.

Gay JE, Taubel JP: Effects of ionizing radiation and magnetic fields on digital data stored on floppy disks, *Radiology* 189:583, 1993.

Giger ML et al: "Intelligent" workstation for computer-aided diagnosis, *Radiographics* 13:647, 1993.

Gonzoley R et al: *Digital image processing,* Reading, Mass, 1977, Addison-Wesley.

Gould RG: Digital hardware in radiography and fluoroscopy, *Appl Radiol* 13:137, 1984.

Greenfield GB, Hubbard LB: *Computers in radiology,* New York, 1984, Churchill Livingstone.

Hendee WR, Ritenour E: *Medical imaging physics,* ed 3, St Louis, 1992, Mosby.

Hiatt M: Computers and the revolution in radiology, *JAMA* 13:273, 1995.

Honeyman JC, Dwyer SJ III: Computers for clinical practice and education in radiology: historical perspective on computer development and glossary of terms, *Radiographics* 13:145, 1993.

Hunter TB: *The computer in radiology,* Rockville, Md, 1986, Aspen.

Kuni CC: *Introduction to computers and digital processing in medical imaging,* St Louis, 1988, Mosby.

Lehr JL: Computer languages and the operating systems, *Appl Radiol* 13:35, 1984.

Lehr JL, editor: *Planning guide for radiologic installations: fascicle 9: computer information systems,* Chicago, 1977, American College of Radiology.

Lehr JL: Software: basics and applications in radiology, *Semin Ultrasound* 4:260, 1983.

Lieberman DE: *Computer methods, the fundamentals of digital nuclear medicine,* St Louis, 1977, Mosby.

Ney D et al: Interactive real-time multiplanar CT imaging, *Radiology* 170:275, 1989.

Novick G: Introduction to computer hardware and internal representation, *Appl Radiol* 12:51, 1983.

Powis RL et al: *A thinker's guide to ultrasonic imaging,* Baltimore, 1984, Urban & Schwarzenberg.

Richardson ML, Gillespy T II: Inexpensive computer-based digital imaging teaching file, *Am J Radiol* 160:1299, 1993.

Robb WL: Future advances and directions in imaging research, *Am J Radiol* 150:39, 1988.

Rowberg AH: Digital hardware in CT and NMR, *Appl Radiol* 13:71, 1984.

Scott R: Artificial intelligence: its use in medical diagnosis, *J Nucl Med* 34:510, 1993.

Seeram E: *Computed tomography technology,* Philadelphia, 1982, WB Saunders.

Simborg DW: Local area networks: why? what? what if? *MD Comput* 1:10, 1984.

Staab EV: Computers for clinical practice and education in radiology: introduction, *Radiographics* 13:143, 1993.

Strong HM, Cerva JR: Image storage and transmission technology, *Semin Ultrasound* 4:270, 1983.

Swett HA et al: Expert system-controlled image display, *Radiology* 172:487, 1989.

Swett HA, Miller PL: ICON: a computer-based approach to differential diagnosis in radiology, *Radiology* 163:555, 1987.

Trux PG: The current state of operating systems: 1983 and 1984, *MD Comput* 1:58, 1984.

Ubaldi S et al: The use of microcomputers in radiologic technology training programs: focus on education, *Radiol Technol* 53:271, 1981.

Verhelle F et al: From archives to picture archiving and communication systems, *Radiology* 78:370, 1995.

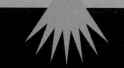

COMPUTED TOMOGRAPHY

LORRIE L. KELLEY

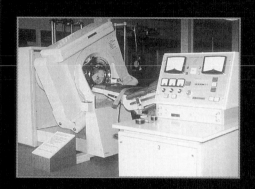

RIGHT: First-generation computed to-mographic scanner from 1971. The operator console *(right)* permitted lit-tle manipulation of the image. The pa-tient couch and gantry *(left rear)* were used to examine a limited area of the brain extending from the skull base to the top of the skull.

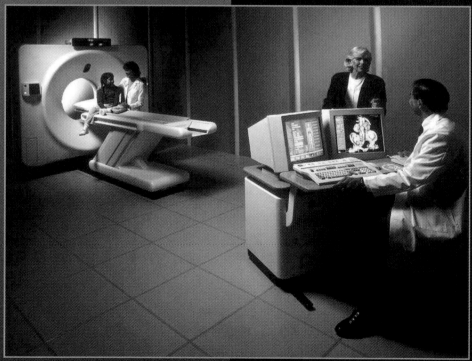

LEFT: Modern gantry *(left)* and opera-tor's control console for computed to-mography. Note the visual display of image on the right monitor and the anatomic selections on the left monitor.

(Courtesy GE Medical Systems, Waukesha, Wisc.)

Fundamentals of Computed Tomography

*Computed tomography (CT)** is the process of creating a cross-sectional tomographic plane of any part of the body (Fig. 33-1). For CT a patient is *scanned* by an x-ray tube rotating about the body part being examined. A *detector assembly* measures the radiation exiting the patient and feeds back the information, referred to as *primary data,* to the host computer. Once the computer has compiled and calculated the data according to a preselected *algorithm,* it assembles the data in a *matrix* to form an *axial* image. Each image, or *slice,* is then displayed on a *cathode ray tube (CRT)* in a cross-sectional format.

---

*Almost all italicized terms are defined at the end of this chapter.

In the early 1970s CT scanning was only used clinically for imaging of the brain. Furthermore, the first CT scanners were capable of producing only axial images and thus were called *CAT (computed axial tomography) units* by the public; this term is no longer accurate because images can now be created in multiple planes. In the past few decades, dramatic technical advancements have led to the development of CT scanners that can be used to image virtually every structure within the human body. Improvements in scanner design and computer science have produced CT units with new imaging capabilities and reconstruction techniques. Three-dimensional reconstruction of images of the internal structures is becoming a popular choice for surgical planning, CT angiography, radiation therapy planning, and virtual reality.

CT-guided biopsies and fluid drainage offer an alternative to surgery for some patients. Although the procedures are considered invasive, they offer shorter recovery periods, no exposure to anesthesia, and less risk of infection. CT is also used in radiation oncology for radiation therapy planning. CT scans taken through the treatment field, with the patient in treatment position, have drastically improved the accuracy and quality of radiation therapy.

Computed Tomography and Conventional Radiography

When a conventional x-ray exposure is made, the radiation passes through the patient and produces an image of the body part. Frequently body structures are superimposed (Fig. 33-2). Visualizing specific structures requires the use of contrast media, varied positions, and usually more than one exposure. Localization of masses or foreign bodies requires at least two exposures and a ruler calibrated for magnification.

In the CT examination, a tightly collimated x-ray beam is directed through the patient from many different angles, resulting in an image that represents a cross section of the area scanned. This imaging technique essentially eliminates the superimposition of body structures. The CT technologist controls the method of acquisition, the slice thickness, the reconstruction algorithm, and other factors related to image quality.

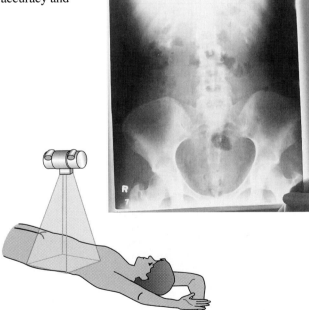

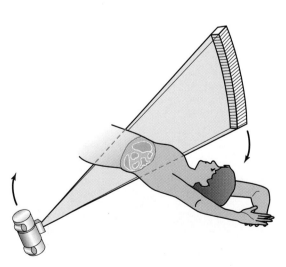

Fig. 33-1 CT scanner provides cross-sectional images by rotating about the patient.

Fig. 33-2 Conventional radiograph superimposes anatomy and yields one diagnostic image with fixed density and contrast.

In the digital radiograph of the abdomen shown in Fig. 33-3, high-density bone and low-density gas are seen, but many soft tissue structures, such as the kidneys and intestines, are not clearly identified. Contrast media are needed to visualize these structures. A CT examination of the abdomen would demonstrate all the structures that lie within the slice. In Fig. 33-4, *A,* the liver, stomach, kidneys, spleen, and aorta can be identified. In addition to eliminating superimposition, CT has the superior capability to differentiate between tissues with similar densities. This differentiation of densities is referred to as *contrast resolution.* The improved contrast resolution with CT is the result of a reduction in the amount of scattered radiation.

Fig. 33-4, *B* is an axial image of the brain that differentiates the gray matter from the white matter and also shows bony structures and cerebrospinal fluid within the ventricles. Because CT can demonstrate subtle differences in various tissues, radiologists are able to diagnose pathologic conditions more accurately than if they were to rely on radiographs alone. Furthermore, because the image is digitized by the computer, numerous image manipulation techniques can be used to enhance and optimize the diagnostic information available to the physician.

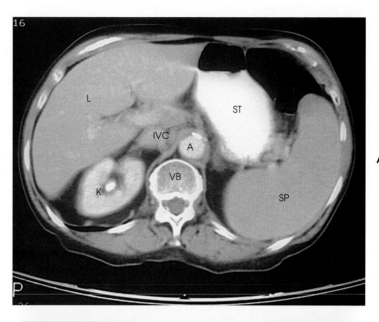

A

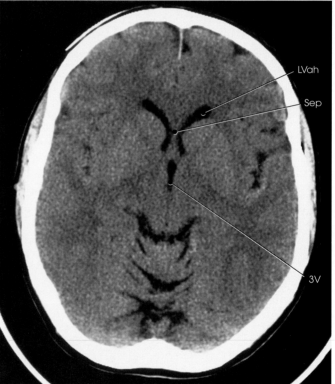

B

Fig. 33-4 A, Axial image of abdomen demonstrating liver *(L),* stomach *(ST),* spleen *(SP),* aorta *(A),* inferior vena cava *(IVC),* vertebral body of thoracic spine *(VB),* and kidney *(K).* **B,** Axial CT scan of lateral ventricles (LVah), septum (Sep), and third ventricle (3V).

(**B,** From Kelly LL, Peterson CM: *Sectional anatomy for imaging professionals,* St Louis, 1997, Mosby.)

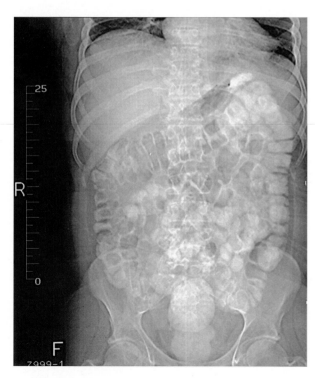

Fig. 33-3 Digital kidney, ureter, and bladder (KUB).

Historical Development

CT was first demonstrated successfully in 1970 in England at the Central Research Laboratory of EMI, Ltd. Dr. Godfrey Hounsfield, an engineer for EMI, and Dr. James Ambrose, a physician at Atkinson Morley's Hospital in London, are generally given credit for the development of CT. For their research they were awarded the Nobel Prize in 1979. After CT was shown to be a useful clinical imaging modality, the first full-scale commercial unit, referred to as a *brain tissue scanner,* was installed in Atkinson Morley's Hospital in 1971. An example of an early dedicated head CT scanner is shown in Fig. 33-5. Physicians recognized its value for providing diagnostic neurologic information, and its use became accepted rapidly. The first CT scanners in the United States were installed in June 1973 at the Mayo Clinic, Rochester, Minn., and later that year at Massachusetts General Hospital, Boston. These early units were also dedicated head CT scanners. In 1974, Dr. Robert S. Ledley of Georgetown University Medical Center, Washington, D. C., developed the first whole-body scanner, which greatly expanded the diagnostic capabilities of CT.

After CT was accepted by physicians as a diagnostic modality, numerous companies in addition to EMI began manufacturing scanners. Although the units differed in the design, the basic principles of operation were the same. CT scanners have been categorized by *generation,* which is a reference to the level of technologic advancement of the tube and detector assembly. There were four recognized generations of CT scanners; newer scanners, however, are no longer categorized by generation but by tube and detector movement.

The early units, referred to as the *first-generation scanners,* worked by a process known as *translation/rotation.* The tube produced a finely collimated beam, or pencil beam. Depending on the manufacturer, one to three *detectors* were placed opposite the tube for radiation detection. The linear tube movement (translation) was followed by a rotation of 1 degree. Scan time was usually 3 to 5 minutes per scan, which required the patient to hold still for extended periods. Because of the slow scanning and reconstruction time, the use of CT was limited almost exclusively to neurologic examinations. A CT image from a first-generation scanner is shown in Fig. 33-6.

The second-generation scanners were considered a significant improvement over first-generation scanners. The x-ray tube now emitted a fan-shaped beam that was measured by approximately 30 detectors placed closely together in a detector array. All subsequent generations would use the fan beam geometry. Tube and detector movement was still translation/ rotation, but the rotation was 10 degrees between each translation. These changes improved overall image quality and decreased scan time to about 20 seconds for a single slice. However, the time required to complete one CT examination remained relatively long.

The *third generation* of scanners introduced a *rotate/rotate movement* in which both the x-ray tube and detector array rotate simultaneously around the patient. An increase in the number of detectors (over 750) and their arrangement in a "curved" detector array considerably improved image quality (Fig. 33-7). Scan times were decreased to 1 to 10 seconds per slice, which made the CT examination much easier for patients and helped to decrease motion artifact. Advancements in computer technology also decreased image reconstruction time, substantially reducing examination time.

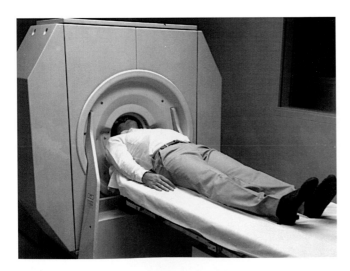

Fig. 33-5 First-generation CT unit: dedicated head scanner.

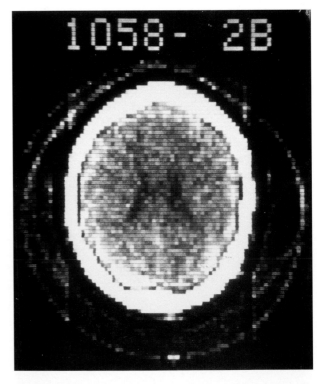

Fig. 33-6 Axial brain image from the first CT scanner in operation in the United States: Mayo Clinic, Rochester, Minn. The 80 × 80 matrix produced a noisy image. The examination was performed in July 1973.

The fourth-generation scanners introduced the *rotate-only movement* in which the tube rotated about the patient, but the detectors were in fixed positions, forming a complete circle within the gantry (Fig. 33-8). The use of stationary detectors required greater numbers of detectors to be installed in a scanner. Fourth-generation scanners tended to yield a higher patient dose per scan than previous generations of CT scanners.

In contemporary CT scanners, both third- and fourth-generation designs incorporate the latest technologic advances and produce similar image quality.

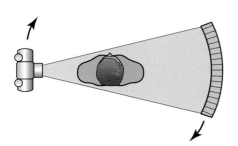

Fig. 33-7 Rotate/rotate movement: tube and detector movement of a third-generation scanner.

Technical Aspects

The axial images acquired by CT scanning provide information about the positional relationships and tissue characteristics of structures within the section of interest. The computer performs a series of steps to generate one axial image when the patient and gantry are perpendicular to each other. The tube rotates around the patient, irradiating the area of interest. For every position of the x-ray tube, the detectors measure the transmitted x-ray values, convert them into an electric signal, and relay the signal to the computer. The measured x-ray transmission values are called *projections (scan profiles)* or *raw data.* Once collected, the electrical signals are digitized, a process that assigns a whole number to each signal. The value of each number is directly proportional to the strength of the signal.

The digital image is an array of numbers arranged in a grid of rows and columns called a *matrix.* A single square, or picture element, within the matrix is called a *pixel.* The slice thickness gives the pixel an added dimension called the *volume element,* or *voxel.* Each pixel in the image corresponds to the volume of tissue in the body section being imaged. The voxel volume is a product of the pixel area and slice thickness (Fig. 33-9). The *field of view (FOV)* determines the amount of data to be displayed on the monitor.

Each pixel within the matrix is assigned a number that is related to the linear attenuation coefficient of the tissue within each voxel. These numbers are called *CT numbers* or *Hounsfield units.* CT numbers are defined as a relative comparison of x-ray attenuation of a voxel of tissue to an equal volume of water. Water is used as reference material because it is abundant in the body and has a uniform density; therefore water is assigned an arbitrary value of 0. Tissues that are denser than water are given positive CT numbers, whereas tissues with less density than water are assigned negative CT numbers. The scale of CT numbers ranges from -1000 for air to $+4000$ for dense bone. Average CT numbers for various tissues are listed in Table 33-1.

For displaying the digital image on the CRT, each pixel within the image is assigned a level of gray. The gray level assigned to each pixel corresponds to the CT number for that pixel.

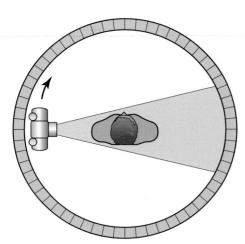

Fig. 33-8 Rotate-only movement: tube movement with stationary detectors of a fourth-generation scanner.

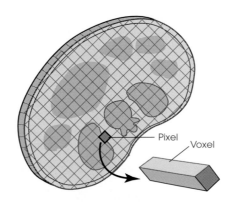

Fig. 33-9 A CT image is composed of a matrix of pixels, with each pixel representing a volume of tissue (voxel).

TABLE 33-1

Average Hounsfield units (HU) for selected substances

Substance	HU
Air	-1000
Lungs	-250 to -850
Fat	-100
Orbit	-25
Water	0
Cyst	-5 to +10
Fluid	0 to +25
Tumor	+25 to +100
Blood (fluid)	+20 to +50
Blood (clotted)	+50 to +75
Blood (old)	+10 to +15
Brain	+20 to +40
Muscle	+35 to +50
Gallbladder	+5 to +30
Liver	+40 to +70
Aorta	+35 to +50
Bone	+150 to +1000
Metal	+2000 to +4000

System Components

The three major components of the CT scanner are (1) the computer, (2) the gantry and table, and (3) the operator's console (Fig. 33-10). Because each component has several subsystems, only a brief description of their main functions is provided in the following sections.

COMPUTER

The computer provides the link between the CT technologist and the other components of the imaging system. The computer system used in CT has four basic functions: control of data acquisition, image reconstruction, storage of image data, and image display.

Data acquisition is the method in which the patient is scanned. The technologist must select among numerous parameters, such as scanning in the conventional or helical mode, before the initiation of each scan. During implementation of the *data acquisition system (DAS)*, the computer is involved in sequencing the generation of x-rays, turning the detectors on and off at appropriate intervals, transferring data, and monitoring the system operation.

The *reconstruction* of a CT image depends on the millions of mathematical operations required to digitize and reconstruct the raw data. This image reconstruction is accomplished using an array processor that acts as a specialized computer to perform mathematical calculations rapidly and efficiently, thus freeing the host computer for other activities. Currently, CT units can acquire scans in less than 1 second and require only a few seconds more for image reconstruction.

The *host computer* in CT has limited storage capacity so image data can be stored only temporarily. Therefore other storage mechanisms are necessary to allow for long-term *data storage* and *retrieval*. After reconstruction, the CT image data can be transferred to either magnetic tapes or optical disks. This allows CT studies to be removed from the limited memory of the host computer and stored independently, a process termed *archiving*.

The reconstructed images are displayed on a CRT or video monitor. At this point the technologist or physician can communicate with the host computer to view specific images, post images on a scout, and/or implement image manipulation techniques such as zoom, control contrast and brightness, and image analysis techniques.

GANTRY AND TABLE

The *gantry* is a circular device that houses the x-ray tube, DAS, and detector array. Newer CT units also house the continuous *slip ring* and high-voltage generator in the gantry. The structures housed in the gantry provide the necessary data to the computer for image reconstruction.

The x-ray tube used in CT is similar in design to the tubes used in conventional radiography, but it is specially designed to handle and dissipate excessive heat units created during a CT examination. Most CT x-ray tubes use a rotating anode to increase heat dissipation. Many CT x-ray tubes can handle around 2.1 million heat units (MHU), whereas advanced CT units can tolerate 4 to 5 MHU.

The detectors in CT function as image receptors. A detector measures the amount of radiation transmitted through the body and then converts the measurement into an electrical signal proportional to the radiation intensity. The two basic detector types used in CT are scintillation (solid state) and ionization (xenon gas) detectors.

The gantry can be tilted forward or backward up to 30 degrees to compensate for body part angulation. The opening within the center of the gantry is termed the *aperture*. Most apertures are about 28 inches (71.1 cm) wide to accommodate a variety of patient sizes as the patient table advances through it.

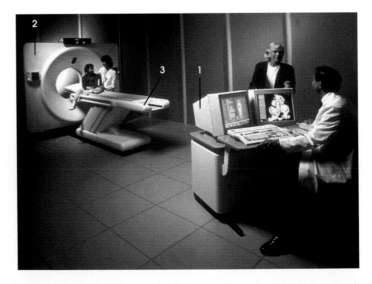

Fig. 33-10 Components of a CT scanner: *1*, Computer and operator's console; *2*, gantry; *3*, patient table.

(Courtesy GE Medical Systems, Waukesha, Wisc.)

For certain head studies, such as those of facial bones, sinuses, or the sella turcica, a combination of patient positioning and gantry angulation results in a *direct coronal* image of the body part being scanned. Fig. 33-11, *A* demonstrates a typical direct coronal image of C1 to C2. In comparison, a computer-reconstructed coronal image created from axial scans through the body part is shown in Fig. 33-11, *B*. Overall image resolution and quality are lost in the reconstructed image as compared with the direct coronal image.

The *table* is an automated device linked to the computer and gantry. It is designed to move in increments *(index)* after every scan according to the scan program. The table is an extremely important part of a CT scanner. Indexing must be accurate and reliable, especially when thin slices (1 or 2 mm) are taken through the area of interest. Most CT tables can be programmed to move in or out, depending on the examination protocol and the patient.

CT tables are made of wood or low-density carbon composite, both of which support the patient without causing image artifacts. The table must be very strong and rigid to handle patient weight and at the same time maintain consistent indexing. All CT tables have a maximum patient weight limit; this limit varies by manufacturer from 300 to 600 lb (136 to 272 kg). Exceeding the weight limit can cause inaccurate indexing, damage to the table motor, and even possible breakage of the tabletop, which could cause serious injury to the patient.

Accessory devices can be attached to the table for a variety of uses. A special device called a *cradle* is used for head CT examinations. The head cradle helps to hold the head still; because the device extends beyond the tabletop, it minimizes artifacts or attenuation from the table while the brain is being scanned. It can also be used in positioning the patient for direct coronal images.

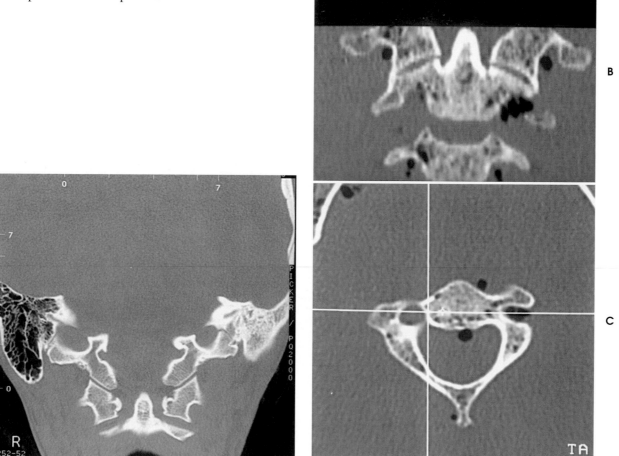

Fig. 33-11 A, Direct coronal image of C1 to C2. **B,** Computed-reconstructed images of C1 to C2. **C,** Axial image for coronal reconstruction.

(Courtesy Siemens Medical Systems, Iselin, N.J.)

OPERATOR'S CONSOLE

The *operator's console* (Fig. 33-12) is the point from which the technologist controls the scanner. A typical console is equipped with a keyboard for entering patient data and a graphic monitor for viewing the images. Other input devices, such as a touch display screen and a computer mouse, may also be used. The operator's console allows the technologist to control and monitor numerous scan parameters. Radiographic technique factors, slice thickness, table index, and reconstruction algorithm are some of the scan parameters that are selected at the operator's console.

Before starting an examination, the technologist must enter the patient information. Therefore a keyboard is still necessary for some functions. Usually the first scan program selected is the scout program from which the radiographer plans the sequence of axial scans. An example of a typical scout image is seen in Fig. 33-3. The operator's console is also the location of the CRT, where image manipulation takes place. Most scanners display the image on the CRT in a 1024 matrix interpolated by the computer from the 512 reconstructed image.

OTHER COMPONENTS
Display monitor

For the CT image to be displayed on a CRT monitor in a recognizable form, the digital CT data must be converted into a *gray-scale image*. This process is achieved by the conversion of each digital CT number in the matrix to an analog voltage. The brightness values of the gray-scale image correspond to the pixels and CT numbers of the digital data they represent.

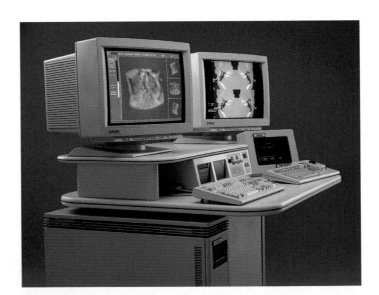

Fig. 33-12 Console with display monitors, keyboards, and workstation for three-dimensional image manipulation.

(Courtesy Picker International, Inc., Highland Heights, Ohio.)

Because of the digital nature of the CT image data, image manipulation can be performed to enhance the appearance of the image. One of the most common image processing techniques is called *windowing,* or *gray-level mapping.* This technique allows the technologist to alter the contrast of the displayed image by adjusting the window width and window level. The *window width* is the range of CT numbers that are used to map signals into shades of gray. Basically, the window width determines the number of gray levels to be displayed in the image. A narrow window width means that there are fewer shades of gray, resulting in higher contrast. Likewise, a wide window width results in more shades of gray in the image, or a longer gray scale. The *window level* determines the midpoint of the range of gray levels to be displayed on the monitor. It is used to set the center CT number within the range of gray levels being used to display the image. The window level should be set to the CT number of the tissue of interest, and the window width should be set with a range of values that will optimize the contrast between the tissues in the image. Fig. 33-13 shows an axial image seen in two different windows: a standard abdomen window and a bone window adjusted for the spine.

The gray level of any image can be adjusted on the CRT to compensate for differences in patient size and tissue densities or to display the image as desired for the examination protocol. Examples of typical window width and level settings are listed in Table 33-2. These settings are averages and usually vary by machine. It is important to note that the level, although an average, is approximately the same as the CT numbers expected for the tissue densities.

TABLE 33-2

Typical window settings

CT examination	Width	Center (level)
Brain	190	50
Skull	3500	500
Orbits	1200	50
Abdomen	400	35
Liver	175	45
Mediastinum	325	50
Lung	2000	-500
Spinal cord	400	50
Spine	2200	400

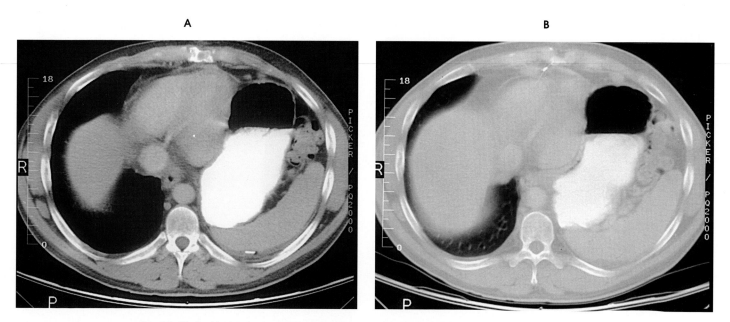

Fig. 33-13 A, Abdominal image, soft tissue window. **B,** Abdominal image: bone window.

System components

Multiplanar reconstruction

Another advantage of the digital nature of the CT image is the ability to reconstruct the axial images into coronal, sagittal, or oblique body planes without additional radiation to the patient. Image reconstruction in a variety of planes is accomplished by stacking multiple contiguous axial images, creating a volume of data. Because the CT numbers of the image data within the volume are already known, a sectional image can be generated in any desired plane by selecting a particular plane of data. This postprocessing technique is termed *multiplanar reconstruction (MPR)*. A sagittal reconstruction of data obtained from axial images is shown in Fig. 33-14, *A*. A coronal reconstruction is seen in Fig. 33-14, *B*.

One of the most important functions of the operator's console is to produce hard copies of axial images in the form of film. The most commonly used filming devices are the matrix camera and the laser printer docked directly to a processor (Fig. 33-15). The matrix camera once was the standard imaging device used in CT. Now the laser printer is the preferred device for imaging, and it should be docked directly to a processor whenever possible.

Diagnostic Applications

CT originally was used primarily for diagnosing neurologic disorders. As scanner technology advanced, the range of applications was extended to other areas of the body. The most commonly requested procedures involve the head, chest, and abdomen. CT is the examination of choice for head trauma; it clearly demonstrates skull fractures and associated subdural hematomas. CT imaging of the central nervous system can demonstrate infarctions, hemorrhage, disk herniations, craniofacial and spinal fractures, and tumors and other cancers. CT imaging of the body excels at demonstrating soft tissue structures within the chest, abdomen, and pelvis. Among the abnormalities demonstrated in this region are metastatic lesions, aneurysms, abscesses, and fluid collections from blunt trauma.

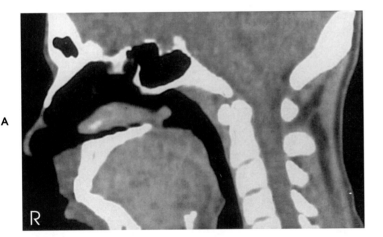

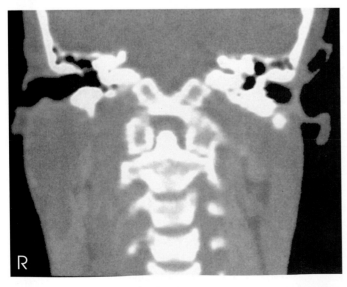

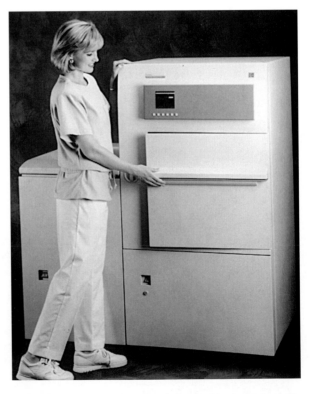

Fig. 33-14 A, Computer-reconstructed sagittal image. **B,** Computer-reconstructed coronal image.

(Courtesy Siemens Medical Systems.)

Fig. 33-15 Laser printer direct-docked to an automatic processor.

(Courtesy Eastman Kodak Company, Rochester, New York.)

CT is also used for numerous interventional procedures such as abscess drainage, tissue biopsy, and cyst aspiration. Fig. 33-16 demonstrates a number of structures and pathologic conditions identified by CT.

For any procedure a protocol is required to maximize the amount of diagnostic information available. Specific examination protocols vary according to the needs of different medical facilities and physicians.

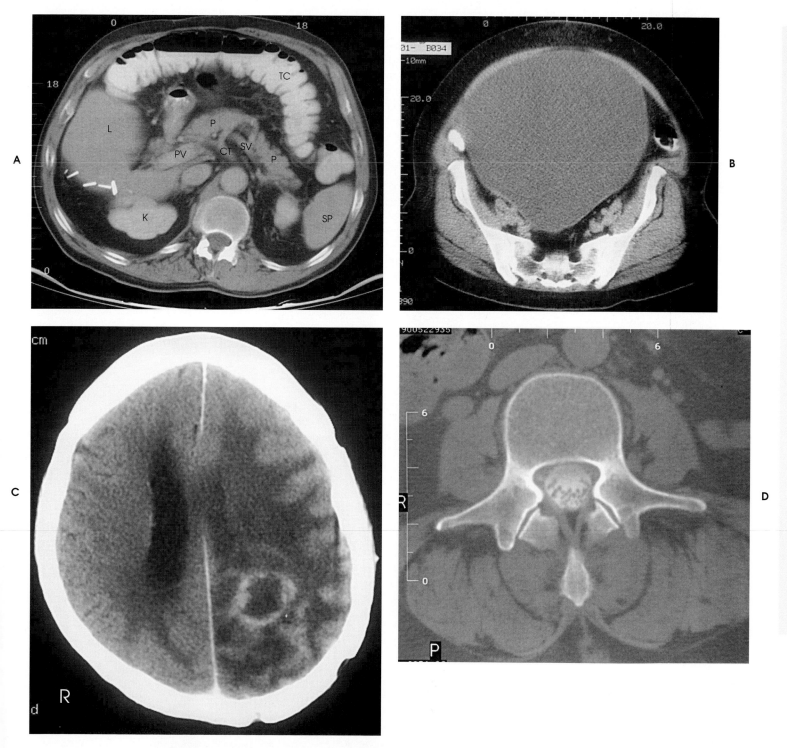

Fig. 33-16 A, Abdominal image demonstrating transverse colon *(TC)* with air-fluid levels; the liver *(L)*, pancreas *(P)*, spleen *(SP)*, kidney *(K)*, portal vein *(PV)*, celiac trunk *(CT)*, and splenic veins *(SV)* are demonstrated with contrast medium. Surgical clips are seen in posterior liver. **B,** Abdominal image demonstrating extremely large ovarian cyst. **C,** Brain image demonstrating parietooccipital mass with characteristic IV contrast ring enhancement. **D,** Image of L3 postmyelogram demonstrating contrast in thecal sac.

Contrast Media

Contrast media is used in CT examinations to help distinguish normal anatomy from pathology and to make various disease processes more visible. Contrast can be administered intravenously, orally, or rectally. Generally, the IV contrast media are the same as those used for excretory urograms. Many facilities use nonionic contrast material for these studies, despite the relatively high cost, because of the low incidence of reaction and known safety factors associated with nonionic contrast. IV contrast media are useful for demonstrating tumors within the head; Fig. 33-17 shows a brain scan with and without contrast. The anterior lesion is evident in the unenhanced scan; in the enhanced scan, the tumor demonstrates characteristic ring enhancement typical of tumors seen in CT scans. IV contrast media is also used to visualize vascular structures in the body.

IV contrast should be used only with approval of the radiologist and after careful consideration of patient history. Many CT examinations can be performed without IV contrast if necessary; however, the amount of diagnostic information available can be limited.

Oral contrast media must be used for imaging the abdomen. When given orally, the contrast material in the gastrointestinal tract helps to differentiate between loops of bowel and other structures within the abdomen. An oral contrast medium is generally a 2% barium mixture. The low concentration prevents contrast artifacts but allows good visualization of the stomach and intestinal tract. An iodinated contrast material such as oral Hypaque can be used, but it must be mixed at low concentrations to prevent contrast artifacts. Rectal contrast is often requested as part of an abdominal or pelvic protocol. Usually mixed in the same concentration as the oral contrast, the rectal contrast material is useful for demonstrating the distal colon relative to the bladder and other structures of the pelvic cavity.

Factors Affecting Image Quality

In CT the technologist has access to numerous scan parameters that can have a dramatic effect on image quality. The four main factors contributing to image quality are spatial resolution, contrast resolution, noise, and artifacts.

SPATIAL RESOLUTION

Spatial resolution describes the amount of blurring in an image. The scan parameters that affect spatial resolution include focal spot size, slice thickness, display FOV, matrix, and reconstruction algorithm. The geometric factor that contributes significantly to spatial resolution is the detector aperture width. The spatial resolution in CT is not as good as in conventional radiography.

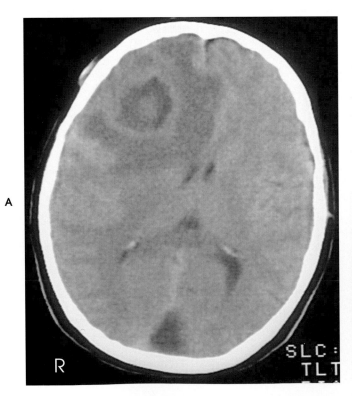
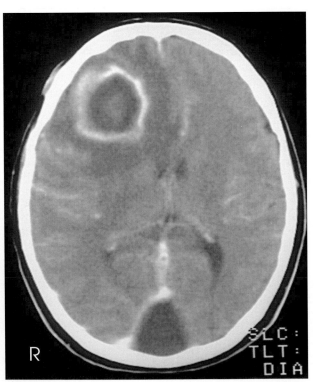

Fig. 33-17 A, Brain image without IV contrast. **B,** Brain image with IV contrast.

CONTRAST RESOLUTION

Contrast resolution is the ability to differentiate between small differences in density within the image. Currently, tissues with density differences of less than 0.5% can be distinguished with CT. The scan parameters that affect contrast resolution are slice thickness, reconstruction algorithm, image display, and x-ray beam energy. The size of the patient and the detector sensitivity also have a direct effect on contrast resolution.

NOISE

The most significant *noise* in CT is *quantum noise.* This type of noise arises from the random variation in photon detection. Noise in a CT image primarily affects contrast resolution. As noise increases in an image, contrast resolution decreases. Noise gives an image a grainy quality or a mottled appearance. Among the scan parameters that influence noise are matrix size, slice thickness, x-ray beam energy, and reconstruction algorithm. Scattered radiation and patient size also contribute to the noise of an image.

ARTIFACTS

Metallic objects, such as dental fillings, pacemakers, and artificial joints, can cause starburst or *streak artifacts,* which can obscure diagnostic information. Dense residual barium from fluoroscopy examinations can cause *artifacts* similar to those caused by metallic objects. Many CT departments do not perform a patient's CT examination until several days after barium studies to allow the body to eliminate the residual barium from the area of interest. Large differences in tissue densities of adjoining structures can cause artifacts that detract from image quality. Bone–soft-tissue interfaces, such as occur with the skull and brain, often cause streak or shadow artifacts on CT images; these artifacts are referred to as *beam hardening.*

OTHER FACTORS
Patient factors

Patient factors also contribute to the quality of an image. If a patient cannot or will not hold still, the scan will likely be non-diagnostic. Body size also can have an effect on image quality. Large patients attenuate more radiation than small patients; this can increase image noise, detracting from overall image quality. An increase in milliampere-seconds (mAs) is usually required to compensate for large body size. Unfortunately, this increase results in a higher radiation dose to the patient. Factors that the radiographer can control include slice thickness, *scan time, scan diameter,* and patient instructions. Slice thickness is usually dictated by image *protocol.* As in tomography, the thinner the slice thickness, the better the image-recorded detail. Thin-section CT scans, often referred to as *high-resolution scans,* are used to better demonstrate structures (Fig. 33-18).

As in conventional radiography, patient instructions are a critical part of a diagnostic examination. Explaining the procedure fully in terms the patient can understand will increase the level of compliance from almost any patient.

Scan times

Scan times are usually preselected by the computer as part of the scan program, but they can be altered by the technologist. When selecting a scan time, the technologist must take into account possible patient motion such as inadvertent body movements, breathing, or peristalsis. A good guideline is to choose a scan time that will minimize patient motion and at the same time provide a quality diagnostic image. When it is necessary to scan an uncooperative patient quickly, using the shortest scan time possible may allow the technologist to complete the examination although the quality of the images obtained will likely be somewhat compromised.

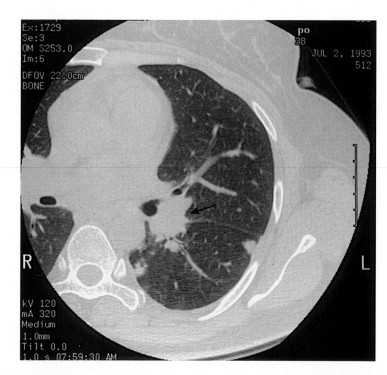

Fig. 33-18 High-resolution 1-mm slice using edge enhancement algorithm, demonstrating nodule in left lung.

Scan diameter

The image that appears on the CRT depends on the *scan diameter.* The technologist can adjust the scan diameter to include the entire cross section of the body part being scanned or to include only a specified region within the part. The anatomy demonstrated is often referred to as the FOV. Like scan time, scan diameter is usually preselected by the computer as part of a scan program, but it can also be adjusted as necessary by the technologist. For most head, chest, and abdomen examinations the selected scan diameter includes all anatomy of the body part to just outside the skin borders. Certain examinations may require the scan diameter to be reduced to include specific anatomy such as the sella turcica, sinuses, one lung, mediastinal vessels, suprarenal glands, one kidney, or the prostate. Decreasing the scan diameter is a way for the operator to magnify an image using scan data; however, as with any image magnification, some loss of resolution occurs.

Special Features
DYNAMIC SCANNING

One of the advantages of CT is that data can be obtained for image reconstruction by the computer. The scanner can be programmed to scan through an area rapidly. In this situation raw data are saved, but image reconstruction after each scan is bypassed to shorten scan time.

Dynamic scanning is based on the principle that after contrast administration, different structures enhance at different rates. Dynamic scanning can consist of rapid sequential scanning at the same level to observe contrast filling within a structure, such as is performed when looking for an aortic aneurysm. Another form of dynamic scanning is incremental dynamic scanning, which consists of rapid serial scanning at consecutive levels during the bolus injection of a contrast medium. This is the preferred method to image the liver. Fig. 33-19 demonstrates the flow of contrast material through the major vessels of the mediastinum.

SPIRAL/HELICAL CT

Spiral CT or *helical CT* are terms used to describe the newest method of data acquisition in CT. During spiral CT, the gantry is rotating continuously while the table moves through the gantry aperture at the same time. The continuous gantry rotation combined with the continuous table movement forms the spiral path from which raw data are obtained. Slip-ring technology has made continuous rotation of the x-ray tube possible by eliminating the cables between the gantry and the generators.

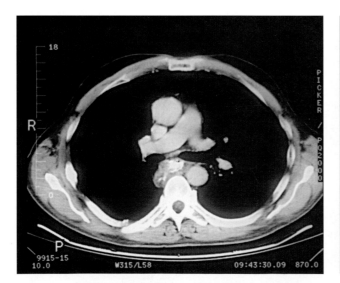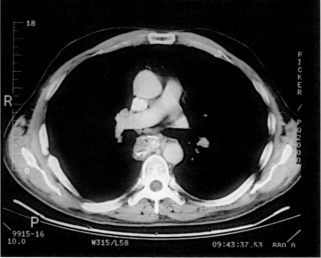

Fig. 33-19 Consecutive dynamic images demonstrating great vessels of mediastinum after bolus injection of 100 ml of IV contrast medium.

One of the unique features of spiral CT is that it scans a volume of tissue rather than a group of individual slices. This method makes it extremely useful for the detection of small lesions because an arbitrary slice can be reconstructed along any position within the volume of raw data. In addition, because a volume of tissue is scanned in a single breath, respiratory motion can be minimized. For a volume scan of the chest such as that shown in Fig. 33-20, the patient was instructed to hold the breath; a tissue volume of 24 mm was then obtained in a 5-second spiral scan.

Two of the resultant images demonstrate a small lung nodule without breathing interference of *image misregistration;* a three-dimensional reconstruction of the lung clearly shows the pathologic condition. Spiral CT is also used to scan noncooperative or combative patients, patients who cannot tolerate lying down for long periods of time, and patients who will not hold still, such as pediatric patients or trauma patients. In some patients, the use of spiral CT decreases the amount of contrast medium necessary to visualize structures; this makes the examination both safer and more cost-effective.

CT ANGIOGRAPHY

CT angiography (CTA) is a relatively new application of spiral CT using three-dimensional imaging techniques. With CTA the vascular system can be viewed in three dimensions. The three basic steps required to generate CTA images are as follows:

1. Design of parameters for IV administration of the *bolus* of contrast medium. (i.e., injection rate, injection duration, and delay between bolus initiation and the start of the scan sequence)
2. Choice of spiral parameters to maximize the contrast in the target vessel (i.e., *scan duration,* collimation, and *table speed)*
3. Reconstruction of two-dimensional image data into three-dimensional image data

Special features

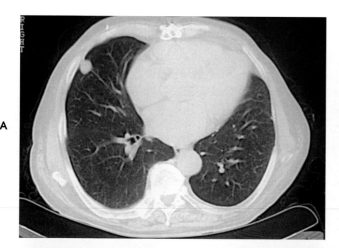

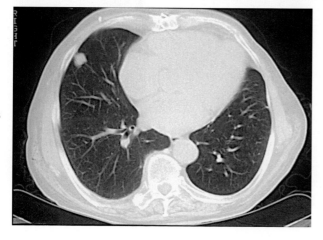

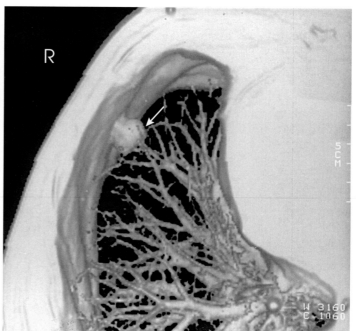

Fig. 33-20 A and **B,** Spiral images of lung demonstrating lung nodule and associated vasculature. **C,** three-dimensional reconstruction of lung nodule *(arrow)* after spiral scan.

(Courtesy Siemens Medical Systems, Iselin, N.J.)

CTA has several advantages over conventional angiography. CTA uses spiral technology; therefore an arbitrary image within the volume of data can be retrospectively reconstructed without exposing the patient to additional IV contrast medium or radiation. Furthermore, during postprocessing of the image data, overlying structures can be eliminated so that only the vascular anatomy is reconstructed. Finally, because CTA is an IV procedure that does not require arterial puncture, only minimal postprocedure observation is necessary.

Currently CTA is not designed to replace angiography as a diagnostic mode; rather, it is a complementary examination that allows image reconstructions of different body planes without further radiation to the patient. Fig. 33-21 demonstrates the vessels of the brain, whereas Fig. 33-22 highlights the great vessels of the heart in a three-dimensional format.

THREE-DIMENSIONAL IMAGING

A rapidly expanding area of CT is three-dimensional imaging. This is a *postprocessing technique* that is applied to the raw data to create realistic images of the surface anatomy to be visualized.

The introduction of advanced computers and faster software programs has dramatically increased the applications of three-dimensional imaging. Two basic techniques are used in creating three-dimensional images: *maximum intensity projection (MIP)* and *shaded surface display (SSD),* which uses segmentation. Both techniques use three initial steps to create the three-dimensional images from the original CT data.

1. Construction of a volume of three-dimensional data from the original two-dimensional CT image data. This same process is used in MPR.
2. *Segmentation* to crop or edit the target objects from the reconstructed data. This step eliminates unwanted information from the CT data.
3. *Rendering* or *shading* to provide depth perception to the final image.

Maximum intensity projection

The MIP technique consists of reconstructing the brightest pixels from a stack of two- or three-dimensional image data into a three-dimensional image. The data are rotated on an arbitrary axis, and an imaginary ray is passed through the data in specific increments. The brightest pixel found along each ray is then *mapped* into a gray-scale image. The MIP technique is commonly used for CTA.

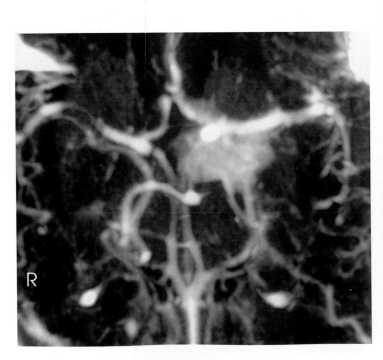

Fig. 33-21 CTA of vessels of the brain.

(Courtesy Picker International, Cleveland, Ohio.)

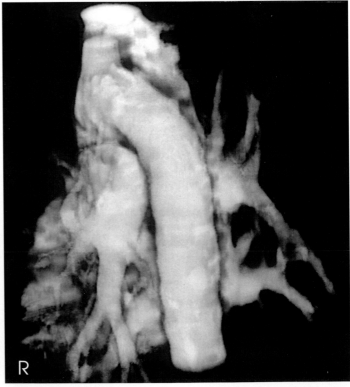

Fig. 33-22 Great vessels of the heart in three-dimensional format.

(Courtesy Picker International, Cleveland.)

Shaded surface display

An SSD image provides a three-dimensional image of a particular structure's surface. Once the original two-dimensional data are reconstructed into three-dimensional information, the different tissue types within the image need to be separated. This process, called segmentation, can be performed by drawing a line around the tissue of interest or more commonly by setting *threshold values*. A threshold value can be set for a particular CT number; the result is that any pixel having an equal or higher CT number than the threshold value will be selected for the three-dimensional image. Once the threshold value is set and the data are reconstructed into a three-dimensional image, a shading technique is applied. The shading or rendering technique provides depth perception in the reconstructed image.

Referring physicians and surgeons use three-dimensional images to clinically correlate CT images to the actual anatomic contours of their patients. These reconstructions are especially useful in surgical procedures. Three-dimensional reconstructions are often requested as part of patient evaluation after trauma and for presurgical planning. Fig. 33-23 shows various anatomic structures in three-dimensional reconstruction.

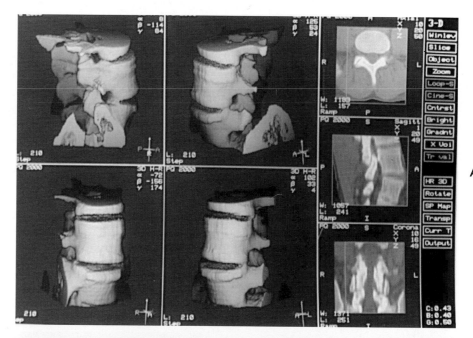

A

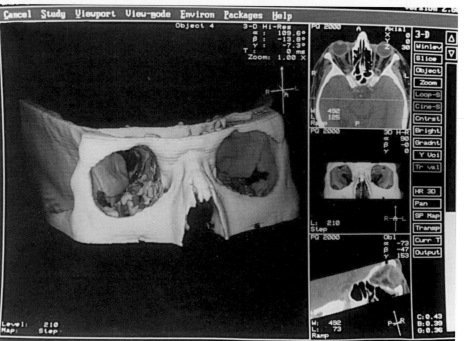

B

Fig. 33-23 Three-dimensional images. **A,** Lumbar spine. **B,** Bony orbits.

(Courtesy Picker International, Cleveland.)

RADIATION TREATMENT PLANNING

Radiation therapy has been used for nearly as long as radiology has been in existence. The introduction of CT has had a major impact on radiation treatment planning. The use of spiral CT in conjunction with MPR provides a three-dimensional approach to radiation treatment planning. This method helps the dosimetrist to plan treatment so that the radiation dose to the target is maximized and the dose to normal tissue is minimized. New three-dimensional simulation software offers the following: volumetric, high-precision localization; calculation of the geometric center of the defined target; patient marking systems; and virtual simulators capable of producing digitally reconstructed radiographs in *real time*. With the new, specially designed software, a single CT simulation procedure can replace a total of three procedures (one conventional CT and two conventional simulations) for radiation treatment planning.

If the CT system is being used for radiation treatment planning, the standard curved couch should not be used. Instead, a flat board should be placed on the couch. In this way the actual therapy delivery can be simulated more accurately. Fig. 33-24 demonstrates the external skin markers and structures that will be in the beam's path.

QUALITY CONTROL

The goal of any quality assurance program in CT is to ensure that the system is producing the best possible image quality with the minimum radiation dose to the patient. A CT system is a complex combination of sensitive and expensive equipment that requires systematic monitoring for performance and image quality. Most CT systems require weekly or biweekly preventative maintenance to assure proper operation.

Preventative maintenance is usually performed by a service engineer from the manufacturer or a private company. Increasingly, however, the technologist is being assigned the responsibility of performing and documenting routine quality assurance tests. Many technologists routinely perform daily test scans on a water phantom to measure the consistency of the CT numbers and to record the standard deviation. As data are recorded over time, the CT scanner's current operating condition, as well as its performance over longer time periods, can be evaluated. Many units are also capable of *air calibrations*, which do not require the water phantom and can be performed between patients for unit self-calibration.

A CT phantom is typically multisectioned and is constructed from plastic cylinders, with each section filled with test objects designed to measure the performance of specific parameters. Some phantoms are designed to allow numerous parameters to be evaluated with a single scan. The recommended quality assurance tests for evaluating routine performance include the following: contrast scale and mean CT number of water, high-contrast resolution, low-contrast resolution, laser light accuracy, noise and uniformity, slice thickness, and patient dose.

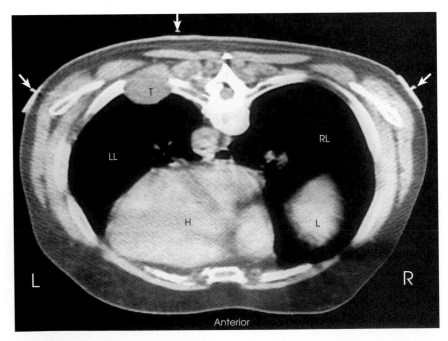

Fig. 33-24 Patient in prone position for radiation treatment planning. Radiopaque markers *(arrows)* demonstrate location of treatment field skin marks: tumor *(T)*, heart *(H)*, liver *(L)*, right lung *(RL)*, and left lung *(LL)*.

Comparison of Computed Tomography and Magnetic Resonance Imaging

As CT was developing and advancing into a significant diagnostic modality, magnetic resonance imaging (MRI) was also progressing. Like CT, MRI was first used to image the brain; whole-body scans were developed shortly afterward. As MRI advanced and the quality of the images improved, it became apparent that MRI images exhibited better low-contrast resolution than CT images. Brain soft tissue detail is not demonstrated as well with CT as with MRI performed at approximately the same level (Fig. 33-25).

The initial introduction of MRI raised concerns that CT scanners would become obsolete. However, each modality has been found to have unique capabilities. Thus CT and MRI are useful for different clinical applications. As previously mentioned, CT does not demonstrate soft tissue as well as MRI; however, CT demonstrates bony structures better than MRI.

Patients often have ferrous metal within their bodies. Such patients cannot be scanned by MRI. CT is one option for these patients. The CT scanner does not affect metal in a patient, but metal can cause artifacts on CT images when the metal lies within the scan plane.

Many patients (especially pediatric and trauma patients) are extremely claustrophobic, combative, or uncooperative. CT is useful for scanning these patients quickly and easily, because of the small gantry, relatively large aperture, and short scan times.

Because equipment costs are lower and a greater number of procedures can be accomplished per day, CT can often be a less costly examination than MRI. Physicians have found that CT and MRI can be complementary examinations. In many situations, both examinations are ordered to provide as much diagnostic information as possible.

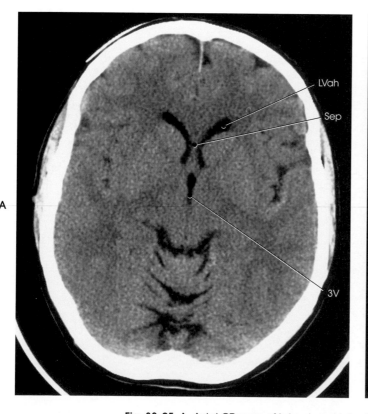
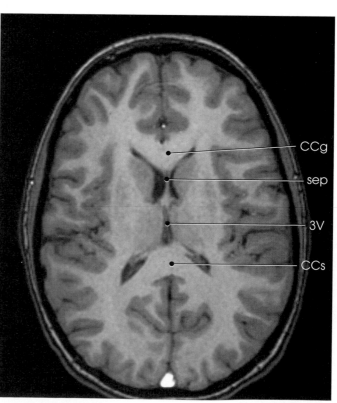

Fig. 33-25 A, Axial CT scan of lateral ventricles (LVah). **B,** Axial MR scan of corpus callosum.

(From Kelly LL, Peterson CM: *Sectional anatomy for imaging professionals,* St Louis, 1997, Mosby.)

The Future

In the last 5 years, CT has significantly increased its diagnostic capabilities. The development of spiral CT was central to the advancement of CT as a discipline. With the rapid advancements in technology, the CT technologist has an increased responsibility to understand contrast dynamics and the new spiral scan parameters of pitch, collimation, scan timing, and table speed.

Advances in computing power and design have provided workstations that can generate three-dimensional models in 30 seconds or less, rotate the models along any axis, and display the models with varying parameters. Digital subtraction CT, multimodality image superimposition, and translucent shading of soft tissue structures are some of the new applications coming from technologic advancements. In the near future, CT will provide image data sets that will allow physicians to manipulate the anatomy on virtual reality and other graphics platforms. As the higher quality images increase the accuracy of diagnosis and treatment, patient care will be improved. Because of CT's superb diagnostic information and cost-effectiveness, this imaging modality will continue to be a highly respected diagnostic tool.

Definition of Terms

air calibration Scan of air in gantry; based on a known value of −1000 for air, the scanner will calibrate itself according to this density value relative to the actual density value measured.

algorithm Mathematic formula designed for computers to carry out complex calculations required for image reconstruction; designed for enhancement of soft tissue, bone, and edge resolution.

aperture Opening of the gantry through which patient passes during scan.

archiving Storage of CT images on long-term storage device such as cassette tape, magnetic tape, or optical disk.

artifact Distortion or error in image that is unrelated to subject being studied.

attenuation coefficient CT number assigned to measured remnant radiation intensity after attenuation by tissue density.

axial Describes plane of image as presented by CT scan; same as *transverse.*

bolus Preset amount of radiopaque contrast medium injected rapidly per IV administration to visualize high-flow vascular structures, usually in conjunction with dynamic scan; most often injected using a pressure injector.

cathode ray tube (CRT) Electronic monitor used for image display or scan protocol display; resolution of a CRT depends on lines per inch; the greater the lines per inch, the better the resolution.

computed tomography (CT) Process by which computer-reconstructed transverse (or axial) image of a patient is created by an x-ray tube and detector assembly rotating 360 degrees about a specified area of the body; also called *CAT (computed axial tomography) scan.*

CT angiography Use of volumetric CT scanning with spiral technique to acquire image data that are reconstructed into three-dimensional CT angiograms.

CT number Arbitrary number assigned by computer to indicate relative density of a given tissue; CT number varies proportionately with tissue density; high CT numbers indicate dense tissue, and low CT numbers indicate less dense tissue. All CT numbers are based on the density of water, which is assigned a CT number of 0; also referred to as a *Hounsfield unit.*

contrast resolution Ability of a CT scanner to demonstrate different tissue densities.

data acquisition system (DAS) Part of detector assembly that converts analog signals to digital signals that can be used by the CT computer.

detector Electronic component used for radiation detection; made of either high-density photoreactive crystals or pressurized stable gases.

detector assembly Electronic component of CT scanner that measures remnant radiation exiting the patient, converting the radiation to an analog signal proportionate to the radiation intensity measured.

direct coronal Describes the position used to obtain images in coronal plane; used for head scans to provide images at right angles to axial images; patient is positioned prone for direct coronal images and supine for reverse coronal images.

dynamic scanning Process by which raw data are obtained by continuous scanning; images are not reconstructed but are saved for later reconstruction; most often used for visualization of high-flow vascular structures; can be used to scan a noncooperative patient rapidly.

field of view (FOV) Area of anatomy displayed by the CRT; can be adjusted to include entire body section or a specific part of the patient anatomy being scanned.

gantry Part of CT scanner that houses x-ray tube, cooling system, detector assembly, and DAS; often referred to as the "doughnut" by patients.

generation Description of significant levels of technologic development of CT scanners; specifically related to tube/detector movement.

gray-scale image Analog image whereby each pixel in the image corresponds to a particular shade of gray.

helical CT Relatively new data acquisition method that combines continuous gantry rotation with continuous table movement to form a helical path of scan data; also called *spiral CT.*

high-resolution scans Use of scanning parameters that enhance contrast resolution of an image, such as thin slices, high matrices, high-spatial frequency algorithms, and small-display FOV.

host computer Primary link between system operator and other components of imaging system.

Hounsfield unit (HU) Number used to describe average density of tissue; term is used interchangeably with *CT number;* named in honor of Godfrey Hounsfield, the man generally given credit for development of the first clinically viable CT scanner.

image misregistration Image distortion caused by combination of table indexing and respiration; table moves in specified increments, but patient movement during respiration may cause anatomy to be scanned more than once or not at all.

index Table movement; also referred to as *table increments.*

mapping Assignment of appropriate gray level to each pixel in an image.

matrix Mathematical formula for calculation made up of individual cells for number assignment; CT matrix stores a CT number relative to the tissue density at that location; each cell or "address" stores one CT number for image reconstruction.

maximum intensity projection (MIP) Reconstruction of brightest pixels from stack of image data into a three-dimensional image.

multiplanar reconstruction (MPR) Postprocessing technique applied to stacks of axial image data that can then be reconstructed into other orientations or imaging planes.

noise Random variation of CT numbers about some mean value within a uniform object; noise produces a grainy appearance in the image.

partial volume averaging Calculated linear attenuation coefficient for a pixel that is a weighted average of all densities in the pixel; the assigned CT number and ultimately the pixel appearance are affected by the average of the different densities measured within that pixel.

pixel (*picture element*) One individual cell surface within an image matrix used for CRT image display.

postprocessing techniques Specialized reconstruction techniques that are applied to CT images to display the anatomic structures from different perspectives.

primary data CT number assigned to the matrix by the computer; the information required to reconstruct an image.

protocol Instructions for CT examination specifying slice thickness, table increments, contrast administration, scan diameter, and any other requirements specified by the radiologist.

quantum noise Any noise in the image that is a result of random variation in the number of x-ray photons detected.

real time Ability to process or reconstruct incoming data in a matter of milliseconds.

reconstruction Process of creating a digital image from raw data.

region of interest (ROI) Measurement of CT numbers within a specified area for evaluation of average tissue density.

rendering Process of changing the shading of a three-dimensional image; commonly used to increase depth perception of an image.

retrieval Reconstruction of images stored on long-term device; can be done for extra film copies or when films are lost.

scan Actual rotation of x-ray tube about the patient; used as a generic reference to one slice or an entire examination.

scan diameter Also referred to as the *zoom* or *focal plane* of a CT scan; predetermined by the radiographer to include the anatomic area of interest; determines FOV.

scan duration Amount of time used to scan an entire volume during a single spiral scan.

scan time X-ray exposure time in seconds.

segmentation Method of cropping or editing target objects from image data.

shaded surface display (SSD) Process used to generate three-dimensional images that show the surface of a three-dimensional object.

shading Postprocessing technique used in three-dimensional reconstructions to separate tissues of interest by applying a threshold value to isolate the structure of interest.

slice One scan through a selected body part; also referred to as a *cut;* slice thickness can vary from 1 mm to 1 cm, depending on the examination.

slip ring Low-voltage electrical contacts within the gantry designed to allow continuous rotation of an x-ray tube without the use of cables connecting internal and external components.

spatial resolution Ability of a CT scanner to demonstrate small objects within the body plane being scanned.

spiral CT Relatively new data acquisition method that combines a continuous gantry rotation with a continuous table movement to form a spiral path of scan data; also called *helical CT.*

streak artifact Artifact created by high-density objects that result in an arc of straight lines projecting across the *FOV* from a common point.

system noise Inherent property of a CT scanner; the difference between the measured CT number of a given tissue and the known value for that tissue; most often evaluated through the use of water phantom scans.

table increments Specific amount of table travel between scans; can be varied to move at any specified increment; most protocols specify from 1 mm to 20 cm, depending on type of examination; also referred to as *indexing.*

table speed Longitudinal distance traveled by the table during one revolution of the x-ray tube.

threshold value CT number used in defining the corresponding anatomy that will comprise a three-dimensional object; any pixels within a three-dimensional volume having the threshold value (CT number) or higher will be selected for the three-dimensional model.

useful patient dose Radiation dose received by the patient that is actually detected and converted into an image.

voxel (*volume element*) Individual pixel with the associated volume of tissue based on the slice thickness.

window Arbitrary numbers used for image display based on various shades of gray; window width controls the overall gray level and affects image contrast; window level (center) controls subtle gray images within a certain width range and ultimately affects the brightness and overall density of an image.

Selected bibliography

Adachi H, Nagai J: *Three-dimensional CT angiography,* Boston, 1995, Little, Brown.

Alexander J et al: *Computed tomography,* Berlin, 1986, Siemens Aktiengesellschaft.

Berland L: *Practical CT: technology and techniques,* New York, 1987, Raven Press.

Bentel GC et al: *Treatment planning and dose calculation in radiation oncology,* Oxford, 1988, Pergamon.

Boethius J et al: CT localization in stereotaxic surgery, *Appl Neurophysiol* 43:164,1980.

Boethius J et al: Stereotaxic computerized tomography with a GE 8800 scanner, *J Neurosurg* 52:794, 1980.

Bushberg et al: *The essential physics of medical imaging,* Baltimore, 1994, Williams & Wilkins.

Bushong: *Radiologic science of technologists: physics, biology, and protection,* ed 16, St Louis, 1997, Mosby.

Chiu LC, Lipcamon JD, Yiu-Chiu VS: *Clinical computed tomography: illustrated procedural guide,* Rockville, Md, 1986, Aspen.

Coulam CM et al, editors: *The physical basis of medical imaging,* New York, 1981, Appleton-Century-Crofts.

Curry TS et al: *Christensen's introduction to the physics of diagnostic radiology,* ed 3, Philadelphia, 1984, Lea & Febiger.

Federle FP et al: *Computed tomography in the evaluation of trauma,* Baltimore, 1982, Williams & Wilkins.

Fishman, Jeffrey RB: *Spiral CT: principles, techniques, and clinical applications,* New York, 1995, Raven Press.

Genant HK, editor: *Computer tomography of the lumbar spine,* San Francisco, 1982, University of California.

Godwin JD, editor: *Computed tomography of the chest,* Philadelphia, 1984, Lippincott.

Haaga JR et al: *Computed tomography of the whole body,* ed 2, vols I and II, St Louis, 1988, Mosby.

Hammerschlag SB et al: *Computed tomography of the eye and orbit,* Norwalk, Conn, 1983, Appleton-Century-Crofts.

Haughton V: *Computed tomography of the spine,* St Louis, 1982, Mosby.

Hendee WR: *The physical principles of computed tomography,* Boston, 1983, Little, Brown.

Kubota K et al: Some devices for computer tomography radiotherapy treatment planning, *J Comput Assist Tomogr* 4:697,1980.

Lee JKT, Sagel SS, Stanley RJ, editors: *Computed body tomography with MRI correlation,* ed 2, New York, 1989, Raven Press.

Lee SH, Rao Krishna CVG, editors: *Cranial computed tomography and MRI,* ed 2, New York, 1987, McGraw-Hill.

Mancuso AA et al: *Computed tomography and magnetic resonance of the head and neck,* ed 2, Baltimore, 1985, Williams & Wilkins.

Marshall, C: *The physical basis of computed tomography,* St Louis, 1982, Warren H. Green. Morgan C: *Basic principles of computed tomography,* Baltimore, 1983, University Park Press.

Moss AA et al: *Computed tomography of the body,* Philadelphia, 1983, WB Saunders.

Naidich DP et al: *Computed tomography of the thorax,* New York, 1984, Raven Press.

Naidich TP et al: Superimposition reformatted CT for preoperative lesion localization and surgical planning, *J Comput Assist Tomogr* 4:693,1980.

Newton TH et al, editors: *Radiology of the skull and brain,* vol 5. *Technical aspects of computed tomography,* St Louis, 1981, Mosby.

Newton TH et al, editors: *Modern neuroradiology,* vol 1. *Computed tomography of the spine and spinal cord,* San Anselmo, Calif, 1983, Clavadel Press.

Post MJD, editor: *Radiographic evaluation of the spine,* New York, 1980, Masson.

Seeram E: *Computed tomography: physical principles, clinical applications, and quality control,* Philadelphia, 1994, WB Saunders.

Sprawls P: *Physical principles of medical imaging,* Rockville, Md, 1987, Aspen.

Stevens JM, Valentine AR, Kendall BE: *Computed cranial and spinal imaging: a practical introduction,* Baltimore, 1988, Williams & Wilkins.

Van Maes PFGM et al: Direct coronal body computed tomography, *J Comput Assist Tomogr* 62:58,1982.

Wegener O: *Whole body computed tomography,* ed 2, Malden, Mass, 1992, Blackwell.

Zeman R et al.: *Helical/spiral CT: a practical approach,* New York, 1995, McGraw-Hill.

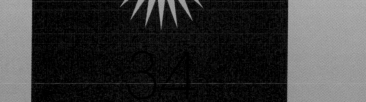

COMPUTED RADIOGRAPHY

REX E. PROFIT

RIGHT: Early attempts to enhance image viewing included the use of stereoscopic, or three-dimensional viewing, such as that provided by this approximate vintage 1920 viewing device. Radiographs were placed on two illuminators. Then each eye viewed a separate image with the intent of creating a three-dimensional mental image.

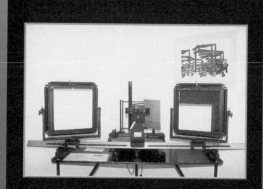

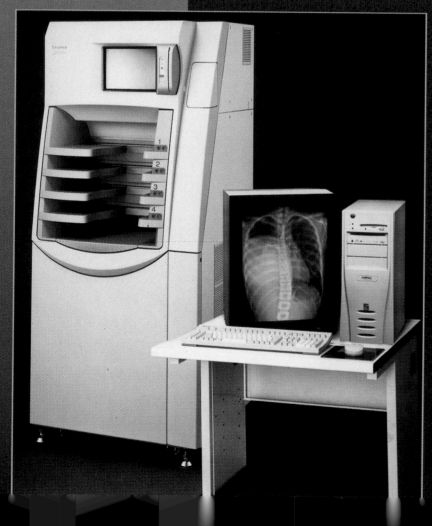

LEFT: The future is digital imaging. Computed radiography systems such as this FCR 5000 reader and workstation acquire and display images in 2K or 4K data sets in less than 30 seconds. Digital imaging provides consistent quality, allows rapid image transmission to multiple sites simultaneously, and gives the user the ability to manipulate the images.

(Courtesy Fuji Medical Systems, USA)

Principles of Computed Radiography

Since the days of Wilhelm Conrad Roentgen, radiography has been continuously improved and diversified. Even in the 1990s the fluorescent x-ray film-screen combination remains the most widely used radiographic method. However, conventional film-screen radiography limits image manipulation to "hot-lighting" or duplication. More recent modalities, such as computed tomography (CT), ultrasonography, and magnetic resonance imaging (MRI), are *digital**; they provide cross-sectional images and allow the image to be manipulated. Conventional projection radiography, which accounts for nearly 70% of a radiology department's volume, remained an *analog* modality until the past decade.

Various methods for enhancing the diagnostic capability of x-ray images have been used over the years. In stereoscopic radiography, for example, two images of the same anatomic structure are obtained, with the x-ray tube shifted 6 degrees for the second image. The two x-ray images are then placed side by side on an illuminator and viewed using a stereoscope. This three-dimensional viewing helps the radiologist to some degree, but the process is operationally cumbersome. An old stereoscopic viewer appears on p. 307.

---

*Almost all italicized terms are defined at the end of this chapter.

ANALOG AND DIGITAL INFORMATION

Analog information is represented in a continuous fashion, whereas digital information is represented in discrete units. An analogy is the difference between oil paints and a box of crayons. The oil paints can be mixed to provide an infinite number of color shades, whereas the box of crayons can provide only the number of colors in the box. The advantage of digital information is that the location and nature of each digital level are known and can be adjusted accordingly. In all digital imaging systems, including CT, MRI, ultrasonography, and computed radiography, information is acquired by a process called *analog-to-digital conversion*. After the x-ray or ultrasound beam has passed through the patient, or is reflected back within the patient for ultrasound, it is still an analog signal. This signal varies smoothly from zero (all the radiation has been absorbed by some part of the patient) to maximum intensity (no radiation has been absorbed).

In a CT scanner the analog-to-digital conversion occurs when the x-ray beam strikes the detector located in the gantry (see Chapter 33). Each detector corresponds to an anatomic location that absorbed the radiation, and the detectors have a limited number of responses. The number of responses the detectors can make is called the *gray-level display* of the system. If the system has 256 gray levels (0 being black, 256 being white), the computer assigns the gray level of these 256 shades that is closest to the intensity of the radiation striking the detector. The system then reproduces the image by combining the responses of all the detectors.

In a computed radiographic system, the analog-to-digital conversion occurs when the exposed image plate is scanned with a laser. At this point the emitted light pattern is converted to digital information by the image reader, as explained later in this chapter.

COMPUTED AND ANALOG RADIOGRAPHY

Computed radiography (often abbreviated *CR*) refers to conventional projection radiography in which the image is acquired in digital format using an imaging plate rather than film. Conventional projection radiography includes all of the radiographic procedures that are now performed using a film-screen system. These procedures include the familiar procedures that comprise the majority of radiographic examinations performed in an imaging facility: chest, abdomen, and orthopedic radiographs as well as contrast-enhanced radiographic studies such as excretory urography and barium studies of the gastrointestinal tract.

The major obstacle to developmental changes in the field of conventional projection radiography has been that one specific medium—x-ray film—serves three distinct functions in the radiographic process: (1) x-ray film is the "sensor" to acquire the diagnostic information; (2) it is used to display the information; and (3) it is used to store the information.

Historical Development

At the 1981 International Congress of Radiology meeting in Brussels, Fuji Photo Film Co., Ltd., introduced the concept of computed radiography employing *photostimulable phosphor* plate technology. In 1983 computed radiography was first used clinically in Japan, and by early 1998 more than 5000 systems were in clinical use worldwide.

Computed radiography using the phosphor plate provides excellent image quality. Computed radiographic technology is digital and supports the development of a variety of computer-based diagnostic information-processing systems. As such, computed radiography provides a missing link for the completely electronic radiographic imaging department and is now a practical imaging modality.

Converting conventional projection radiography into a digital format can be accomplished (1) by digitizing the standard radiographic film images or (2) by acquiring a digital image directly by having the x-rays strike an electronic sensor or an image intensifier or by using an imaging plate that is then scanned with a laser and the emitted light read by an electronic sensor. The second technique is currently the best option for computed radiography when a reusable imaging plate is used. In the remainder of this chapter, computed radiography refers to imaging performed using imaging plates.

Unlike scanned projection radiography or intensifier-based systems, which require that images be acquired on dedicated equipment, the reusable photostimulable phosphor plate system can be used with standard radiographic imaging equipment. The key to computed radiography's development is separation of the functions of sensing, displaying, and storing information. Each function uses separate media and devices, and each function can be separately manipulated; however, central control of the final image is maintained through computer technology.

Operational Components: Separation of Functions

IMAGE ACQUISITION FUNCTIONS

The image acquisition or "sensor" function is served by the photostimulable phosphor *imaging plate,* which, like x-ray film, receives the portion of the x-ray beam that has passed through the patient. This imaging plate looks much like an intensifying screen (Fig. 34-1) and is placed in a cassette similar in external appearance to an x-ray film cassette. The cassette consists of a frame of either lightweight aluminum or rigid steel, with the x-ray tube side composed of honeycombed carbon fiber to produce a low x-ray attenuation surface. The back of the cassette is lined with a thin layer of lead to absorb backscatter radiation. The primary function of the cassette is to protect the imaging plate, not to control light.

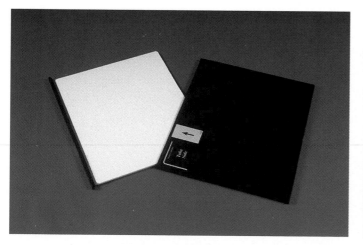 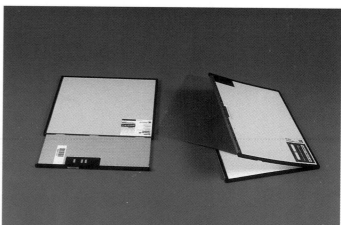

A   B

Fig. 34-1 A, Tube side of computed radiography cassette with imaging plate partially inserted. **B,** Back side of the CR cassette *(left)* and older film-screen cassette *(right).*

The imaging plate contains a layer of europium-doped barium fluorohalide (BaFX:Eu²⁺) crystals (the photostimulable phosphor). When x-rays strike the crystals, BaFX is changed to a new semistable state. The distribution of these semistable molecules forms the *latent image.* The BaFX:Eu²⁺ phosphor is applied to a polyester support base and then coated with a clear protective layer composed of fluorinated polymer material (Fig. 34-2). A supporting layer protects the phosphor layer from external shocks. The supporting layer also prevents reflection of the laser light. Next is a backing layer that protects the imaging plate from scratches during transfer and storage. Last is a bar code label that contains a number assigned to the imaging plate. This bar code provides a mechanism for associating each imaging plate with patient identification and related examination and positioning information.

The imaging plate is flexible and less than 1 mm thick. A unique property of the phosphor material is its "memory" capability: it can maintain a latent image for a certain period of time after exposure to x-rays. Although some image degradation occurs as time elapses, the plate retains a diagnostic image for at least 24 hours.

A valuable characteristic of the imaging plate is its extreme *dynamic range.* The imaging plate demonstrates an excellent linear response to the intensity of x-ray exposure over a broad range. When the imaging plate response is compared with the characteristic H&D curve of radiographic film (Fig. 34-3), the imaging plate shows superior performance capability in that it provides far more information in the low- and high-exposure regions of the image.

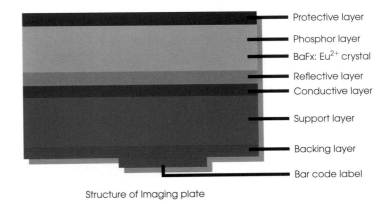

Structure of Imaging plate

Fig. 34-2 Schematic diagram showing layered composition of photostimulable imaging plate.

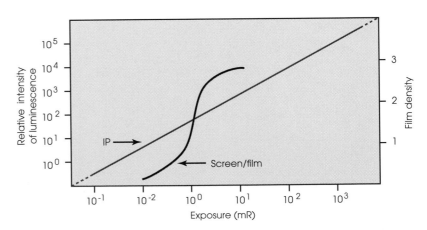

Fig. 34-3 Comparison of radiographic film H&D response curve to linear plate response.

The *image plate reader* is another important component of the image acquisition control in computed radiography (Fig. 34-4). The image reader converts the continuous analog information (latent image) on the imaging plate to a digital format. As the imaging plate is scanned by the laser in the image reader, the portion of the plate struck by a laser emits light. This emitted light is directed by high-efficiency light guides to photomultiplier tubes where it is converted to digital electric signals.

The first reader systems became available in 1983 and were capable of processing only 40 plates per hour. Reader systems today are more compact and are capable of processing approximately 110 to 140 plates per hour. Several image readers can be interfaced to each other or to laser printers, computer workstations, or digital archives. For high-volume applications such as chest radiography, stand-alone systems with integrated image processors are available. In any of the reader systems the imaging plate is transported internally through all the various stages of processing, which are transparent to the operator.

DISPLAY FUNCTIONS

The display of computed radiography data is basically the result of *spatial frequency response* and *gradation processing*. Spatial frequency response controls the contrast (sharpness) of the boundaries between two structures of different densities. Gradation processing controls the range of densities used to display structures on the image; it is similar to the window settings used in CT for display. The two different characteristics—contrast and density—are optimized by the digital image processor for the specific anatomic region being studied.

To produce an image for viewing, the computed radiography computer system constructs (formats) the image from the raw data set as read from the photostimulable plate. Because the computed radiographic image is in a digital format, the primary image data can be manipulated to accentuate or suppress various features of the image. Consequently the image can be tailored to a specific clinical task. This is similar to the operation of other digital imaging modalities such as CT, in which the window and level setting of the image can be changed to visualize a specific structure such as the liver or lung.

If no special parameters are specified by the user, the image is reconstructed using the *default* (preset) settings that the specific medical center has decided produce the images of the best quality. If special image characteristics are desired to highlight specific structures, the reconstruction factors can be changed by the radiographer or other user. The final image can be displayed on a monitor or produced as a hard-copy image on film or another medium. Unlike the CT scan, the computed radiographic image is reconstructed each time from the primary data. If the image is displayed on a monitor, the image characteristics can be adjusted visually by the user to examine all features of the image to best advantage. Various workstations with high-resolution *cathode ray tube (CRT)* monitors can be directly interfaced to the computed radiography unit to assist in the display process.

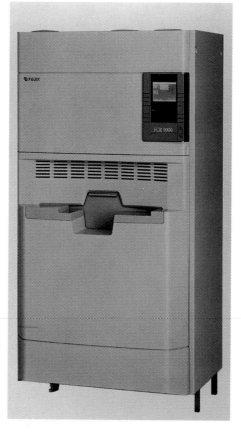

Fig. 34-4 Example of two computed radiography readers. These image readers can process between 110 and 140 imaging plates per hour in either 2K × 2K or 4K × 4K acquisitions.

Operational components: separation of functions

The electronic workstation undoubtedly represents the alternator (viewbox) of the future. Workstations may be linked to a central image archive (an "electronic file room") and also to the text data from the radiology and hospital information systems to provide a central clearing area for all information (images and text) needed by the imaging specialist. The functions for these workstations, which continue to be expanded (Box 34-1), allow the user to alter the image display to best advantage for interpretation. The gradational (contrast) and spatial frequency (sharpness) enhancement can be varied on the workstation; this is similar to formatting the hard-copy image. If, for example, two images have been taken sequentially or using different energy characteristics (see the discussion of dual-energy subtraction), the images can be subtracted much as in angiography with the use of radiographic film and digital subtraction systems. The image also can be magnified, rotated, flipped, or inverted. Statistical analyses can be performed on portions of the image by calculating surface areas and estimated volumes or by characterizing the change in density in a part of the image. Most important for daily operations, however, is the fact that the workstation contains a database that enables the user to easily locate images and create lists of images for conferences, interpretation, and teaching files.

The number of CRT monitors required for an interpretation workstation is still under review. However, it is clear that at least two monitors are needed. The monitor resolution factor remains a point of contention among experts in this field. Currently, 1K × 1K *matrix* monitors are generally used. The resolution is adequate for most studies, and the cost is within reason. However, 2K × 2K monitors are the norm for primary review workstations. With 2K × 2K resolution, all studies can be appropriately displayed with little or no loss of diagnostic information. Finally, the use of 4K × 4K monitors is under discussion. These monitors require that the image acquisition be of 4K × 4K architecture. If the data are acquired in a 4 K × 4 K data set, they can be fully displayed on 4K × 4K monitors. Cost remains a major consideration in the use of these very costly high-resolution monitors.

Computed radiography also offers several options for film-based display. Fig. 34-5 shows a 2-on-1 format of an identical shoulder image. The image on the left demonstrates the shoulder with display factors similar to those of a conventional film-screen radiograph. An *edge-enhanced* image is also automatically displayed, as seen in the right image. Certain studies and the imaging of some pathologic conditions benefit from this enhanced image.

STORAGE FUNCTIONS

Computed radiography decreases image archive storage space requirements by reducing the size of films stored or by converting bulky film storage to electronic storage. Benefits include tremendous space savings, reduction in image retrieval time, and decreased film loss.

Several points about the design of electronic image archive devices must be considered. Flexibility is important. The device should interface with desired modalities and should be expandable. The amount of storage on the electronic image archive should be adequate for the amount of data to be stored. The storage capacity of an electronic image archive depends on several variables, including the size of the basic storage unit (i.e., optical disk, magnetic tape), the number of units on-line, and the ratio of data compression that is used.

BOX 34-1

Workstation functions

Gradation enhancement
Spatial frequency enhancements
Statistical analysis
Rotation/inversion
Anatomic measurements
Short-term database functions
Dynamic range control
Magnification

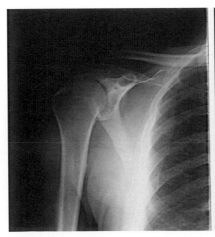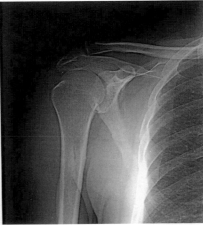

Fig. 34-5 CR image of a shoulder with conventional *(left)* and edge-enhanced *(right)* display parameters.

Magnetic tape and optical disk are currently the storage media of choice for computed radiographic images. These images contain more total data per individual image than the images of other digital modalities, including CT and ultrasonography (Table 34-1). Each computed radiographic image contains about 8 megabytes (MB) of data. For example, a PA or lateral chest image contains about 16 MB of data; that amount of data requires the same electronic storage as the first four volumes of digital text from the *Encyclopaedia Britannica.* One 5¼-inch dual-sided optical disk has the capacity to store up to 3000 computed radiographic images with reversible compression. Optical disks clearly provide a space-savings benefit.

With optical electronic storage, digital data do not deteriorate. When such data are retrieved at a later date for image review and/or for copying on film, the reproduced image will be an exact duplicate of the initial image. In addition, any number of copies may be made using the original data, and each copy will be an original image. With this storage medium, computed radiographic image data can be searched for, retrieved, transmitted, or processed with tremendous ease.

Other large-capacity memory devices can be used for digital data storage. Magnetic tape and optical disk can serve these storage needs with high degrees of efficiency. Naturally, x-ray film can still be used to store visual analog patterns for image-data filing purposes.

With a computed radiography system, flexibility can exist with the three primary options of (1) maintaining an active image file for display and storage purposes, (2) reviewing data on workstations and using long-term archiving devices for permanent electronic files, and (3) employing a combination of these methods to accommodate individual preferences.

Characteristics of a Computed Radiographic Image

Three factors are directly responsible for computed radiography image resolution: (1) dimension of the crystals in the imaging plate, (2) size of the laser beam in the reader, and (3) image-reading matrix. Although computed radiography currently offers greater contrast resolution than conventional film, it provides slightly less *spatial resolution* than film. The resolution with computed radiography averages from 2 to 5 line pairs per millimeter (lp/mm), whereas standard film can demonstrate 3 to 6 lp/mm. With further advances in imaging plate phosphor quality, a reduction in the microbeam laser size, and an increase in matrix dimension and image, spatial resolution with computed radiography could become inherently superior to that of conventional film-screen techniques. Present-day diagnoses are not hampered by the current resolution factors. However, chest imaging and mammography will further benefit from the increased spatial resolution that these examinations demand.

TABLE 34-1

Capacities of various electronic data storage medium

Medium	Capacity
DLT magnetic tape	35-GB
Optical disk	
5¼-inch single disk	4-GB
5¼-inch dual disk	8 G-bytes
Multiple-platter optical jukebox	5-10 T-bytes

Clinical Applications

The sequence of events in computed radiographic imaging in the clinical environment is shown in Fig. 34-6. The process begins at the reception desk, where demographic information (patient name, birthdate, sex, identification [ID] number, and examination ordered) is entered into a reception terminal. Transfer of this information to the computed radiography processor may be accomplished directly via a radiology information system (RIS) or health information system (HIS) interface, bar code, magnetic card, or optical scanner.

The radiographer exposes the imaging plate in the same manner as when a conventional film-screen cassette is used. The exposure may be made using a tabletop, mobile, or table/wall Bucky technique. The exposed imaging plate cassette is taken to the control terminal of the computed radiography reader unit. There, the patient demographic and examination information is entered, and the cassette is scanned with the bar code reader. In this way, each specific exposed imaging plate is linked to the correct patient and image data. This step replaces the typical ID camera step in film radiography.

The radiographer inserts the exposed cassette into the computed radiography reader. Once inside, the cassette is automatically opened, and the imaging plate is removed. The imaging plate is scanned, erased, and returned to the cassette or an internal stacker for use on another patient (Figs. 34-6 and 34-7).

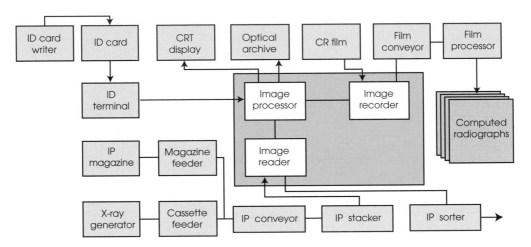

Fig. 34-6 Computed radiography sequence flowchart. (*IP,* Image processor.)

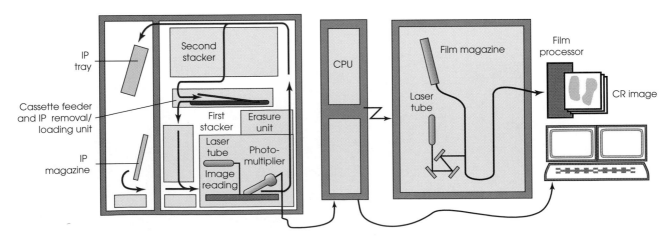

Fig. 34-7 Generalized internal functions and components of a computed radiography system. (*IP,* Image processor.)

The internal functions of a computed radiography system are illustrated in Fig. 34-7. Inside the system and not apparent to the radiographer is the image plate reader assembly, which scans the imaging plate. The plate is transported through the system at right angles to a red *helium-neon (633 nm) laser* beam or a visible-light semiconductor (680-nm) laser beam until the entire plate is sequentially scanned. When the $BaFx:Eu^{2+}$ crystals on the photostimulable plate are exposed to the laser beam, the crystal layer emits the energy in the form of light, which was retained in its "memory" after x-ray exposure. The light intensity emitted is proportional to the amount of x-rays that initially excited the crystal layer. Tracking with the laser beam is a light guide that focuses the emitted light from the imaging plate to a photomultiplier tube. The emitted light energy is converted to an electric signal and is sent to an amplifier and then on to an analog/digital convertor where the analog is converted to a digital data set. The digital data set is related spatially and is proportional in intensity to the original x-ray exposure in each *pixel* of the imaging plate (Fig. 34-8).

The imaging plates offer wide exposure latitude. During the scanning process a sensitivity adjustment is made to make effective use of this latitude. The data from the imaging plate, as well as the anatomic menu, are examined to analyze the image characteristics and determine the reading sensitivity and exposure latitude. This entire process allows for the wide exposure latitude in computer radiographic imaging.

Errors in technical exposure factors are virtually eliminated. Exposure factors 500% greater than or 80% less than that which would normally be used to present the information aesthetically on a conventional film-screen system can be corrected using the computed radiography system. Although these examples are obviously the extreme limits of correction and rarely occur, it must be realized that even gross technical errors are correctable with the computed radiography system.

Technical corrections are achieved with computer-aided auto-ranging techniques. Optimized computed radiography display parameters are achieved through *histogram* analysis in proportion to the linear dynamic range of the imaging plates and tailoring the final image characteristics to an agreed-on subjective H&D curve for best display of the anatomic structure(s) of interest.

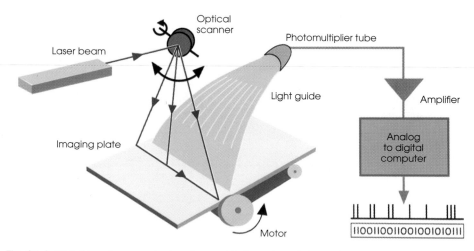

Fig. 34-8 Reading of computed radiographic imaging plate and conversion to digital information.

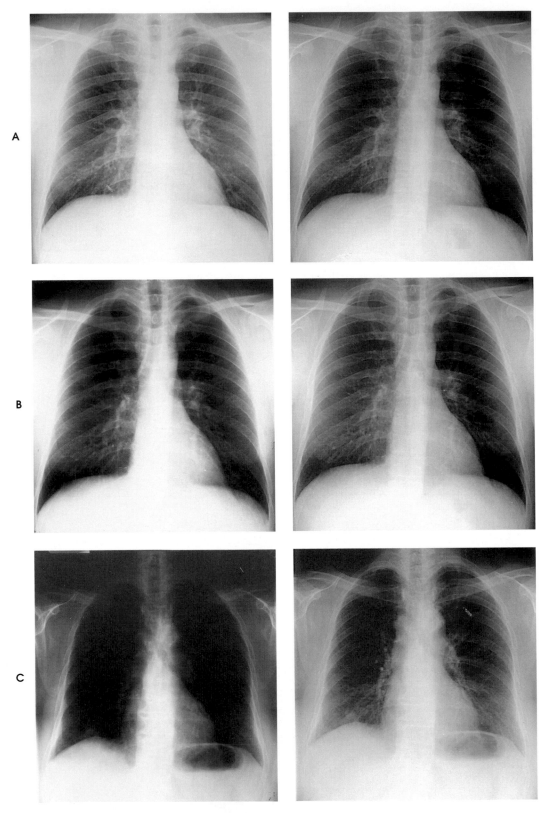

Fig. 34-9 Six images showing pairs of analog *(left)* and computed radiographs *(right)* acquired simultaneously. Note that despite the widely differing exposure factors, the computed radiographic images do not vary in quality, although the analog radiographs are clearly suboptimal in quality. **A**, Analog radiograph *(left)* and computed radiographic image *(right)*, both using exposure factors of 125 kVp, 1 mAs. **B**, Analog radiograph *(left)* and computed radiographic image *(right)*, both using 125 kVp, 2.5 mAs. **C**, Analog radiograph *(left)* and computed radiographic image *(right)*, both using 125 kVp, 6.3 mAs.

A review of the chest radiographs in Fig. 34-9 is helpful in understanding the effects of this process. Analog and computed radiographic images were simultaneously obtained using a cassette containing both a radiographic film and an imaging plate. Despite technique factors that produced inadequate analog radiographs, all of the computed radiographic images are of consistent and appropriate penetration and quality. The "sampling" process normalized the image for the particular anatomic region being studied.

After the exposure of the imaging plate and its subsequent scanning by the laser beam, the image on the plate is erased. The energy remaining on the imaging plate after reading is completely eliminated by exposing the plate to a uniform and specific light source. This light source is either a bright sodium-vapor or high-brightness fluorescent light with both filtered and nonfiltered ultraviolet components. The plates are reusable for thousands of times. In fact, plates may well be mechanically destroyed or damaged before any degradation of the crystalline structure is realized.

Other Techniques to Improve Diagnostic Efficacy

In addition to the manipulation of images on a workstation, several other techniques can be used to improve the diagnostic power of computed radiography. These techniques include dynamic range control and energy subtraction.

Dynamic range control (DRC) is a processing protocol to set optical density of certain anatomic regions that normally appear as overexposed or underexposed. These regions might exist in high-density or low-density areas. The computer generates a filter (mask) image from the original, and the filter is then superimposed on the original. The result of DRC is better visualization of the mediastinum in chest imaging and better soft tissue display in shoulder and knee images.

Energy subtraction is a recently developed type of processing. It requires the use of two imaging plates with a 1-mm copper filter sandwiched between them. The full-energy spectrum of the radiation beam is recorded by the first plate. Radiation that passes through the first plate undergoes low-energy filtration (beam hardening) by the copper filter before it enters the second plate. The image recorded by the second plate consists primarily of the high-energy component of the beam; therefore the bone/calcium contrast is markedly reduced over that in the image recorded on the first plate.

A subtraction process, aided by the computer, takes place twice. This provides one image of the soft tissue and a second image of the bone and calcium. In all, three PA chest images are produced: a standard radiograph image, a soft tissue image and a bone/calcium image. Fig. 34-10 shows a standard image and a soft tissue image.

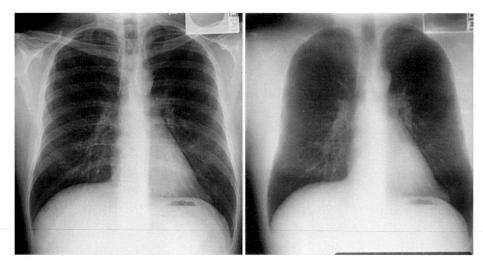

Fig. 34-10 Standard computed radiographic chest image *(left)* and soft tissue image *(right)* of only lung tissue using the energy subtraction process.

Clinical Acceptance

Computed radiography is being used in private offices, medical centers, and hospitals for all applications in which conventional projection radiography can be used, including chest, bone, and mobile radiography. It is also being used for contrast-enhanced examinations such as excretory urography and gastrointestinal radiography. Angiographic applications are primarily performed using digital radiography (see Chapter 35).

Quality Assurance Concerns

A positive design feature of a computed radiography system is its ability to minimize image *artifacts,* whether induced from system irregularities or operator errors. Periodic failures in these safeguards, however, are inevitable and affect image quality.

System *noise,* artifacts, and unevenness in an image are determined by the noise inherent in the imaging plate (structure noise) and reader system (quantum noise). Digital processing errors can create artifacts and density irregularities.

Several *artifacts* can be controlled by the operator. Dust on the imaging plate can be seen on the resulting image. It is therefore important to maintain a periodic schedule of cleaning the imaging plate surfaces for quality assurance, just as a similar program of quality control maintenance is used for radiographic intensifying screens. In addition, grids of a particular ratio and line factor are recommended for various examinations. If these recommendations are not followed, a *moiré* pattern of laser light scanning lines or data loss can occur. Scatter radiation is detrimental to the quality of both computed radiographic and conventional film-screen images. Grids must be used when warranted by the examination or the patient's body habitus.

Although computed radiography systems are able to correct for gross technical errors, there is a limit to the minimum dosage required for appropriate penetration and a diagnostic image. Each computed radiography operating institution must establish radiation dose reduction limits. Inadequate radiation doses result in images that demonstrate quantum mottle or areas devoid of data.

Pitfalls

Correctly produced computed radiography images have few undesirable characteristics, and these will not cause diagnostic problems, even with a relatively inexperienced computed radiography operator. Edge-enhancement artifacts are the primary problems in this type of imaging. In certain circumstances, edge enhancement creates an appearance that may be confused with a pathologic disorder. On the edge-enhanced image a dark band may appear at the interface between structures that differs widely in density. This effect is primarily seen in computed radiographic images involving metal prostheses and barium contrast studies. The dark line of the edge-enhancement artifact is always perfectly symmetric around the dense object, which makes it relatively easy to distinguish from a lesion causing lucency.

Benefits

When a computed radiography system is used, several benefits are readily apparent. These benefits are discussed in the following sections.

IMPROVED DIAGNOSTIC ACCURACY AND EXPANDED DIAGNOSTIC SCOPE

With the storage of laser-scanned x-ray images on high-sensitivity imaging plates, minute differences in x-ray absorption are detected, providing highly detailed and easily readable diagnostic information. The wide exposure latitude permits diagnosis of an entire area of interest, allowing imaging from bones to soft tissue with a single exposure. Computer analysis of images can provide increased diagnostic information to assist in the medical treatment of a patient.

X-RAY DOSAGE REDUCTION

The imaging plate coupled with efficient readout of the high-precision laser scanner can help to reduce the exposure in certain instances. This dose reduction depends on the type of film-screen system and the technical factors employed by the imaging facility. The actual dose reduction varies with the type of examination and the institution. Table 34-2 shows approximate dose reductions by type of examination.

TABLE 34-2

Radiation dose for diagnostic-quality images obtained by computed radiography compared with standard radiography

Procedure	Relative decrease in dose (%)
Chest radiography	5
Upper gastrointestinal series	5
Excretory urography	10
Pediatric examinations	15-30

REPEAT RATE REDUCTION

Because of the wide technique latitude of the computed radiography system, technical errors are easily corrected to provide prime diagnostic information. When a film-screen combination is used, technical errors in either direction can markedly degrade the image quality. Technical errors have much less effect on the final quality of a computed radiographic image. This benefit obviously increases *throughput* and reduces the patient's discomfort because it lessens the need to repeat the examination. The technical latitude of computed radiography is a tremendous asset in the area of mobile or portable radiography.

TELERADIOGRAPHIC TRANSMISSION

Image plate reader devices can be linked via dedicated phone lines, microwave transmission, or other *teleradiographic* means to centralize the review of image data. This means of image sharing is an obvious benefit to affiliated hospitals or clinics that are separated by large geographic distances but share professional staff. Teleradiology could also provide immediate consultation with specialists, which benefits not only the patient but also the level of efficiency of the institution.

Many radiology departments are contemplating the installation of a *picture archive and communication system (PACS)* for the immediate or near future. Many others, however, are hesitating to implement PACS because of concerns about multimodality/multivendor interfacing as well as the requirement that conventional projection radiography (which represents approximately 60% to 70% of a radiology department's volume) be digital format compatible. Computed radiography is the link needed for PACS. With computed radiography, all imaging modalities can be integrated and can share processing, display, and archiving ventures.

DEPARTMENT EFFICIENCY

The computed radiography system eliminates all darkroom work. This factor plus the previous benefits ultimately increase departmental efficiency.

Conclusion

Computed radiography will improve both the operational and diagnostic efficiency of radiology departments. With the placement of conventional projection radiography in digital format, computed radiography forms the keystone for PACS. Computed radiography improves the efficiency of conventional projection radiography by providing consistent image quality, decreasing repeat exposure rate, minimizing patient radiation exposure, and decreasing lost images. By realizing such benefits, many departments have already found that computed radiography is a justifiable long-term investment.

Appreciation is extended to Rebecca Schodt-Lupo for her assistance and expert guidance regarding computed radiography.

Definition of Terms

analog Any information represented in continuous fashion rather than discrete units.

analog-to-digital conversion Process of converting a continuous (analog) signal to discrete (digital) units.

artifacts Observable, undesirable image features resulting from faulty image processing techniques.

barium fluorohalide (BaFX:Eu²) Barium florohalide with europium, the photostimulable phosphor used on CR image plates.

cathode ray tube (CRT) Electron tube (like a television tube) that makes the computer output visible; sometimes called a *video display unit (VDU)*.

computed radiography (CR) Digital imaging process using a photostimulable chemical plate for initial acquisition of image data; the display parameters of the image can be manipulated by a computer at a later time.

default Parameters by which the system operates; if no changes in instructions are made by the operator, the preset operating parameters or controls of the system prevail.

digital Any information represented in discrete units (also see *analog*).

dual energy imaging X-ray imaging technique in which two x-ray exposures are taken of the same body part using two different kilovoltages; the two images are processed to remove image contrast resulting from either soft tissue or bone.

dynamic range Orders of magnitude over which the system can accurately portray information.

dynamic range control Image-processing algorithm for image enhancement that provides a wide diagnostic field, allowing visualization of bone and soft tissue in a single image display.

edge enhancement Technique of setting the spatial frequency response so that structures of a given type, usually bones, stand out in bold relief.

energy subtraction Processing techniques used in computed radiography that include a dual-exposure method, which requires irradiation with two different x-ray energies, and a single-exposure method, which requires only one x-ray irradiation but in which the x-ray energies are separated by inserting a copper filter between two imaging plates.

gradation processing Technique of setting the range of values over which an image is displayed; similar to the window setting in CT; allows selection of a wide range of values to display structures with widely differing densities or a narrow range to display structures close together in density; for example, a body part such as the mediastinum.

gray-level display Number of possible shades of gray in a digital image; this number depends on the pixel depth of the digital acquisition devices and the display units. Acquisition devices and display units with 8-bit pixel depth capabilities give 256 possible shades of gray, whereas units with 10 bit pixel depth give 1024 possible shades of gray.

helium-neon (633-nm) laser Intense, coherent beam of light in the red wavelength

histogram Graphic representation of the frequency distribution of gray levels, which represent the anatomy in a computed radiographic image (see Chapter 32, Fig. 32-13, for an example).

image plate reader Component of the computed radiography system that scans the image plate with a laser and converts the analog information on the image plate into an electric signal; an analog-to-digital converter then changes the electric signal to a digital signal.

imaging plate Image capture portion of computed radiography; appears the same as a screen in the film-screen environment except that the imaging plate is a photostimulable phosphor with the ability to "capture" an x-ray image as electrons are stored in stable traps within the phosphor compound.

latent image Nonobservable representation of a structure such as the varied energy changes inherent in the crystalline structure of imaging plates.

matrix Gridlike pattern of an image composed of a certain number of pixels both in the horizontal and the vertical planes.

megabyte (MB) 1000 bytes.

moiré Fine network of wavy lines that have a watered appearance on the displayed image.

noise Image appearance as graininess on monitors and printed radiographic images.

photostimulable phosphor Special luminescent material that stores x-ray energy and emits light proportional to the stored x-ray energy when stimulated by energy such as visible light from a laser.

picture archive and communication system (PACS) System of computers linked together via a network to store and transmit digital images throughout the network; can be within a hospital but may also include remote sites.

pixels (*picture elements*) Small squares that form the image; pixels have depth in bits usually 8, 12, 15; the greater the pixel depth, the larger the gray scale.

spatial frequency response Sharpness of image that controls how prominently the "edges" are seen in one structure of one density compared with the "edges" in an adjacent structure of another density. In the computed radiography system the technique is called "unsharp masking"; an unsharp (blurred) image is used as the mask image to enhance the spatial frequency response.

spatial resolution How small an object that can be detected by an imaging system and how close together two similar objects can be and still be identified as separate objects; unit of measure usually used is line pairs per millimeter (lp/mm); for example, if the spatial resolution is 10 lp/mm, it means that 10 lines per millimeter can be distinguished as discrete lines, but if there are more than 10 lines per millimeter, some lines will "run together" and appear to be a single line.

teleradiography Ability to send and receive radiographic images over telephone lines from one institution to another.

throughput Rate at which items can be processed through a system; originally a systems analysis term but now commonly used in medicine. If a radiology department can perform a maximum of 60 chest radiographs per hour, this is the maximum throughput for chest radiographs.

Selected bibliography

Anasuma K: Technical trends of the CR system. In Tateno Y, Linuma T, Takano M, editors: *Computed radiography*, Tokyo, 1988, Springer-Verlag.

Andriole K: Wide exposure latitude sets CR apart from x-ray diagnostic imaging, *Comput Radiol* 6, Supplement to Diagnostic Imaging, 1997.

Barnes GT, Sones RA, Tesic MM: Digital chest radiography: performance evaluation of a prototype unit, *Radiology* 154:801, 1985.

Ergon DL et al: Single exposure dual energy computed radiography: improved detection and processing, *Radiology* 174:243, 1993.

Fraser RG, Breatnach E, Barnes GT: Digital radiography of the chest: clinical experience with a prototype unit, *Radiology* 148:1, 1983.

Hindel R: Review of optical storage technology for archiving digital medical images, *Radiology* 161:257, 1986.

Huebener KH: Scanned projection radiography of the chest versus standard film radiography: a comparison of 250 cases, *Radiology* 148:363, 1983.

Ikezoe J et al: Dynamic range control processing of digital chest images: a clinical evaluation, *Acta Radiol* 37:107, 1996.

Ito W et al: Improvement of detection in computed radiography by new single exposure and dual energy subtraction, *Proc SPIE* 1652:386, 1992.

Johnson GA, Ravin CE: A survey of digital chest radiography, *Radiol Clin North Am* 21: 655, 1983.

Kuni CC: *Introduction to computers and digital processing in medical imaging*, St Louis, 1988, Mosby.

Long BW: Computed tomography: photo stimulable phosphor image plate technology, *Radiol Technol* 61:107, 1989.

Long BW: Image enhancement using computed radiography, *Radiol Technol* 61:276, 1990.

McAdams HP et al: Histogram-directed processing of digital chest images, *Invest Radiol* 21:253, 1986.

Sakuma H et al: Plain chest radiograph with computed radiography: improved sensitivity for the detection of coronary artery calcification, *AJR* 151:27, 1988.

Tateno Y: An introduction to clinical utilization of CR. In Tateno Y, Linuma T, Takeno M, editors: *Computed radiography*, Tokyo, 1987, Springer-Verlag.

Templeton AW et al: A digital radiology imaging system: description and clinical evaluation, *AJR* 149:847, 1987.

Tesic MM et al: Digital radiography of the chest: design features and considerations for a prototype unit, *Radiology* 148:259, 1983.

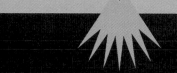

DIGITAL ANGIOGRAPHY AND DIGITAL SPOT IMAGING

WALTER W. PEPPLER

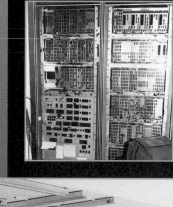

RIGHT: Early-prototype image-processing system for digital subtraction angiography, 1976.

(Courtesy Charles Mistretta, University of Wisconsin—Madison, Madison, Wis.)

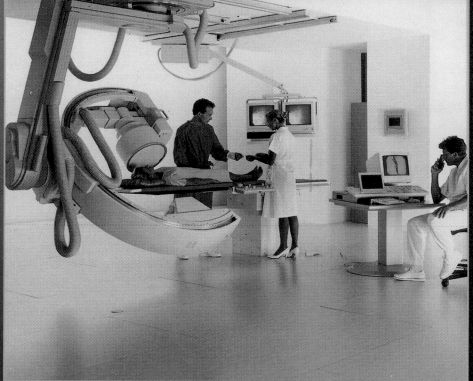

LEFT: Digital fluoroscopy unit and operators control panel, 1999.

(Courtesy Philips Medical Systems, Shelton, Conn.)

Principles of Digital Angiography and Digital Spot Imaging

Digital electronic technology has increased the speed of image processing and decreased costs to the point where totally electronic radiographic image detection, storage, and display have largely replaced film in a number of procedures. More importantly, radiographic images stored in a digital memory can be manipulated in ways that are impossible with traditional film-screen technology. Such manipulation enables the radiologist to isolate image information that is too low in image contrast to be recognized on a conventional radiograph. The ability to "see" what previously had been invisible has opened new areas for radiographic study.

Historical Development

The acquisition of digital images from a combination *image intensifier/television (II/TV)* system was first introduced as *digital subtraction angiography*[1] *(DSA)*. DSA was developed during the 1970s by groups at the University of Wisconsin, the University of Arizona, and the Kinderklinik at the University of Kiel, Germany. This work led to the development of commercial systems, which were introduced in 1980. Within the next few years many manufacturers of x-ray equipment introduced DSA products. After several years of rapid change the systems evolved to those available today. The primary changes since the introduction of DSA include improved image quality, a larger pixel *matrix* (up to 1024 × 1024), and fully digital systems.

---

[1]Almost all italicized terms are defined at the end of this chapter.

INTRAVENOUS VERSUS INTRAARTERIAL INJECTION

The most notable change in DSA was not in equipment design but in clinical practice. The initial success and promise of DSA were predicated on the IV injection of contrast media. IV procedures were less risky and less expensive than the intraarterial procedures used for conventional angiography, and they could be performed on an outpatient basis. This was advantageous because conventional intraarterial film *angiography* usually required an overnight hospital stay. In addition, IV DSA was less painful for the patient.

However, IV DSA did have serious drawbacks. Cardiac motion, diaphragmatic motion, bowel peristalsis, swallowing, and coughing all caused image *artifacts*. In patients with decreased cardiac output, the contrast bolus became seriously diluted; as a result, examinations were frequently nondiagnostic. In addition, large volumes of contrast material were required for the IV method of DSA, and contrast toxicity became a serious consideration. Finally, because all arteries in the region of interest (ROI) were opacified, superimposition made the diagnosis of arterial pathology difficult.

The standard of practice quickly evolved to performing DSA using intraarterial injection of contrast material. Because the examination was performed intraarterially, a smaller volume of more dilute contrast medium was required. With the contrast material injected intraarterially near the ROI, patient motion and the attendant image degradation occurred less frequently. The evolution of smaller catheters (4 to 5 Fr) allowed outpatient arteriography to be performed safely. After the introduction of *nonionic contrast media,* patients experienced less discomfort (nausea and vomiting); the incidence of severe life-threatening reactions also decreased significantly, with nephrotoxicity remaining about the same.

However, the main reason for the transition to intraarterial injection is the very significant improvement in image quality. IV injection of contrast media produces not only poorer image quality but also more variable results than those obtained routinely using intraarterial injections.

DIGITAL SPOT IMAGING

Image quality has improved to the point that the digital imaging system, originally developed for subtraction images, now has sufficient image quality for *unsubtracted imaging* applications. In the general radiographic/fluoroscopic (R/F) suite, unsubtracted digital images are of sufficient image quality to replace traditional spot-film devices based on film. In addition to the excellent image quality, the ease of use and rapid display of images on a digital system are extremely advantageous. Images are available on the monitor immediately, with no need to wait for film to be processed or cassettes to be changed. The digital nature of the image data also lends itself to electronic archiving and transmission of the images. Digital spot radiography is on the verge of becoming commonplace. In the digital angiography suite, subtraction is now viewed as an important but optional adjunct to image processing.

Digital imaging suites can also serve multiple purposes. X-ray equipment manufacturers are producing equipment that can be used, depending on optional components, for general R/F, angiographic, and interventional procedures. The equipment requirements for unsubtracted applications are virtually identical to those for DSA except that many of the *postprocessing* options are not necessary. However, regardless of the added features, the systems share the same basic image acquisition equipment and image quality, which are described in the next section.

Equipment and Apparatus

An II/TV system (fluoroscopy) can be used to form images with little electrical interference, to provide moderate resolution, and to yield diagnostic-quality images when combined with a high-speed *image processor* in a digital angiography (DA) system (Fig. 35-1).

The procedure room is much like a standard angiographic suite, and the fluoroscopic equipment operates in the conventional way. However, the following brief review helps to explain the DA system. The input surface of the *image intensifier* is coated with an x-ray–sensitive phosphor, typically cesium iodide (CsI). The phosphor is contained within a vacuum and enclosed in glass. X-rays that are absorbed by the CsI *input phosphor* emit visible light that is converted to electrons within the image intensifier. The electrons, proportional to the amount of radiation absorbed, are electronically amplified and accelerated across the image tube and are then absorbed by the *output phosphor* of the image intensifier. The output phosphor, approximately 1 inch (2.5 cm) in diameter, emits light when it absorbs electrons. The resulting light intensity is 5000 to 10,000 times brighter than if the CsI phosphor had been used alone.

The television camera is focused onto the image-intensifier output phosphor and converts the light intensity into an electrical signal. The camera forms an image by electronically scanning a photosensitive *semiconductor,* called the *target,* on which the light has been focused. The presence of light on a small portion of the target changes the electrical properties in that target region. These changes are detected by the television camera.

An image is synthesized line by line by the scanning of a narrow electron beam across the television target in up to 1024 parallel lines every one thirtieth of a second. With normal fluoroscopic operation the video image is displayed on a television monitor. The scanning rate is so fast that the human eye does not notice the scanning process but sees a two-dimensional image on the television screen. The images are called *frames* and are presented at a rate of 30 per second.

In a digital imaging system each of the television lines is further divided into segments called *pixels* (*pic*ture *el*ements). The electronic video signal corresponding to each pixel is *digitized* and stored in a digital memory. Typically each line is divided into 512 or 1024 pixels, and the digitized value (gray level) assigned to each pixel is usually in the range of 0 (representing black) to 1023 (white). The image in *memory,* which is made up of a total of 512×512 pixels or 1024×1024 pixels (the number of lines multiplied by the number of pixels per line), is also stored on a digital disk for later review, manipulation, and analysis.

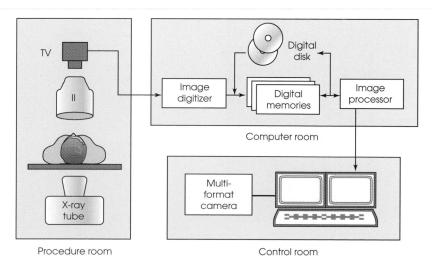

Fig. 35-1 Block diagram of a digital angiography (DA) system.

The *image processor* consists of a computer and image processing hardware. The computer controls the various components (e.g., memories, image processing hardware, and x-ray generator), and the image-processing hardware gives the system the speed to do many image processing operations in *real time.* The computer and the operator communicate via a keyboard with special function keys, a mouse, and/or a touch-sensitive screen.

The control room is usually separated from the procedure room and has a leaded glass window for observation (Fig. 35-2). Typically one video monitor is located on the operator's console, and another one is in the procedure room next to the fluoroscopic monitor. A computer monitor at the operator's console is used for communicating with the computer. The video monitors display the images in real time as the images are obtained during the imaging sequence. At a later time, images *(hard copies)* are produced using a multiformat camera or laser imager.

Performing Digital Subtraction Angiographic Procedures

A DSA study begins with catheter placement performed in the same manner as for conventional angiography. Injection techniques vary, but typically 15 to 20 ml of iodinated contrast medium is injected at a rate of 10 ml/sec. An automatic pressure injector is used to ensure consistency of injection and to facilitate computer control of injection timing and image acquisition.

The intravascular catheter is positioned using conventional fluoroscopic apparatus and technique, and a suitable imaging position is selected. At this point an image that does not have a large dynamic range should be established; no part of the image should be significantly brighter than the rest of the image. This can be accomplished by proper positioning, but it often requires the use of compensating filters. The filters can be bags of saline or thin pieces of metal inserted in the imaging field to reduce the intensity of bright regions. Metal filters are often part of the collimator, and water or saline bags are placed directly on or adjacent to the patient.

If proper placement of compensating filters is not performed, image quality is reduced significantly. The reason is that the video camera operates most effectively with video signals that are at a fixed level. Automatic controls in the system adjust the exposure factors so that the brightest part of the image is at that level. An unusually bright spot satisfies the automatic controls and causes the rest of the image to lie at significantly reduced levels, where the camera performance is worse. An alternative to proper filter placement is to adjust the automatic sensing region, similar to automatic exposure control (AEC) for conventional radiography, to exclude the bright region. This solution is less desirable than the use of compensating filters, and it is not always effective for some positions of the bright spot on the image.

As the imaging sequence begins, an image that will be used as a subtraction mask (without contrast medium) is digitized and stored in the digital memory. This mask image and those that follow are produced when the x-ray tube is energized and x-rays are produced, usually one exposure per second at 65 to 95 kVp and between 5 and 150 mAs. The radiation dose received by the patient for each image is approximately the same as that used for a conventional radiograph. Images can be acquired at variable rates, from one image every 2 to 3 seconds up to 30 images per second.

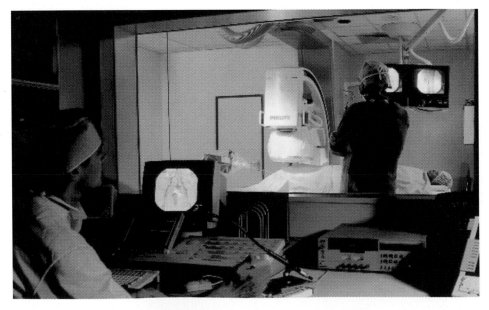

Fig. 35-2 Operator console of digital angiography system with procedure room in the background.

(Courtesy Philips Medical Systems, Shelton, Conn.)

The *acquisition rate* can also be varied during a run. Most commonly, images are acquired at a faster rate during the passage of iodine contrast medium through the arteries and then at a reduced rate in the venous phase, during which the blood flow is much slower. This procedure minimizes the radiation exposure to the patient but provides a sufficient number of images to demonstrate the clinical information. Each of these digitized images is electronically *subtracted* from the mask, and the subtraction image is amplified (contrast enhanced) and displayed in real time so that the subtraction images appear essentially instantaneously during the imaging procedure (Fig. 35-3). The images are simultaneously stored on a *digital disk* or *videotape recorder.* Videotape recorders are often used when images are acquired at a rate of 30 per second. Real-time digital disks capable of recording images at a rate of 30 per second are expensive and are usually restricted to cardiac applications, in which high imaging rates are more common.

Some DSA equipment allows the table or the II/TV system to be moved during acquisition. The movement is permitted in order to "follow" the flow of iodine contrast material as it passes through the arteries. Sometimes called the "bolus chase" method, this technique is particularly useful for evaluating the arteries in the pelvis and lower limb. Previously, several separate imaging sequences would be performed with the II/TV positioned in a different location for each sequence, but this method required an injection of iodine contrast material for each sequence. The bolus chase method requires only one injection of iodine, and the imaging sequence follows (or "chases") the iodine as it flows down the limb. The imaging sequence may be followed by a duplicate sequence without iodine injection to enable subtraction.

Misregistration, a major problem in DSA, occurs when the mask and the images displaying the vessels filled with contrast medium do not exactly coincide. Misregistration is sometimes caused by voluntary movements of the patient, but it is also caused by involuntary movements such as bowel peristalsis or heart contractions. Preparing the patient by describing the sensations associated with contrast-medium injection and the importance of holding still can help to eliminate voluntary movements. It is also important to have the patient suspend respiration during the procedure. Compression bands, glucagon, and cardiac gating can be effective in reducing misregistration caused by involuntary movement.

During the imaging procedure the subtraction images appear on the display monitor. Often a preliminary diagnosis can be made at this point or as the images are reviewed immediately after each exposure sequence. However, a formal reading session occurs after the patient study has been completed; at that time the final diagnosis is made.

Some *postprocessing* (described in the next section) is performed after each exposure sequence to improve visualization of the anatomy of interest or to correct misregistration. More involved postprocessing, including quantitative analysis, is performed after the patient study has been completed. The processed images are available on the computer monitor for review by the radiologist. Because the images are digital, it is possible to store them in a *picture archive and communication system (PACS).* With PACS, images can be archived in digital format on various computer devices, including magnetic tape and optical disk. The images can also be transmitted via a computer network throughout the hospital or to remote locations for consultation with an expert or the referring physician. As an alternative to digital storage and reading, hard-copy images may be produced using a *laser printer* or *multiformat camera,* with several images appearing on each radiograph. When produced, they are normally used for the formal reading session and are also kept for archival purposes.

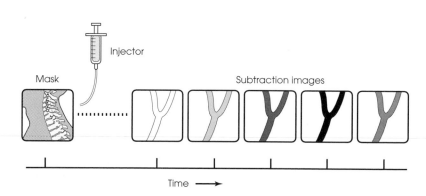

Fig. 35-3 Schematic representation of a DSA imaging sequence.

Image Postprocessing

CONTRAST AND BRIGHTNESS ADJUSTMENT

After the images have been obtained and stored on a disk, several methods can be used to manipulate, or postprocess, the images. The most common is to adjust the contrast and brightness to produce an optimum display of the image. The contrast and brightness adjustments are equivalent to the window and level adjustments performed on CT images (see Chapter 33) or MRI images (see Chapter 36). The terms *contrast* and *brightness* are often used for DSA because of the similarity to adjusting these elements on a television set.

REMASKING

Another common postprocessing task is correction of misregistered images. The most effective way to fix misregistration is simply to *remask* the image. In remasking, another mask image is chosen that is properly registered with the image of interest. The procedure is usually simple. Rather than choosing new masks one at a time (which may or may not work), the operator selects as the mask the image that contains the maximum iodine signal. Then the operator looks for a "live" image (in this case, without iodine) that subtracts from the mask without misregistration. The reversal of the role of the images changes the polarity of the subtraction image (i.e., from white contrast to black contrast). However, the original polarity can be restored by pressing the contrast inversion button. This procedure usually produces an acceptable image with minimal effort (Fig. 35-4).

PIXEL SHIFTING

In some runs an acceptable mask cannot be found. One way to salvage such runs is by *pixel shifting*. In this technique one of the images is shifted with respect to the other to compensate for the movement of the patient between the two images. In many cases, shifts of a fraction of a pixel are necessary to obtain proper registration. Most processors allow at least horizontal and vertical translation, and some also permit rotation. Pixel shifting can be a tedious procedure that requires a great deal of patience. In addition to many possible pixel shifts, several combinations of mask and live images may have to be tried. Pixel registration routines that automatically register (shift) the images are available.

UNSUBTRACTED IMAGES

Obtaining adequate registration of the mask and iodinated images may be impossible in some situations, such as when patients are uncooperative or bowel peristalsis causes problems. In such cases, the use of unsubtracted images may be the best approach. Unsubtracted images are planned from the outset for certain imaging sequences, such as pulmonary angiography, in which motion cannot be completely eliminated. In these cases, contrast injection with a greater iodine concentration or volume may be used.

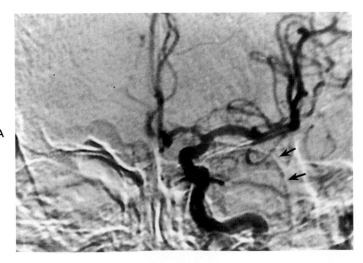
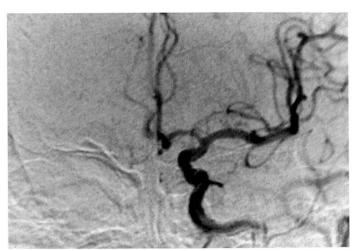

Fig. 35-4 Intraarterial DSA angiogram of the intracranial arteries, **A,** Misregistration artifacts. **B,** Same image after remasking. Note the significant improvement in misregistration artifacts, particularly in the region of the orbit *(arrows)*.

VIEW TRACING

A series of images acquired during the passage of contrast medium can be combined into one image that reveals the entire flow of iodine. First the series of images must be selected. The chosen beginning image is one in which the iodine has first reached the artery, and the last image is one showing that the iodine has filled the distal parts of the arterial tree. The *view trace* function takes the images from the first to the last and, for each pixel in the image, finds the maximum contrast for that pixel. The composite image then displays each pixel at the maximum contrast it contained during the chosen sequence. The resulting image looks as though the contrast material is spread throughout the entire arterial structure simultaneously.

EDGE ENHANCEMENT

Using *edge enhancement,* also called *unsharp masking*, the edges of vessels can be accentuated (or enhanced) so that small details can be made more obvious. Various amounts of edge enhancement can be obtained. However, greater amounts of edge enhancement also accentuate the noise in the image.

IMAGE ZOOM

Another postprocessing option is to magnify, or *zoom,* the image. Zooming the image increases the size of a part of the image to make some subtle feature more visible. One option is to zoom a part of the image to occupy the entire screen. The image can be "panned" in all directions so that the parts of the image outside the screen area can be seen. Another option is to display a magnifying glass region on the image. The part of the image within this region appears larger, as if viewed through a magnifying glass placed on the screen (Fig. 35-5). The size of the magnifying region is adjustable, and the region can be moved about the image. It should be noted that neither of the methods increases the image resolution. They simply present the same information as a larger image.

LANDMARKING

In *landmarking,* a small amount of the original image is put back into the subtraction image. This common procedure gives surgeons anatomic landmarks so that they can more accurately locate structures in the image. Without the landmark information it is difficult to locate the structures because the background has been so effectively eliminated. Only a fraction of the mask is added, however, so that the mask does not overwhelm the subtraction image. As an alternative to landmarking, an unsubtracted image may be printed on the same film as the subtraction images and used as a reference.

ANALYTIC TOOLS

Most image processors have a wide variety of analytic tools, including methods to measure distances, quantitate vessel stenoses, calculate ventricular ejection fraction, and measure blood flow. These tools are used regularly for cardiac studies. They are also used often for neurologic studies and occasionally for vascular studies.

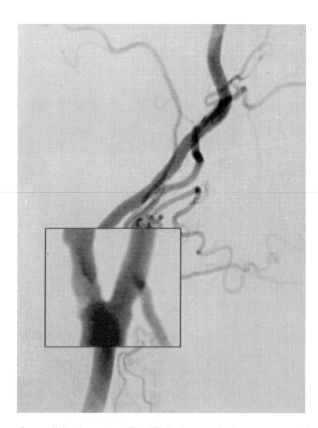

Fig. 35-5 Image of carotid artery (see Fig. 35-6) demonstrating a magnifying-glass type of image zoom.

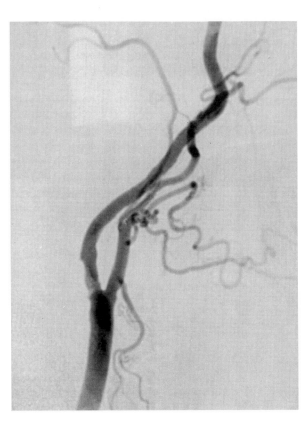

Fig. 35-6 DSA image of common carotid artery, demonstrating stenosis of internal carotid artery.

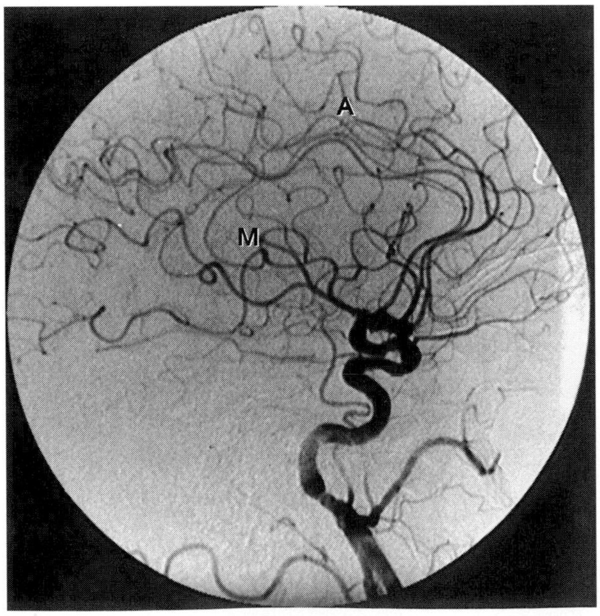

Clinical Applications
INTRAARTERIAL DIGITAL SUBTRACTION ANGIOGRAPHY

Nearly all peripheral and cerebrovascular arteriography is performed with intraarterial DSA (Figs. 35-6 to 35-8). Digital unsubtracted imaging is used whenever misregistration is a problem. For example, in patients with gastrointestinal bleeding, diaphragmatic motion or bowel peristalsis can cause severe image degradation of subtracted images.

Patients with peripheral vascular disease typically undergo intraarterial DSA examination of the infrarenal abdominal aorta, pelvic vessels, and runoff vessels. The intraarterial DSA method permits the identification of small vessels in the lower limbs of patients with severe peripheral vascular disease (Fig. 35-9). Some of these patients have been able to undergo a distal bypass procedure or angioplasty rather than amputation.

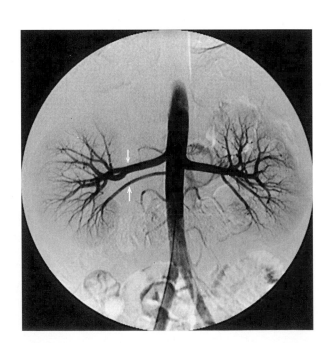

Fig. 35-7 Intraarterial DSA image of the intracranial vasculature showing patent anterior (A) and middle (M) cerebral arteries.

Fig. 35-8 Intraarterial DSA image of abdominal aorta, showing one renal artery on the left and two renal arteries on the right (arrows). All renal arteries are widely patent.

The intraarterial DSA approach can also be applied to pulmonary arteriography. For this examination a catheter is placed within the main pulmonary artery. Consequently, only a small amount of contrast medium must be injected, and a rapid framing sequence (6 frames/sec to 15 frames/sec) is often used. Alternatively, electrocardiographic triggering can be used with lower imaging rates. This application of the intraarterial DSA approach is particularly helpful in the patient with severe pulmonary arterial hypertension who is at significant risk from the high-rate, high-volume contrast injection used for standard pulmonary arteriography.

ROAD MAPPING

The intraarterial DSA approach has also resulted in the evolution of the *road map technique*. Most angiographic/interventional radiologists use this technique routinely in the performance of angioplasty. The intraarterial road map technique provides the angiographer with a real-time continuous subtraction on the fluoroscopic monitor during a procedure. Contrast medium is injected while the subtraction mask is obtained; then the fluoroscopic images are subtracted continuously from the mask. The stationary anatomy is canceled, but the iodinated arteries remain. When the catheter is advanced, it appears on the monitor along with the iodinated arteries, which act as a road map to guide the catheter (Fig. 35-10). The road map technique is often used during catheterization of a patient with a high-grade stenosis or an occlusion within a peripheral runoff vessel. Likewise, the intraarterial road map technique is also applied in *superselective catheterization* and as a monitor during arterial embolization.

INTRAVENOUS DIGITAL SUBTRACTION ANGIOGRAPHY

Currently, IV DSA is performed infrequently. In patients with groin hematomas or possible cellulitis, an IV DSA is helpful in excluding a pseudoaneurysm or mycotic aneurysm of the artery. When the radiologist has difficulty catheterizing the artery, an IV DSA examination may be helpful in determining the anatomy of the vessel and in facilitating subsequent catheter placement.

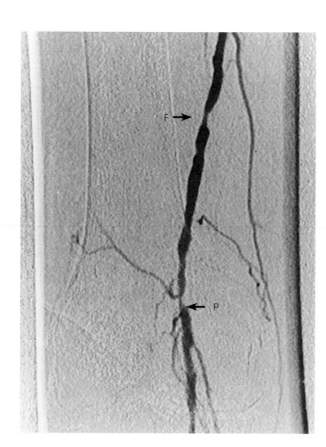

Fig. 35-9 Intraarterial DSA image of distal superficial femoral *(F)* and popliteal *(P)* arteries, showing diffuse, near occlusive disease *(arrows)*.

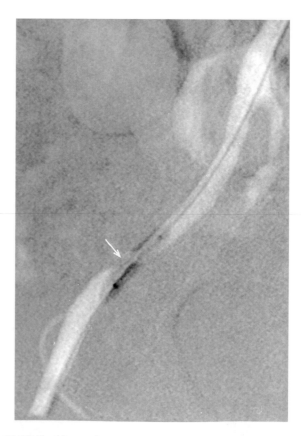

Fig. 35-10 Road map image of right external iliac artery during balloon angioplasty. The roadmap image was helpful in crossing the stenosis and correctly centering the angioplasty balloon at the stenosis *(arrow)*.

DIGITAL SPOT IMAGING

Digital imaging equipment can be used for many imaging situations in which the subtraction capabilities and rapid acquisition capabilities used for angiography are not necessary. The digital spot imaging equipment is well suited for most R/F applications, including gastrointestinal, genitourinary, myelographic, arthrographic, and even skeletal examinations. For example, Fig. 35-11 shows a barium study demonstrating the distal part of the stomach and the duodenum.

Conclusion

DSA has had a great impact on diagnostic radiology. Its advantages over film angiography are its much greater contrast sensitivity, its lower cost, and the immediate availability of results. The digital nature of the data also permits quantitative analysis of DSA images; this has proved valuable, particularly in cardiac applications. The increased contrast sensitivity has permitted lower total volumes and concentrations of contrast media to be used. As a result, patients experience less discomfort, and toxicity is a less frequent problem.

The digital imaging system, originally developed for subtraction images, now has sufficient image quality for unsubtracted imaging applications. In the general R/F suite, unsubtracted digital images are of sufficient quality to replace traditional spot-film devices based on film-screen technology. In addition to excellent image quality, the ease of use and rapid display of images on a digital system are extremely advantageous. Images are available on the monitor immediately, eliminating the need to wait while film is processed or cassettes are changed. The digital nature of the image data also lends itself to electronic archiving and transmission of the images. Digital spot radiography is on the verge of becoming commonplace.

The author thanks John C. McDermott, M.D., of the University of Wisconsin at Madison, for his assistance in developing this chapter.

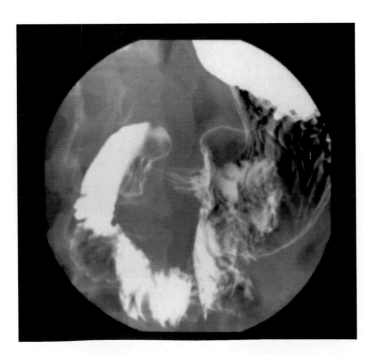

Fig. 35-11 Digital spot image from a barium study, demonstrating lower stomach (antrum) and duodenum.

Definition of Terms

acquisition rate Rate, in images per second, that x-ray images are produced.

angiography Producing x-ray images of the blood vessels after injection of contrast medium.

artifact Any undesirable side effect resulting from an image-processing technique.

digital Information stored in discrete units, called *bits,* which are used to form a binary code for representing information.

digital disk Circular plate coated with magnetic material and used to store digital data.

digital subtraction angiography (DSA) Use of digitally recorded x-ray images to produce subtraction images of vessels.

digitize Process of converting a continuous analog voltage signal into a discrete digital value.

edge enhancement Making the edges of anatomic structures more clearly visualized through intentional unsharp masking and/or computer manipulation.

frame Single image from sequence of images.

hard copy Copy of video image on film.

image intensifier Imaging device that converts an x-ray distribution (image) to an optical image with a large increase in brightness.

II/TV Image intensifier/television unit.

image processor Special-purpose computer designed to operate on images in a short time.

input phosphor Material coated on the input surface of an image intensifier tube; emits light in response to the absorption of x-rays.

landmarking Process in which a reduced-contrast mask image is superimposed on a subtraction image so that the arteries can be seen in relation to the local anatomy. Without landmarking the arteries appear on a completely blank background.

laser printer Device that uses a scanning laser beam to produce a copy of images on film.

mask Image in which the arteries do not contain iodine; the image is subtracted from images with iodine in the arteries.

matrix Two-dimensional array of pixel values that make up an image.

memory Portion of an image processor in which the numbers that represent an image are stored.

misregistration Occurs when the two images used to form a subtraction image are slightly displaced from one another.

multiformat camera Device that produces copies of images on a single film.

nonionic contrast medium Contrast agent that does not ionize in solution and is safer, less painful, and better tolerated by the patient than ionic contrast medium.

output phosphor Material that is coated on the output surface of an image intensifier; emits light (an image) in response to being struck by electrons.

picture archive and communication system (PACS) System of computers linked together via a network to store and transmit digital images throughout the network. The network can be within a hospital institution but may also include remote sites.

pixel (*picture element*) One of the small cells an image breaks into when it is digitized; each cell represents only a small fraction of an entire picture.

pixel shifting Shifting of a digital image to compensate for misregistration marks caused by patient motion; an alternative to remasking.

postprocessing Image-processing operations performed when reviewing an imaging sequence.

real time Any image-processing technique that can be performed within a time frame that is so short as to appear instantaneous.

remask Repeating the masking process by choosing a different mask image to correct misregistration marks.

road map technique Image of the contrast-filled arteries is superimposed on the fluoroscopic image and acts as a road map to guide catheter placement.

semiconductor Solid-state material used in the construction of electronic devices such as transistors or integrated circuits.

subtracted When the mask image is used to remove the scout image (via electronic superimposition) from the postinjection angiographic image.

superselective When the catheter is advanced past the main arteries into smaller, more distal, branches.

unsharp masking Process in which a blurred copy of an image is subtracted from the original image to produce edge enhancement.

unsubtracted image Image that has not been subtracted from a mask image.

video tape recorder A device that uses magnetic tape to record video images.

view trace Process in which several images, with contrast in different parts of the arteries, are added together to produce one image with contrast in all parts of the arteries.

zoom Magnification of an image via interpolation or pixel duplication; resolving power remains unchanged.

Selected bibliography

American Association of Physicists in Medicine: *Performance evaluation and quality assurance in digital subtraction angiography,* Report No. 15, New York, 1985, American Institute of Physics.

Balter S: Fundamental properties of digital images, *Radiographics* 13:129, 1993.

Brennecke R et al: Computerized video-image pre-processing with applications to cardioangiographic roentgen-image series. In Nagel HH, editor: *Digital image processing,* Berlin, 1977, Springer-Verlag.

Carmody RF et al: Digital subtraction angiography: update 1986, *Invest Radiol* 21:899, 1986.

Coltman JW: Fluoroscopic image brightening by electronic means, *Radiology* 51:359, 1948.

Crummy AB et al: Computerized fluoroscopy: digital subtraction for intravenous angiocardiography and arteriography, *AJR* 135:1131, 1980.

Crummy AB: Digital subtraction angiography. In Taveras JM and Ferrucci JT, editors: *Radiology: diagnosis-imaging-intervention,* Philadelphia, 1992, Lippincott.

Crummy AB et al: Digital subtraction angiography "road map" for transluminal angioplasty, *Semin Interv Radiol* 1:247, 1984.

Ludwig JW et al: *Digital subtraction angiography in clinical practice,* Best, Netherlands, 1986, Philips Medical Systems.

Fink U et al: Peripheral DSA with automated stepping, *Eur J Radiol* 13:50, 1991.

Foley WD et al: Intravenous DSA examination of patients with suspected cerebral ischemia, *Radiology* 151:651, 1984.

Heintzen PH, Brennecke R, Bursch JH: Computer quantitation of angiocardiographic images. In Miller HA, Schmidt EV, Harrison DC, editors: *Noninvasive cardiovascular measurements,* vol 167, Bellingham, Wash, 1978, Society of Photooptical Industrial Engineers.

Hillman BJ: Digital radiology of the kidney, *Radiol Clin North Am* 23:211, 1985.

Katzen BT: Current status of digital angiography in vascular imaging, *Radiol Clin North Am* 33:1, 1995.

Kruger RA, Riederer SJ: *Basic concepts of digital subtraction angiography,* Boston, 1984, GK Hall.

Kruger RA et al: A digital video image processor for real time subtraction imaging, *Opt Engineering* 17:652, 1978.

Kruger RA et al: Computerized fluoroscopy in real time for noninvasive visualization of the cardiovascular system, *Radiology* 130:49, 1979.

Malden ES et al: Peripheral vascular disease: evaluation with stepping DSA and conventional screen-film angiography, *Radiology* 191:149, 1994.

Meaney TF et al: Digital subtraction angiography of the human cardiovascular system, *AJR* 135:1153, 1980.

Mistretta CA, Crummy AB: Diagnosis of cardiovascular disease by digital subtraction angiography, *Science* 214:761, 1981.

Mistretta CA, Crummy AB: Digital fluoroscopy. In Coulam CM et al, editors: *The physical basis of medical imaging,* New York, 1981, Appleton-Century-Crofts.

Mistretta CA et al: Multiple image subtraction technique for enhancing low contrast periodic objects, *Invest Radiol* 8:43, 1973.

Mistretta CA et al: *Digital subtraction arteriography: an application of computerized fluoroscopy,* St Louis, 1982, Mosby.

Moodie DS, Yiannikas J: *Digital subtraction angiography of the heart and lungs,* Orlando, Fla, 1986, Grune & Stratton.

Morgan RH, Sturm RE: Johns Hopkins fluoroscopic screen intensifier, *Radiology* 57:556, 1951.

Norman D et al: Intraarterial digital subtraction imaging cost considerations, *Radiology* 156:33, 1985.

Ovitt TW et al: Intravenous angiography using digital video subtraction: x-ray imaging system, *AJR* 135:1141, 1980.

Picus D et al: Comparison of non-subtracted digital angiography and conventional screen-film angiography for the evaluation of patients with peripheral vascular disease, *J Vasc Interv Radiol* 2:359, 1991.

Seeley GW et al: Computer controlled video subtraction procedures for radiology, *Proc Soc Photooptical Instrumentation Engineers* 206:183, 1979.

Strother CM et al: Clinical applications of computerized fluoroscopy: the extracranial carotid arteries, *Radiology* 136:781, 1980.

MAGNETIC RESONANCE IMAGING

LUANN J. CULBRETH

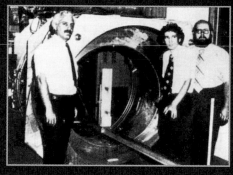

RIGHT: First nuclear magnetic resonance scanner for humans. (*Left to right,* R. Damadian, L. Minkhoff, M Goldsmith, 1988).

(From Eisenberg RL: *Radiology: an illustrated history,* ed 1, St. Louis, 1992, Mosby.)

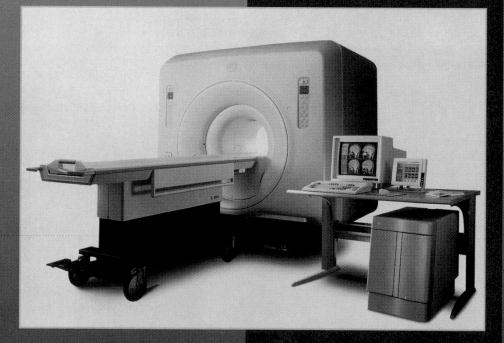

LEFT: Modern magnetic resonance scanner creates images in all planes. The operating control panel shown on the right.

(Courtesy General Electric Medical Systems.)

Principles of Magnetic Resonance Imaging

*Magnetic resonance imaging (MRI)** has generated a great deal of interest among medical workers and the general public because it is an examination technique that provides both anatomic and physiologic information noninvasively. Like computed tomography (CT) (see Chapter 33), MRI is a computer-based cross-sectional imaging modality. However, the physical principles of MRI image production are totally different from those of CT and conventional radiography in that no x-rays are used to generate the MRI image. Indeed, no ionizing radiation of any kind is used in MRI. Instead, MRI creates images of structures through the interactions of magnetic fields and radio waves with tissues.

MRI was originally called *nuclear magnetic resonance (NMR)*. The word "nuclear," indicating that the nonradioactive atomic nucleus played an important role in the technique, has since been disassociated from MRI because of public apprehension about nuclear energy and nuclear weapons—neither of which is associated with MRI in any way (unless by coincidence a nuclear power plant is supplying electricity to an MRI unit). In addition, some forms of MRI do not involve the atomic nucleus and may, in the future, be used for imaging under the "magnetic resonance" umbrella.

---

*Almost all italicized terms are defined at the end of this chapter.

Comparison of Magnetic Resonance Imaging and Conventional Radiography

Because MRI provides sectional images, it serves as a useful adjunct to conventional x-ray techniques. On a radiograph, all body structures exposed to the x-ray beam are superimposed into one "flat" image. In many instances, multiple projections or contrast agents are required to clearly distinguish one anatomic structure or organ from another. Sectional imaging techniques such as ultrasonography, CT, and MRI more easily separate the various organs because there is no superimposition of structures. However, multiple *slices* (cross sections) are required to cover a single area of the body.

In addition to problems with overlapping structures, conventional radiography is relatively limited in its ability to distinguish types of tissue. In radiographic techniques, *contrast* (the ability to discriminate two different substances) depends on differences in x-ray *attenuation* within the object and the ability of the recording medium (e.g., film) to detect these differences.

Radiographs cannot detect small attenuation changes. In general, conventional radiographs can distinguish only air, fat, soft tissue, bone, and metal because of the considerable difference in attenuation with each group. Most organs, such as the liver and kidneys, cannot be separated by differences in x-ray attenuation alone unless the differences are magnified through the use of contrast agents.

CT is much more sensitive to small changes in x-ray attenuation than is plain-film radiography. Thus CT can distinguish the liver from the kidneys on the basis of their different x-ray attenuation, as well as by position.

Like CT, MRI can resolve relatively small contrast differences among tissues. It should be emphasized, however, that these tissue differences are unlike the differences in x-ray attenuation and the exiting radiation that produces the image. Contrast in MRI depends on the interaction of matter with electromagnetic forces other than x-rays.

Historical Development

The basic principle of MRI (discussed more fully in the next section) is that protons in certain atomic nuclei, if placed in a magnetic field, can be stimulated by (absorb energy from) radio waves of the correct frequency. After this stimulation the protons relax while energy is induced into a receiver antenna (the MRI signal), which is then digitized into a viewable image. *Relaxation times* represent the rates of signal decay and the return of protons to equilibrium.

The properties of magnetic resonance were first discovered in the 1940s by separate research groups headed by Bloch and Purcell. Their work led to the use of MRI *spectroscopy* for the analysis of complex molecular structures and dynamic chemical processes. In 1952 Bloch and Purcell were jointly awarded the Nobel Prize in physics, and spectroscopic MRI is still in use today.

Nearly 20 years after the properties of MRI were discovered, Damadian showed that the relaxation time of water in a tumor differed from the relaxation time of water in normal tissue. This finding suggested that images of the body might be obtained by producing maps of relaxation rates. In 1973 Lauterbur published the first cross-sectional images of objects obtained with MRI techniques. These first images were crude, and only large objects could be distinguished. Since that time, MRI technology has developed so much that tiny structures can be imaged rapidly with increased resolution and contrast.

Physical Principles

SIGNAL PRODUCTION

The structure of an atom is often compared to that of the solar system, with the sun representing the central atomic *nucleus*. The planets orbiting the sun represent the electrons circling around the nucleus. MRI depends on the properties of the nucleus. Currently, most MRI scanners use the element hydrogen, the nucleus of which is a single proton, to generate a *signal*. Hydrogen nuclei are the strongest nuclear magnets on a per-nucleus basis; thus they emit the strongest MRI signal. Also, hydrogen is the most common element in the body, which is another reason that it gives off the strongest signal. Strong signals are important to produce satisfactory images.

Many but not all atomic nuclei have magnetic properties, which means they act like tiny bar magnets (Fig. 36-1). Normally the magnetic protons point in random directions, as shown in Fig. 36-2. However, if these nuclei are placed in a strong, uniform magnetic field, they attempt to line up with the direction of the magnetic field, much as iron filings line up with the field of a toy magnet. The word *attempt* is appropriate because the protons do not line up precisely with the external field but at an angle to the field, and they rotate about the direction of the magnetic field in a manner similar to the wobbling of a spinning top. This wobbling motion, depicted in Fig. 36-3, is called *precession* and occurs at a specific *frequency* (rate) for a given atom's nucleus in a magnetic field of a specific strength. These precessing protons can absorb energy if they are exposed to *radiofrequency (RF) pulses,* which are very fast bursts of radio waves, provided that the radio waves and nuclear precession are of the same frequency. This absorption of energy occurs through the process of *resonance.*

The resonant frequency varies depending on the field strength of the MRI scanner. For example, at a field strength of 1.5 *tesla* the frequency is approximately 63 MHz; at 1 tesla, the frequency is approximately 42 MHz; at 0.5 tesla, the frequency is approximately 21 MHz; and at 0.2 tesla, the frequency is approximately 8 MHz.

Before exposure to the RF pulse, the bulk of the hydrogen protons are oriented with the direction of the magnetic field. This causes the tissues to be magnetized in the longitudinal direction, which is also parallel to the magnetic field. When the RF pulse is applied and the protons absorb the energy, the result is a reorientation of the bulk of the tissue magnetization into a plane perpendicular to the main field. This is known as the *transverse plane.* The magnetization in the transverse plane also precesses at the same resonant frequency. The precessing transverse magnetization in the tissues then creates an electrical current in the receiving *antenna.* This follows Faraday's law of induction, in which a moving magnetic field induces electrical current in a coil of wire. The electrical current in this application is measured as the MRI signal, which is much like the broadcasting radio waves that induce current in a car radio antenna.

The MRI signal is picked up by a sensitive antenna, amplified, and processed by a computer to produce a sectional image of the body. This image, like the image produced by a CT scanner, is an electronic image that can be viewed on a television monitor and adjusted to produce the most information. If desired, the image can be photographed for further study.

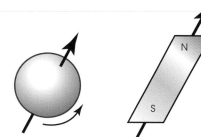

Fig. 36-1 A proton with magnetic properties can be compared to a tiny bar magnet. The *curved arrow* indicates that a proton spins on its own axis; this motion is different from that of precession.

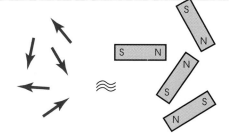

Fig. 36-2 In the absence of a strong magnetic field, the protons (*arrows*) point in random directions and cannot be used for imaging.

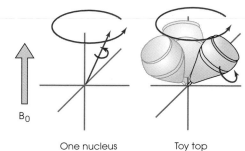

Fig. 36-3 Precession. Both the protons (*arrow*) and the toy top spin on their own axes. Both also rotate (*curved arrows*) around the direction of an external force in a wobbling motion called *precession*. Precessing protons can absorb energy through resonance. B_0 represents the external magnetic field acting on the nucleus. The toy top precesses under the influence of gravity.

Many other nuclei in the body are potential candidates for use in imaging. Nuclei from elements such as phosphorus and sodium may provide more useful or diagnostic information than hydrogen nuclei, particularly in efforts to understand the metabolism of normal and abnormal tissues. Metabolic changes may prove to be more sensitive and specific in detecting abnormalities than the more physical and structural changes recognized by hydrogen-imaging MRI or by CT. However, the MRI signal from nonhydrogen nuclei is weak, imaging requires more elaborate equipment, and to date anatomic detail produced with sodium and phosphorus MRI is less complete than that produced with hydrogen MRI. Nonhydrogen nuclei may be of particular importance for combined imaging and spectroscopy, in which small volumes of tissue may be analyzed for chemical content.

SIGNIFICANCE OF THE SIGNAL

Conventional radiographic techniques, including CT, produce images based on a single property of tissue: x-ray attenuation or density. MRI images are more complex because they contain information about three properties of tissue: nuclear density, relaxation rates, and flow phenomena. Each property contributes to the overall strength of the MRI signal. Computer processing converts signal strength to a shade of gray on the image. Strong signals are represented by white in the image, and weak signals are represented by black.

One determinant of signal strength is the number of precessing nuclei (spin density) in a given volume of tissue. The signal produced by the excited nuclei is proportional to the number of nuclei present. Therefore signal strength depends on the nuclear concentration, or density. Because the hydrogen nucleus is a single proton, its nuclear concentration is often referred to as *proton density*. Most soft tissues, including fat, have a similar number of protons per unit volume; therefore the use of proton density poorly separates most tissues. However, some tissues have few hydrogen nuclei per unit of volume; examples include the cortex of bone and air in the lungs. These have a weak signal as a result of low proton density and can be easily distinguished from other tissues.

MRI signal intensity also depends on the relaxation times of the nuclei. One component of *relaxation* is the release of energy by the excited protons, which occurs at different rates in different tissues. Excited nuclei relax through two processes. The process of nuclei releasing their excess energy to the general environment or lattice (the arrangement of atoms in a substance) is called *spin-lattice relaxation*. The rate of this relaxation process is measured by *T1*. *Spin-spin relaxation* is the release of energy by excited nuclei through interaction among themselves. The rate of this process is measured by *T2*.

The rates of relaxation (T1 and T2) of a hydrogen nucleus depend on the chemical environment in which the nucleus is located. Chemical environment differs among tissues. For example, the chemical environment of a hydrogen nucleus in the spleen differs from that of a hydrogen nucleus in the liver. Therefore the relaxation rates of these nuclei differ, and the MRI signals created by these nuclei differ. The different relaxation rates in the liver and spleen result in different signal intensities and appearances on the image, enabling the viewer to discriminate between the two organs. Similarly, fat can be separated from muscle and many tissues can be distinguished from others, based on the relaxation rates of their nuclei. Indeed, the most important factor in tissue discrimination is the relaxation time.

The signals produced by MRI techniques contain a combination of proton density and T1 and T2 information. However, it is possible to obtain images weighted toward any one of these three parameters by stimulating the nuclei with certain specific radio-wave *pulse sequences*. In most imaging sequences a short T1 (fast spin-lattice relaxation rate) produces a high MRI signal in T1-weighted images. Conversely, a long T2 (slow spin-spin relaxation rate) generates a high signal in T2-weighted images.

The final property that influences image appearance is flow. For complex physical reasons, moving substances usually have weak MRI signals. (With some specialized pulse sequences, the reverse may be true; see the discussion of magnetic resonance angiography [MRA] later in the chapter.) With standard pulse sequences, flowing blood in vessels produces a low signal and thus is easily discriminated from surrounding stationary tissues without the need for the contrast agents required by regular radiographic techniques. Stagnant blood, such as an acute blood clot, typically has a high MRI signal in most imaging schemes as a result of its short T1 and long T2. The flow sequences of MRI may facilitate the assessment of vessel patency or the determination of the rate of blood flow through vessels (Fig. 36-4).

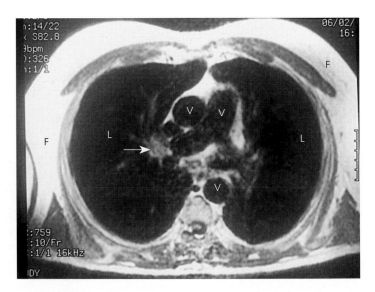

Fig. 36-4 Axial 1.5-tesla T1-weighted MRI scan through the upper chest. Lungs (*L*) have low signal as a result of low proton density. Fat (*F*) has high signal because of its short T1 relaxation rate. Moving blood in vessels (*V*) has low signal from the flow phenomenon. Hilar tumor (*arrow*) is easily identified, outlined against the low signal intensity of the lung and the vessels.

Equipment

Like CT, MRI requires a patient area (magnet room), a computer room, and an operator's console. A separate diagnostic workstation is optional.

CONSOLE

The operator's console is used to control the computer. The computer initiates the appropriate radio-wave transmissions and then receives and analyzes the data. Images are viewed on the operator's console to ensure that the proper part of the patient is being evaluated (Fig. 36-5). Images may be printed, most often on special medical film using a laser or multiimage camera.

The independent diagnostic workstation may be used to perform the same functions as those of the operator's console, depending on system configuration. However, usually only the operator's console can control the actual imaging process.

COMPUTER ROOM

The computer room houses the electronics necessary for transmitting the radio-wave pulse sequences and for receiving and analyzing the MRI signal. The *raw data* and the computer-constructed images can be stored on a computer disk temporarily but are usually transferred to a magnetic tape or an optical disk for permanent storage and retrieval.

MAGNET ROOM

The magnet is the major component of the MRI system in the scanning room. This magnet must be large enough to surround the patient and any antennas that are required for radio-wave transmission and reception. Antennas are typically wound in the shape of a positioning device for a particular body part. These are commonly referred to as *coils*. The patient is usually placed within the coil. Surface coils are placed directly on the patient and are used in the imaging of superficial structures. However, the patient and coil must still be within the magnet to be exposed to the proper magnetic field for imaging. The patient lies on the table and is advanced into the imaging magnetic field (Fig. 36-6).

Various magnet types and strengths may be used to provide the strong uniform magnetic field required for imaging.

Resistive magnets are simple but large electromagnets consisting of coils of wire. A magnetic field is produced by passing an electric current through the wire coils. High magnetic fields are produced by passing a large amount of current through a large number of coils. The electrical resistance of the wire produces heat and limits the maximum magnetic field strength of resistive magnets. The heat produced is conducted away from the magnet by a cooling system.

Superconductive (cryogenic) magnets are also electromagnets. However, their wire loops are cooled to very low temperatures with liquid helium and liquid nitrogen to reduce electrical resistance. This permits higher magnetic field strengths than those produced by resistive magnets.

Permanent magnets are a third source for producing the magnetic field. A permanent magnet has a constant field that does not require additional electricity or cooling. The early permanent magnets were extremely heavy, even when compared to the massive superconductive and resistive units; because of their weight these magnets were difficult to place for clinical use. With improvements in technology, permanent magnets have become more competitive with the other magnet types. For example, the magnetic field of permanent magnets does not extend as far away from the magnet (*fringe field*) as do the magnetic fields of other types of magnets. Fringe fields are a problem because of their effect on nearby electronic equipment.

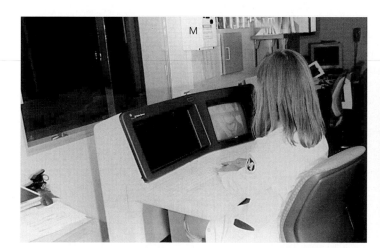

Fig. 36-5 Operator's console. This device controls the imaging process and allows visualization of images on a television monitor. Note the monitor *(M)* for magnet-room oxygen concentration.

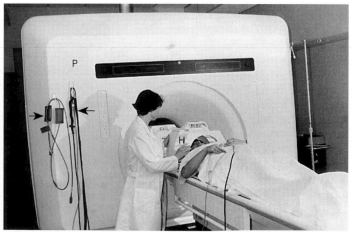

Fig. 36-6 Patient prepared for MRI. A protective housing *(P)* covers the magnet. The antenna coil for head imaging *(H)* is placed over the patient's head before both are advanced into the magnet. The head coil is removed when body imaging is performed. Note probes *(arrows)* for physiologic monitoring and gating.

Various MRI systems operate at different magnetic field strengths. The choice of optimum field strength for imaging is controversial. Magnetic field strength is measured in tesla or *gauss (G)*. Most MRI has been performed with field strengths ranging from 0.2 to 1.5 tesla. Resistive systems generally do not exceed 0.15 tesla, and permanent magnet systems do not exceed 0.3 tesla. Higher field strengths require superconductive technology. However, the U.S. Food and Drug Administration currently limits clinical MRI systems to a maximum field strength of up to 2 tesla. Most research has concluded that field strengths in this range do not produce any substantial harmful effects.

Regardless of magnet type, MRI units remain relatively difficult to install in hospitals. Current units are quite heavy—up to 10 tons for resistive and superconductive magnets and approximately 100 tons for some permanent magnets. Some institutional structures cannot support these weights without reinforcement. In addition, choosing a location for an MRI unit can be difficult because of fringe fields. With resistive and superconductive magnets, the fringe field extends in all directions and thus may interfere with nearby electronic or computer equipment, such as television monitors and computer tapes. In addition, metal objects moving through the magnetic fringe field, such as automobiles or elevators, may cause ripples in the field, similar to the ripples caused by a pebble thrown into a pond. These ripples can be carried into the center of the magnet, where they distort the field and ruin the images. Thus MRI sites must be located far enough away from moving metal objects. Efforts continue to be made to find more ways to shield the magnetic fringe field to prevent its extension beyond the patient area.

Stray radio waves present another difficulty in the placement of MRI units. The radio waves used in MRI may be the same as those used for other nearby radio applications. The stray radio waves can be picked up by the MRI antenna coils and interfere with normal image production. Many MRI facilities require specially constructed rooms to shield the antenna from outside radio interference, thus adding to the cost of the installation.

Safety of Magnetic Resonance Imaging

MRI is generally considered safe. It is often preferred over CT for the imaging of children because it does not use ionizing radiation, which has known potential adverse health effects. The young and growing child's body is thought to be more susceptible to the effects of ionizing radiation. Nevertheless, a number of potential safety issues concerning MRI must be raised, some related to potential direct effects on the patient from the imaging environment, and others related to indirect hazards.

Opinions differ about the safety of the varying magnetic and RF fields to which the patient is directly exposed. Many studies in which experimental animal and cell culture systems were exposed to these fields over long periods have reported no adverse effects, whereas others have reported changes in cell cultures and embryos. Some energy is deposited in the patient during imaging and is dissipated in the body as heat. The resulting changes appear to be less than the levels considered clinically significant, even in areas of the body with poor heat dissipation such as the lens of the eye. The significance of direct short-term exposure (i.e., exposure of a patient) and long-term exposure (i.e., exposure of an employee who works with MRI) is not clear. No clear association of MRI with adverse effects in humans has been proved, but research is continuing.

A number of hazards related to MRI have, however, been well documented. Objects containing magnetic metals (e.g., iron, nickel, cobalt) in various combinations may be attracted to the imaging magnet with sufficient force to injure patients or personnel who may be interposed between them. Scissors, oxygen tanks, and patient gurneys are among the many items that have been drawn into the magnetic field at MRI sites. Metallic implants within patients or personnel can become dislodged within the body and cause injury if they are in delicate locations.

Examples include prosthetic heart valves, intracranial aneurysm clips, auditory implants, and metallic foreign bodies in the eye. On the other hand, long-standing, firmly bound surgical clips, such as those from a cholecystectomy, do not pose problems. Electronic equipment can malfunction when exposed to strong magnetic fields. The most critical items in this category are cardiac pacemakers and the similar automatic implantable cardiac defibrillators. Therefore patients, visitors, and personnel should be screened to ensure that they do not have metallic objects on or in their bodies that could be adversely affected by exposure to strong magnetic fields.

Patients have received local burns from wires, such as electrocardiographic (ECG or EKG) leads, and other monitoring devices touching their skin during MRI examinations. These injuries have resulted from electrical burns caused by currents induced in the wires or thermal burns caused by heating of the wires. Such burns can be prevented by checking wires for frayed insulation, ensuring that no wire loops are within the magnetic field, and placing additional insulation between the patient and any wires exiting the MRI system.

The varying magnetic forces in an MRI unit act on the machine itself, causing knocking or banging sounds. These noises can be loud enough to produce temporary or permanent hearing damage. The use of earplugs or nonmagnetic headphones can be helpful in preventing auditory complications.

Claustrophobia can be a significant impediment to MRI in up to 10% of patients (Fig. 36-7). Patient education is perhaps most important in preventing this problem, but tranquilizers, appropriate lighting and air movement within the magnet bore, and mirrors or prisms that enable a patient to look out of the imager may be helpful. Claustrophobia can also be prevented by having a family member or friend accompany the patient and be present in the room during the scan.

In superconductive magnet systems, rapid venting of the supercooled liquid gases (helium and/or nitrogen) from the magnet or its storage containers into the surrounding room space is a rare but potential hazard because the relative concentration of oxygen in the air could be reduced to unsafe levels. Unconsciousness or asphyxiation could result. Oxygen monitoring devices in the magnet or cryogen storage room can signal personnel when the oxygen concentration falls too low. Personnel may then evacuate the area and activate ventilation systems to exchange the escaped gas for fresh air.

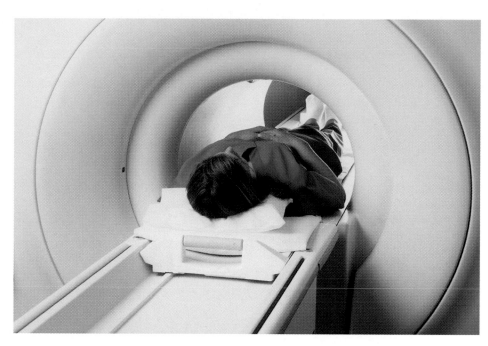

Fig. 36-7 Patient inside a superconducting 1.5-tesla magnet. Some patients cannot be scanned because of claustrophobia.

(Courtesy General Electric Medical Systems.)

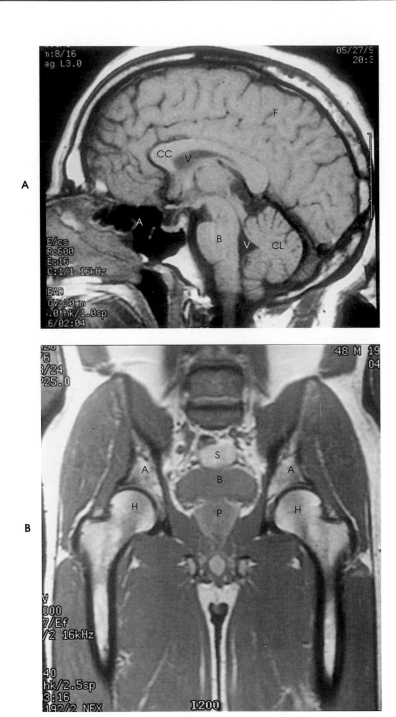

Fig. 36-8 Two images (different patients) from a 1.5-tesla superconductive MRI scanner, showing excellent resolution of images. **A,** This image shows remarkable anatomic detail in a midsagittal image of the head. Normal folds *(F)* on the inner surface of the brain are identified. *CC,* Corpus callosum; *CL,* cerebellum; *B,* brainstem; *V,* ventricle; *A,* air in sinuses. **B,** This coronal image of the pelvis shows anatomic relationships of the prostate *(P),* which is enlarged and elevating the bladder *(B).* Hips *(H)* and acetabula *(A)* are also shown. A loop of the sigmoid *(S)* colon is on top of the bladder. This degree of resolution in coronal or sagittal images would be difficult to obtain by reformatting a series of transverse CT slices.

Examination Protocols

IMAGING PARAMETERS

The availability of many adjustable parameters makes MRI a complex imaging technique. Knowledge of the patient's clinical condition or probable disease is important in choosing the proper technique and in imaging the correct area of the body.

The operator may choose to obtain MRI images in sagittal, coronal, transverse, or oblique planes. These are independently acquired images with equal resolution in any plane (Fig. 36-8). In contrast, data can be obtained only in the transverse plane with CT. Sagittal and coronal CT images can then be generated by reformatting the data from a series of transverse slices, usually with a loss of resolution.

Another MRI technique, especially when a large number of thin slices and/or multiple imaging planes are desired, is three-dimensional imaging. In this technique, MRI data are collected simultaneously from a three-dimensional block of tissue rather than from a series of slices. Special data collection techniques and subsequent computer analysis allow the images from the single imaging sequence to be displayed in any plane (Fig. 36-9).

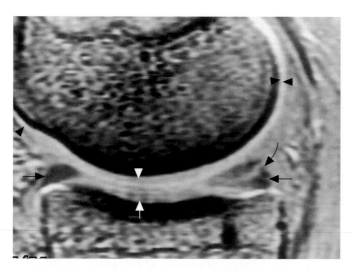

Fig. 36-9 Single slice from a three-dimensional acquisition of the knee on a 1.5-tesla MRI unit. Data from an entire volume within the imaging coil are obtained concurrently. The data may then be reconstructed into thin slices in any plane, such as the sagittal image shown here. This imaging sequence shows hyaline cartilage *(arrowheads)* as a fairly high signal intensity rim overlying the bone. Meniscal fibrocartilage *(arrows)* has low signal intensity. High signal intensity from joint fluid in a tear *(curved arrow)* within the posterior meniscus is visualized.

Slice thickness is important in the visualization of pathology. More MRI signal is available from a thicker slice than a thinner slice, so thicker slices may provide images that are less grainy. However, small pathologic lesions may be hidden by the surrounding tissues in the thicker slices. Therefore slice thickness may need to be adjusted based on the type of lesion under investigation.

Another important MRI parameter is overall imaging time. As imaging time (per slice) is lengthened, more MRI signal is available for analysis. Image quality thus improves with increased signal. However, fewer patients can be imaged when extended data acquisitions are performed. In addition, patient motion increases with prolonged imaging times; as a result, image quality is reduced.

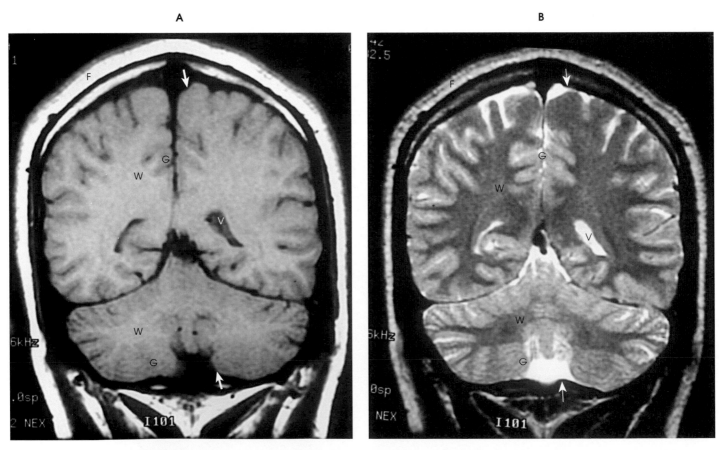

A
B

Fig. 36-10 Coronal 1.5-tesla images through a normal brain. **A,** The T1-weighted image shows relatively low differentiation of gray matter *(G)* and white matter *(W)* within the brain. **B,** The heavily T2-weighted image shows improved differentiation between gray and white matter. Cerebrospinal fluid (CSF) around the brain *(arrows)* and within the ventricles *(V)* also changes in appearance with change in pulse sequence (low signal on T1-weighted image); fat *(F)* normally shows high signal intensity, whereas on the T2-weighted image, the signal intensity of fat is less than that of CSF.

The imaging sequence is a crucial parameter in MRI. Depending on the choice of pulse sequence, the resulting images may be more strongly weighted toward proton density, T1, or T2 information. Depending on the relative emphasis given to these factors, normal anatomy (Fig. 36-10) or a pathologic lesion (Fig. 36-11) may be easily recognized or difficult to see. It is not unusual for a lesion to stand out dramatically when one pulse sequence is used, yet be nearly invisible (same MRI signal as surrounding normal tissue) with a different pulse sequence. Considerable research continues to determine the optimum pulse sequences for scanning various patient problems.

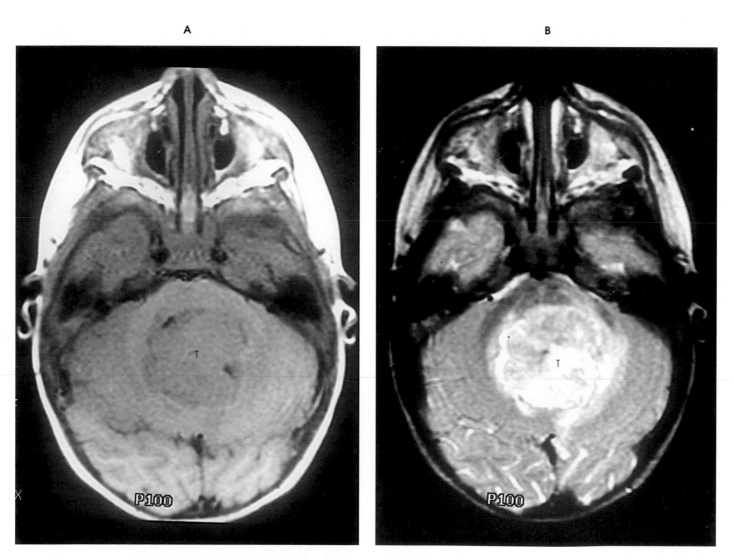

Fig. 36-11 Axial MRI scans using two different pulse sequences in a child with a medulloblastoma. **A,** The T1-weighted image shows limited contrast exists between the tumor (*T*) and normal brain. **B,** The lesion becomes dramatically more obvious using the pulse sequence of the T2-weighted image. Choice of pulse sequence is critical. These images also demonstrate how the lack of bone artifact makes MRI superior to CT for the imaging of posterior fossa lesions.

Although varying the timing parameters of an individual pulse sequence can alter the relative weighting of information received, certain classes of pulse sequences tend to emphasize information about proton density, T1, T2, and even flow. *Spin echo* sequences are the classic imaging sequences usually used with timing parameters to yield T1-weighted images, but they can also provide proton density–weighted images and T2-weighted images. *Inversion recovery* is a sequence that accentuates T1 information but can also provide a special result in that the timing parameters can be chosen to minimize signal intensity in a particular tissue. Fat is usually the tissue chosen to have its intensity minimized, and so-called *fat-suppressed images* can be useful when the high signal from extensive fat overwhelms small signal intensity differences in the tissues of interest. However, techniques to suppress the signal from fat have been developed for pulse sequences other than inversion recovery, and these newer techniques have generally replaced inversion recovery sequences for this purpose.

Standard imaging sequences such as spin echo and inversion recovery are relatively time consuming and slow patient "throughput," or productivity regarding the number of procedures per unit of time. Therefore MRI engineers and physicists have developed faster pulse sequences to speed up examinations. The oldest and most common type of faster imaging sequence is the *gradient echo* pulse sequence. In the early 1990s a fast spin-echo pulse sequence, known as *rapid acquisition recalled echo,* was created. In recent years an even faster sequence, called *echo planar imaging,* has been implemented. Some imaging sequences are short enough that imaging can be accomplished during a breath hold. Many of the fast pulse sequences are sensitive to flow and may be used to provide images of blood vessels. (See the discussion of MRA later in this chapter.)

POSITIONING

Patient positioning for MRI is usually straightforward. In general, the patient lies supine on a table that is subsequently advanced into the magnetic field. As previously discussed, it is important to ensure that the patient has no contraindications to MRI, such as a cardiac pacemaker or intracranial aneurysm clips. As previously noted, claustrophobia may be a problem for some patients because the imaging area is tunnel shaped in most MRI system configurations (see Fig. 36-7).

COILS

The body part to be examined determines the shape of the antenna coil that is used for imaging (Fig. 36-12). Most coils are round or oval in shape, and the body part to be examined is inserted into the coil's open center. Some coils, rather than encircling the body part, are placed directly on the patient over the area of interest. These surface coils are best for the imaging of thin body parts, such as the limbs, or superficial portions of a larger body structure, such as the orbit within the head or the spine within the torso. Another form of surface coil is the endocavitary coil, which is designed to fit within a body cavity such as the rectum. This enables a receiver coil to be placed close to some internal organs that may be distant from surface coils applied to the exterior body. Endocavitary coils also may be used to image the wall of the cavity itself (Fig. 36-13).

PATIENT MONITORING

Although most MRI sites are constructed so that the operator can see the patient during imaging, the visibility is often limited; thus the patient is relatively isolated within the MRI room (see Fig. 36-7). At most sites, intercoms are used for verbal communication with the patient, and some units have "panic buttons" with which the patient may summon assistance. However, these devices may be insufficient to monitor the health status of a sedated, anesthetized, or unresponsive patient. MRI-compatible devices now exist to monitor multiple physiologic parameters such as heart rate, respiratory rate, blood pressure, and oxygen concentration in the blood. Typically, leads from probes placed on extend to the operator's room, where the data are displayed on a monitor (see Fig. 36-6). Local policy and patient condition dictate which physiologic parameters are monitored.

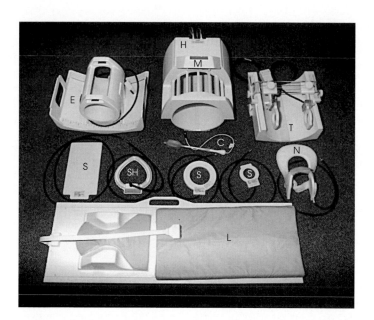

Fig. 36-12 Various coils used in MRI. The "extremity" coil (E) is used for knees and ankles. The head coil (H) has an open construction and a mirror (M); these factors allow the patient to see through the coil and out of the machine, thereby reducing claustrophobia. The shoulder coil (SH) fits over the shoulder. The neck coil (N) fits around the neck. Surface coils in a special holder (T) are used to image temporomandibular joints. Various shapes of general purpose surface coils (S) may be applied directly over the superficial part to be imaged, such as the wrist, orbit, or spine. The patient lies on a larger specialized surface coil (L) for extensive spine imaging. An endocavitary coil (C) can be placed in the rectum. All coils shown, except those used for head and limb imaging, are surface coils because the antenna does not encircle the imaged part. Any coil can act as both a radio-wave transmitter and receiver, though often an encircling coil is used as a transmitter when surface coils are used as receivers.

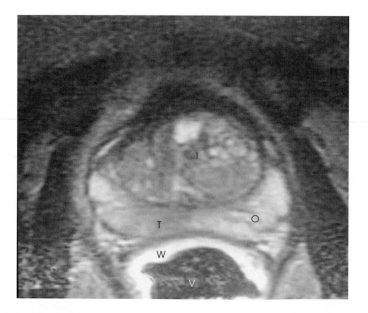

Fig. 36-13 Axial image of the prostate obtained with an endorectal coil. The mixed signal intensity in the inner gland region (I) of the prostate results from benign prostatic hyperplasia. The high-intensity outer gland (O) is interrupted by a low intensity region representing prostatic carcinoma (T). The close proximity of the endorectal coil to the area of the desired imaging improves resolution. V, Signal void from rectum (coil itself is not imaged); W, rectal wall.

CONTRAST MEDIA

Contrast agents that widen the signal differences in MRI images between various normal and abnormal structures are the subjects of a continuing research and development. A good orally administered agent for identifying bowel loops in MRI scans has not yet been identified. In CT scanning, the use of high-attenuation orally administered contrast medium allows clear differentiation of the bowel from surrounding lower-attenuation structures. However, in MRI scans, the bowel may lie adjacent to normal or pathologic structures of low, medium, and high signal intensity, and these intensities may change as images of varying T1 and T2 weighting are obtained. It is difficult to develop an agent that provides good contrast between the bowel and all other structures under these circumstances. Air, water, fatty liquids (e.g., mineral oil), dilute iron solutions (e.g., Geritol), gadolinium compounds designed for IV use, barium sulfate, kaolin (a clay), and a variety of miscellaneous agents have all been used—none with complete success.

At this time the only IV MRI contrast agents approved in the United States for routine clinical use in the whole body are gadolinium-containing compounds. Gadolinium is a metal with *paramagnetic* effects. Pharmacologically, an intravenously administered gadolinium compound acts in a manner similar to radiographic iodinated IV agents: it distributes through the vascular system, its major route of excretion is the urine, and it respects the blood-brain barrier (i.e., it does not leak out from the blood vessels into the brain substance unless the barrier has been damaged by a pathologic process). Gadolinium compounds have lower toxicity and fewer side effects than the IV iodinated contrast media used in radiography and CT.

Gadolinium compounds are used most commonly in evaluation of the central nervous system (CNS). The most important clinical action of gadolinium compounds is the shortening of T1. In T1-weighted images, this provides a high-signal, high-contrast focus in areas where gadolinium has accumulated by leaking through the broken blood-brain barrier into the brain substance (Fig. 36-14). Furthermore, in gadolinium-enhanced T1-weighted images, brain tumors or metastases are better distinguished from their surrounding edema than in routine T2-weighted images.

Gadolinium improves the visualization of small tumors or tumors that have a signal intensity similar to that of a normal brain, such as meningiomas. IV injections of gadolinium also have been used in dynamic imaging studies of body organs such as the liver and kidneys, similar to techniques using standard radiographic iodinated agents in CT.

A number of novel contrast agents for MRI are under development, but many of them are not yet approved for routine clinical use. A new manganese-based paramagnetic liver contrast agent (Teslascan) is now available. This IV-administered agent is used in the detection, characterization, localization, and evaluation of lesions of the liver. An iron oxide mixture (Feridex) is the only *superparamagnetic* contrast agent currently available. This contrast agent is also used to detect and diagnose liver lesions.

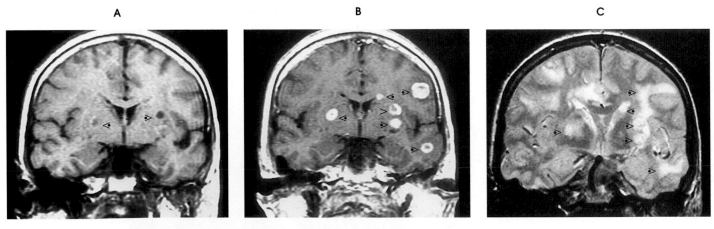

A **B** **C**

Fig. 36-14 Use of IV-administered gadolinium contrast medium for lesion enhancement in coronal images of the brain. **A,** T1-weighted sequence. Two brain metastases *(arrowheads)* are identified as focal areas of low signal. **B,** Image obtained using similar parameters after IV administration of gadolinium contrast material. Previously seen metastases are more conspicuous, and additional metastases are visualized. **C,** T2-weighted image. High signal areas *(arrowheads)* represent metastases and surrounding edema; focal lesion size and precise location are more difficult to identify. Additional high signal intensity areas on T2-weighted image represent edema from focal lesions seen on other slices in the gadolinium-enhanced series.

Contrast media currently in development include agents that are specifically designed to enhance the blood. Imaging using these agents may allow estimates of tissue perfusion and ischemia. Enhancement of heart muscle could assist in differentiating healthy, ischemic, or infarcted myocardial tissue. Contrast agents selectively taken up in the liver may improve the detection of liver tumors or metastases. Selective enhancement of lymph nodes may allow tumor involvement to be detected directly, obviating the need to rely on crude size criteria for abnormality. The production of contrast agents with an affinity for specific tumors may also be possible. Radioactive-labeled antibodies against tumors are available for use in nuclear medicine, and appropriately labeled antibodies could carry paramagnetic compounds to tumor sites.

GATING

Gated imaging is another technique for improving image quality in areas of the body in which involuntary patient motion is a problem. A patient can hold the head still for prolonged data acquisition, but the heartbeat and breathing cannot be suspended for the several minutes required for standard MRI studies. Even fast pulse sequences are susceptible to motion *artifact* from the beating heart. This is a problem when images of the chest or upper abdomen are desired. If special techniques are not used, part of the MRI signal may be obtained when the heart is contracted (systole) and part when the heart is relaxed (diastole). When information is combined into one image, the heart appears blurred. This problem is analogous to photographing a moving subject with a long shutter speed. Similar problems in MRI occur with the different phases of respiration.

Gating techniques are used to organize the signal so that only the signal received during a specific part of the cardiac or respiratory cycle is used for image production (Fig. 36-15). Gated images may be obtained in one of two ways. In one technique of cardiac gating, the imaging pulse sequence is initiated by the heartbeat (usually monitored by an ECG). Thus the data collection phase of the pulse sequence occurs at the same point in the cardiac cycle. Another method is to obtain data throughout the cardiac cycle but record the point in the cycle that each group of data was obtained. After enough data are collected, the data are reorganized so all data recorded within a certain portion of the cardiac cycle are collated together; for example, data collected during the first eighth of the cycle, second eighth of the cycle, etc. Each grouping of data can be combined into a single image, producing multiple images at different times in the cycle.

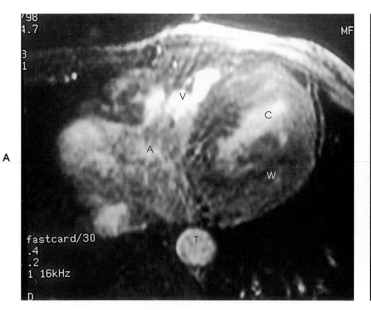
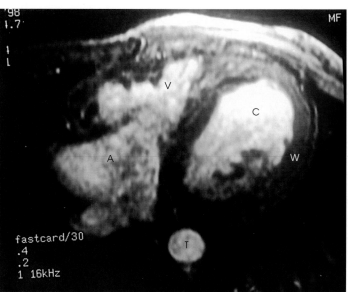

A

B

Fig. 36-15 Gated axial image of the heart in two phases of the cardiac cycle. Imaging was obtained continuously, with incoming data subdivided into various portions of the cardiac cycle. Selected images shown were obtained in systole **(A)** and diastole **(B)**. Note the reduction in the size of the left ventricular cavity (C) and the thickening of the left ventricular wall (W) during systole compared with diastole. Also shown at this level are the chambers of the right atrium (A) and right ventricle (V) and thoracic aorta (T). Note that moving blood has a high signal intensity on this cardiac pulse sequence.

The gating techniques are analogous to obtaining high-quality pictures of eight children on a spinning merry-go-round with a video camera in which the image from a single frame is of insufficient quality. If an image of only one of the children is desired, one video frame could be shot each time the child came into the video viewfinder. Later all the frames could be combined into one high-quality image. This is equivalent to the first gating technique. Alternately, if pictures of all the children are desired, the video camera could be run continuously, with documentation of which frames have which child in them. Later all the frames showing the first child could be matched together, all the frames showing the second child could be matched, and so forth. The result would be eight pictures, each showing one of the children. This is equivalent to the second gating technique.

OTHER CONSIDERATIONS

When MRI was introduced, quite long imaging times were required to obtain enough information to reconstruct the sectional images. For most routine imaging this remains the standard. With advances in technology, however, it has become possible to quickly (within seconds) obtain enough data to reconstruct an image by using special fast-imaging pulse sequences. These fast-imaging pulse sequences are becoming more popular for specialized applications such as the obtainment of a dynamic series of images after IV administration of contrast agents. In many such sequences, fluid has a high signal intensity. This can produce a myelogramlike effect in studies of the spine or an arthrogramlike effect in evaluation of joint fluid (see Fig. 36-9).

Quality assurance is important in a complex technology such as MRI. Calibration of the unit is generally performed by service personnel. However, routine scanning of phantoms can be useful for detecting any problems that may develop.

Clinical Applications
CENTRAL NERVOUS SYSTEM

MRI is superior to CT for imaging the posterior fossa, which is the portion of the brain that includes the cerebellum and brainstem. Artifact from the dense bone of the surrounding skull obscures this area in CT. This area is artifact-free with MRI because there is little MRI signal from bone (see Fig. 36-11).

In general the absence of bone artifact with MRI is a distinct advantage over CT. However, the inability to image calcified structures can be a disadvantage when the lesion is more easily recognized because of its calcium content. Calcified granulomas of the lung or calcifications in certain other tumors are more difficult to detect with MRI than with CT.

MRI is playing an increasing role in the routine examination of the brain. Because of the more natural contrast among tissues with MRI than with CT, the differentiation of gray matter from white matter in the brain is better with MRI (see Fig. 36-10). This enables MRI to be more sensitive than CT in detecting white matter disease such as multiple sclerosis.

Primary and metastatic brain tumors, pituitary tumors, and acoustic neuromas (tumors of the eighth cranial nerve) are generally better demonstrated by MRI than by CT. The use of gadolinium-based contrast agents has improved the ability of MRI to identify meningiomas (Fig. 36-16). MRI can detect cerebral infarction earlier than CT, but both tests provide similar information in subacute and chronic strokes.

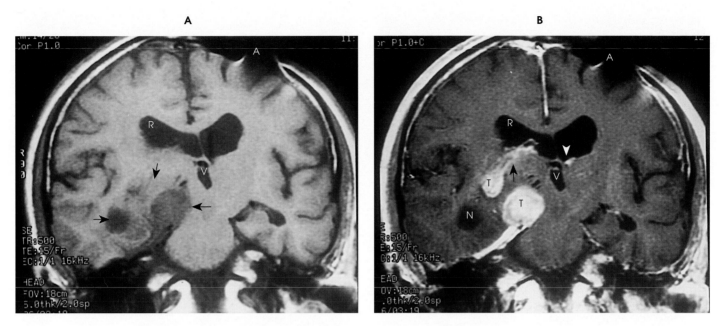

Fig. 36-16 Coronal MRI scan of the brain in a patient with a meningioma arising from the tentorium cerebelli. **A,** The precontrast T1-weighted image shows an inhomogeneous area of abnormality *(black arrows),* with mass effect elevating the right lateral ventricle *(R)* and midline shift of the third ventricle *(V).* **B,** This image was obtained at the same level after gadolinium enhancement. Active tumor *(T)* demonstrates high signal intensity, and the area of necrosis *(N)* does not enhance. Additional spread of tumor toward the ventricle *(arrows)* is visualized only after contrast enhancement. Choroid plexus *(white arrowhead)* enhances. Note that cerebrospinal fluid in the ventricles does not enhance. *(A),* Artifact from metal in skull defect from previous surgery.

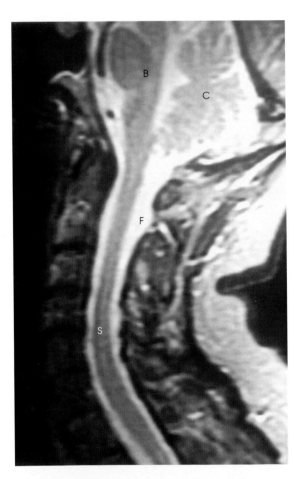

Fig. 36-17 Sagittal T2-weighted MRI scan through the upper cervical spine and brainstem. The high signal from cerebrospinal fluid *(F)* outlines the normal brain stem *(B)*, cerebellum *(C)*, and spinal cord *(S)*, giving a myelogram-like effect without the use of contrast agents.

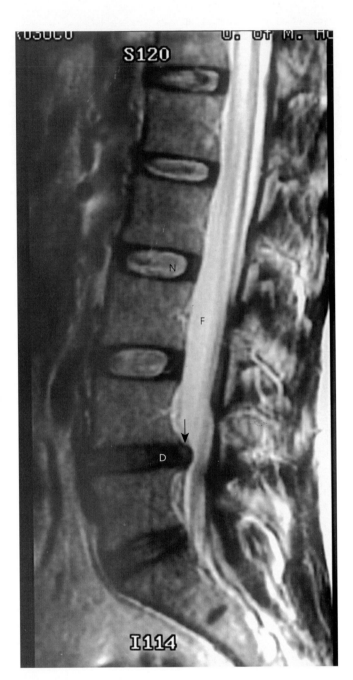

Fig. 36-18 Sagittal T2-weighted image of the lumbar spine. The spinal canal is filled with high signal intensity cerebrospinal fluid *(F)* except for low signal intensity linear nerve roots running within the spinal canal. Normal vertebral disks have a high signal intensity nucleus pulposus *(N)*. Desiccated disks *(D)* show low signal intensity. At L4-L5, note the herniated disk *(arrow)* protruding into the spinal canal and compressing the nerve roots.

MRI has been successfully used to image the spinal cord. The absence of bone artifact allows excellent visualization of the contents of the neural canal. In addition, the technique can separate the spinal cord from the surrounding cerebrospinal fluid (CSF) without the use of the contrast agents (as required for CT) injected directly into the CSF during radiographic myelography (Fig. 36-17). MRI is sensitive in detecting spinal cord tumors and cystic changes of the spine (syringomyelia). MRI is also valuable in the detection of degenerated and herniated vertebral disks (Fig. 36-18).

CHEST

The chest would seem to be an ideal area for MRI examination because of its anatomy. The lungs have low signal as a result of low proton density, and the flowing blood in the great vessels of the chest also has a low MRI signal when standard pulse sequences are used. The heart muscle is well outlined by the lung and moving blood within the chambers. Furthermore, examination of the mediastinum is potentially fruitful because the normal structures of blood vessels and airways are of low signal. Any tumors of the mediastinum are easily seen as areas of MRI signal standing out against the normal low-signal surroundings (see Fig. 36-4). In addition, the ability of MRI to image in multiple planes may be helpful in evaluating tumor spread in the thoracic inlet, chest wall, or brachial plexus region (Fig. 36-19).

Nonetheless, difficulties with chest imaging remain because of cardiac and respiratory motion. Cardiac gating has markedly improved visualization of the heart with demonstration of septal defects and the cardiac valve leaflets. This is of great value in the study of congenital heart disease. Evaluation of the heart muscle for ischemia or infarction may require MRI contrast agents. Respiratory gating should help chest images.

A

B

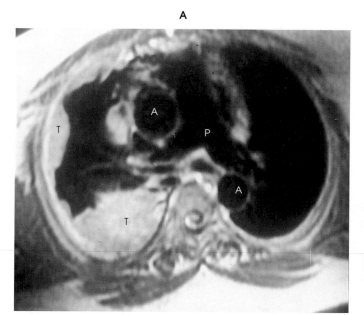
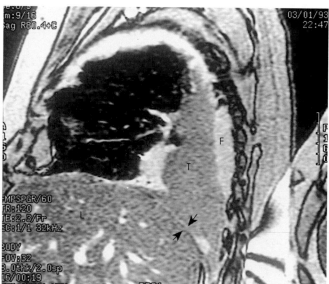

Fig. 36-19 MRI chest images in a patient with extensive mesothelioma. **A,** Image shows axial proton density-weighted image through the middle mediastinum. Because of flow void phenomenon, the ascending and descending aorta (A) and pulmonary artery (P) are well visualized. Extensive rind of tumor (T) is visualized. **B,** This sagittal fast sequence image was obtained with breath holding. Although this is a somewhat more noisy image, the lack of motion artifact allows evaluation of the diaphragm. A thin line of diaphragm and fluid (arrows) is intact between the liver (L) and tumor (T), indicating that the tumor has not invaded through the diaphragm. Some pleural fluid (F) is visualized around the tumor in the pleural space.

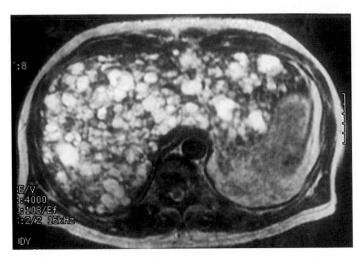

Fig. 36-20 Axial heavily T2-weighted MRI scan through the liver in a patient with hemangiocarcinoma. The multiple lesions of this tumor have virtually replaced the entire liver. No contrast agents were required to demonstrate these multiple liver lesions.

ABDOMEN

Respiratory and cardiac motion also detract from upper abdominal images. Again, gating should be of assistance. Evidence exists that MRI is more sensitive than CT in detecting primary and metastatic tumors of the liver (Fig. 36-20). The suprarenals, kidneys, and retroperitoneal structures such as lymph nodes are seen well with MRI. However, limited evidence exists that MRI is superior to CT for abdominal imaging, particularly general screening for abnormalities. Visualization of the normal pancreas has been difficult with MRI.

MRI has some ability to predict the histologic diagnosis of certain abnormalities. For example, hepatic hemangiomas (common benign tumors of the liver) have a distinctive MRI appearance that can be helpful in ruling out other causes of hepatic masses. Patterns of enhancement with gadolinium-based contrast agents can assist in evaluating various tumors (Fig. 36-21).

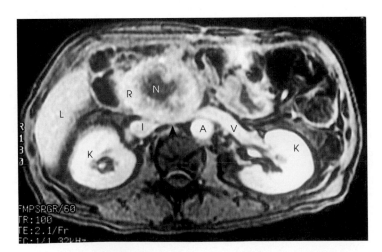

Fig. 36-21 Axial fast sequence MRI of the central abdomen in a patient with a pancreatic islet cell tumor after gadolinium injection. Enhancement of the rim of the mass *(R)* indicates necrosis *(N)* in a central portion of mass that does not enhance. Also well visualized is the relationship of the mass to vessels, such as compression *(arrowhead)* of left renal vein *(V)*. A, Aorta; *I,* inferior vena cava; *K,* kidney; *L,* lower tip of liver.

PELVIS

Respiratory motion has little effect on the structures in the pelvis. As a result, these structures can be better visualized than those in the upper abdomen. The ability of MRI to image in the coronal and sagittal planes is helpful in examining the curved surfaces in the pelvis. For example, bladder tumors are shown well, including those at the dome and base of the bladder that can be difficult to evaluate in the transverse dimension. In the prostate (see Fig. 36-13) and female genital tract (Fig. 36-22), MRI is useful in detecting neoplasm and its spread.

MUSCULOSKELETAL SYSTEM

MRI produces excellent images of the limbs because involuntary motion is not a problem and MRI contrast among the soft tissues is excellent. The lack of bone artifact in MRI permits excellent visualization of the bone marrow (Fig. 36-23). In plain-film radiography and occasionally in CT, dense cortical bone is often hidden in the marrow space. However, as previously stated, calcium within tumors is better visualized with CT because of the lower MRI signal from calcium.

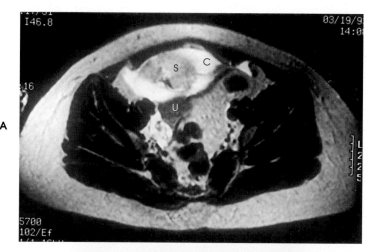

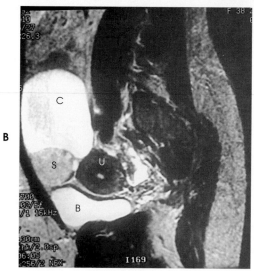

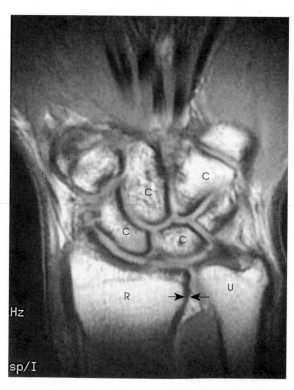

Fig. 36-22 T2-weighted images through the pelvis of a woman. **A,** Axial image. **B,** Sagittal image. Both images show solid (S) and cystic (C) components of a large ovarian tumor. The relationship to the uterus (U) and bladder (B) is also shown well using multiple imaging planes.

Fig. 36-23 Coronal MRI scan of the wrist using a surface coil to improve visualization of superficial structures. Marrow within the carpal bones (C), radius (R), and ulna (U) has high signal as a result of its fat content. A thin black line of low-signal cortex (arrows) surrounds the marrow cavity of each bone, and trabecular bone can be seen as low signal detail interspersed within marrow.

Overall, the ability to image in multiple planes, along with excellent visualization of soft tissues and bone marrow, has rapidly expanded the role of MRI in musculoskeletal imaging. MRI is particularly valuable for the study of joints, and it is replacing arthrography and to a lesser extent arthroscopy in the evaluation of the injured knee (see Fig. 36-9), ankle, and shoulder. Small joints also are well evaluated with MRI. Local staging of soft tissue and bone tumors is best accomplished with MRI (Fig. 36-24). Early detection of ischemic necrosis of bone is another strength of MRI (Fig. 36-25).

VESSELS

The contrast between soft tissue structures and the typical low signal of flowing blood using standard pulse sequences gives MRI the ability to visualize thrombosis within major vessels such as the venae cavae or the tumor invasion of these vessels. Vascular anomalies, dissections, and coarctations also can be well evaluated by MRI. Special pulse sequences allow MRI visualization of moving blood within the vascular system (Fig. 36-26). These noninvasive angiogramlike images of the vessels (magnetic resonance angiograms) improve the visualization of vascular lesions.

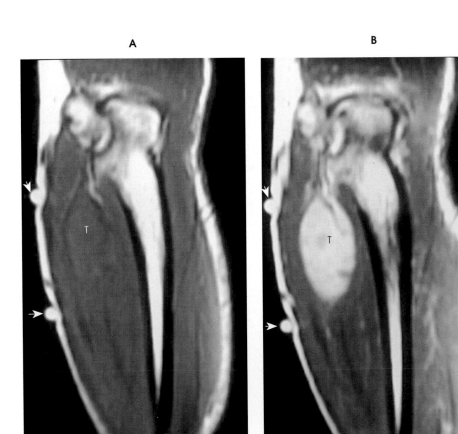
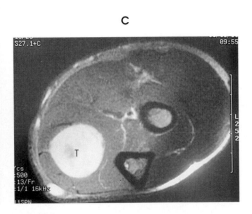

Fig. 36-24 Coronal and axial images of the arm obtained with T1 weighting. **A,** Image obtained before contrast administration. **B** and **C,** Images obtained after IV gadolinium injection. Little contrast between neurofibroma (*T*) and normal tissue is seen before enhancement; the tumor is markedly enhanced after gadolinium injection. The location of the tumor is evident before contrast injection, only because the palpable mass is marked externally with vitamin E capsules (*arrowheads*). The relationship of the tumor to muscles and bone is evident in the coronal and axial sections.

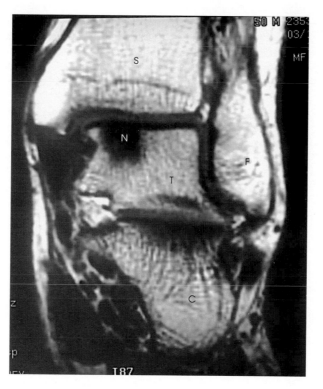

Fig. 36-25 Coronal T1-weighted image of the ankle. The bone marrow demonstrates high signal intensity because of fat. A focal area *(N)* of devascularization at the dome of the talus *(T)* shows low signal intensity. However, the overlying bony cortex and cartilage are intact. *S,* Tibia; *F,* fibula; *C,* calcaneus.

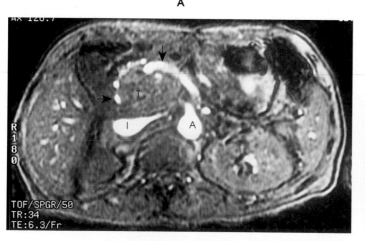

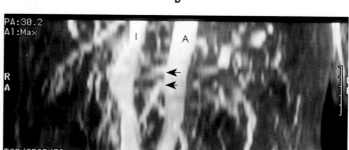

Fig. 36-26 MRA images obtained in the midabdomen. Time-of-flight sequence was used to demonstrate vessels. Blood shows high signal intensity. However, the contrast of non-moving soft tissues is reduced. **A,** This image demonstrates vessels *(arrows)* displaced around the pancreatic islet cell tumor *(T)* in the same patient as in Fig. 36-21. **B,** This image represents superimposition of multiple axial images and is viewed from an oblique coronal projection. The inferior vena cava *(I),* aorta *(A),* and their branches are demonstrated. The *upper arrow* marks the celiac artery, and the *lower arrow* marks the superior mesenteric artery.

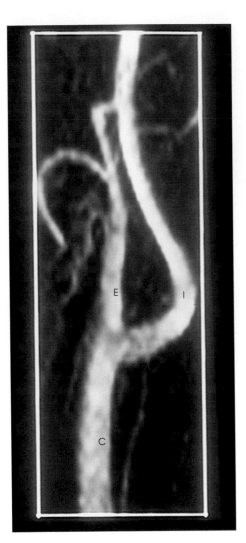

The carotid arteries in the neck (Fig. 36-27) and their intracranial branches (Fig. 36-28) can be studied for aneurysms, arteriovenous malformations, plaques, stenoses, and occlusions. Small arteries in the peripheral vascular system also can be studied. Flow studies of the thoracic and abdominal vessels are more difficult, but specialized fast sequences permit cardiac gated images to be obtained during a single breath hold. Typical uses include evaluation of the thoracic aorta for dissections, the abdominal aorta for aneurysms, and the renal arteries for stenoses.

Two common techniques to obtain images of flowing blood are time-of-flight and phase-contrast MRA. Using either of these techniques, magnetic resonance angiograms can be obtained in two-dimensional (obtaining a series of slices) or three-dimensional images. In time-of-flight imaging, a special pulse sequence is used that suppresses the MRI signal from the anatomic area under study (see Fig. 36-27). Consequently, an MRI signal is given only by material that is outside the area of study when the signal-suppressing pulse occurs. Thus incoming blood makes vessels appear bright, whereas stationary tissue signal is suppressed. Phase-contrast imaging takes advantage of the shifts in phase, or orientation, experienced by magnetic nuclei moving through the MRI field (see Fig. 36-28). Special pulse sequences enhance these effects in flowing blood, producing a bright signal in vessels when the unchanging signal from stationary tissue is subtracted.

Gadolinium-based contrast agents also can be useful in MRA studies. Many MRA schemes use fast pulse sequences to reduce overall imaging time, particularly with three-dimensional vascular imaging. For better contrast in images obtained with fast sequences, a gadolinium-based intravascular contrast agent may be injected to shorten the T1 of blood in order to increase its signal intensity.

Fig. 36-27 Two-dimensional time-of-flight image of the carotid bifurcation. The normal appearance of the common (C), internal (I), and external (E) carotid arteries is well demonstrated. Slight ribbed irregularity of the edges is present because the image is constructed from a series of two-dimensional images.

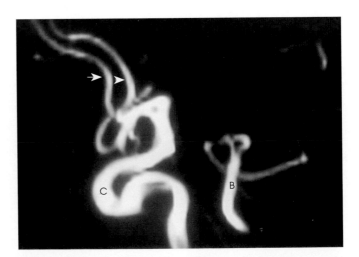

Fig. 36-28 Sagittal image of the cerebral circulation obtained by a three-dimensional phase-contrast pulse sequence. The image displays the midline and right-sided vessels. The left-sided vessels have been electronically removed for clarity. The carotid artery (C) and its major branches, including the anterior cerebral arteries (arrows), are well visualized. The basilar artery (B) and its branches are also demonstrated.

DIFFUSION AND PERFUSION

The sensitivity of MRI to motion can be both a handicap and a potential source of information. For example, motion artifacts interfere with upper abdominal images that are affected by heart and diaphragmatic motion, yet flow-sensitive pulse sequences can image flowing blood in blood vessels.

Specialized techniques that can image the *diffusion* and *perfusion* of molecules within matter are currently under investigation. Molecules of water undergo random motion within tissues, but the rate of this diffusion is affected by cellular membranes and macromolecules as well as by temperature. Molecules are also moving slowly through tissues with the perfusion of blood into the small capillary vessels.

Tissues have structure, and this structure affects both the rates of diffusion and perfusion and their direction; in other words, diffusion and perfusion are not entirely random in a structured tissue. These microscopic motions can be detected by specialized MRI pulse sequences that can image their rate and direction. Diffusion and perfusion motion differ between tissue types. For example, diffusion patterns of gray matter in the brain differ from the diffusion patterns in more directionally oriented fiber tracts of white matter. For technical reasons, most diffusion and perfusion imaging research has focused on the central nervous system.

Diffusion and perfusion imaging can produce clinically significant images that may help in the understanding of white matter degenerative diseases (e.g., multiple sclerosis, ischemia, infarction), the development of possible therapies to return blood flow to underperfused brain tissue, and the characterization of brain tumors. Similar applications for the rest of the body may be developed if technical difficulties, particularly those related to patient motion such as breathing, can be overcome.

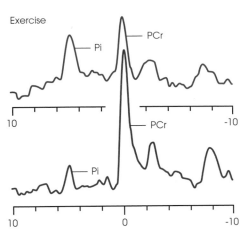

Exercise

Pi

PCr

10   PCr   -10

Pi

10   0   -10

Fig. 36-29 Spectra from human muscle before *(red line)* and during *(blue line)* exercise. The thin horizontal lines represent separate baselines for each spectrum. Each peak represents a different chemical species, and the area under the peak down to the baseline indicates the amount of substance present. The inorganic phosphate *(Pi)* peak increases with exercise as energy-rich phosphocreatine *(PCr)* is used to provide energy for muscle contraction.

Spectroscopy

With MRI it is generally assumed that each nucleus in a specific small area in space is exposed to the same magnetic field and thus precesses at a particular frequency and releases energy of that frequency. If the magnetic field varies across the imaging volume in a known way, frequency can be used as one determinant of the location from which a signal is originating. A one-to-one relationship between frequency and location is an integral part of creating the image in MRI. In actuality, however, each nucleus in a small area in space does not detect precisely the same magnetic field. The externally imposed field is the same, but the magnetic environments of the nuclei differ, depending on the magnetic effects of other nearby atoms. These differences in frequencies are small and generally do not affect the image significantly; each signal is still placed in the correct position in the image. In magnetic resonance spectroscopy a detailed graph of signal strength against frequency is produced instead of an image. The graphs produced are called *spectra*.

Spectroscopy is essentially a tool for clinical analysis that can determine the relative quantity of chemical substances within a volume of tissue. Because the frequency differences are small and electronic noise is relatively high, large volumes of tissue must be studied to receive enough total signal to produce useful spectra. Nevertheless, it is possible to obtain spectra from organs (e.g., muscle, liver) or large masses to examine normal physiologic changes (e.g., with exercise), chemical alterations in persons with metabolic diseases, or differences in chemical composition between normal tissue and tumors or other pathologic processes (Fig. 36-29). Spectroscopy of the CNS is now widely accepted and routinely used (Fig. 36-30).

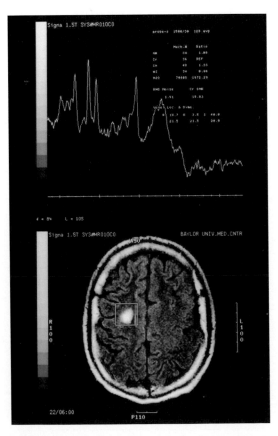

Fig. 36-30 Routine spectroscopy technique in a 31-year-old male patient. The study shows toxoplasmosis with schizencephaly and pachygyria.

Conclusion

MRI is an exciting form of imaging that examines properties of tissue never before visualized. Thousands of publications have attested to the effectiveness of MRI for evaluating various clinical conditions. However, it is more difficult to prove that MRI is clinically superior to all other imaging modalities. Although comparative studies have been completed for some clinical situations, more extensive research is needed for others. In some cases, various imaging modalities are complementary.

MRI is an expensive imaging technology. With the recent increased emphasis on cost constraints, the use of MRI will not expand as quickly as it otherwise might have. MRI will also have to compete with other modalities for an imaging "niche." Nevertheless, MRI is clearly the technique of choice in many clinical situations. MRI applications continue to increase, in part because of the extreme flexibility of this imaging modality. New pulse sequences can be programmed into the computer, and new contrast agents are under development; both provide new information about anatomy and pathology. Thus, despite cost constraints, the depth and breadth of the role of MRI in diagnostic imaging continue to increase.

Definition of Terms

antenna Device for transmitting or receiving radio waves.

artifact Spurious finding in or distortion of an image.

attenuation Reduction in energy or amount of a beam of radiation when it passes through tissue or other substances.

coil Single or multiple loops of wire (or another electrical conductor such as tubing) designed to produce a magnetic field from current flowing through the wire or to detect a changing magnetic field by voltage induced in the wire.

contrast Degree of difference between two substances in some parameter. The parameter varying depending on the technique used; for example, attenuation in radiographic techniques or signal strength in MRI.

cryogenic Relating to extremely low temperature (see *superconductive magnet*).

diffusion Spontaneous random motion of molecules in a medium; a natural and continuous process.

echo planar imaging Fast pulse sequence that can be used to create magnetic resonance images within a few seconds.

frequency Number of times that a process repeats itself in a given period; for example, the frequency of a radio wave is the number of complete waves per second.

fringe field That portion of the magnetic field extending away from the confines of the magnet that cannot be used for imaging but can affect nearby equipment or personnel.

gating Organizing the data so that the information used to construct the image comes from the same point in the cycle of a repeating motion, such as a heartbeat. The moving object is "frozen" at that phase of its motion, reducing image blurring.

gauss (G) Unit of magnetic field strength (see *tesla*).

gradient echo Fast pulse sequence that is often used with three-dimensional imaging to generate T2-weighted images.

inversion recovery Standard pulse sequence available on most MRI imagers, usually used for T1-weighted images. The name indicates that the direction of longitudinal magnetization is reversed (inverted) before relaxation (recovery) occurs.

magnetic resonance (MR) Process by which certain nuclei, when placed in a magnetic field, can absorb and release energy in the form of radio waves. This technique can be used for chemical analysis or for the production of cross-sectional images of body parts. Computer analysis of the radio wave data is required.

noise Random contributions to the total signal that arise from stray external radio waves, imperfect electronic apparatus, etc. Noise cannot be eliminated, but it can be minimized; it tends to degrade the image by interfering with accurate measurement of the true MRI signal, similar to the difficulty in maintaining a clear conversation in a noisy room.

nuclear magnetic resonance (NMR) Another name for magnetic resonance.

nucleus Central portion of an atom, composed of protons and neutrons.

paramagnetic Referring to materials that alter the magnetic field of nearby nuclei. Paramagnetic substances are not themselves directly imaged by MRI but instead change the signal intensity of the tissue where they localize, thus acting as MRI contrast agents. Paramagnetic agents shorten both the T1 and T2 of the tissues they affect, actions that tend to have opposing effects on signal intensity. In clinical practice, agents are administered in a concentration in which either T1 or T2 shortening predominates (usually the former) to provide high signal on T1-weighted images.

perfusion Flow of blood through the vessels of an organ or anatomic structure; usually refers to blood flow in the small vessels (e.g., capillary perfusion).

permanent magnet Object that produces a magnetic field without requiring an external electricity supply.

precession Rotation of an object around the direction of a force acting on that object. This should not be confused with the axis of rotation of the object itself; for example, a spinning top rotates on its own axis, but it may also precess (wobble) around the direction of the force of gravity that is acting on it.

proton density Measure of proton (i.e., hydrogen, because its nucleus is a single proton) concentration (number of nuclei per given volume). One of the major determinants of MRI signal strength in hydrogen imaging.

pulse See *radiofrequency (RF) pulse*.

pulse sequence Series of radio-wave pulses designed to excite nuclei in such a way that their energy release has varying contributions from proton density, T1, or T2 processes.

rapid acquisition recalled echo Commonly known as *fast,* or *turbo, spin echo;* a fast pulse sequence used to rapidly create spin-echolike T2-weighted images.

raw data Information obtained by radio reception of the MRI signal as stored by a computer. Specific computer manipulation of these data is required to construct an image from them.

radiofrequency (RF) pulse A short burst of radio waves. If the radio waves are of the appropriate frequency, they can give energy to nuclei that are within a magnetic field by the process of *magnetic resonance.* The length of the pulse determines the amount of energy given to the nuclei.

relaxation Return of excited nuclei to their normal, unexcited state by the release of energy.

relaxation time Measure of the rate at which nuclei, after stimulation, release their extra energy.

resistive magnet Simple electromagnet in which electricity passing through coils of wire produces a magnetic field.

resonance Process of energy absorption by an object that is tuned to absorb energy of a specific frequency only. All other frequencies will not affect the object; for example, if one tuning fork is struck in a room full of tuning forks, only those forks tuned to that identical frequency will vibrate (resonate).

signal In MRI, the induction of current into a receiver coil by the precessing magnetization.

slice Cross-sectional image; can also refer to the thin section of the body from which data are acquired to produce the image.

spectroscopy Science of analyzing the components of an electromagnetic wave, usually after its interaction with some substance (to obtain information about that substance).

spin echo Standard MRI pulse sequence that can provide T1-, T2-, or proton density–weighted images. The name indicates that a declining MRI signal is refocused to gain strength (like an echo) before it is recorded as raw data.

spin-lattice relaxation Release of energy by excited nuclei to their general environment. One of the major determinants of MRI signal strength. T1 is a rate constant measuring spin-lattice relaxation.

spin-spin relaxation Release of energy by excited nuclei as a result of interaction among themselves; one of the major determinants of MRI signal strength. T2 is a rate constant measuring spin-spin relaxation.

superconductive magnet Electromagnet in which the coils of wire are cooled to extremely low temperature so that the resistance to the conduction of electricity is nearly eliminated (superconductive).

superparamagnetic Material that has a greater effect with a magnetic field; it can dramatically decrease the T2 of tissues, causing a total loss of signal by the absorbing structures.

T1 Rate constant measuring spin-lattice relaxation.

T2 Rate constant measuring spin-spin relaxation.

tesla (T) Unit of magnetic field strength; 1 tesla equals 10,000 gauss or 10 kilogauss (other units of magnetic field strength). The Earth's magnetic field approximates 0.5 gauss.

Selected bibliography

Atlas SW et al, eds: Gadolinium contrast agents in neuro-MRI, *J Comput Assist sTomogr* 17:S1,1993.

Axel L, ed: *Glossary of MRI terms*, ed 3, Reston, Va, 1991, American College of Radiology.

Bellon EM et al: Magnetic resonance imaging of internal derangements of the knee, *Radiographics* 8:95,1988.

Bloch F: Nuclear induction, *Physiol Rev* 70:460,1946.

Boechat MI et al: MR imaging of the abdomen in children, *AJR, Am J Roentgenol* 152:1245,1989.

Bottomley PA: Human in vivo NMR spectroscopy in diagnostic medicine: clinical tool or research probe? *Radiology* 170:1,1989.

Brant-Zawadzki M: MR imaging of the brain, *Radiology* 166:1,1988.

Brasch RC: New directions in the development of MR imaging contrast media, *Radiology* 183:1,1992.

Bushong SC: *MRI physical and biological principles,* ed 2, St Louis, 1996, Mosby.

Chenevert TL et al: Anisotropic diffusion in human white matter: demonstration with MR techniques in vivo, *Radiology* 177:401,1990.

Chezmar JL et al: Liver and abdominal screening in patients with cancer: CT versus MR imaging, *Radiology* 168:43,1988.

Chien D et al: Basic principles and clinical applications of magnetic resonance angiography, *Semin Roentgenol* 27:53,1992.

Council on Scientific Affairs, American Medical Association: Magnetic resonance imaging of the abdomen and pelvis, *JAMA* 261:420,1989.

Damadian R: Tumor detection by nuclear magnetic resonance, *Science* 171:1151, 1971.

Ehman RL et al: MR imaging of the musculoskeletal system: a 5-year appraisal, *Radiology* 166:313,1988.

Ellis JH et al: Resistive magnet systems: an MRI "whether" report, *Diagn Imaging* 6:60,1984.

Ellis JH et al: NMR physics for physicians, *Indiana Med* 78:20,1985.

Elster AD: *Questions and answers in MRI,* St Louis, 1994, Mosby.

Evens RG et al: Economic and utilization analysis of MR imaging units in the United States in 1987, *Radiology* 166:27,1988.

Francis IR et al: Integrated imaging of adrenal disease, *Radiology* 184:1,1992.

Glazer GM: MR imaging of the liver, kidneys, and adrenal glands, *Radiology* 166:303, 1988.

Haughton VM: MR imaging of the spine, *Radiology* 166:297,1988.

Heiken JP et al: MR imaging of the pelvis, *Radiology* 166:11,1988.

Hendrick RE et al: Basic physics of MR contrast agents and maximization of image contrast, *J Mag Reson Imaging* 3:137,1993.

Kanal E et al: Safety considerations in MR imaging, *Radiology* 176:593,1990.

Kanal E et al: Patient monitoring during clinical MR imaging, *Radiology* 185:623,1992.

Kanzer GK et al: Magnetic resonance imaging of diseases of the liver and biliary system, *Radiol Clin North Am* 29:1259,1991.

Kelley LL: *Sectional anatomy for imaging professionals,* St Louis, 1997, Mosby.

Kneeland JB et al: High-resolution MR imaging with local coils, *Radiology* 171:1,1989.

Lauterbur PC: Image formation by induced local interactions: examples employing nuclear magnetic resonance, *Nature* 242:190, 1973.

LeBihan D et al: Diffusion MR imaging: clinical applications, *AJR, Am J Roentgenol* 159:591,1992.

Lee SH et al, eds: Imaging in neuroradiology I and II, *Radiol Clin North Am* 26:701,1988.

Mitchell DG et al: The biophysical basis of tissue contrast in extracranial MR imaging, *AJR, Am J Roentgenol* 149:831,1987.

Moser RP, editor: Imaging of bone and soft tissue tumors, *Radiol Clin North Am* 31:237, 1993.

Nghiem HV et al: The pelvis: T2-weighted fast spin-echo MR imaging, *Radiology* 185:213, 1992.

Owen RS et al: Symptomatic peripheral vascular disease: selection of imaging parameters and clinical evaluation with MR angiography, *Radiology* 187:627,1993.

Potchen EJ, ed: Magnetic resonance angiography, *Semin Ultrasound CT MR* 13:225, 1992.

Purcell EM et al: Resonance absorption by nuclear magnetic moments in a solid, *Physiol Rev* 69:37,1946.

Sartoris DJ et al: MR imaging of the musculoskeletal system: current and future status, *AJR, Am J Roentgenol* 149:457,1987.

Shellock FG: MR *Bioeffects, safety, and patient management,* ed 2, Philadelphia, 1996, Lippincott-Raven.

Stehling MJ et al: Whole-body echo-planar MR imaging at 0.5 T, *Radiology* 170:257,1989.

Turner R et al: Echo-planar imaging of intravoxel incoherent motion, *Radiology* 177:407,1990.

Webb WR et al: MR imaging of thoracic disease: clinical uses, *Radiology* 182:621, 1992.

Wehrli FW: *Fast-scan magnetic resonance: principles and applications,* New York, 1991, Raven Press.

Woodward P: *MRI for technologists,* New York, 1995, McGraw-Hill.

Young SW: *Magnetic resonance imaging: basic principles,* ed 2, New York, 1988, Raven Press.

37

DIAGNOSTIC ULTRASOUND

SANDRA L. HAGEN-ANSERT

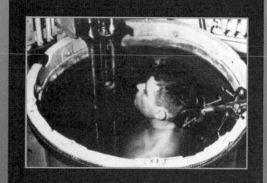

RIGHT: Scanning position for a patient in the fluid-filled B-29 gun turret scanner, 1954. On a transverse cross section of the neck, the 2-inch (6-cm) focus transducer is just below the water level. The transducer carriage travels around the tank on the outside track.

(From Holmes JH: Diagnostic ultrasound historical perspective. In King DL, editor: *Diagnostic ultrasound,* St. Louis, 1974, Mosby.)

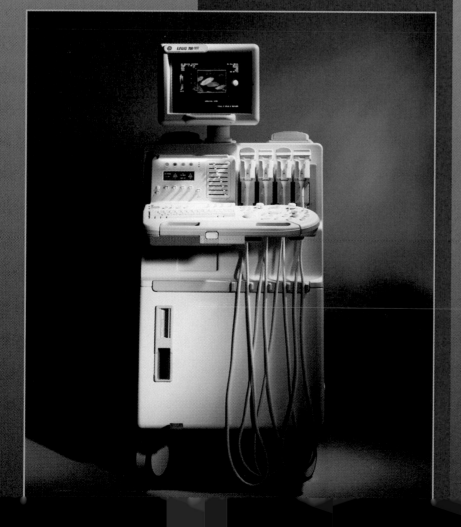

LEFT: Modern ultrasound equipment produces images with nonionizing radiation.

(Courtesy General Electric Medical Systems.)

Principles of Diagnostic Ultrasound

Diagnostic *ultrasound,*[1] sometimes called *diagnostic medical sonography, sonography, ultrasonography, vascular sonography,* or *echocardiography,* has become a clinically valuable imaging technique over the past four decades. Ultrasound differs from diagnostic radiography in that it uses nonionizing, high-frequency sound waves to generate an image of a particular structure in the body. Radiography is useful for visualizing dense bony structures and air-filled or contrast-filled structures such as the lungs, stomach, colon, or small bowel. In contrast, ultrasound is employed for visualization of soft tissue interfaces of homogeneous, fluid-filled, or solid organs, tumor masses, and muscles located within the body.

The blood flow velocities of a vessel may be calculated with the *Doppler* technique. *Pulsed-wave, continuous-wave (CW),* and *color-flow mapping* techniques have been shown to be clinically useful in determining not only the direction of blood flow within vessels but also the resistance, turbulence, or regurgitation of flow.

Diagnostic ultrasound has many advantages over other imaging techniques. One advantage is its mobility. The ultrasound system may be easily moved into the surgical suite, emergency room, neonatal nursery, or intensive care unit. The ultrasound system may also be wheeled onto a van to provide services for small hospitals and clinics that may not be able to employ a full-time sonographer. Ultrasound is more cost-effective than computed tomography (CT), magnetic resonance imaging (MRI), and angiography (see Chapters 33, 36, and 26, respectively). The versatility of ultrasound equipment allows flexibility in hospital schedules. Furthermore, minimal supplies are needed to run the ultrasound laboratory, and equipment costs much less than for other imaging modalities.

---

[1]Almost all italicized terms are defined at the end of this chapter.

Ultrasound, once considered a *noninvasive technique,* now includes examinations that involve transvaginal, transrectal, and transesophageal transducers. Intraluminal transducers have given cardiovascular surgeons an advanced "window" for viewing the intima of the vascular system such as during a cardiac catheterization or during an open surgical case. Three-dimensional reconstruction has produced exquisite images of the intracardiac structures. Contrast media for further enhanced visualization of the pancreas, and the small and large bowel are presently being evaluated clinically.

SONOGRAPHER

The diagnostic medical sonographer performs ultrasound studies and gathers diagnostic imaging data under the direct or indirect supervision of a physician. The sonographer has the ability to "look" inside organs such as the liver, gallbladder, pancreas, spleen, and kidney.

The sonographer approaches the evaluation of the patient in a manner very different from the radiographer. The principal difference lies in the sonographer's knowledge of detailed anatomy and pathophysiology. An understanding of the three-dimensional anatomy and reconstruction of the sonographic image is necessary for the sonographer to produce an adequate image.

The sonographer must have intellectual curiosity because the examination of each patient can present special challenges. This imaging professional needs to have an analytic capability coupled with perseverance to obtain high-quality images. Furthermore, the sonographer must enjoy both working with complex equipment and communicating with patients.

On a daily basis the sonographer works directly with patients and members of the health care team. Tasks include reviewing the patient's medical chart to record pertinent information before the ultrasound examination, determining the equipment to use and the image planes that will yield the most information, and explaining the details of the examination to the patient. Throughout the examination the sonographer reviews image quality to select the appropriate images for interpretation.

Educational opportunities are available for the sonographer in baccalaureate programs or community colleges. A nationally accredited educational program in ultrasound requires graduation from a 2-year, accredited allied health program, in which prerequisites are completed in anatomy and physiology, algebra, biology, communication, and medical terminology. Then specialized education in ultrasound is necessary. The formal educational program requires a minimum of 18 months. However, the actual length of the ultrasound education program varies. Sonography is a career in which specialized skills and abilities make a difference. Many sonographers work in hospitals or clinics. Others have found productive careers with companies in product design, marketing, research, or education. Some work as technical field application specialists. Sonography is a respected field, and professionals in the field often have positions of authority. Their work provides day-to-day variety and often allows a flexible schedule. Many employment opportunities are available, and salaries are attractive. On the job sonographers have opportunities to be creative and solve problems, involving quite diverse human conditions.

Of course, sonography is not a flawless profession. The work may be stressful and demanding particularly in situations in which patient loads are increased and staff members are reduced. The lack of cure for certain diseases may lead to frustration, and daily contact with high-risk obstetric patients may lead to depression. Job tasks can be physically demanding. Constant manipulation of patients and position of the transducer may lead to muscle fatigue and stress-related inflammation problems.

RESOURCE ORGANIZATIONS

Resource organizations devoted to ultrasound include the American Society of Echocardiography (ASE), the Society of Diagnostic Medical Sonographers (SDMS), the American Institute of Ultrasound in Medicine (AIUM), and the Society of Vascular Technology (SVT).

Historical Development

The development of *sonar*, along with certain materials and testing techniques, provided major impetus for the development of diagnostic ultrasound. Sonar equipment was initially constructed for the defense efforts during World War II to detect the presence of submarines. Various investigators later proved that ultrasound had a valid contribution to make in medicine.

In 1947 Dussick positioned two transducers on opposite sides of the head to measure ultrasound transmission profiles. He also discovered that tumors and other intracranial lesions could be detected by this technique. In the early 1950s Dussick, with Heuter, Bolt, and Ballantyne, continued to use *through-transmission* techniques and computer analysis to diagnose brain lesions in the intact skull. However, they discontinued their studies after concluding that the technique was too complicated for routine clinical use.

In the late 1940s Douglas Howry (a radiologist), John Wild (a diagnostician interested in tissue characterization), and George Ludwig (interested in reflections from gallstones) independently demonstrated that when ultrasound waves generated by a piezoelectric crystal transducer were transmitted into the human body, these waves would be returned to the transducer from tissue interfaces of different *acoustic impedances*. At this time, research efforts were directed toward transforming naval sonar equipment into a clinically useful diagnostic tool.

In 1948 Howry developed the first ultrasound scanner, consisting of a cattle watering tank with a wooden rail anchored along the side. The transducer carriage moved along the rail in a horizontal plane, while the object to be scanned and the transducer were positioned inside the water tank. (An early ultrasound scanner is shown on the title page of this chapter.)

Echocardiographic techniques were developed by Hertz and Edler in 1954 in Sweden. These investigators were able to distinguish normal heart valve motion from the thickened, calcified valve motion seen in patients with rheumatic heart disease. Then in 1957 an early obstetric contact-compound scanner was built by Tom Brown and Ian Donald in Scotland. This scanner was used primarily to evaluate the location of the placenta and to determine the gestational age of the fetus.

Further developments have resulted in the real-time ultrasound instrumentation used in hospitals and clinics today. High-frequency transducers with improved *resolution* now allow the sonographer to accumulate several images per second at a rate of up to 30 frames per second. Diagnostic ultrasound as used in clinical medicine has not been associated with any harmful biologic effects and is generally accepted as a safe modality.

Physical Principles
PROPERTIES OF SOUND WAVES

An acoustic *wave* is a propagation of energy that moves back and forth or vibrates at a steady rate. Sound waves are mechanical oscillations that are transmitted by particles in a gas, liquid, or solid medium. Generated by an external source, ultrasound is the transmission of high-frequency mechanical vibrations greater than 20 kHz through a medium.

Ultrasound refers to sound waves beyond the audible range (16,000 to 20,000 cycles/second). Diagnostic applications of ultrasound use frequencies of 1 to 10 million cycles/second, or 1 to 10 MHz. The ultrasound beam is produced from a transducer by the *piezoelectric effect*. The Curie brothers described the piezoelectric effect in 1880, when they observed that when certain crystals such as quartz undergo mechanical deformation a potential difference develops across the two surfaces of the crystals.

Acoustic impedance

The *ultrasound wave* is similar to a light beam in that it may be *focused, refracted, reflected,* or *scattered* at interfaces between different media. At the junction of two media of different acoustic properties, an ultrasound beam may be reflected, depending on the difference in acoustic impedance between the two media and the angle at which the beam hits the interface (Fig. 37-1).

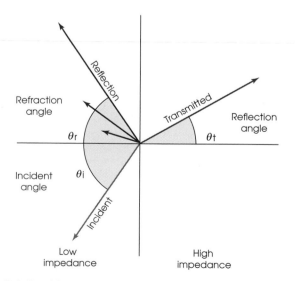

Fig. 37-1 Relationship among incident, reflected, and transmitted waves.

Velocity of sound

The *velocity of sound* in a *medium* is determined by the *density* and elastic properties of the medium. The velocity of sound differs greatly among air, bone, and soft tissue, but varies only slightly from one soft tissue to another. Sound transmission is impeded by air-filled structures such as the lungs and stomach or by gas-filled structures such as the bowel. However, sound is *attenuated* through most bony structures.

REAL-TIME IMAGING, DOPPLER EFFECT, AND COLOR FLOW DOPPLER

Real-time imaging is the presentation of multiple image frames per second over selected areas of the body. The *transducer* may be composed of several elements that can be electronically focused and fired in rapid sequence to produce a real-time image. Thus structures are visible as they change position in time. With this dynamic imaging it is possible to see, for example, pulsatile vascular and cardiac structures, diaphragm motion, and peristalsis in the bowel and stomach.

The *Doppler effect* refers to a change in *frequency* when the motion of laminar or turbulent flow is detected within a vascular structure. *Color flow Doppler* is a technique that assigns a color scale to the change in frequency or Doppler shift. Generally, red signifies a shift toward the transducer, whereas blue signifies a shift away from the transducer.

Anatomic Relationships and Landmarks

The ability of the sonographer to understand anatomy as it relates to the *sectional, coronal,* and *oblique planes* is critical to the performance of a high-quality sonogram (Figs. 37-2 to 37-4). Normal anatomy varies in size and position, and the sonographer must be able to demonstrate these findings on the sonogram. To complete this task, the sonographer must have a thorough understanding of anatomic relationships and their variations.

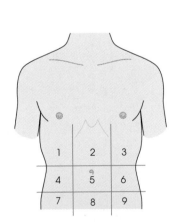

Fig. 37-2 Transverse scans of the upper abdomen are made over the nine regions of the anterior abdominal wall: *1,* right hypochondrium; *2,* epigastrium; *3,* left hypochondrium; *4,* right lumbar region; *5,* umbilical region; *6,* left lumbar region; *7,* right iliac fossa; *8,* hypogastrium; *9,* left iliac fossa.

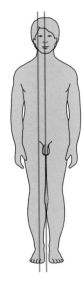

Fig. 37-3 Anterior view of the body in the anatomic position. The midsagittal plane *(blue)* bisects the umbilicus; a sagittal plane *(green)* is any plane parallel to this axis.

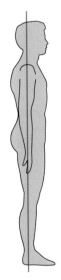

Fig. 37-4 Lateral view of the body. The line demonstrates the transducer axis to obtain a coronal view of the abdomen.

Clinical Applications

ABDOMEN AND RETROPERITONEUM

The upper abdominal ultrasound examination generally includes a survey of the abdominal cavity from the diaphragm to the level of the umbilicus (Fig. 37-5). Specific protocols are followed to image the texture, borders, anatomic relationships, and blood flow patterns within the liver, biliary system, pancreas, spleen, vascular structures, retroperitoneum, and kidneys. Patients may be examined in the supine, decubitus, upright, or prone positions.

Most often, optimum resolutions requires the use of a high-frequency (3.5-MHz) transducer. However, a lower-frequency transducer may be used to increase depth information in obese patients, and a higher frequency transducer may be used to improve the resolution of tissue structures in pediatric patients.

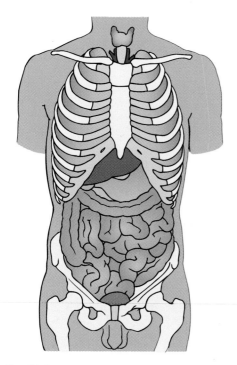

Fig. 37-5 Anteroposterior view of the abdomen showing most of the organs posterior to the costal margin *(cm)*, or transverse colon, *(TC)*.

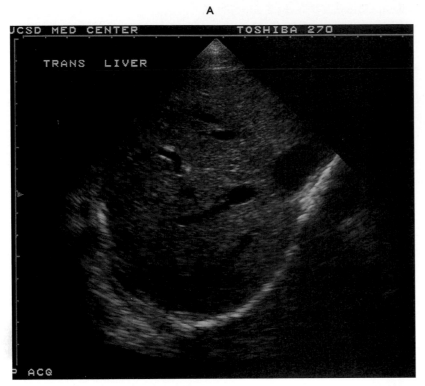

Air and gas in the abdominal cavity may obstruct the ultrasound beam. Consequently, the upper abdominal ultrasound examination is best performed after a patient has been fasting for at least 6 hours. Reducing or eliminating gas and air in the abdomen allows maximum visualization of the biliary system in its distended state. Specific images of the abdominal cavity are made, with the vascular structures serving as the primary landmarks for the abdominal organs. Scanning is performed in the transverse, oblique, sagittal, coronal, and subcostal planes (Figs. 37-6 and 37-7).

The left upper quadrant may be obscured secondary to air in the stomach or gas in the overlying bowel, making it difficult to image the spleen, left kidney, tail of the pancreas, and suprarenal area. A liquid such as degassed water, tomato juice, or ultrasound contrast material may be given to dilate the stomach and fill the duodenum in an effort to improve visualization of the structures in the left upper quadrant.

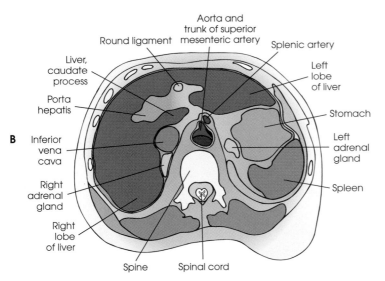

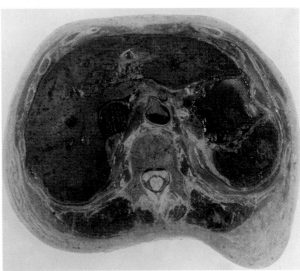

Fig. 37-6 A, Transverse sonogram of the right upper quadrant over the right lobe of the liver. **B,** Line drawing of the gross anatomic section. **C,** Gross anatomic section at approximately the same level as **A.**

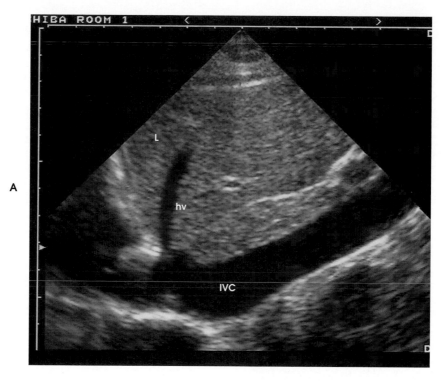

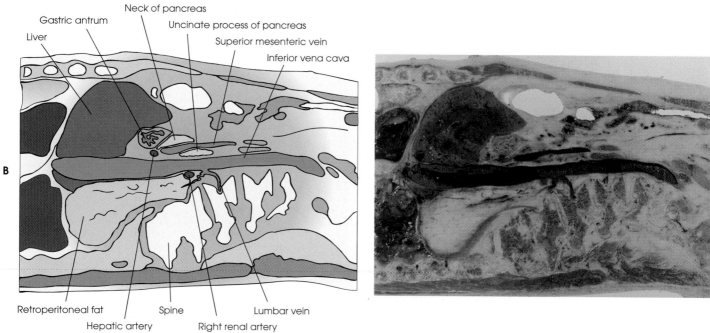

Fig. 37-7 A, Sagittal sonogram of the right upper quadrant over the medial segment of the left lobe of the liver, *(L),* the hepatic vein *(hv),* and the inferior vena cava *(IVC).* **B,** Line drawing of the gross anatomic section. **C,** Gross anatomic section at approximately the same level as **A.**

The sonographer must have an understanding of the patient's clinical history and symptoms to produce an adequate survey of the abdominal cavity. The normal sonographic patterns of all the abdominal organs and vascular structures must be adequately imaged to detect any pathologic condition that may require further investigation (Figs. 37-8 and 37-9). Although ultrasound cannot diagnose the specific pathology of a lesion, the clinical picture may lead to a more specific differential diagnosis to rule out infection, diffuse disease, hematoma, tumor, or an infiltrative process.

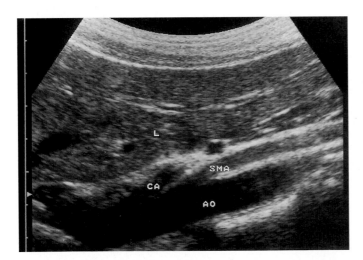

Fig. 37-8 Sagittal scan of the midline of the abdomen over the left lobe of the liver (L), the aorta (AO), the celiac axis (CA), and the superior mesenteric artery (SMA).

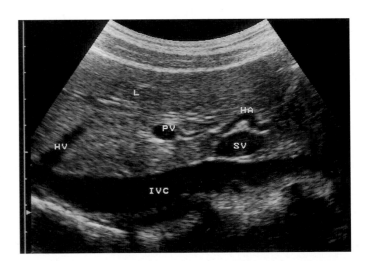

Fig. 37-9 Sagittal scan of the midline of the abdomen over the medial segment of the left lobe of the liver (L), the inferior vena cava (IVC), the hepatic vein (HV), the portal vein (PV), the hepatic artery (HA), and the splenic vein (SV).

The liver and spleen are evaluated to assess the size and homogeneity of tissues. The texture of these organs is normally uniform *(homogeneous)* throughout with the exception of the vascular structures that enter the hilus and branch into the surrounding tissue (Fig. 37-10). Abnormalities in this texture pattern enable the sonographer to determine if the organ has any of the following: fat infiltration, abscess, hematoma, cystic displacement, diffuse disease, or tumor invasion (Fig. 37-11). The presence or absence of vascular structures within the hepatosplenic organs helps the sonographer determine if portal hypertension, thrombosis, or diffuse disease is present. The combined use of color flow and Doppler helps to determine the direction of vascular flow or the presence of thrombus within the portal system or hepatic veins.

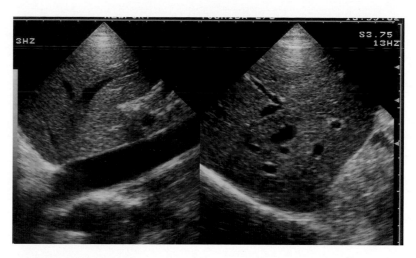

Fig. 37-10 Sagittal scans of the right upper quadrant demonstrating the homogeneity of the liver texture, with the vascular structures representing hepatic veins as draining toward the inferior vena cava and portal veins as they enter the liver at the porta hepatis.

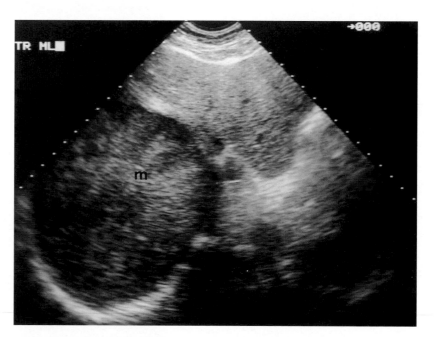

Fig. 37-11 Transverse scan over the inhomogeneous right lobe of the liver showing a huge complex mass *(m)* diagnosed as hepatocellular carcinoma.

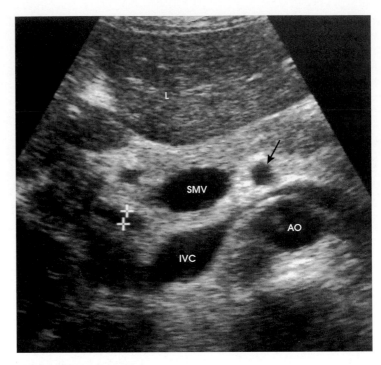

Fig. 37-12 Transverse scan over the epigastric region of the abdomen demonstrating a normal pancreas. The left lobe of the liver *(L)*, is seen anterior to the pancreas. The aorta *(AO)*, and inferior vena cava *(IVC)*, superior mesenteric artery *(arrow)*, and superior mesenteric vein *(SMV)*, are the posterior borders.

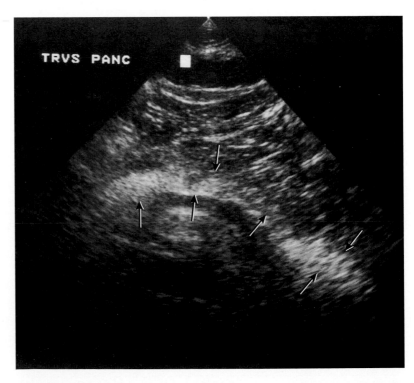

Fig. 37-13 Transverse scan over the pancreas area showing bright, echogenic reflections *(arrows)* that represent chronic, fibrotic pancreatitis.

The pancreas is a retroperitoneal gland. Its head lies in the curve of the duodenum, and its body and tail lie posterior to the antrum of the stomach. The texture of the pancreas varies, depending on the amount of fat that is interspersed throughout its islets of Langerhans. The aorta, inferior vena cava, superior mesenteric artery, and vein serve as the posterior landmarks for the pancreas (Fig. 37-12). Ultrasound examination of the pancreas can demonstrate inflammation (acute or chronic), tumor, abscess, or retroperitoneal bleed (Figs. 37-13 and 37-14).

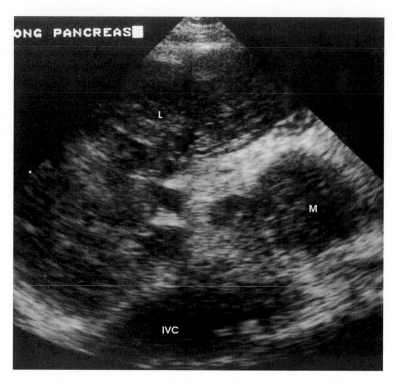

Fig. 37-14 Sagittal scan over the area of the pancreas in a 65-year-old female patient with a history of back pain, weight loss, and jaundice. A large hypoechoic mass *(M)*, is seen in the head of the pancreas, anterior to the inferior vena cava *(IVC)*, and inferior to the liver *(L)*.

Clinical applications

375

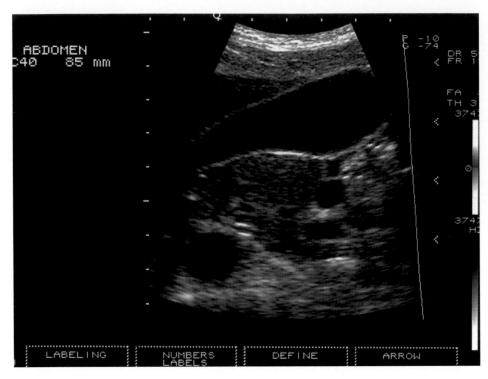

Fig. 37-15 Sagittal scan over the right upper quadrant showing a well-distended gallbladder with thin walls.

On ultrasound examination the gallbladder and bile ducts are seen just inferior to the right lobe of the liver and anterior to the right kidney (Fig. 37-15). The intrahepatic bile duct runs slightly anterior to the portal vein as it drains bile from the liver into the storage cistern (gallbladder) via the cystic duct (Fig. 37-16). Bile is released into the common bile duct, where it joins the pancreatic duct secretions to drain into the duodenum at a small raised area called the duodenal papilla. The biliary system is evaluated with ultrasound to assess size and wall thickness and to detect sludge, stones, polyps, or other masses (Figs. 37-17 and 37-18).

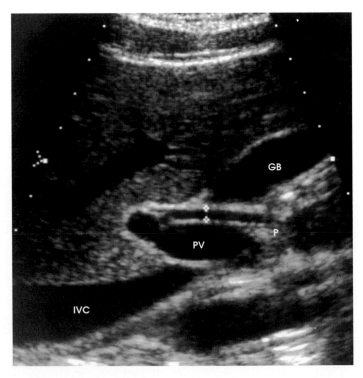

Fig. 37-16 The common bile duct (denoted by calipers) may be seen as it rests anterior to the portal vein *(PV)*, before it enters the posterior border of the pancreas, *P. IVC,* Inferior vena cava; *GB,* gallbladder.

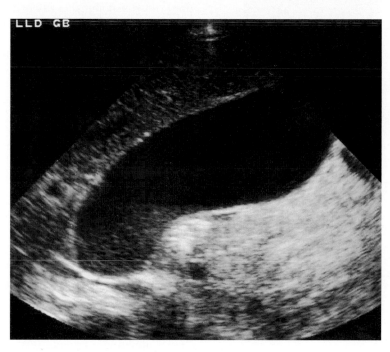

Fig. 37-17 Sagittal image of the distended gallbladder. Low-level echoes near the neck *(bottom left of image)* represent sludge.

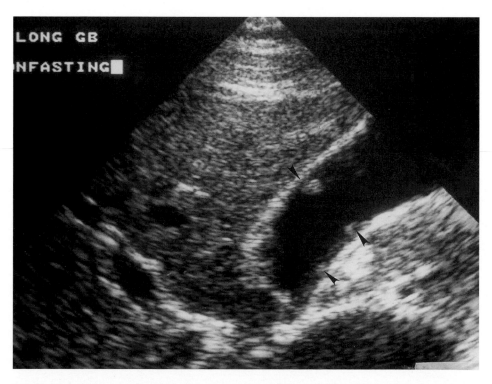

Fig. 37-18 Small polyps *(arrows)* attached to the inflamed gallbladder wall. These polyps do not shadow and do not move with change of position.

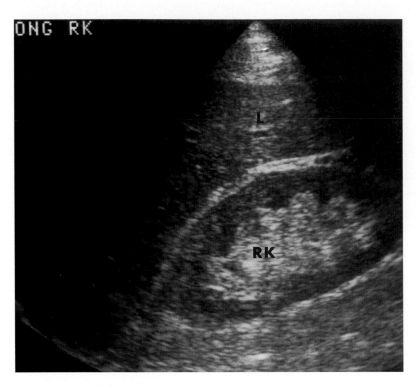

Fig. 37-19 Sagittal scan of the right kidney *(RK),* as it lies posterior to the inferior border of the right lobe of the liver *(L).*

The kidneys rest on the posterior surface of the abdominal cavity in an oblique plane lateral to the psoas muscles (Fig. 37-19). The large right lobe of the liver causes the right kidney to be slightly lower than the left kidney. The kidneys are assessed for size, dilation of calyces structures (hydronephrosis), or abnormal texture pattern secondary to a cyst, a tumor, an abscess, an infarct, a hematoma, or an infiltrative process (Figs. 37-20 and 37-21). Ultrasound is also useful for denoting the exact location and depth of the lower pole of the kidney; the urologist can then use this information in performing a renal biopsy. The transplanted kidney is placed in the iliac fossa, just superficial to the muscle layer. Ultrasound is very useful in measuring the size of the transplanted kidney, imaging the organ's texture to detect abnormal patterns that may suggest rejection, or evaluating the transplant recipient for hydronephrosis. Fluid collections (i.e., lymphocele, seroma, abscess, hematoma) that surround the renal transplant may also be evaluated with ultrasound. The anterior and posterior pararenal spaces may be evaluated for the presence of abnormal fluid or ascites, hematoma, or tumor invasion.

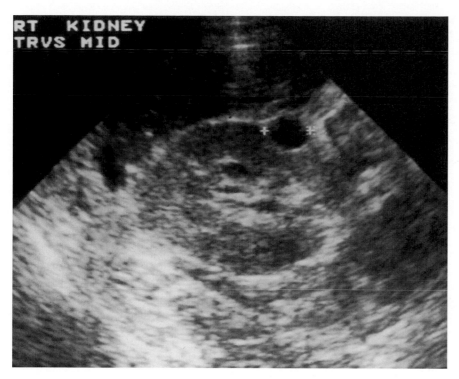

Fig. 37-20 Transverse scans of the right kidney with a small renal cyst located on the outer margin of the renal parenchyma (denoted by calipers).

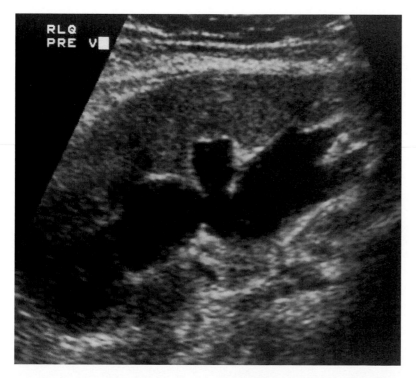

Fig. 37-21 In hydronephrosis of the kidney the dilated pyelocaliceal system appears as a separation of the renal sinus echoes by fluid-filled areas that conform anatomically to the infundibula, calyces, and pelvis.

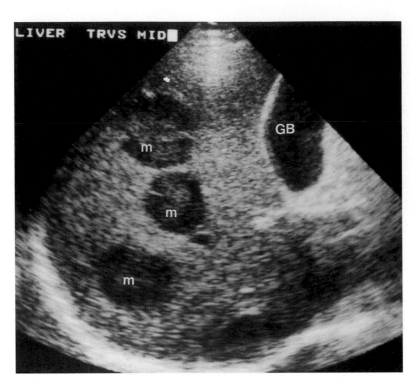

Fig. 37-22 Transverse scan of the right lobe of the liver showing multiple hypoechoic areas with a central-core echo pattern suggestive of metastatic disease *(m)* from adenocarcinoma of the colon. The gallbladder *(GB)*, is shown along the upper right border.

The sonographer must be able to analyze a mass to determine if its borders are smooth, irregular, poorly defined, thin, or thick to further define its characteristics. Once a mass is suspected, the sonographer must evaluate its acoustic properties to determine if it is *heterogeneous,* homogeneous, *hypoechoic, hyperechoic, isoechoic,* or *anechoic.* A hypoechoic lesion is characterized by very low-level echoes and good through-transmission of sound (Fig. 37-22). A hyperechoic mass may represent a tumor, thrombus, or calcification; the lesion presents with bright *echo* reflectors and possibly shadowing beyond it (Figs. 37-23 and 37-24). An isoechoic mass shows nearly the same texture pattern as the surrounding parenchyma with no significant change in the through transmission. An anechoic mass shows no internal echoes, has smooth walls, and displays increased through transmission (Fig. 37-25).

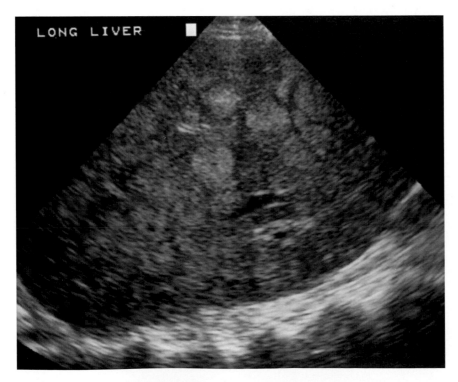

Fig. 37-23 Sagittal scan of the right lobe of the liver showing another pattern of metastatic liver disease with diffuse hyperechoic lesions throughout the liver parenchyma.

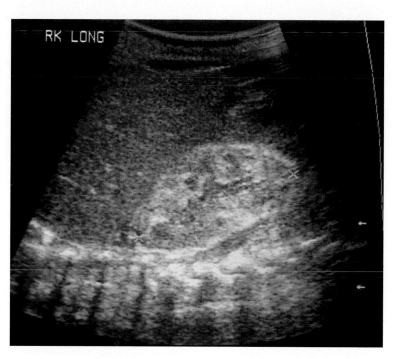

Fig. 37-24 Sagittal scan of the right upper quadrant showing the renal parenchyma to be more hyperechoic than the liver parenchyma. This represents renal failure from neuropathy associated with the acquired immunodeficiency syndrome.

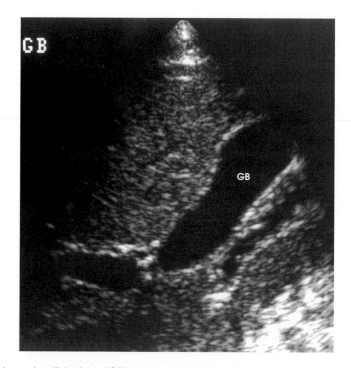

Fig. 37-25 Normal gallbladder *(GB)* is an excellent example of an anechoic structure without internal echoes.

A mass that shows characteristics of more than one pattern is considered complex. Examples include an abscess, a necrotic tumor with hemorrhage, a decomposing thrombus, a cyst with septations, and an abscess (Fig. 37-26).

Once a mass has been localized, ultrasound may aid the clinician in the aspiration or biopsy procedure. The sonographer may locate the site of the lesion, calculate its depth, and determine the direction and angulation of needle placement for the procedure.

A small calculus within a structure, such as a gallstone or renal stone, produces a sharp, well-defined acoustic shadow as the sound is attenuated beyond its calcified border (Fig. 37-27). The transducer must be perpendicular to the calculus for it to appear sharply marginated on the image. A new thrombus within a vessel may produce a low-level echo pattern within the vascular structure. Color flow Doppler is then used to further outline the patency of the lumen as the thrombus obstructs the flow of blood.

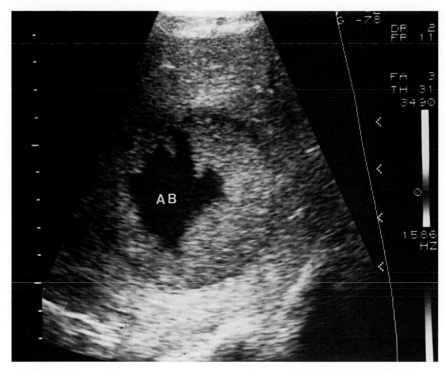

Fig. 37-26 Complex amebic abscess (*AB*) of the right lobe of the liver in a patient who had recently returned from a vacation in Mexico.

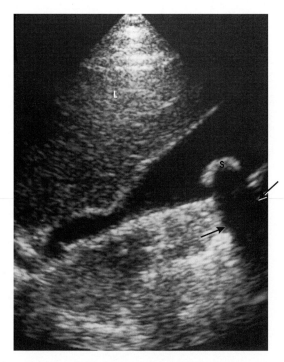

Fig. 37-27 Sagittal scan of the right upper quadrant showing the anechoic gallbladder with a large echogenic focus (gallstone, *S*) causing a large acoustic shadow posterior to its border (*arrows*).

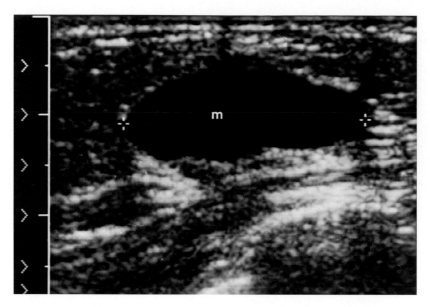

Fig. 37-28 A large anechoic mass *(M)* in the right breast parenchyma just anterior to the pectoralis major muscle.

SUPERFICIAL STRUCTURES

Superficial structures such as the thyroid, breast, scrotum, and penis are imaged very well with ultrasound using high-frequency transducers. Routine ultrasound examination demonstrates minute structures such as the lactiferous ducts within the breast and the spermatic cord within the testes. Pathologic hypoechoic and hyperechoic areas within the structures (e.g., cyst, adenoma, carcinoma, hydrocele, torsion) may be demonstrated with high-resolution ultrasound instrumentation (Figs. 37-28 to 37-31).

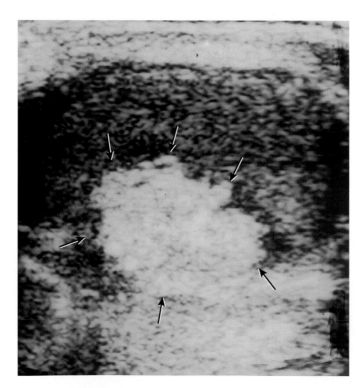

Fig. 37-29 Large echogenic hemorrhagic adenoma of the thyroid gland *(arrows)*.

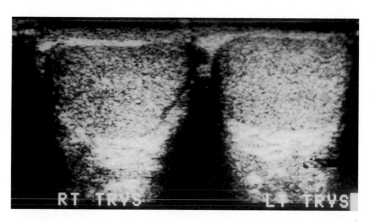

Fig. 37-30 Transverse sonogram showing symmetry in the size and texture of the testicles.

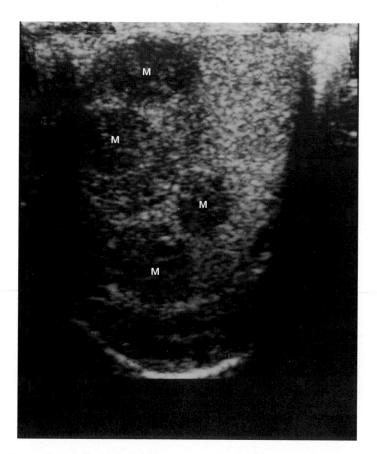

Fig. 37-31 Sonogram of the right testicle, which contains diffuse well-defined hypoechoic tumors *(m)* later diagnosed as seminoma.

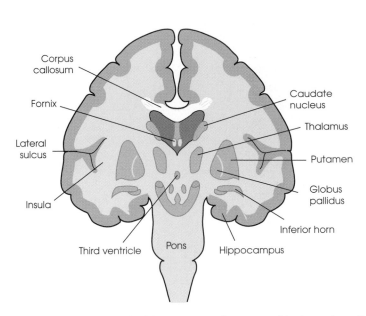

Fig. 37-32 Prenatal development of the corpus callosum, ventricular system, thalamus, and pons.

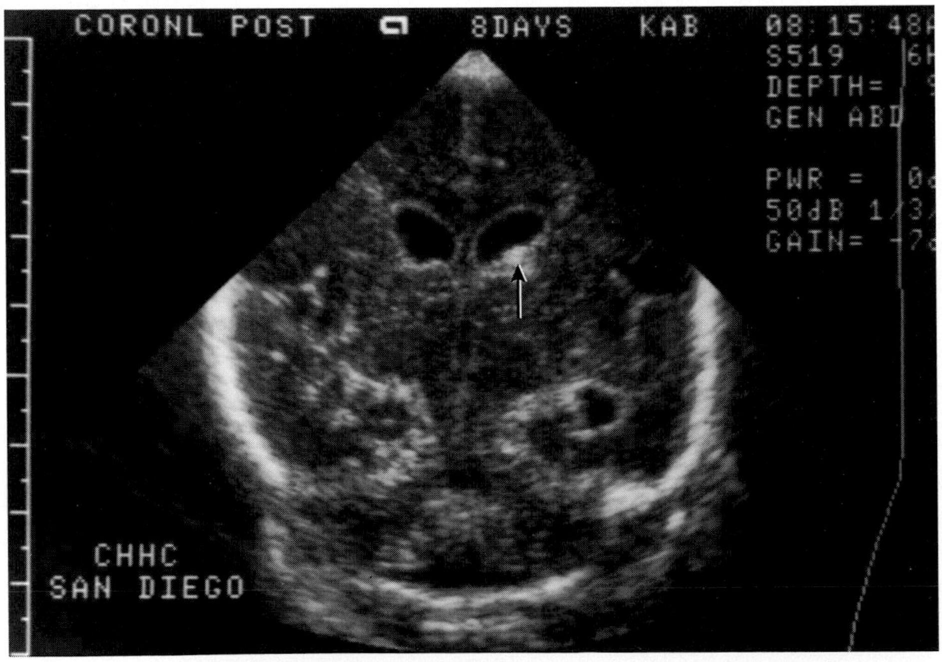

NEONATAL NEUROSONOGRAPHY

The premature infant is susceptible to intracranial hemorrhage during the stress of delivery and the struggle to survive. The internal anatomy of the neonatal brain may be well imaged through the coronal suture with high-frequency ultrasound. Structures such as the ventricular system, septum pellucidum, corpus callosum, choroid plexus, posterior fossa, vermis, and cerebrum are visualized with detailed resolution (Fig. 37-32). The infant may be examined in the special-care nursery using special petite transducers that adapt to the neonatal skull.

Sonography is the preferred clinical diagnostic tool to evaluate the premature infant for intracranial hemorrhage, infection, or shunt drainage for ventriculomegaly (Figs. 37-33 to 37-35). Other pathologic condition that ultrasound examination can detect within the neonatal skull include meningomyelocele, Arnold-Chiari deformity, hydrocephalus or ventriculomegaly, Dandy-Walker deformity, agenesis of the corpus callosum, and arteriovenous malformation.

Fig. 37-33 Posterior coronal image of an 8-day-old premature infant with a bilateral grade III bleed. The ventricles are slightly dilated, and a subependymal bleed *(arrow)* extends into the ventricular cavity.

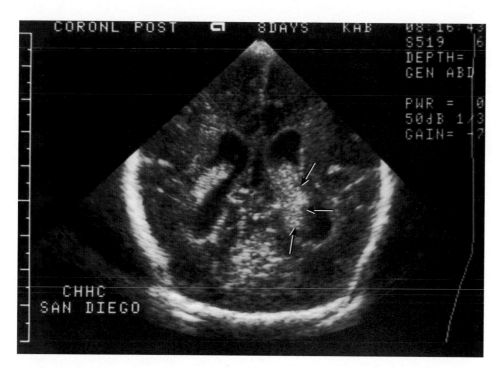

Fig. 37-34 Posterior coronal image of the full choroid plexus secondary to the hemorrhage (*arrows*) in the patient shown in Fig. 37-33.

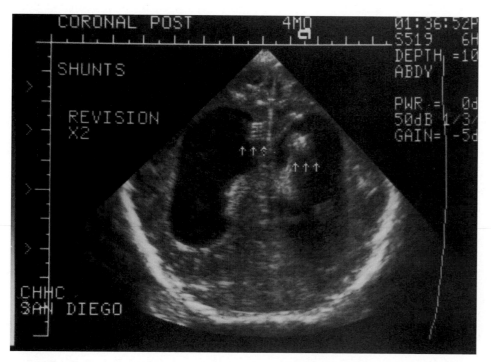

Fig. 37-35 Posterior coronal image of a patient with a ventricular shunt in place (*upper left arrows*) for draining cerebrospinal fluid and stent (*lower right arrows*) within the lateral ventricle.

GYNECOLOGIC APPLICATIONS

Anatomic features of the pelvis

The pelvis is divided into the greater and lesser pelvic cavity, with the pelvic brim being the circumference of a plane dividing the two cavities. The greater pelvic cavity, or "false" pelvis, is superior to the pelvic brim and is bounded on each side by the ileum. The lesser pelvic cavity, or "true" pelvis, is caudal to the pelvic brim. The walls of the pelvic cavity are formed by several muscles collectively called the *pelvic diaphragm*. These muscles include the levator ani, piriformis, and coccygeus muscles.

The female peritoneal cavity extends inferiorly into the lesser pelvis and is bounded by the peritoneum, which covers the rectum, bladder, and uterus. In the female, the peritoneum descends from the anterior abdominal wall to the level of the pubic bone onto the superior surface of the bladder (Fig. 37-36). It then passes from the bladder to the uterus to form the vesicouterine pouch. The rectouterine pouch, or pouch of Douglas, lies between the uterus and the rectum. Free fluid accumulates in this area before it moves cephalad to fill the gutters of the abdominal cavity.

Sonography of the female pelvis

A complete transabdominal examination of the female pelvis includes visualization of the distended urinary bladder, uterus, cervix, endometrial canal, vagina, ovaries, and supporting pelvic musculature. The full bladder helps to push the small bowel superiorly out of the pelvic cavity, flattens the body of the uterus, and serves as a *sonic window* to image the pelvic structures (Fig. 37-37). The rectum and other bowel structures may also be seen and must be distinguished from the normal pelvic structures. The sonographer may distinguish the bowel by watching for peristalsis or changes in fluid patterns throughout the examination. The fallopian tubes and broad ligaments are usually seen only when the patient presents with excessive free fluid or ascites within the pelvic cavity.

Endovaginal ultrasound has now become the preferred procedure for imaging the myometrium and ovaries. A high-frequency transducer is inserted into the vagina to image the uterus, cervix, fallopian tubes, ovaries, and adnexal area in coronal and sagittal planes (Fig. 37-38).

Sonography of the pelvis is clinically useful for imaging normal anatomy (Fig. 37-39), identifying the size of ovarian follicles as part of an infertility workup, measuring endometrial thickness, evaluating the texture of the myometrium, determining if a pregnancy is intrauterine or extrauterine, detecting tumors or abscess formations, and localizing an intrauterine contraceptive device.

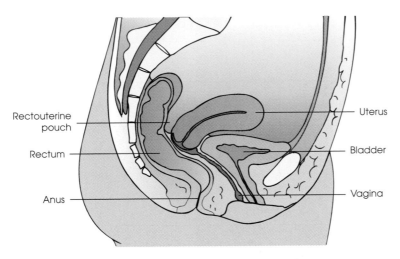

Fig. 37-36 Line drawing of the sagittal female pelvis.

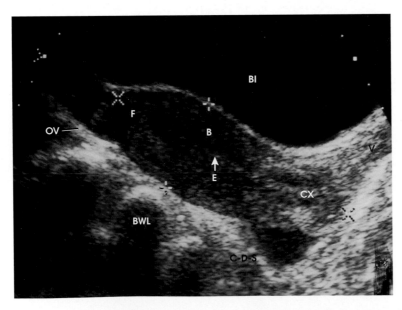

Fig. 37-37 Normal sagittal sonogram of the midline of the pelvic cavity. The distended urinary bladder *(Bl)* is shown anterior to the uterus. The endometrium appears as the bright linear echo within the uterus. The myometrium is the homogeneous smooth echo tissue surrounding the endometrium *(E)* of the uterus. The cervix *(CX)* and vagina (V) are well seen.

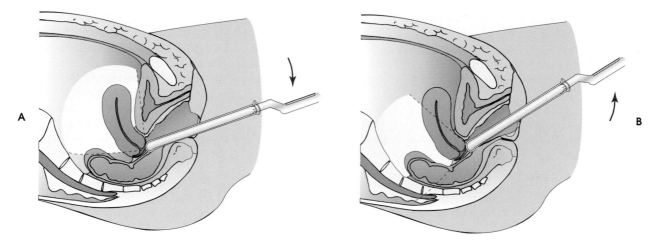

Fig. 37-38 A, Transvaginal sagittal scan with anterior angulation to better visualize the fundus of a normal anteflexed uterus. **B,** Transvaginal sagittal scan with posterior angulation to better visualize the cervix and rectouterine recess.

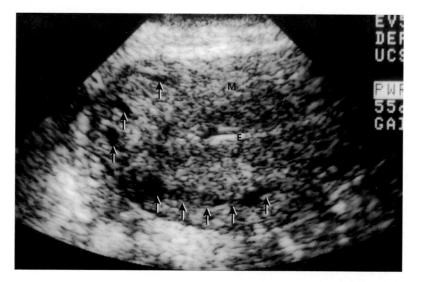

Fig. 37-39 Transvaginal midline sagittal image of the uterus. The arcuate vessels *(arrows)* are seen in the periphery of the homogeneous myometrium *(M)*; *(E),* endometrium.

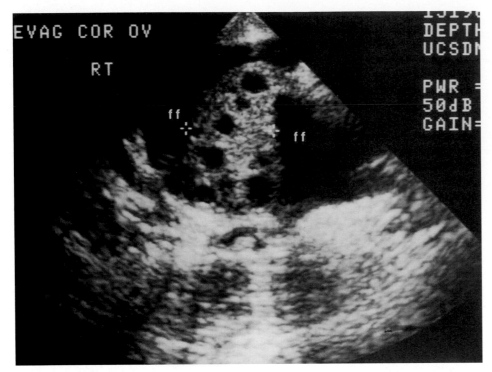

Fig. 37-40 Transvaginal sagittal image of the right ovary with multiple follicles, showing free fluid *(FF)* surrounding the ovary.

Distinct echo patterns of an enlarged uterus allow the sonographer to distinguish a leiomyoma from endometriosis or from a gestational sac (Fig. 37-40). The sonographer is able to identify the characteristic patterns of a pelvic mass to distinguish if it is cystic, solid, or complex. The ultrasound interpretation, correlated with the patient's history and clinical symptoms, helps to provide a differential diagnosis for the clinician.

Sonography of the follicles within the ovary has been used to follow infertile women to monitor the correct time to receive fertility medication (Fig. 37-41). A large follicular cyst may be an indication that the egg is ready for stimulation with high doses of human chorionic gonadotropin (HcG) and subsequent fertilization.

In postoperative patients with a fever of unknown origin, sonography may play a role in excluding abscess formation that may form in the cul-de-sac, the peripheral margins, or the gutters of the abdomen or perirenal space.

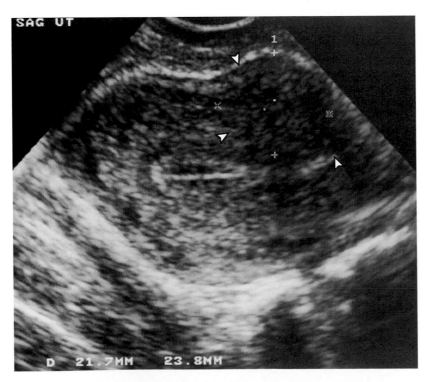

Fig. 37-41 Transvaginal sagittal scan of the uterus demonstrating a small hypoechoic intramural fibroid *(arrows).*

OBSTETRIC APPLICATIONS

The pregnant woman is the ideal candidate for an ultrasound examination. The amniotic fluid enhances the sound penetration to differentiate fetal anatomy, umbilical cord, placenta, and amniotic membranes within the uterine cavity. *Endovaginal ultrasound* is the procedure of choice during the first trimester of pregnancy to delineate the gestational sac with the embryo, yolk sac, chorion, and amniotic cavities. The gestational sac may be visualized as early as 4 weeks from the date of conception (Figs. 37-42 and 37-43). The embryo, heartbeat, and site of the placenta may be seen at 5 weeks of gestation.

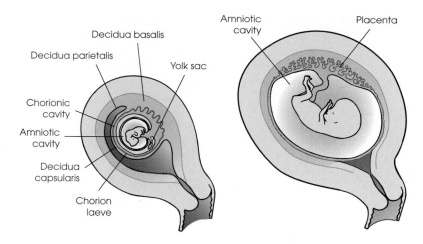

Fig. 37-42 First trimester representation of the developing embryo and yolk sac within the amniotic and chorionic cavities of the uterus.

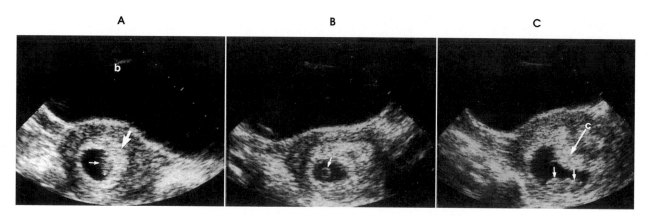

Fig. 37-43 A, Transabdominal sonograms of the first trimester pregnancy demonstrating the distended urinary bladder *(B),* gestational sac *(large arrow),* and embryo *(small arrow).* **B,** Small yolk sac *(small arrow).* **C,** Beginning of the placenta *(C)* and embryo *(small arrows).*

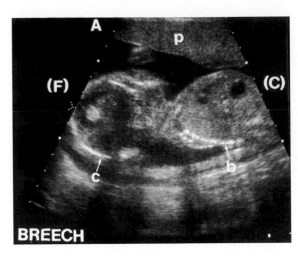

Fig. 37-44 Breech presentation of the fetus in the second trimester. The body (*B*), is closest in proximity to the direction of the cervix (*C*), and the cranium (*c*), is directed toward the uterine fundus (*F*).

The beginning of the second trimester (13 to 28 weeks of gestation) allows the sonographer to image the detailed anatomy of the fetus (Fig. 37-44). Structures such as the brain, face, limbs, neck, abdominal wall, liver, gallbladder, kidneys, stomach, pancreas, bowel, heart, lungs, and bladder may be seen with high-resolution transducers (Figs. 37-45 and 37-46). Heart motion, fetal size and position, and number of fetuses may be easily assessed with sonography. Serial examinations provide information relevant to normal or abnormal growth of the fetus and placenta.

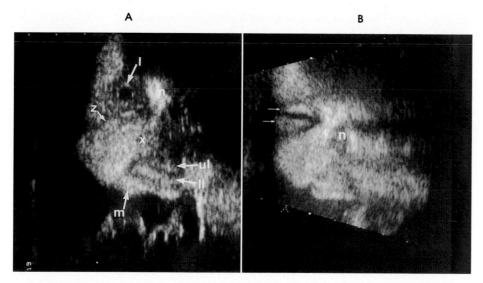

Fig. 37-45 A, Coronal image showing facial features. *L,* lens; *Z,* zygomatic bone; *X,* maxilla; *UL,* upper lip; *LL,* lower lip; *M,* mandible; *N,* nasal bones. **B,** A more anterior coronal scan in the same fetus, showing the upper and lower eyelids *(arrows)* and the nose *(n).*

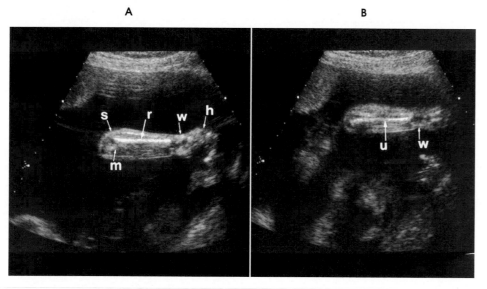

Fig. 37-46 A, The forearm is observed in a sagittal view. Note the medially positioned radius, *r.* The skin line, *s;* muscle, *m;* wrist, *w;* and hand, *h,* are in view. **B,** By rotating laterally, the ulna *(u)* comes into view; *w,* wrist.

NORMAL VENTRICLES

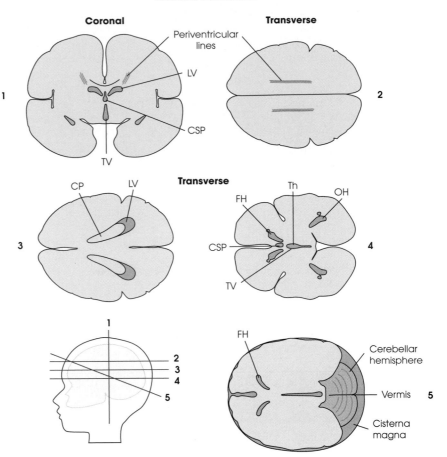

Fig. 37-47 Schematic of the normal fetal head: *LV,* lateral ventricle; *CSP,* cavum septum pellucidum; *TV,* Third ventricle; *CP,* choroid plexus; *FH,* frontal horn; *Th,* thalamus; *OH,* occipital horn.

The location and homogeneity of the placenta may be accurately defined in a patient who, presenting with clinical signs of pain and bleeding, may be diagnosed with placenta previa or abruptio placentae. With ultrasound the lower extent of the placenta may be seen in relation to the cervical os to determine if placenta previa is present. The sonographer may provide support to the perinatologist by helping localize the position of the placenta and fetus in amniocentesis, chorionic villus sampling, fetal blood sampling, or cord transfusion procedures. Color flow Doppler has been useful in defining the vascularity of the placenta in difficult cases such as placenta previa or placenta accreta.

A patient who presents with a uterus larger than expected for the weeks of gestation may be scheduled for an ultrasound examination to assess fetal growth and fluid accumulation. The examination can also assess the patient for the presence of multiple gestation, the development of a hydatidiform mole, or the growth of a fibroid or extrauterine mass secondary to the pregnancy.

The fetal *biparietal diameter* (measurement taken perpendicular to the falx of the midline of the skull) may be measured after the twelfth week of gestation. Along with the fetal abdomen, femur, and head circumference, the biparietal diameter is useful in monitoring fetal growth by serial evaluations and measurements (Figs. 37-47 and 37-48).

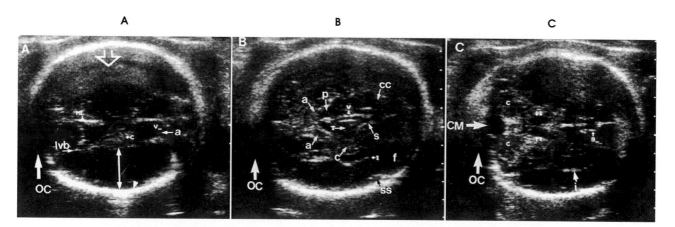

Fig. 37-48 A, Anatomic depiction at the ventricular level at 27 weeks of gestation. The *open arrow* points to a reverberation artifact in the proximal cranial hemisphere. The *double-ended* arrows point to fetal brain tissue. *OC,* Occiput; *ML,* interhemispheric fissure/falx; *LVB,* lateral ventricular border; *C,* choroid plexus; *V,* ventricular cavity; *A,* anterior chamber of the ventricle. Note the lateral ventricular border, which appears to lie less than halfway between the interhemispheric fissure and inner skull table *(arrowhead).*
B, Anatomic depiction at the thalamic level in a 31-week fetus: *T,* thalamus; *P,* cerebral peduncles; *V,* third ventricle; *S,* cavum septum pellucidum; *CC,* area of corpus callosum; *I,* insula; *C,* choroid plexus; *A,* ambient cisterns; *F,* frontal lobe; *SS,* subarachnoid space; *OC,* occiput. **C,** Anatomic depiction at the skull base in a 31-week fetus. The double arrows indicates the cerebral peduncles. *C,* Cerebellum; *CM,* cisternal magna; *I,* insula; *S,* cavum septum pellucidum; *OC,* occiput.

A   B

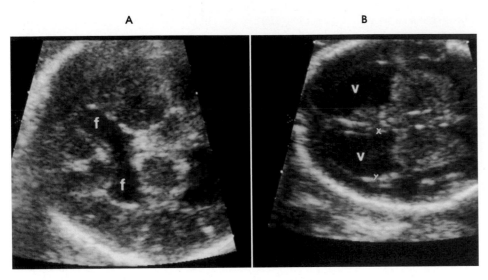

Ultrasound is helpful for defining both normal and abnormal development of anatomy. A detailed ultrasound examination can assess complications of pregnancy such as neural tube defects, skeletal or limb anomalies, cardiac defects, gastrointestinal and genitourinary defects, and head anomalies (Figs. 37-49 to 37-52).

Fig. 37-49 **A,** Frontal horn dilation *(F),* in a fetus with ventriculomegaly. **B,** In the same fetus, celpocephaly or dilation of the occipital ventricular horns *(V),* is observed bilaterally. Ventricular width was 17 mm. After birth the neonate was found to have fetal alcohol syndrome.

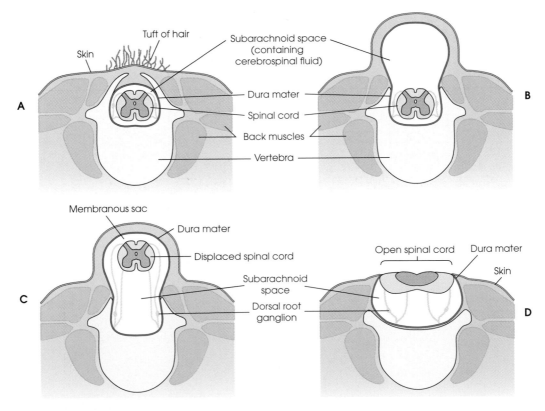

Fig. 37-50 Diagrammatic sketches illustrating the various types of spina bifida and the common associated malformations of the nervous system. **A,** Spina bifida occulta. About 10% of people have this vertebral defect in L5 and/or S1. It usually causes no back problems. **B,** Spina bifida with meningocele. **C,** Spina bifida with meningomyelocele. **D,** Spina bifida with myeloschisis. The types illustrated in **B** to **D** are often referred to collectively as *spina bifida cystica* because of the associated cystic sac.

(From Moore KL: *The developing human, clinically oriented embryology,* ed 6, Philadelphia, 1998, WB Saunders.)

A   B

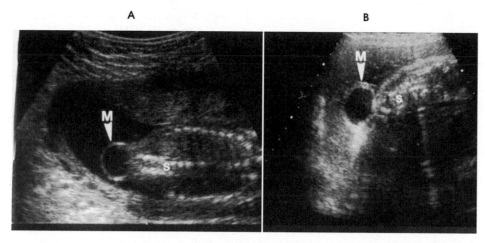

Fig. 37-51 A, Skin-covered meningocele *(M)*, in a 20-week-old fetus. A small head size and normal ventricles with a hypoplastic cerebellum were also found: *s*, spine. **B,** In the same fetus, sacral spina bifida *(M)*, at 37 weeks of gestation. Note the thickened appearance of the meningocele, which may suggest a skin-covered lesion.

A   B

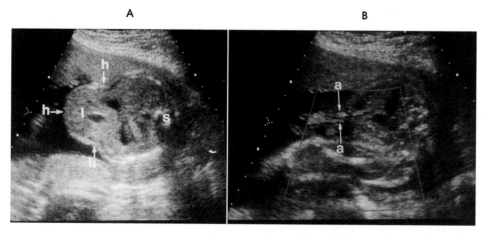

Fig. 37-52 A, Umbilical hernia *(H* and *arrows)* observed in a fetus with Carpenter's syndrome, or acrocephalopolysyndactyly, type II (see Fig. 30-31); *l,* liver; *S,* spine. **B,** Scan in the same fetus, performed at the cord insertion level using color imaging; the umbilical arteries *(a)* are observed entering the abdomen in a normal location, a finding that excludes the diagnosis of omphalocele.

VASCULAR APPLICATIONS

The use of ultrasound and color flow Doppler has enhanced the ability to image peripheral vascular structures in the body. The common carotid artery with its internal and external branches and the vertebral artery are well seen with high-frequency ultrasound (Fig. 37-53). The detection of plaque formation, thrombus, obstruction, or stenosis is documented with both color and spectral Doppler waveforms.

The ultrasound facilitates good visualization of the common femoral artery and vein and their branches as they extend into the calf (Fig. 37-54). Thrombus within a distended venous structure is identified when the sonographer is unable to compress the vein with the transducer. Color flow Doppler is also useful for denoting an absence of flow within a vessel. Arterial and venous structures may be reliably mapped using the ultrasound vascular mapping technique.

Ultrasound is also useful for imaging the patency of other vascular structures, such as the jugular vein, the subclavian artery and vein, the brachial artery and vein, and radial grafts.

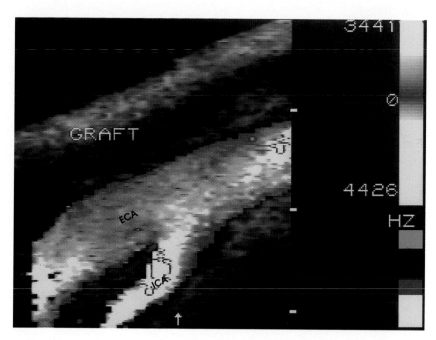

Fig. 37-53 Postoperative image of the carotid graft with a reimplanted external carotid artery, ECA.

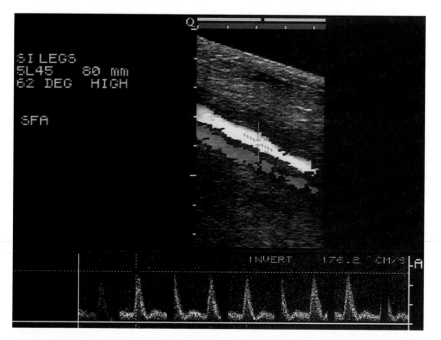

Fig. 37-54 Longitudinal image of the superficial femoral artery with a normal spectral waveform.

Cardiologic Applications

Real-time two-dimensional echocardiography of the fetal, neonatal, pediatric, and adult heart has proved to be a tremendous diagnostic aid for the cardiologist and internist. A complete two-dimensional study of the heart uses real-time color flow Doppler with pulsed and continuous wave Doppler spectral tracings. With echocardiography, it is possible to image cardiac structures in detail, including the four chambers of the heart, the four heart valves (mitral, tricuspid, aortic, and pulmonic), the interventricular and interatrial septa, the muscular wall of the ventricles, the papillary muscles, and the chordae tendineae cordis. Difficult cases can be imaged using a transesophageal technique in which the transducer is passed from the mouth, through the esophagus, to the orifice of the stomach. This high-frequency transducer uses the "window" of the stomach and esophagus to exquisitely image intracardiac structures.

PROCEDURE FOR ECHOCARDIOGRAPHY

The echocardiographic examination begins with the patient in a left lateral decubitus position. This position allows the heart to move away from the sternum and fall closer to the chest wall, thereby providing a better cardiac "window," or open area for the sonographer to image. The transducer is placed in the third, fourth, or fifth intercostal space to the left of the sternum. The protocol for a complete echocardiographic examination includes images in the long axis, short axis, apical, and suprasternal windows (Fig. 37-55).

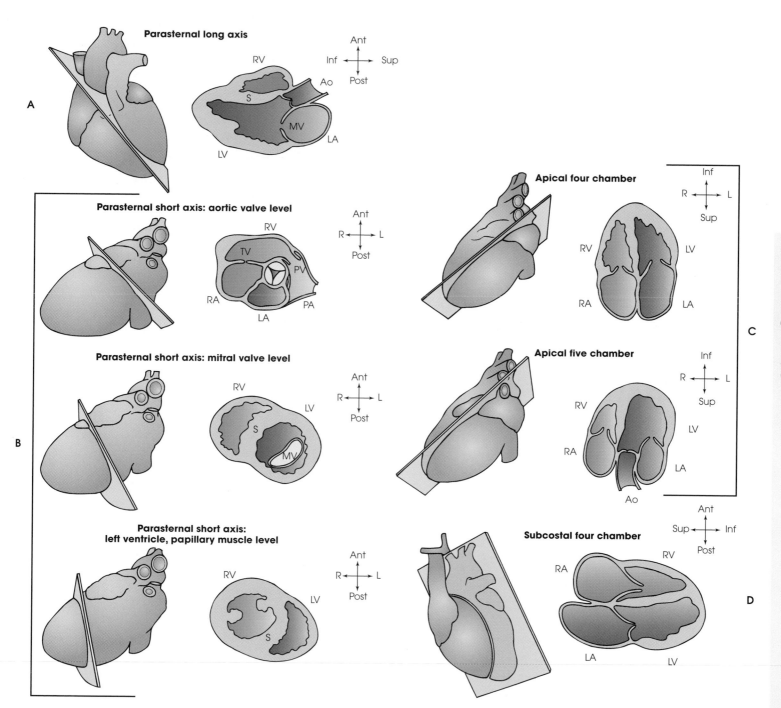

Fig. 37-55 A, Parasternal long axis drawing: *RV,* right ventricle; *Ao,* aorta; *LV,* left ventricle; *LA,* left atrium, *S,* septum, *MV,* mitral valve. **B,** Parasternal short axis drawings at various levels. *Aortic valve level: RA,* right atrium; *LA,* left atrium; *TV,* tricuspid valve; *RV,* right ventricle; *Ao,* aorta; *PV,* pulmonic valve; *PA,* pulmonary artery. *Mitral valve level: RV,* right ventricle; *S,* septum; *LV,* left ventricle; *MV,* mitral valve. *Left ventricle, papillary muscle level: RV,* right ventricle; *S,* septum; *LV,* left ventricle. **C,** Apical four-chamber image: *RV,* right ventricle; *LV,* left ventricle; *RA,* right atrium; *LA,* left atrium. Apical five-chamber image: *RA,* right atrium; *RV,* right ventricle; *LV,* left ventricle; *LA,* left atrium; *Ao,* aorta. **D,** Subcostal four chamber image: *RA,* right atrium; *RV,* right ventricle; *LA,* left atrium; *LV,* left ventricle.

Cardiologic applications

CARDIAC PATHOLOGY

Echocardiography is used to evaluate many cardiac conditions. Atherosclerosis or previous rheumatic fever may lead to scarring, calcification, and thickening of the valve leaflets. With these conditions, valve tissue destruction continues, causing stenosis and regurgitation of the leaflets and subsequent chamber enlargement.

The effects of subbacterial endocarditis can also be evaluated with echocardiography. With this infectious process, multiple small vegetations form on the endocardial surface of the valve leaflets. This causes the leaflets to tear or thicken, with resultant severe regurgitation into subsequent cardiac chambers. The echocardiogram of a patient with congestive cardiomyopathy shows generalized four-chamber enlargement, valve regurgitation, and the threat of thrombus formation along the nonfunctioning ventricular wall. The pericardial sac surrounds the ventricles and right atrium and may fill with fluid, impairing normal cardiac function.

The analysis of ventricular function and the serial evaluation of patients after a myocardial infarction are accomplished with two-dimensional echocardiography and, in some cases, stress dobutamine echocardiography. For the latter evaluation, as the patient is monitored with electrocardiographic leads, dobutamine is administered intravenously at 5-minute increments. Multiple images of the left ventricle are simultaneously made by the cardiac sonographer and recorded on a four-quadrant viewing panel. After the examination is completed, the images are carefully reviewed to determine the left ventricular wall motion abnormalities (Fig. 37-56).

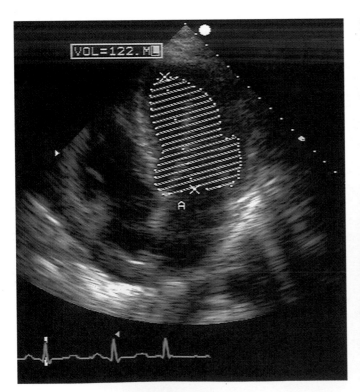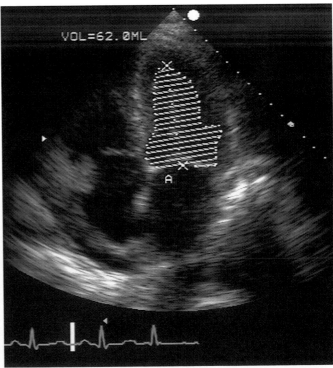

Fig. 37-56 In calculating ejection fractions, volumes are obtained from two-dimensional echocardiographic images. The images needed to obtain these volumes depends on the algorithm used. Most commercial cardiac ultrasound units have on-line calculations for ejection fractions. Volumes are obtained by tracing the endocardium of end-diastolic and end-systolic frames. The modified Simpson's algorithm is used here to calculate the volumes from the apical (A) images.

Complications of myocardial infarction (MI) may include rupture of the ventricular septum, development of a left ventricular aneurysm in the weakest area of the wall, or coagulation of thrombus in the akinetic or immobile apex of the left ventricle (Figs. 37-57 and 37-58).

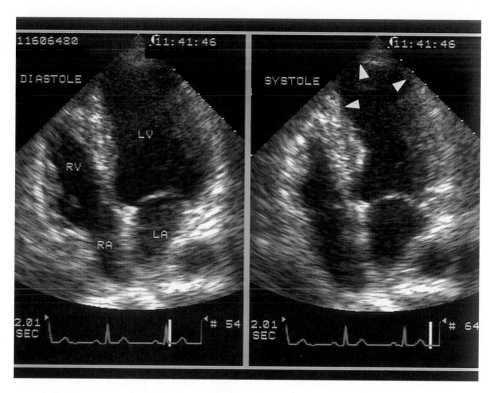

Fig. 37-57 Localized apical chamber dilation with reduced myocardial wall thickness and regional dyskinetic motion in systole are the criteria for diagnosing apical aneurysms. Comparison of a systolic frame (right panel) with a diastolic frame (left panel) shows an apical aneurysm (arrows). In systole the apex moves outward when the base and mid-portions of the left ventricle contract inward.

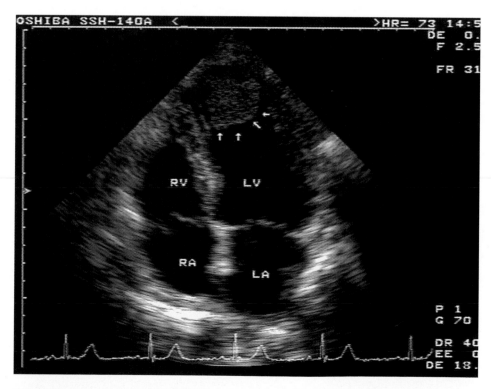

Fig. 37-58 Apical four-chamber image with a large apical thrombus. This thrombus *(arrows)* is distinguished from an artifact because it is located in a region with abnormal wall motion, is attached to the apical endocardium, has well-defined borders, and moves in the same direction as the apex. *RV,* Right ventricle; *LV,* left ventricle; *RA,* right atrium *LA,* left atrium.

Congenital heart lesions

Echocardiography has been used to diagnose congenital lesions of the heart in fetuses, neonates, and young children. The cardiac sonographer is able to assess abnormalities of the four cardiac valves, determine the size of the cardiac chambers, assess the interatrial and interventricular septum for the presence of shunt flow, and identify the continuity of the aorta and pulmonary artery with the ventricular chambers to look for abnormal attachment relationships (Fig. 37-59).

The premature infant has an improved chance of survival if the correct diagnosis is made early. If the neonate is cyanotic, congenital heart disease or respiratory failure may be rapidly diagnosed with echocardiography. Critical cyanotic disease in the premature infant may include hypoplastic left heart syndrome, transposition of the great vessels with pulmonary atresia, or severe tetralogy of Fallot (Figs. 37-60 and 37-61).

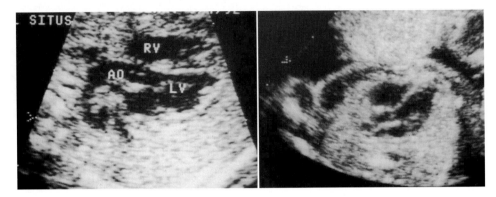

Fig. 37-59 Five-chamber image of the fetal heart in a normal 18-week-old fetus shows the aorta *(AO)*, right ventricle *(RV)*, and left ventricle *(LV)*.

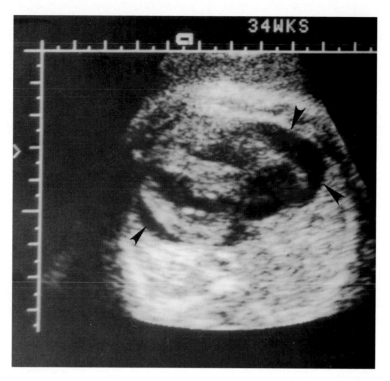

Fig. 37-60 Large pericardial effusion *(arrows)* surrounding the ventricular and right atrial cavities in a 34-week-old fetus.

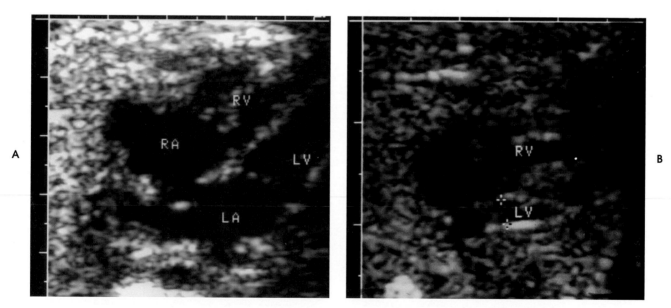

Fig. 37-61 A, Normal four-chamber image of the fetal heart showing the communication through the patent foramen ovale from the right atrium to the left atrium. **B,** Four-chamber image in a fetus with a hypoplastic (underdeveloped) left heart. The dilated right ventricle is shown anterior to the left ventricle. *RV,* right ventricle; *RA,* right atrium; *LV,* left ventricle; *LA,* left atrium.

Conclusion

Diagnostic ultrasound has continued to improve the differential diagnosis of diseases and the subsequent management of patients. The contributions of ultrasound have been facilitated by technologic advances in instrumentation and transducer design, increased ability to process the returned echo information, and improved technology for the three-dimensional reconstruction of images. The development of high-frequency *endovaginal, endorectal*, and *transesophageal transducers* with *endoscopic* imaging has aided the visualization of previously difficult areas. Improved computer capabilities have enabled the sonographer to obtain more information and process multiple data points to obtain a comprehensive report from the ultrasound study. Color flow Doppler has made it possible for the sonographer to distinguish the direction and velocity of arterial and venous blood flow from other structures in the body. Furthermore, Doppler has allowed the sonographer to determine the exact area of obstruction or leakage and to determine precisely the degree of turbulence present.

Continued improvements in transducer design have improved resolution in superficial structures, muscles, and tendons. Advancements in equipment design have also improved the results of ultrasound examinations in neonates and children. Increased sensitivity allows the sonographer to define the texture of organs and glands with more detail and greater tissue differentiation. The improvements in resolution have aided the visualization of small cleft palate defects, abnormal development of fingers and toes, and small spinal defects. The ability to image the detail of the fetal heart has facilitated the early diagnosis of congenital heart disease.

Advanced research and development of the computer analysis and tissue characterization of echo reflections should further contribute to the total diagnostic approach using ultrasound. Various abdominal contrast agents are being investigated to improve visualization of the stomach, pancreas, and small and large intestine. Cardiac contrast agents are already being used to improve the visualization of viable myocardial tissue within the heart. Furthermore, saline and other contrast agents are being injected into the endometrial cavity to outline the lining of the endometrium for the purpose of distinguishing polyps and other lesions from the endometrial stripe.

Ultrasound has rapidly emerged as a useful, noninvasive, high-yield clinical diagnostic examination for various applications in medicine. Expected advancements include further developments in transducer design, image resolution, tissue characterization applications, color flow sensitivity, and three-dimensional reconstruction of images.

Definition of Terms

acoustic impedance Ratio of acoustic pressure to particle velocity at any point in the acoustic field.

acoustic shadow Loss of acoustic power of structures lying behind an attenuating or reflecting target.

A-mode (amplitude) Method of acoustic echo display in which time is represented along the horizontal axis and echo amplitude is displayed along the vertical axis.

anechoic Property of being free of echoes or without echoes.

angle of incidence Angle at which the ultrasound beam strikes an interface with respect to normal (perpendicular) incidence.

artifact An echo that does not correspond in distance or direction to a real target.

attenuation Reduction of acoustic amplitude along propagation pathway as a result of diffraction, absorption, scattering, reflections, or any other process that redirects the signal away from the receiver.

attenuation compensation Compensation for attenuation of acoustic signals along the propagation pathway as a result of losses and geometric divergence. When accomplished electronically, this is called *time-gain compensation (TGC)*.

backscatter Part of the acoustic energy reflected from a small (compared with wavelength) target back toward the source.

biparietal diameter (BPD) Largest dimension of the fetal head perpendicular to the midsagittal plane; measured by ultrasonic visualization and used to measure fetal development.

B-mode (brightness) Method of acoustic display on an oscilloscope in which the intensity of the echo is represented by modulation of the brightness of the spot and in which the position of the echo is determined from the position of the transducer and the transit time of the acoustic pulse; displayed in the x-y plane.

color flow Doppler Velocity in each direction is quantified by allocating a pixel to each area; each velocity frequency change is allocated a color.

continuous wave ultrasound Waveform in which the amplitude modulation factor is less than or equal to a small value.

coronal image plane Anatomic term used to describe a plane perpendicular to both the sagittal and transverse planes of the body.

cross-sectional display Display that presents ultrasound interaction echo data from a single plane within a tissue. It is produced by sweeping the ultrasound beam through a given angle, by translating it along a line, or by some combination of linear and angular motions. The depth in the tissue is represented along one coordinate, and the position in the scan is represented by the second coordinate. The plane of the section may be sagittal, coronal, or transverse. The lateral resolution is determined by the beam width of the transducers.

decibel Unit used for expressing the ratio of two quantities of electrical signal or sound energy.

density Mass divided by volume.

Doppler effect Shift in frequency or wavelength, depending on the conditions of observation; caused by relative motions among the sources, receivers, and medium.

Doppler ultrasound Application of the Doppler effect to ultrasound to detect movement of a reflecting boundary relative to the source, resulting in a change of the wavelength of the reflected wave.

dynamic imaging Imaging of an object in motion at a frame rate sufficient to cause no significant blurring of any one image and at a repetition rate sufficient to adequately represent the movement pattern. This is frequently referred to as *imaging at a real-time (frame) rate.*

echo Reflection of acoustic energy received from scattering elements or a specular reflector.

echogenic Refers to a medium that contains echo-producing structures.

endorectal transducer High-frequency transducer that can be inserted into the rectum to visualize the bladder and prostate gland.

endovaginal transducer High-frequency transducer (and decreased penetration) that can be inserted into the vagina to obtain high-resolution images of the pelvic structures.

focus To concentrate the sound beam into a smaller beam area than would exist without focusing.

frequency Number of cycles per unit of time, usually expressed in Hertz (Hz) or megahertz (MHz; a million cycles per second).

gray scale Property of the display in which intensity information is recorded as changes in the brightness of the display.

hard copy Method of image recording in which data are stored on paper, film, or other recording material.

heterogenous Having a mixed composition.

homogeneous Having a uniform composition.

hyperechoic Producing more echoes than normal.

hypoechoic Producing fewer echoes than normal.

isoechoic Having a texture nearly the same as that of the surrounding parenchyma.

medium Material through which a wave travels.

M-mode (motion) Method in which tissue depth is displayed along one axis and time is displayed along the second axis.

noninvasive technique A procedure that does not require the skin to be broken or an organ or cavity to be entered (e.g., taking the pulse).

oblique plane A slanting direction or any variation that is not starting at a right angle to any axis.

piezoelectric effect Conversion of pressure to electrical voltage or conversion of electrical voltage to mechanical pressure.

pulse wave ultrasound Sound waves produced in pulse form by applying electrical pulses to the transducer.

real-time imaging Imaging with a real-time display whose output keeps pace with changes in input.

reflection Acoustic energy reflected from a structure with a discontinuity in the characteristic acoustic impedance along the propagation path.

refraction Phenomenon of bending wave fronts as the acoustic energy propagates from the medium of one acoustic velocity to a second medium of differing acoustic velocity.

resolution Measure of the ability to display two closely spaced structures as discrete targets.

scan Technique for moving an acoustic beam to produce an image for which both the transducer and display movements are synchronized.

scattering Diffusion or redirection of sound in several directions on encountering a particle suspension or rough surface.

sectional plane Plane corresponding to transverse or sagittal plane.

sonar Instrument used to discover objects under the water and to show their location.

sonic window Sonographer's ability to visualize a particular area. For example, the full urinary bladder is a good sonic window to image the uterus and ovaries in a transabdominal scan. The intercostal margins may be a good sonic window to image the liver parenchyma.

through transmission Process of imaging by transmitting the sound field through the specimen and picking up the transmitted energy on a far surface or a receiving transducer.

transducer Device that converts energy from one form to another.

ultrasound Sound with a frequency greater than 20 kHz.

velocity of sound Speed with direction of motion specified.

wave Acoustic wave is a mechanical disturbance that propagates through a medium.

Selected bibliography

Allan LD: *Manual of fetal echocardiography,* Lancaster, England, 1986, MTP Press.

Babcock DS, Han BK: *Cranial ultrasonography of infants,* Baltimore, 1981, Williams & Wilkins.

Callen PW: *Ultrasonography in obstetrics and gynecology,* ed 3, Philadelphia, 1994, WB Saunders.

Cooperberg P et al: Advances in ultrasonography of the gallbladder and biliary tract, *Radiol Clin North Am* 20:611, 1982.

Fink B: *Congenital heart disease,* ed 3, St Louis, 1991, Mosby.

Hagen-Ansert SL: *Abdominal ultrasound study guide and exam review,* St Louis, 1996, Mosby.

Hagen-Ansert SL: *Textbook of diagnostic ultrasonography,* vols I and II, ed 4, St Louis, 1995, Mosby.

Hatle L, Angelsen B: *Doppler ultrasound in cardiology: physical principles and clinical applications,* Philadelphia, 1982, Lea & Febiger.

Holmes JH: Perspectives in ultrasonography: early diagnostic ultrasonography, *J Ultrasound Med* 2:33, 1983.

Jeffrey RB, Ralls PW: *Sonography of the abdomen,* New York, 1995, Raven Press.

Kurtz AB, Middleton WD: *Ultrasound: the requisites,* St Louis, 1996, Mosby.

Lerski RA: Ultrasonic tissue characterization, *Diagn Imaging* 51:238, 1982.

McDicken WN: *Diagnostic ultrasonics: principles and use of instruments,* London, 1976, Granada.

Mittelstaedt CA: *Abdominal ultrasound,* New York, 1987, Churchill Livingstone.

Nyberg DA, Mahony BS, Pretorious DH: *Diagnostic ultrasound of fetal anomalies: text and atlas,* Chicago, 1990, Yearbook.

Oh JK, Seward JB, Tajik AJ: *The echo manual,* Boston, 1994, Little, Brown.

Powis RL: *Ultrasound physics for the fun of it,* Denver, 1978, Unirad Corp.

Rumack CM, Johnson ML: *Perinatal and infant brain imaging,* Chicago, 1984, Yearbook.

Sanders RC, James AE: *The principles and practice of ultrasonography in obstetrics and gynecology,* New York, 1990, Appleton-Century-Crofts.

Siegel MJ: *Pediatric sonography,* New York, 1991, Raven.

Zweibel WJ, editor: *Introduction to vascular ultrasonography,* New York, 1993, Grune & Stratton.

38

NUCLEAR MEDICINE

NANCY L. HOCKERT

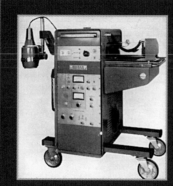

RIGHT: First-generation nuclear medicine rectilinear scanner, 1950s.

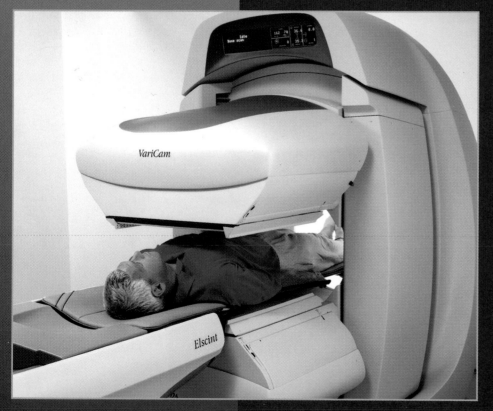

LEFT: Modern dual-head gamma camera capable of single photon emission computed tomography, simultaneous posterior whole-body and planar imaging, and coincidence (positron emission tomography) imaging.

(Courtesy Elscint, Inc.)

Principles of Nuclear Medicine

Nuclear medicine is a medical specialty that focuses on the use of *radioactive* materials called *radiopharmaceuticals** for diagnosis, therapy, and medical research. Unlike radiologic procedures, which determine the presence of disease based on structural appearance, nuclear medicine studies determine the cause of a medical problem based on organ or tissue *function* (physiology).

In a nuclear medicine test the radioactive material, or *tracer,* is generally introduced into the body by injection, swallowing, or inhalation. Different tracers are used to study different parts of the body. Tracers are selected that localize in specific organs or tissues. The amount of radioactive tracer material is selected carefully to provide the lowest amount of radiation exposure to the patient and still ensure a satisfactory examination or therapeutic goal. Radioactive tracers produce *gamma-ray* emissions from within the organ being studied. A special piece of equipment, known as a *gamma* or *scintillation camera,* is used to transform these emissions into images that provide information about the function and anatomy of the organ or system being studied. The camera records this information on a computer or on film.

Nuclear medicine tests are performed by a team of specially educated professionals: a nuclear medicine physician, a specialist with extensive education in the basic and clinical science of medicine who is licensed to use radioactive materials; a nuclear medicine technologist, who performs the tests and is educated in the theory and practice of nuclear medicine procedures; a physicist who is experienced in the technology of nuclear medicine and the care of the equipment, including computers; and a pharmacist or specially prepared technologist who is qualified to prepare the necessary radioactive pharmaceuticals.

---

*Almost all italicized terms are defined at the end of this chapter.

History

John Dalton is considered the father of the modern theory of *atoms* and molecules. In 1803, this English schoolteacher stated that all atoms of a given element are chemically identical, are unchanged by chemical reaction, and combine in a ratio of simple numbers. Dalton measured atomic weights in reference to hydrogen, to which he assigned the value of 1 (the atomic number of this element).

The discovery of x-rays by Wilhelm Conrad Röntgen in 1895 was a great contribution to physics and the care of the sick. A few months later another physicist, Henri Becquerel, discovered naturally occurring radioactive substances. In 1898 Marie Curie discovered two new elements in the uranium ore pitchblende. Curie named these trace elements *polonium* (after her homeland, Poland) and *radium.* Curie also coined the terms *radioactive* and *radioactivity.*

In 1913 Georg de Hevesy, often called the "father of nuclear medicine," developed the tracer principle. He coined the term *radioindicator* and extended his studies from inorganic to organic chemistry. The first radioindicators were naturally occurring substances such as radium and radon. The invention of the *cyclotron* by Ernest Lawrence in 1931 made it possible for de Hevesy to expand his studies to a broader spectrum of biologic processes by using phosphorus-32, sodium-22, and other cyclotron-produced radioactive tracers.

Radioactive elements began to be produced in *nuclear reactors* developed by Enrico Fermi and his colleagues in 1946. The nuclear reactor greatly extended the ability of the cyclotron to produce radioactive tracers. A key development was the introduction of the *gamma camera* by Hal Anger in 1958. Another major event that contributed to the development of molecular nuclear medicine was the invention of the Univac digital computer, which was able to perform 5000 calculations per second. These advances, together with the invention of transistors, magnetic tape, and printed circuits, made feasible the continued growth of nuclear medicine.

The thyroid was one of the first organs to be examined by nuclear medicine studies using *external radiation detectors.* In the 1940s investigators found that the rate of incorporation of radioactive iodine by the thyroid gland was greatly increased in hyperthyroidism (overproduction of thyroid hormones) and greatly decreased in hypothyroidism (underproduction of thyroid hormones). Over the years tracers and instruments were developed to allow almost every major organ of the body to be studied by application of the tracer principle. Images subsequently were made of structures such as the liver, spleen, brain, and kidneys. Today the emphasis of nuclear medicine studies is more on function and chemistry than anatomic structure.

Physical Principles

An understanding of radioactivity must precede an attempt to grasp the principles of nuclear medicine and how images are created using radioactive compounds. The term *radiation* is taken from the Latin word *radii,* which refers to the spokes of a wheel leading out from a central point. The term *radioactivity* is used to describe the radiation of energy in the form of high-speed *alpha* or *beta particles* or waves (gamma rays), from the nucleus of an atom.

BASIC NUCLEAR PHYSICS

The basic components of an atom include the nucleus, which is composed of varying numbers of *protons* and *neutrons,* and the orbiting *electrons,* which revolve around the nucleus in discrete energy levels. Protons have a positive electric charge, electrons have a negative charge, and neutrons are electrically neutral. Both protons and neutrons have masses nearly 2000 times the mass of the electron; therefore, the nucleus composes most of the mass of an atom. This configuration can be described by the Bohr atomic model (Fig. 38-1). The total number of protons, neutrons, and electrons in an atom determines its characteristics, including its stability.

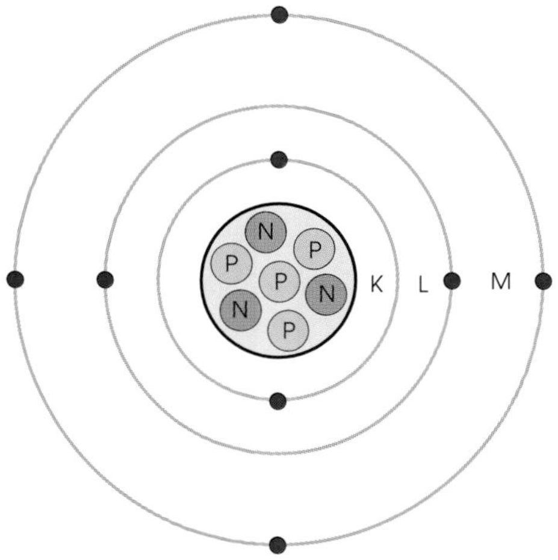

The term *nuclide* is used to describe an atomic species with a particular arrangement of protons and neutrons in the nucleus. Elements with the same number of protons but a different number of neutrons are referred to as *isotopes.* Isotopes have the same chemical properties as one another because the total number of protons and electrons is the same. They differ simply in the total number of neutrons contained in the nucleus. The neutron-to-proton ratio in the nucleus determines the stability of the atom. At certain ratios, atoms may be unstable, and a process known as spontaneous *decay* can occur as the atom attempts to regain stability. Energy is released in various ways during this decay, or return to *ground state.*

Radionuclides decay by the emission of alpha, beta, and gamma radiation. Most radionuclides reach ground state through various decay processes, including alpha, beta, or positron emission and *electron capture,* as well as several other methods. These decay methods determine the type of particles or gamma rays given off in the decay.

Fig. 38-1 Diagram of Bohr atom containing a single nucleus of protons (*P*) and neutrons (*N*) with surrounding orbital electrons of varying energy levels (*K, L, M . . .*).

To better explain this process, investigators have created decay schemes to show the details of how a *parent* nuclide decays to its *daughter* or ground state (Fig. 38-2, *A*). Decay schemes are unique for each radionuclide and identify the type of decay, the energy associated with each process, the probability of a particular decay process, and the rate of change into the ground state element, commonly known as the *half-life* of the radionuclide.

Radioactive decay is considered a purely random and spontaneous process that can be mathematically defined by complex equations and represented by average decay rates. The term *half-life (T)* is used to describe the time it takes for a quantity of a particular radionuclide to decay to one half of its original activity. This radioactive decay is a measure of the physical time it takes to reach one half of the original number of atoms through spontaneous disintegration. The rate of decay has an exponential function, which can be plotted on a linear scale (Fig. 38-2, *B*). If plotted on a semilogarithmic scale, the decay rate would be represented as a straight line. Radionuclide half-lives range from milliseconds to years. The half-lives of most radionuclides used in nuclear medicine range from several hours to several days.

NUCLEAR PHARMACY

The radionuclides used in nuclear medicine are produced in reactors, or *particle accelerators*. Naturally occurring radionuclides have very long half-lives (i.e., thousands of years). These natural radionuclides are unsuitable for nuclear medicine imaging because of limited availability or the high absorbed dose the patient would receive. Thus the radionuclides for nuclear medicine are produced in a particle accelerator through nuclear reactions created between a specific target chemical and high-speed charged particles. The number of protons in the target nuclei is changed when the nuclei are bombarded by the high-speed charged particles, and a new element or radionuclide is produced. Radionuclides can be created in nuclear reactors either by inserting a target element into the reactor core where it is irradiated or by separating and collecting the *fission* products.

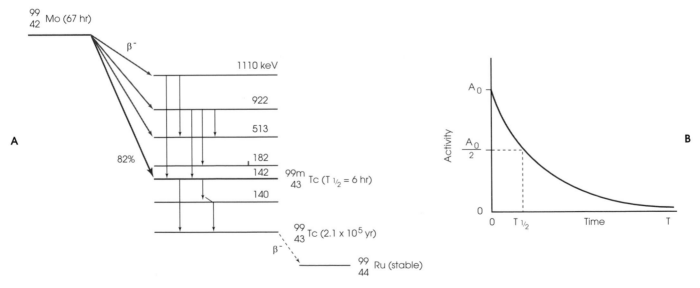

Fig. 38-2 A, Decay scheme illustrating the method by which radioactive molybdenum (^{99}Mo) decays to radioactive technetium (^{99m}Tc), one of the most commonly used radiopharmaceuticals in nuclear medicine. **B,** Graphic representation showing the rate of physical decay of a radionuclide. The y (vertical) axis represents the amount of *radioactivity* and the x (horizontal) axis represents the time at which a specific amount of activity has decreased to *one half* of its initial value. Every radionuclide has an associated half-life that is representative of its rate of decay.

The most commonly used radionuclide in nuclear medicine today is technetium-^{99m}Tc, which is produced in a generating system. This system makes available desirable short-lived radionuclides—the *daughters*—which are formed by the decay of relatively longer-lived radionuclides—the *parents*. The generator system uses molybdenum-99 as the parent. 99Mb has a half-life of 66.7 hours and decays (86%) to a daughter product known as *metastable* technetium (^{99m}Tc). Because technetium and molybdenum are chemically different, they can easily be separated through an ion-exchange column. ^{99m}Tc exhibits nearly ideal characteristics for use in nuclear medicine examinations, including a relatively short physical half-life of 6.04 hours and a high-yield (98.6%) 140-keV gamma photon (see Fig. 38-2, *A*).

Because radiopharmaceuticals are administered to patients, they need to be sterile and *pyrogen free*. They also need to undergo all of the quality control measures required of conventional drugs. A radiopharmaceutical generally has two components: a *radionuclide* and a *pharmaceutical*. The pharmaceutical is chosen on the basis of its preferential localization or participation in the physiologic function of a given organ. A radionuclide is tagged to a pharmaceutical. After the radiopharmaceutical is administered, the target organ is localized and the radiation emitted from it can be detected by imaging instruments.

The following characteristics are desirable in an imaging radiopharmaceutical:
- Ease of production and ready availability
- Low cost
- Lowest possible radiation dose
- Primary photon energy between 100 and 400 keV
- Physical half-life greater than the time required to prepare the material for injection
- Effective half-life longer than the examination time
- Suitable chemical forms for rapid localization
- Different uptake in the structure to be detected than in the surrounding tissue
- Low toxicity in the chemical form administered to the patient
- Stability or near-stability

^{99m}Tc can be bound to biologically active compounds or drugs to create a radiopharmaceutical that localizes in a specific organ system or structure when the radionuclide is administered intravenously or orally. A commonly used radiopharmaceutical is ^{99m}Tc tagged to a macroaggregated albumin (MAA). After IV injection, this substance follows the pathway of blood flow to the lungs, where it is distributed throughout and trapped in the small pulmonary capillaries (Fig. 38-3). Blood clots along the pathway prevent this radiopharmaceutical from distributing in the area beyond the clot. As a result the image shows a void or clear area, often described as *photopenia* or a *cold spot*. More than 30 different radiopharmaceuticals are used in nuclear medicine (Table 38-1).

Radiopharmaceutical doses vary, depending on the radionuclide used, the examination to be performed, and the size of the patient. The measure of radioactivity is expressed as either the *becquerel (Bq),* which corresponds to the decay rate, expressed as one disintegration per second, or as the *curie (Ci),* which equals 3.7×10^{10} disintegrations per second, relative to the number of decaying atoms in 1 g of radium.

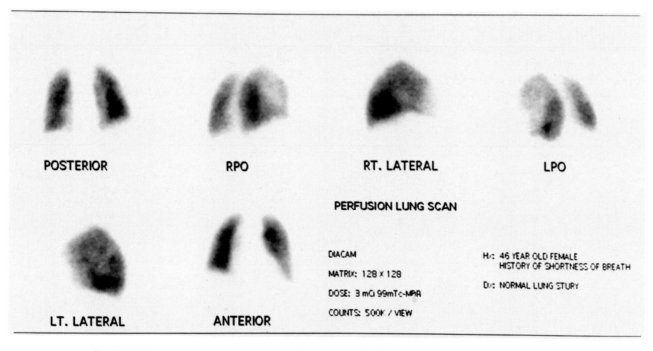

Fig. 38-3 Normal perfusion lung scan using 3 mCi of ^{99m}Tc tagged to a macroaggregated albumin (^{99}Tc MAA) on a large field-of-view gamma camera approximately 5 minutes after injection of the radiopharmaceutical. *RPO,* Right posterior oblique; *LPO,* left posterior oblique; *RT,* right; *LT,* left.

(Courtesy Siemens Medical Systems, Iselin, NJ.)

TABLE 38-1

Radiopharmaceuticals used in nuclear medicine

Radionuclide	Symbol	Physical half-life	Chemical form	Diagnostic use
Chromium	^{51}Cr	27.8 days	Sodium chromate	Red blood cell volume and survival
			Albumin	Gastrointestinal protein loss
Cobalt	^{57}Co	270 days	Cyanocobalamin (vitamin B_{12})	Vitamin B_{12} absorption
	^{58}Co	72 days	Cyanocobalamin (vitamin B_{12})	Vitamin B_{12} absorption
Gallium	^{67}Ga	77 hours	Gallium citrate	Inflammatory process and tumor imaging
Indium	^{111}In	67.4 hours	Diethylenetriamine penta-acetic acid (DTPA)	Cerebrospinal fluid imaging
			OncoScint (satumomab pendetide)	Colorectal or ovarian cancer
			OctreoScan (pentetreotide)	Neuroendocrine tumors
			ProstaScint (capromab pendetide)	Prostrate cancer
			Oxine	White blood cell/abscess imaging
Iodine	^{123}I	13.3 hours	Sodium iodide	Thyroid function and imaging
	^{125}I	60 days	Triiodothyronine	Thyroid hormone assay
			Thyroxine	Thyroid hormone assay
			Other hormones or drugs	Radioassays
			Human serum albumin	Plasma volume
	^{131}I	8 days	Sodium iodide	Thyroid function, imaging, and therapy
			Hippurate	Renal function
Technetium	^{99m}Tc	6 hours	Sodium pertechnetate	Imaging of brain, thyroid, scrotum, salivary glands, renal perfusion, and pericardial effusion; evaluation of left-to-right cardiac shunts
			Sulfur colloid	Imaging of liver and spleen and renal transplants, lymphoscintigraphy
			Macroaggregated albumin	Lung imaging
			Sestamibi	Cardiovascular imaging, myocardial perfusion
			DTPA	Brain and renal imaging
			Dimercaptosuccinic acid (DMSA)	Renal imaging
			Mertiatide (MAG_3)	Renal imaging
			Diphosphonate	Bone imaging
			Pyrophosphate	Bone and myocardial imaging
			Red blood cells	Cardiac function imaging
			Hexamethylpropyleneamine-oxime (HMPAO)	Functional brain imaging
			Iminodiacetic (IDA) derivations	Liver function imaging
			Neurolite (Bicisate)	Brain imaging
			Myoview (Tetrofosmin)	Myocardial ischemia
			CEA-scan (Arcitumomab)	Gastrointestinal tract
			Verluma (NR-LU-10)	Small cell lung cancer
Thallium	^{201}Tl	73.5 hours	Thallous chloride	Myocardial imaging
Xenon	^{133}Xe	5.3 days	Xenon gas	Lung ventilation imaging

Radiation Safety in Nuclear Medicine

The radiation protection requirements in nuclear medicine differ from the general radiation safety measures used for diagnostic radiography. The radionuclides employed in nuclear medicine are in liquid, solid, or gaseous form. Because of the nature of radioactive decay, these radionuclides continuously emit radiation after administration (unlike diagnostic x-rays, which can be turned on and off mechanically). Therefore special precautions are required.

In general, the quantities of radioactive tracers used in nuclear medicine present no significant hazard. Nonetheless, care must be taken to reduce unnecessary exposure. The high concentrations or activities of the radionuclides used in a nuclear pharmacy necessitate the establishment of a designated preparation area that contains isolated ventilation, protective lead or glass shielding for vials and syringes, absorbent material, and gloves. The handling and administering of diagnostic doses to patients warrants the use of gloves and a lead syringe shield at all times (Fig. 38-4). Any radioactive material that is spilled continues to emit radiation and therefore must immediately be cleaned up and contained. Because radioactive material that contacts the skin can be absorbed and may not be easily washed off, it is very important to wear protective gloves when handling radiopharmaceuticals.

Technologists and nuclear pharmacists are required to wear appropriate radiation monitoring (dosimetry) devices, such as film badges and thermoluminescent dosimetry (TLD) rings, to monitor radiation exposure to the body and hands. The ALARA (*as low as reasonably achievable*) program applies to all nuclear medicine personnel.

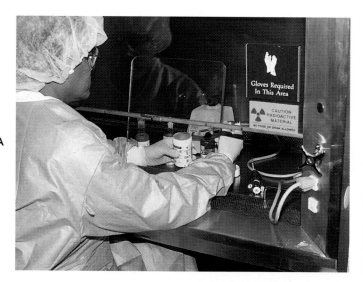
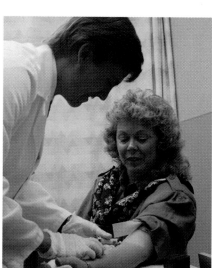

Fig. 38-4 A, Area in a radiopharmacy in which doses of radiopharmaceuticals are prepared in a clean and protected environment. **B,** Nuclear medicine technologist administering a radiopharmaceutical intravenously using appropriate radiation safety precautions, including gloves and a syringe shield.

Instrumentation

RADIOACTIVE DETECTORS

Gas-filled detectors

For radioactivity to be detected, it must first interact with matter and release energy. When radioactivity strikes matter, as with gas molecules inside a detector, the gas ionizes (becomes charged), creating a voltage potential between two electrodes. This voltage potential is then used as a measure of the radioactivity present.

Two gas-filled radiation detectors are commonly used to detect and estimate the amount of radiation present. One is the Geiger-Mueller survey meter, usually called the *Geiger counter* (Fig. 38-5, *A*). The other is the dose calibrator, which is an ionization chamber used to measure the amount of radioactivity in a sample, such as a syringe, vial, or test tube (Fig. 38-5, *B*).

Scintillation detectors

The term *scintillate* means to emit light photons. Becquerel discovered that ionizing radiation caused certain materials to glow. A *scintillation detector* is a sensitive element used to detect ionizing radiation by observing the emission of light photons induced in a material. When a light-sensitive device is affixed to this material, the flash of light can be changed into small electrical impulses. The electrical impulses are then amplified so that they may be sorted and counted to determine the amount and nature of radiation striking the scintillating materials. Scintillation detectors were used in the development of the first-generation nuclear medicine scanner, the *rectilinear scanner,* which was built in 1950.

Modern-day gamma camera

Rectilinear scanners have evolved into complex imaging systems known today as *gamma cameras* (because they detect gamma rays). These cameras are still scintillation detectors that use a thallium-activated sodium iodide crystal to detect and transform radioactive emissions into light photons. Through a complex process, these light photons are amplified and their locations are electronically recorded to produce an image that is displayed as a hard copy or on computer output systems. Scintillation cameras with single or multiple crystals are used today.

Gamma cameras can be either stationary or mobile. Mobile gamma cameras are used to perform bedside studies on patients who cannot be transported to the nuclear medicine department. The mobile cameras can be moved throughout the hospital, or they may be transported to other sites using a cross-country truck unit. Mobile gamma cameras typically have limitations, including a smaller field of view and less detector shielding; thus the types and quality of examinations that can be performed are restricted. The gamma camera has many components that work together to produce an image (Fig. 38-6).

A

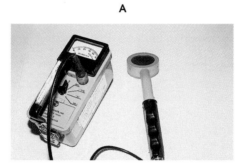

B

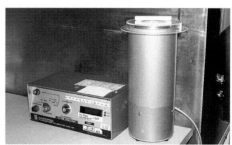

Fig. 38-5 A, Geiger-Mueller survey meter used to detect and determine the relative amount of radioactivity present. **B,** Dose calibrator used to determine the amount of radioactivity in syringes or vials.

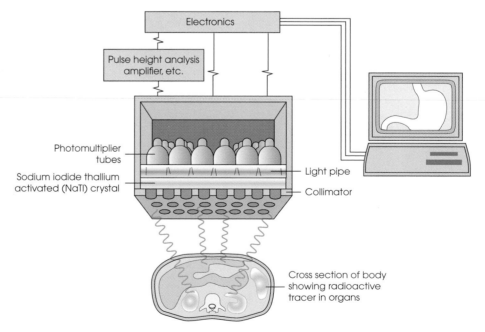

Fig. 38-6 Typical gamma camera system, which includes complex computers and electronic mechanical components for acquiring, processing, displaying, and analyzing nuclear medicine images.

Collimator

Located at the face of the detector, where photons from radioactive sources first enter the camera, is a *collimator*. The collimator is used to separate gamma rays and keep scattered rays from entering the scintillation crystal. *Resolution* and *sensitivity* are terms used to describe the physical characteristics of collimators. Collimator sensitivity is determined by the fraction of photons that are actually transmitted through the collimator and strike the face of the camera crystal. Spatial resolution is the capability of a system to produce an image in which the small details are observable.

Collimators are usually made of a material with a high atomic number, such as lead. Different collimators are used for different types of examinations, depending on photon energy and the desired level of sensitivity and resolution.

Crystal and light pipe

The scintillation crystals commonly used in gamma cameras are made of sodium iodide with trace quantities of thallium added to increase light production. This crystal composition is effective for stopping most common gamma rays emitted from the radiopharmaceuticals used in nuclear medicine.

The thickness of the crystal varies from $\frac{1}{4}$ to $\frac{1}{2}$ inch (0.6 to 1.3 cm). Thicker crystals are better for imaging radiopharmaceuticals with higher energies (more than 180 keV) but have decreased resolution. Thinner crystals provide improved resolution but cannot efficiently image photons with a higher kiloelectron voltage.

A *light pipe* may be used to attach the crystal to the *photomultiplier tubes (PMTs)*. The light pipe is a disk of optically transparent material that helps direct photons from the crystal into the PMTs.

Detector electronics

An array of PMTs are attached to the back of the crystal or light pipe. Inside the detector are PMTs used to detect and convert light photons emitted from the crystal into an electronic signal that amplifies the original photon signal by a factor of as much as 10^7. A typical gamma camera detector head contains 80 to 100 PMTs.

The PMTs send the detected signal through a series of processing steps, which include determining the location (x, y) of the original photon and its amplitude or energy (z). The x and y values are determined by where the photon strikes the crystal. Electronic circuitry known as a *pulse height analyzer* is used to eliminate the z signals that are not within a desired preset energy range for a particular radionuclide. This helps reduce scattered lower energy, unwanted photons ("noise") that generally would degrade resolution of the image. Once the information has been processed, the signals are transmitted to the display system, which includes a cathode ray tube and a film imaging system or computer to record the image.

Multihead gamma camera systems

The standard gamma camera is a single detector that can be moved in various positions around the patient. Gamma camera systems may include as many as three detectors (heads). Dual-head gamma camera systems allow simultaneous anterior and posterior imaging and may be used for whole-body bone or tumor imaging. Triple-head systems may be used for brain and heart studies. Although these systems are primarily suited for single photon emission computed tomography (SPECT), they can also provide multiplanar images.

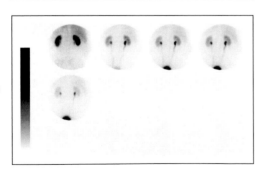

A

B

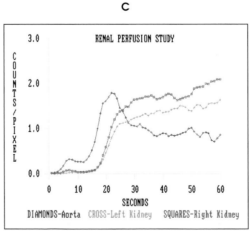

C

D

Cortical Analysis			
	Left Kidney	Right Kidney	Bladder
Appearance time in collecting system	2.7 min	2.7 min	3.8 min
Time to peak	2.7 min	2.5 min	
20 min counts / peak counts	21.7 %	21.2 %	
T 3/4 clearance	4.0 min	4.2 min	
T 1/2 clearance	6.5 min	6.7 min	

Lt   Rt

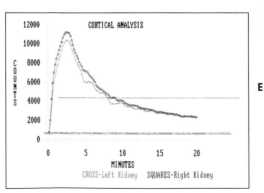

CROSS-Left Kidney   SQUARES-Right Kidney

E

Fig. 38-7 A, Posterior renal blood flow in an adult patient using 10 mCi of ^{99m}Tc with diethylenetriamine pentaacetic acid (DTPA) imaged at 3 seconds per frame. The image in the lower right corner is a blood-pool image taken immediately after the initial flow sequence. Together the images demonstrate normal renal blood flow to both kidneys. **B,** Normal, sequential dynamic 20-minute ^{99m}Tc with mertiatide (MAG$_3$) images. **C,** Renal arterial perfusion curves showing minor renal blood flow asymmetry. **D,** Renal cortical analysis curves showing rapid uptake and prompt parenchymal clearance. **E,** Quantitative renal cortical analysis indices showing normal values.

COMPUTERS

Computers have become an integral part of the nuclear medicine imaging system. Computer systems are used to acquire and process data from gamma cameras. They allow data to be collected over a specific time frame or to a specified number of counts; the data can then be analyzed to determine functional changes occurring over time (Fig. 38-7, *A* and *B*). A common example is the renal study, in which the radiopharmaceutical that is administered is cleared by normally functioning kidneys in about 20 minutes. The computer can collect images of the kidney during this period and analyze the images to determine how effectively the kidneys clear the radiopharmaceutical (Fig. 38-7, *C, D,* and *E*). The computer also allows the operator to enhance a particular structure by adjusting the contrast and brightness of the image.

Electronically stored records can decrease reporting turnaround time, physical image storage requirements, and the use of personnel for record maintenance and retrieval. Long-term computerized records can also form the basis for statistical analysis to improve testing methods and predict disease courses.

Computerization of the nuclear pharmacy operation also has become an important means of record keeping and quality control. Radioactive dosages and dose volumes can be calculated more quickly by computer than by hand. The nuclear pharmacy computer system may be used to provide reminders and keep records as required by the Nuclear Regulatory Commission (NRC), the U.S. Food and Drug Administration (FDA), and individual state regulatory agencies. Computers can also assist in the scheduling of patients, based on dose availability and department policies.

Computers are necessary to acquire and process SPECT images, to be discussed in the next section. SPECT uses a scintillation camera that moves around the patient to obtain images from multiple angles for tomographic image reconstruction. SPECT studies are complex and, like magnetic resonance imaging (MRI) studies, require a great deal of computer processing to create images in transaxial, sagittal, or coronal planes. Rotating three-dimensional images can also be generated from SPECT data (Fig. 38-8).

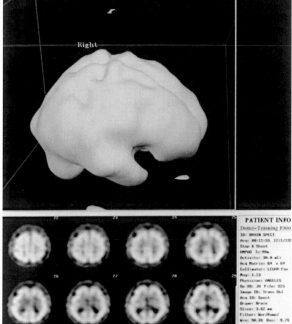
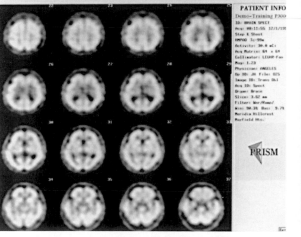

A

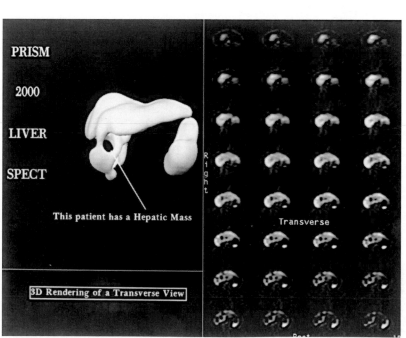

B

Fig. 38-8 A, Three-dimensional single photon emission computed tomography (SPECT) brain study using 30 mCi of ^{99m}Tc with hexamethylpropyleneamine-oxime (HMPAO). Three-dimensional representation of a normal brain *(top)* and transaxial slices shown *(bottom)*. **B,** Three-dimensional SPECT liver study using 8 mCi of ^{99m}Tc sulfur colloid. A mass is seen on both the three-dimensional image *(top)* and the transaxial images *(bottom)*.

Computer networks are becoming an integral part of the way a department communicates information within and among institutions. In a network, several or many computers are connected so that they all have access to the same files, programs, printers, etc. Networking allows the movement of both image-based and text-based data to any computer or printer in the network. Networking improves the efficiency of a nuclear medicine department. A computer network can serve as a vital component, reducing the time expended on menial tasks while allowing retrieval and transferal of information. Consolidation of all reporting functions in one area eliminates the need for the nuclear medicine physician to travel between departments in order to read studies. Centralized archiving, printing, and retrieval of the majority of image-based and nonimage-based data have increased the efficiency of data analysis, reduced the cost of image hard copy, and permitted more sophisticated analysis of image data than would routinely be possible.

QUANTITATIVE ANALYSIS

Many nuclear medicine procedures require some form of quantitative analysis to provide physicians with numeric results based on and depicting organ function. Specialized software allows computers to collect, process, and analyze functional information obtained from nuclear medicine imaging systems. Cardiac ejection fraction is one of the more common quantitation studies (Fig. 38-9). In this dynamic study of the heart's contractions and expansions, the computer accurately determines the ejection fraction, or the amount of blood pumped out of the left ventricle with each contraction.

Imaging Methods

A wide variety of diagnostic imaging examinations are performed in nuclear medicine. These examinations can be described on the basis of the imaging method used: static, whole body, dynamic, SPECT, and positron emission tomography (PET) (see Chapter 40).

STATIC IMAGING

Static imaging is the acquisition of a single image of a particular structure. This image can be thought of as a "snapshot" of the radiopharmaceutical distribution within a part of the body. Examples of static images include lung scans, spot bone scan images, and thyroid images. Static images are usually obtained in various orientations around a particular structure to demonstrate all aspects of that structure. Anterior, posterior, and oblique images are often obtained.

In static imaging, low radiopharmaceutical activity levels are used to minimize radiation exposure to the patients. Because of these low activity levels, images must be acquired for a preset time or a minimum number of counts or radioactive emissions. This time frame may vary from a few seconds to several minutes to acquire 100,000 to more than 1 million counts. Generally, it takes 30 seconds to 5 minutes to obtain a sufficient number of counts to produce a satisfactory image.

A

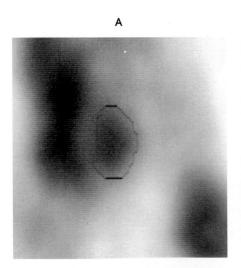

B

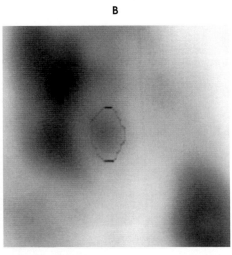

C

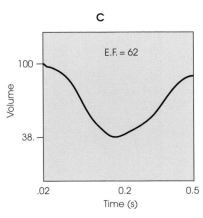

Fig. 38-9 **A,** Cardiac-gated study showing heart wall motion and quantitative results, including the cardiac ejection fraction. This is an LAO image of the left ventricle at end-diastole (relaxed phase), with a region of interest drawn around the left ventricle. **B,** Same LAO image showing end-systole (contracted phase). **C,** Curve representing the volume change in the left ventricle of the heart before, during, and after contraction. This volume change is referred to as the *ejection fraction (EF),* with a normal value being approximately 64% ± 10%.

WHOLE-BODY IMAGING

Whole-body imaging uses a specially designed moving detector system to produce an image of the entire body or a large body section. In this type of imaging, the gamma camera collects data as it passes over the body. Earlier detector systems were smaller and required as many as two or three incremental passes to encompass the entire width of the body.

During the past several years the detector width for whole-body systems has been increased to allow for a single head-to-foot pass that encompasses the entire body from side to side. These systems may also include dual heads for simultaneous anterior and posterior imaging. Whole-body imaging systems are used primarily for whole-body bone scans, whole-body tumor or abscess imaging, and other clinical and research applications (Fig. 38-10).

DYNAMIC IMAGING

Dynamic images display the distribution of a particular radiopharmaceutical over a specific period. A dynamic or "flow" study of a particular structure is generally used to evaluate blood perfusion to the tissue. This can be thought of as a sequential or time-lapse image. Images may be acquired and displayed in time sequences as short as one tenth of a second to longer than 10 minutes per image. Dynamic imaging is commonly used for first-pass cardiac studies, hepatobiliary studies, and gastric emptying studies.

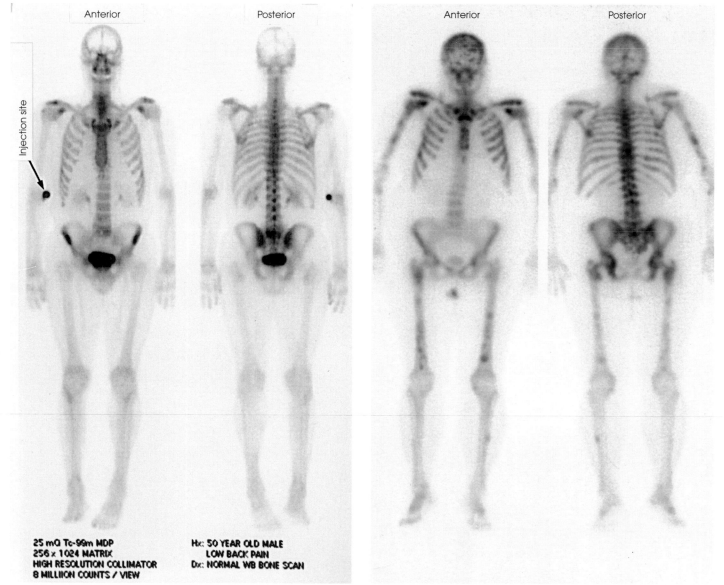

A

Anterior Posterior

Injection site

25 mCi Tc-99m MDP
256 × 1024 MATRIX
HIGH RESOLUTION COLLIMATOR
8 MILLION COUNTS / VIEW

Hx: 50 YEAR OLD MALE
     LOW BACK PAIN
Dx: NORMAL WB BONE SCAN

B

Anterior Posterior

Fig. 38-10 A, Whole-body bone scan performed using ^{99m}Tc with methylene diphosphonate (MDP) in a 50-year-old male patient with low back pain. The study was normal. Note the injection site in the right antecubital fossa. **B,** Whole-body scan on a 67-year-old female patient with breast cancer. The study demonstrates numerous foci of increased uptake in the axial and appendicular skeleton, consistent with bony metastases. Metastases are seen in the calvarium, both humeri and femurs, the entire spine, the ribs, and the pelvis.

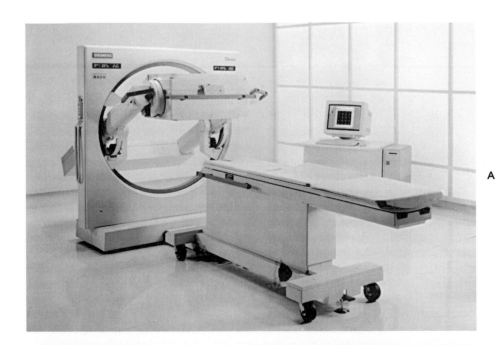

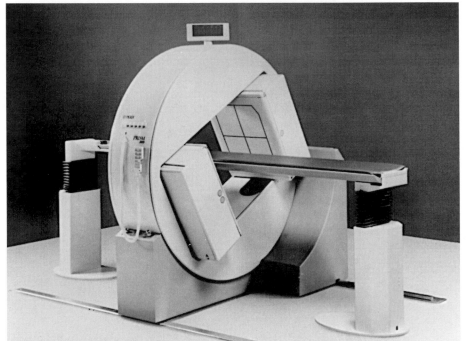

Fig. 38-11 Single photon emission computed tomography (SPECT) camera systems. **A,** Single-head system. **B,** Dual-headed system. **C,** Triple-headed system.

(Courtesy Picker International and Siemens Medical Systems.)

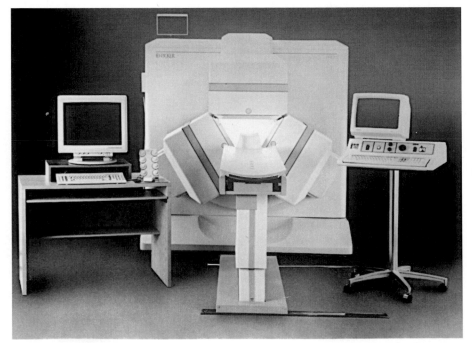

SINGLE PHOTON EMISSION COMPUTED TOMOGRAPHY

SPECT produces images similar to those obtained by CT or MRI in that a computer creates thin slices through a particular organ. This imaging technique has proved very beneficial for delineating small lesions within tissues, and it can be used on virtually any structure or organ. Improved clinical results with SPECT are due to improved target-to-nontarget ratios. Planar images record and demonstrate all radioactivity emitting from the patient above and below the region of interest, causing degradation of the image. In contrast, SPECT eliminates the unnecessary information.

With SPECT, one to three gamma detectors may be used to produce tomographic images (Fig. 38-11). Tomographic systems are designed to allow the detector heads to rotate as much as 360 degrees around a patient's body to collect "projection" image data. The image data are reconstructed by a computer in several formats, including transaxial, sagittal, coronal, planar, and three-dimensional representations. The computer-generated images allow for the display of thin slices through different planes of an organ or structure, thereby helping to identify small abnormalities.

The most common uses of SPECT include cardiac perfusion, brain, liver (see Fig. 38-8, *B*), and bone studies. An example of a SPECT study is the myocardial perfusion thallium study, which is used to identify perfusion defects in the left ventricular wall. Radioactive thallium is injected intravenously while the patient is being physically stressed on a treadmill or is being infused with a vasodilator. The radiopharmaceutical distributes in the heart muscle in the same fashion as blood flows to the tissue. An initial set of images is acquired immediately after the stress test. A second set is obtained several hours later when the patient is rested (when the thallium has redistributed to viable tissue) to determine whether any blood perfusion defects that were seen on the initial images have resolved. By comparing the two image sets, the physician may be able to tell whether the patient has damaged heart tissue resulting from a myocardial infarction or myocardial ischemia (Fig. 38-12).

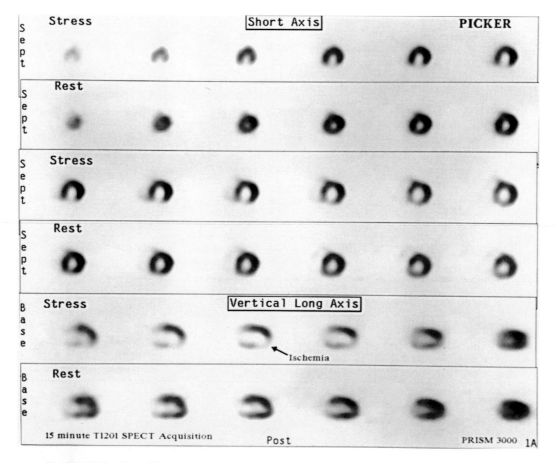

Fig. 38-12 Thallium-201 myocardial perfusion study comparing stress and redistribution (resting) images in various planes of the heart (short axis and long axis). A perfusion defect is identified in the stress images but not seen in the redistribution (rest) images. This finding is indicative of ischemia.

POSITRON EMISSION TOMOGRAPHY

PET imaging uses positron emissions from particular radionuclides to produce detailed functional images within the body. PET is unique in that its images are of blood flow or metabolic processes at the cellular level rather than the more conventional anatomic images produced by x-ray, CT, MRI, or even SPECT. A positron emitter releases two identical photons that travel in exactly opposite directions. These photons are of high energy (511 keV) and require special imaging by two opposing detectors. Because the positron radiopharmaceuticals generally have short half-lives of anywhere from a few seconds to a few hours, they must be produced in a cyclotron located near the imaging facility or through a specially designed generator system. One of the more common PET procedures uses fluorine-18 fluorodeoxyglucose to measure glucose metabolism in the brain (Fig. 38-13). PET is also frequently used to detect tumors in the body, which generally have a very high rate of glucose uptake. (For additional discussion, see Chapter 40.)

Clinical Nuclear Medicine

The term *in vivo* means "within the living body." Because all diagnostic nuclear medicine imaging procedures are based on the distribution of radiopharmaceuticals within the body, they are classified as *in vivo* examinations.

Patient preparation for nuclear medicine procedures is minimal, with most tests requiring no special preparation. Patients usually remain in their own clothing. However, all metal objects outside or inside the clothing must be removed because they may mimic pathologic conditions on nuclear medicine imaging. The waiting time between dose administration and imaging varies with each study. After completion of a routine procedure, patients may resume all normal activities.

Following are technical summaries of some of the more commonly performed nuclear medicine procedures. After each procedure summary is a list, by organ or system, of many common studies that may be done in an average nuclear medicine department.

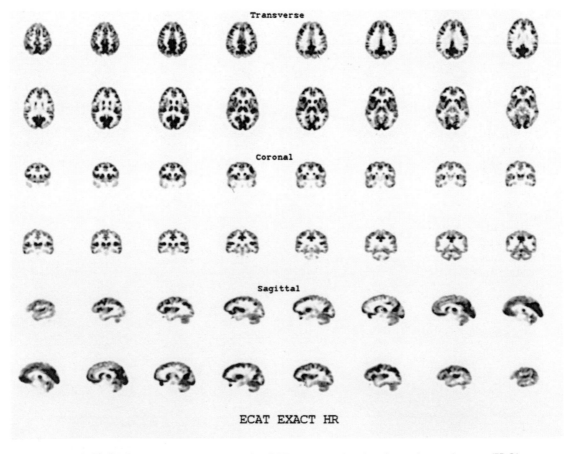

ECAT EXACT HR

Fig. 38-13 Positron emission tomography (PET) brain study using fluorodeoxyglucose (FDG) to measure metabolic changes in the brain.

BONE SCINTIGRAPHY

Bone scintigraphy is generally a survey procedure to evaluate patients with malignancies, diffuse musculoskeletal symptoms, abnormal laboratory results, and hereditary or metabolic disorders. Tracer techniques have been used for many years to study the exchange between bone and blood. Radionuclides have played an important role in understanding both normal bone metabolism and the metabolic effects of pathologic involvement of bone. Radiopharmaceuticals used for bone imaging can localize in bone and also in soft tissue structures. Skeletal areas of increased uptake are commonly a result of tumor, infection, or fracture.

Bone scan
Principle

It is not entirely clear how ^{99m}Tc-labeled diphosphonates are incorporated into bone at the molecular level; however, it appears that regional blood flow, osteoblastic activity, and extraction efficiency are the major factors that influence the uptake. In areas in which osteoblastic activity is increased, active hydroxyapatite crystals with large surface areas appear to be the most suitable sites for uptake of the diphosphonate portion of the radiopharmaceutical.

Radiopharmaceutical

The adult dose of 20 mCi (740 MBq) of ^{99m}Tc hydroxymethylene diphosphonate (HDP) or 20 mCi (740 MBq) of ^{99m}Tc methylene diphosphonate (MDP) is injected intravenously. The pediatric dose is adjusted according to the patient's weight.

Scanning

A routine survey begins 2 to 3 hours after the injection and takes 30 to 45 minutes. The number of camera images acquired depends on the indication for the examination.

Bone (skeletal) studies

Bone scan, bone marrow scan, joint scan

NUCLEAR CARDIOLOGY

Nuclear cardiology has experienced rapid growth in recent years and currently composes a significant portion of daily nuclear medicine procedures. These noninvasive studies assess cardiac performance, evaluate myocardial perfusion, and measure viability and metabolism. Advances in computers and scintillation camera technology have facilitated the development of a quantitative cardiac evaluation unequaled by any other noninvasive or invasive methods. The stress test is performed with the patient using a treadmill or stationary bicycle. During the stress test the patient's heart rate, electrocardiogram (ECG or EKG), blood pressure, and symptoms are continuously monitored. Some patients cannot exercise because of peripheral vascular disease, neurologic problems, or musculoskeletal abnormalities. In these patients, a pharmacologic intervention can be used in place of the exercise test to alter the blood flow to the heart in a way that simulates exercise, allowing the detection of myocardial ischemia. Three procedures are discussed in the following sections.

Exercise radionuclide angiography
Principle

Gated radionuclide angiography (RNA) can be used to measure left ventricular ejection fraction and evaluate left ventricular regional wall motion. RNA requires that the blood be labeled with an appropriate tracer such as ^{99m}Tc. For optimum image quality in RNA, the patient must be in normal sinus rhythm so that successive cardiac cycles can be accurately summed. The technique is based on imaging the left ventricle for a large number of beats and summing the image data from each beat to produce a composite beat with adequate counting statistics for analysis. RNA requires simultaneous acquisition of the patient's ECG and images of the left ventricle.

Radiopharmaceutical

The adult dose is 30 mCi (1110 MBq) of ^{99m}Tc-labeled red blood cells. The pediatric dose is adjusted according to the patient's weight.

Scanning

Imaging can begin immediately after the injection and takes about 1 hour. Studies of the heart should be obtained in the anterior, left lateral, and left anterior oblique positions.

^{201}Tl myocardial perfusion study
Principle

The stress thallium-20 study has high sensitivity (about 90%) and specificity (about 75%) for the diagnosis of coronary artery disease. This study also has been useful for assessing myocardial viability in patients with known coronary artery disease and for evaluating patients after revascularization. At rest, symptoms may not be apparent. ^{201}Tl is an analog of potassium and has a high rate of extraction by the myocardium over a wide range of metabolic and physiologic conditions. ^{201}Tl is distributed in the myocardium in proportion to regional blood flow and myocardial cell viability. Under stress, myocardial ^{201}Tl uptake peaks within 1 minute. ^{201}Tl uptake in the heart ranges from about 1% of the injected dose at rest to about 4% with maximum exercise. Regions of the heart that are infarcted or underperfused at the time of injection appear as areas of decreased activity (photopenia).

Radiopharmaceutical

The adult dose for a stress study is 3 mCi (111 MBq) of ^{201}Tl thallous chloride administered intravenously at peak stress; 1 mCi (37 MBq) of ^{201}Tl is administered intravenously before the delayed study. The adult dose for a rest study is 4 mCi (148 MBq) of ^{201}Tl administered intravenously before the rest study. The minimum dose recommended for pediatric patients is 300 μCi (11.1 MBq) of ^{201}Tl thallous chloride. Whenever possible, ^{99m}Tc sestamibi should be used in place of ^{201}Tl in obese patients.

Scanning

The images obtained include the anterior planar image of the chest and heart, followed by a 180-degree SPECT study (45 degrees right anterior oblique to 45 degrees left posterior oblique).

^{99m}Tc sestamibi myocardial perfusion study
Principle

Like ^{201}Tl, ^{99m}Tc sestamibi is a cation; however, it has a slightly lower fractional extraction than thallium, particularly at high flow rates. ^{99m}Tc sestamibi has favorable biologic properties for myocardial perfusion imaging. It is used to assess myocardial salvage resulting from therapeutic intervention in acute infarction, to determine the myocardial blood flow during periods of spontaneous chest pain, and to diagnose coronary artery disease in obese patients. A first-pass flow study can be performed with a rest or stress ^{99m}Tc sestamibi myocardial perfusion scan. A first-pass study evaluates heart function during the short time (in seconds) that it takes the injected bolus to travel through the left ventricle.

Radiopharmaceutical

The adult dose for the stress study is 10 to 30 mCi (370 to 1100 MBq) of ^{99m}Tc sestamibi administered intravenously at peak stress. The adult dose for rest study is 10 to 30 mCi (370 to 1100 MBq) of ^{99m}Tc sestamibi administered intravenously before the rest study.

Scanning

SPECT imaging should be performed 30 to 60 minutes after injection of the stress dose. Although SPECT imaging should be performed 30 to 60 minutes after injection of the rest dose, it may be done as long as 6 hours after injection. A 2-day protocol provides optimum image quality, but the 1-day protocol is more convenient for patients, technologists, and physicians.

Cardiovascular studies

Aortic/mitral regurgitant index, cardiac shunt study, dobutamine multiple gated acquisition (MUGA), rest MUGA, rest MUGA-ejection fraction only, exercise MUGA, stress testing (myocardial perfusion), ^{201}Tl myocardial perfusion scan, ^{99m}Tc sestamibi first-pass study, ^{99m}Tc sestamibi myocardial perfusion scan, ^{99m}Tc pyrophosphate (PYP) myocardial infarct scan, rest ^{201}Tl scan with infarct quantitation

CENTRAL NERVOUS SYSTEM

The central nervous system (CNS) consists of the brain and spinal cord. For patients with diseases of the central or peripheral nervous systems, nuclear medicine techniques can be used to assess the effectiveness of surgery or radiation therapy, document the extent of involvement of the brain by tumors, and determine progression or regression of lesions in response to different forms of treatment. Brain perfusion imaging is useful in the evaluation of patients with stroke, transient ischemia, and other neurologic disorders such as Alzheimer's disease, epilepsy, and Parkinson's disease. Radionuclide cisternography is particularly useful in the diagnosis of meningitis, hemorrhage, tumors, CSF leakage after trauma or surgery, and normal-pressure hydrocephalus. Recent studies indicate that documented lack of cerebral blood flow should be the criterion of choice to confirm brain death when clinical criteria are equivocal, when a complete neurologic examination cannot be performed, or when patients are younger than 1 year.

Brain SPECT study
Principle

Some imaging agents are capable of penetrating the intact *blood-brain barrier*. After a radiopharmaceutical crosses the blood-brain barrier, it becomes trapped inside the brain. The regional uptake and retention of the tracer are related to the regional perfusion. Note that before the imaging agent is injected, the patient is placed in a quiet, darkened area and instructed to close the eyes. These measures are helpful in reducing uptake of the tracer in the visual cortex.

Radiopharmaceutical

The adult dose is 20 mCi (740 MBq) of ^{99m}Tc ethylcysteinate diamer (ECD) or ^{99m}Tc hexamethylpropyleneamine-oxime (HMPAO).

Scanning

The pediatric dose is based on body surface area. Imaging begins 10 to 15 minutes after ^{99m}Tc ECD injection or 1 hour after ^{99m}Tc HMPAO injection. Tomographic images of the brain are obtained.

Central nervous system studies

Brain perfusion imaging–SPECT study, brain imaging–acetazolamide challenge study, CNS shunt patency, CSF imaging–cisternography/ventriculography, ^{201}Tl scan for recurrent brain tumor, ^{99m}Tc HMPAO scan for determination of brain death

ENDOCRINE SYSTEM

The endocrine system organs, located throughout the body, secrete hormones into the bloodstream. Hormones have profound effects on overall body function and metabolism. The endocrine system consists of the thyroid, parathyroid, pituitary, and suprarenal glands, the islet cells of the pancreas, and the gonads. Nuclear medicine procedures have played a significant part in the current understanding of the function of the endocrine glands and their role in health and disease. These procedures are useful for monitoring treatment of endocrine disorders, especially in the thyroid gland. Thyroid imaging is performed to evaluate the size, shape, nodularity, and functional status of the thyroid gland. Imaging is used to screen for thyroid cancer and to differentiate hyperthyroidism, nodular goiter, solitary thyroid nodule, and thyroiditis.

Thyroid scan
Principle

^{99m}Tc pertechnetate is trapped by the thyroid gland but, unlike iodine-131, is not organified *into* the gland. It offers the advantages of low radiation dose to the patient, no particulate radiation (unlike ^{131}I), and well-resolved images. Imaging is used to determine the relative function in different regions within the thyroid, with special emphasis on the function of nodules compared to the rest of the gland. Scanning can also determine the presence and site of thyroid tissue in unusual areas of the body, such as the tongue and anterior chest (ectopic tissue).

Radiopharmaceutical

The adult dose is 5 mCi (185 MBq) of ^{99m}Tc pertechnetate administered intravenously. The pediatric dose is adjusted according to the patient's weight. Uptake may be affected by thyroid medication and by foods or drugs, including some iodine-containing contrast agents used for renal radiographic imaging and CT scanning.

Scanning

Scanning should start 10 to 15 minutes after the injection. A gamma camera with a pinhole collimator is used to obtain anterior, left oblique, and right anterior oblique thyroid images and a 6-inch (15-cm) anterior neck image. The pinhole collimator is a thick, conical collimator that allows for magnification of the thyroid.

^{131}I thyroid uptake measurement
Principle

Radioiodine is concentrated by the thyroid gland in a manner that reflects the ability of the gland to handle stable dietary iodine. Therefore ^{131}I uptake is used to estimate the function of the thyroid gland by measuring its avidity for administered radioiodine. The higher the uptake of ^{131}I, the more active the thyroid; conversely, the lower the uptake, the less functional the gland. Uptake conventionally is expressed as the percentage of the dose in the thyroid gland at a given time after administration. ^{131}I uptake measurement is of value in distinguishing between thyroiditis (reduced uptake) and Graves' disease or toxic nodular goiter (Plummer's disease) (increased uptake). It is also used to determine the appropriateness of a therapeutic dose of ^{131}I in patients with Graves' disease, residual or recurrent thyroid carcinoma, or thyroid remnant after thyroidectomy.

Radiopharmaceutical

All doses of ^{131}I sodium iodide are administered orally. The exact activity administered depends on the type of uptake measurement and the presence of residual activity from previous ^{131}I uptake or scan procedures and is specified by the nuclear medicine physician. The adult dose for a standard uptake test is 4 to 6 μCi (148 to 222 kBq) of ^{131}I. The pediatric dose is adjusted according to the patient's weight.

Measurements are obtained using an uptake probe consisting of a 2 × 2 inch (5 × 5 cm) sodium iodide/photomultiplier tube assembly fitted with a flat-field lead collimator (Fig. 38-14). Uptake readings are acquired at 6 and 24 hours.

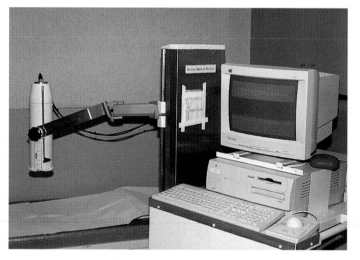

Fig. 38-14 Uptake probe used for thyroid uptake measurements over the extended neck area.

Neck/total-body ^{131}I scan

Principle

A neck or total-body ^{131}I scan is recommended for locating residual thyroid tissue or recurrent thyroid cancer cells in patients with thyroid carcinoma. Most follicular or papillary thyroid cancers concentrate radioiodine; other types of thyroid cancer do not. A neck scan is usually performed 1 to 3 months after a thyroidectomy to check for residual normal thyroid tissue. After the residual thyroid tissue has been ablated (destroyed), a total-body ^{131}I scan is performed to check for the metastatic spread of the cancer.

Radiopharmaceutical

The adult dose for a total-body ^{131}I scan is generally 3 mCi (111 MBq) of ^{131}I sodium iodide administered orally. The adult dose for a neck scan is 1 mCi (37 MBq) of ^{131}I sodium iodide administered orally. The pediatric dose is adjusted according to the patient's weight.

Scanning

Neck imaging starts 24 hours after administration of the dose. Total-body imaging begins 48 hours after dose administration. Images are obtained of the anterior planar neck. Total-body images are of the anterior and posterior whole body.

Endocrine studies

Adrenal cortical scan (NP-59), adrenal medullary scan (mIBG), ectopic thyroid scan (^{131}I/^{123}I), thyroid scan (^{99m}Tc pertechnetate), ^{131}I thyroid uptake measurement, ^{123}I thyroid uptake/scan, ^{131}I neck/total body iodine scan, parathyroid scan, indium-11 pentetreotide scan

GASTROINTESTINAL SYSTEM

The gastrointestinal system, or alimentary canal, consists of the mouth, oropharynx, esophagus, stomach, small bowel, colon, and several accessory organs (salivary glands, pancreas, liver, and gallbladder). The liver is the largest internal organ of the body. The portal venous system brings blood from the stomach, bowel, spleen, and pancreas to the liver.

Liver/spleen scan

Principle

Liver and/or spleen scanning is used to evaluate the liver for functional disease (e.g., cirrhosis, hepatitis, metastatic disease) and to look for residual splenic tissue following splenectomy. Imaging techniques such as ultrasonography, CT, and MRI provide excellent information about the anatomy of the liver, but nuclear medicine studies can assess the *functional* status of this organ. Liver and spleen scintigraphy is also useful for detecting hepatic lesions, performing biopsies, and evaluating hepatomegaly, jaundice, ascites, and liver enzyme abnormalities of unknown causes. It is also used to determine whether certain lesions found with other methods may be benign (e.g., focal nodular hyperplasia), thereby obviating the need for biopsy. Uptake of a radiopharmaceutical in the liver, spleen, and bone marrow depends on blood flow and the functional capacity of the phagocytic cells. In normal patients, 80% to 90% of the radiopharmaceutical is localized in the liver, 5% to 10% in the spleen, and the rest in the bone marrow.

Radiopharmaceutical

Adults receive 6 mCi (222 MBq) of ^{99m}Tc sulfur colloid or ^{99m}Tc albumin colloid injected intravenously. The pediatric dose is adjusted according to the patient's weight.

Scanning

Images obtained may be planar standard, life-size, or SPECT.

Gastrointestinal studies

Anorectal angle study, colonic transit study, colorectal/neorectal emptying study, esophageal scintigraphy, gastroesophageal reflux (adults and children) study, gastric emptying study, hepatic artery perfusion scan, hepatobiliary scan, hepatobiliary scan with gallbladder ejection fraction, evaluation of human serum albumin for protein-losing gastroenteropathy, liver/spleen scan, liver hemangioma study, Meckel's diverticulum scan, salivary gland study, small-bowel transit study

GENITOURINARY NUCLEAR MEDICINE

Genitourinary nuclear medicine studies are recognized as reliable, noninvasive procedures for evaluating the anatomy and function of the systems in nephrology, urology, and kidney transplantation. These studies can be accomplished with minimum risk of allergic reactions, unpleasant side effects, or excessive radiation exposure to the organs.

Dynamic renal scan

Principle

Renal scanning is used to assess renal perfusion and function, particularly in renal failure and renovascular hypertension and after renal transplantation. ^{99m}Tc mertiatide (MAG$_3$) is highly protein-bound, is secreted primarily by the proximal renal tubules, and is not retained in the parenchyma of normal kidneys.

Radiopharmaceutical

The adult dose is 10 mCi (370 MBq) of ^{99m}Tc MAG$_3$. The pediatric dose is adjusted according to the patient's weight.

Scanning

Imaging is initiated immediately after the injection. Because radiographic contrast media may interfere with kidney function, renal scanning should be delayed for 24 hours after contrast studies. Images are often taken over the posterior lower back, centered at the level of the twelfth rib. Transplanted kidneys are imaged in the anterior pelvis. Patients need to be well hydrated before all renal studies.

Genitourinary studies

Dynamic renal scan, dynamic renal scan with furosemide, dynamic renal scan with captopril, dynamic renal scan with glomerular filtration rate/effective renal plasma flow, pediatric furosemide renal scan, ^{99m}Tc dimercaptosuccinic acid (DMSA) renal scan, residual urine determination, testicular scan, voiding cystography

IN VITRO AND IN VIVO HEMATOLOGIC STUDIES

In vitro and in vivo hematologic studies have been performed in nuclear medicine for many years. Quantitative measurements are made after a radiopharmaceutical has been administered, often at predetermined intervals. The two types of nonimaging nuclear medicine procedures are as follows:

- *In vitro* radioimmunoassay for quantitating biologically important substances in the serum or other body fluids.
- *In vivo* evaluation of physiologic function by administering small tracer amounts of radioactive materials to the patient and subsequently counting specimens of urine, blood, feces, or breath. A wide variety of physiologic events may be measured, including vitamin B12 absorption (Schilling test), fat absorption, ability to deconjugate bile acids, red cell survival and sequestration, red cell mass, plasma volume, various body space measurements, ferrokinetics, and total body water.

Hematologic studies

Plasma volume measurement, Schilling test, red cell mass, red cell survival, red cell sequestration

IMAGING FOR INFECTION

Imaging for infection is another useful nuclear medicine diagnostic tool. Inflammation, infection, and abscess may be found in any organ and at any location. Recent dental extractions, IV drug abuse, and infections from other areas of the body can precede and cause bacterial endocarditis (infection of the valves of the heart). Lung abscesses can result from certain types of pneumonia or from chronic lung disease. A pelvic abscess can occur from pelvic inflammatory disease, ruptured diverticulum of the colon, appendicitis, regional enteritis, or prior surgery. Imaging procedures such as gallium-67 scans, ^{111}In-labeled white cell scans, radiolabeled antibody procedures, planar and SPECT studies, and PET scans aid in the localization and identification of inflammatory and tumor disorders.

Infection studies

[67]Ga gallium scan, white blood cell scans with ^{111}In oxine, ^{99m}Tc HMPAO, and ^{111}In tropolone

RESPIRATORY IMAGING

Respiratory imaging commonly involves the demonstration of pulmonary perfusion using limited, transient capillary blockade and the assessment of ventilation using an inhaled radioactive gas or aerosol. Lung imaging is most commonly performed to evaluate pulmonary emboli, chronic obstructive pulmonary disease, chronic bronchitis, emphysema, asthma, and lung carcinoma. It is also used for lung transplant evaluation.

[133]Xe lung ventilation scan
Principle

Lung ventilation scans are used in combination with lung perfusion scans. The gas used for a ventilation study must be absorbed significantly by the lungs and diffuse easily. Xenon-133 has adequate imaging properties, and less than 15% of the gas is usually absorbed by the body.

Radiopharmaceutical

The adult dose is 15 to 30 mCi (555 to 1,110 MBq) of ^{133}Xe gas administered by inhalation.

Scanning

Imaging starts immediately after inhalation of the xenon gas begins in a closed system to which oxygen is added and carbon dioxide is withdrawn. When ^{133}Xe gas is used, the ventilation study must precede the ^{99m}Tc perfusion scan. Posterior images are obtained for the first breath, equilibrium, and *washout*. If possible, left and right posterior oblique images should be obtained between the first breath and equilibrium.

[99m]Tc macroaggregated albumin lung perfusion scan
Radiopharmaceutical

The adult dose is 4 mCi (148 MBq) of ^{99m}Tc MAA. The pediatric dose is adjusted according to the patient's weight.

Scanning

Imaging starts 5 minutes after the injection. Eight images should be obtained: anterior, posterior, right and left lateral, right and left anterior oblique, and right and left posterior oblique. The nuclear medicine physician may need additional images. All patients should have a chest radiograph within 24 hours of the lung scan. The chest radiograph is required for accurate interpretation of the lung scans, to determine the probability for pulmonary embolism.

Respiratory studies

[99m]Tc DTPA lung aerosol scan, ^{99m}Tc MAA lung perfusion scan, ^{133}Xe lung ventilation scan

THERAPEUTIC NUCLEAR MEDICINE

The potential that radionuclides have for detecting and treating cancer has been recognized for decades. Radioiodine is a treatment in practically all adults with Graves' disease, except those who are pregnant or breast-feeding. High-dose ^{131}I therapy (30 mCi or more) is used in patients with residual thyroid cancer or thyroid metastases. Phosphorus-32 in the form of sodium phosphate can be used to treat polycythemia, a disease characterized by the increased production of red blood cells. [32]P chromic phosphate colloid administered into the peritoneal cavity is useful in the postoperative management of ovarian and endometrial cancers because of its effectiveness in destroying many of the malignant cells remaining in the peritoneum. Skeletal metastases occur in more than 50% of patients with breast, lung, or prostate cancer in the end stages of the disease. Strontium-99 is often useful for managing patients with bone pain from metastases when other treatments have failed.

Therapeutic procedures

[131]I therapy for hyperthyroidism and thyroid cancer, ^{32}P therapy for polycythemia, ^{32}P intraperitoneal therapy, ^{32}P intrapleural therapy, ^{89}Sr bone therapy

SPECIAL IMAGING PROCEDURES

Special imaging procedures include dacryoscintigraphy, LeVeen shunt patency test, and lymphoscintigraphy of the limbs.

TUMOR STUDIES

[67]Ga tumor scan, lymphoscintigraphy for melanoma and/or breast cancer, ^{99m}Tc sestamibi breast scan, [111]In OncoScint (satumomab pendetide) scan, [111]In ProstaScint (capromab pendetide) scan, ^{99m}Tc CEA gastrointestinal scan, and ^{99m}Tc verluma for small cell lung cancer

Bone Mineral Density

Information on bone mineral loss is clinically important for the monitoring of age-related bone loss, the diagnosis and monitoring of bone loss resulting from metabolic bone disease, the assessment of drug effects on bone mineralization, and the accurate assessment of fracture risk at specific sites. An awareness of bone density is important because *osteoporosis* (severe progressive bone loss) affects more than 20 million women and 5 million men in the United States. Women experience normal bone loss after menopause as a result of a decrease in estrogen. Osteoporosis may not have symptoms because it is a progressive disease. The decrease in bone density is gradual and can lead to fractures of the hip, spine, or wrist. The broken bones result in pain, height loss, difficulty in mobility, a deformed backbone that curves forward (sometimes called "dowager's hump"), and possibly permanent disability and dependence. Hip fracture is responsible for considerable mortality in the elderly. (See Chapter 39 for a more complete description of bone mineral densitometry.)

Measurements may be performed to assess cortical or trabecular bone mineral loss resulting from accelerated bone resorption or decreased bone formation, to predict total body calcium, and to provide a quantitative result that can be used as a predictor of fracture risk.

Several types of devices are available for the measurement of bone density; all are painless, noninvasive, and safe (Fig. 38-15). *Dual-energy x-ray absorptiometry (DXA)* is the diagnostic method currently preferred by many experts because it provides the best resolution and reproducibility. Bone mineral analysis studies are done on the spine, hip, or wrist, the most common sites of osteoporosis-related fractures. Measurements are compared with expected values for populations of the patient's age, sex, and size and with the estimated peak bone density of a healthy young adult of the same sex. Routine radiographs are not sensitive enough to detect osteoporosis until 25% to 40% of bone mass has been lost and the disease is well advanced.

The most common bone density measurement techniques are as follows:

- DXA, also known as *DEXA*, is the most accurate and advanced technique. A focused x-ray beam is used to scan in a rectilinear fashion and to record separate low- and high-energy transmitted photon energy values through the bone. The study is based on the principle that normal healthy bone containing adequate mineral blocks x-ray better than weak, undermineralized bone. DXA scans of the hip and spine take 5 to 15 minutes.
- Dual photon absorptiometry (DPA), an earlier generation of DXA, is now in limited use.
- Single-energy x-ray absorptiometry (SXA) uses a very low-dose x-ray source and measures bone in the wrist or heel. Single photon absorptiometry (SPA) is an earlier version of SXA.
- Quantitative computed tomography (QCT) uses a conventional CT scanner with special computer software. Although QCT provides an effective measurement of the spine, it emits a higher radiation dose than DXA and is usually more costly.
- Radiographic absorptiometry (RA) uses a specialized x-ray technique of the hand to calculate bone density.

The total-body method is the fastest growing area of densitometry in the United States and worldwide. The increasing interest in body composition, pediatric applications, and sports medicine has been a strong factor in this growth. Densitometer sales have been continuous during the past few years, with about half of these devices being installed in radiology practices. The introduction of new drugs for the treatment of osteoporosis has also increased the demand for patient studies.

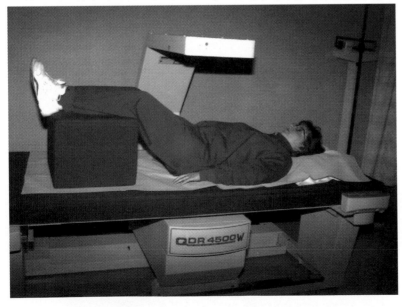

Fig. 38-15 Bone mineral measurements are painless, noninvasive, and safe.

Conclusion

Nuclear medicine technology is a multidisciplinary field in which medicine is linked to quantitative sciences, including chemistry, radiation biology, physics, and computer technology. During the past 100 years, nuclear medicine has expanded to include molecular nuclear medicine, in vivo and in vitro chemistry, and physiology. The spectrum of nuclear medicine technology skills and responsibilities varies. The scope of nuclear medicine technology includes patient care, quality control, diagnostic procedures, computer data acquisition and processing, radiopharmaceuticals, radionuclide therapy, and radiation safety. Many clinical procedures currently are performed in nuclear medicine departments across the country and throughout the modern world. Nuclear medicine procedures complement other imaging methods in radiology and pathology departments.

The future of nuclear medicine may lie in its unique ability to identify functional or physiologic abnormalities. With the continued development of new radiopharmaceuticals and imaging technology, nuclear medicine will continue to be a unique and valuable tool for diagnosing and treating disease.

Definition of Terms

alpha particle Nucleus of a helium atom, consisting of 2 protons and 2 neutrons, having a positive charge of 2.

atom Smallest division of an element that exhibits all the properties and characteristics of the element; composed of neutrons, electrons, and protons.

becquerel (Bq) Unit of activity in the International System of Units; equal to one disintegration per second (dps): 1 Bq = 1 dps.

beta particle Electron whose point of origin is the nucleus; electron originating in the nucleus by way of decay of a neutron into a proton and an electron.

blood-brain barrier Anatomic and physiologic feature of the brain thought to consist of walls of capillaries in the CNS and surrounding glial membranes. The barrier separates the parenchyma of the central nervous system from blood. The blood-brain barrier prevents or slows the passage of some drugs and other chemical compounds, radioactive ions, and disease-causing organisms such as viruses from the blood into the CNS.

cold spot Lack of radiation being received or recorded, thus not producing any image and resulting in an area of no, or very light, density. May be caused by disease or artifact.

collimator Shielding device used to limit the angle of entry of radiation; usually made of lead.

curie Standard of measurement for radioactive decay; based on the disintegration of 1 gram of radium at 3.7×10^{10} disintegrations per second.

cyclotron Device for accelerating charged particles to high energies using magnetic and oscillating electrostatic fields. As a result, particles move in a spiral path with increasing energy.

daughter Element that results from the radioactive decay of a parent element.

decay Radioactive disintegration of the nucleus of an unstable nuclide.

dual-energy x-ray absorptiometry (DXA) Currently the most accurate and advanced technique for measuring bone mineral density. It uses a very small dose of radiation emitted through a highly focused beam.

electron Negatively charged elementary particle that has a specific charge, mass, and spin.

electron capture Radioactive decay process in which a nucleus with an excess of protons brings an electron into the nucleus, creating a neutron out of a proton, thus decreasing the atomic number by 1. The resulting atom is often unstable and gives off a gamma ray to achieve stability.

external radiation detector Instrument used to determine the presence of radioactivity from the exterior.

fission Splitting of a nucleus into two or more parts with the subsequent release of enormous amounts of energy.

gamma camera Device that uses the emission of light from a crystal struck by gamma rays to produce an image of the distribution of radioactive material in a body organ.

gamma ray High-energy, short-wavelength electromagnetic radiation emanating from the nucleus of some nuclides.

ground state State of lowest energy of a system.

half-life ($T^1/_2$) Term used to describe the time elapsed until some physical quantity has decreased to half of its original value.

in vitro Outside a living organism.

in vivo Within a living organism.

isotope Nuclide of the same element with the same number of protons but a different number of neutrons.

light pipe A tubelike structure attached to the scintillation crystal to convey the emitted light to the photomultiplier tube.

metastable Describes the excited state of a nucleus that returns to its ground state by emission of a gamma ray; has a measurable lifetime.

neutron Electrically neutral particle found in the nucleus; has a mass of 1 mass unit.

nuclear reactor Device that under controlled conditions is used for supporting a self-sustained nuclear reaction.

nuclide General term applicable to all atomic forms of an element.

parent Radionuclide that decays to a specific daughter nuclide either directly or as a member of a radioactive series.

particle accelerator Device that provides the energy necessary to enable a nuclear reaction.

pharmaceutical Relating to a medicinal drug.

photomultiplier tube Electronic tube that converts light photons to electric pulses.

photopenia Lack of radiation being received or recorded, thus not producing any image and resulting in an area of no, or very light, density. May be caused by disease or artifact.

proton Positively charged particle that is a fundamental component of the nucleus of all atoms. The number of protons in the nucleus of an atom equals the atomic number of the element.

pulse height analyzer Instrument that accepts input from a detector and categorizes the pulses on the basis of signal strength.

pyrogen free Free of a fever-producing agent of bacterial origin.

radiation Emission of energy; rays of waves.

radioactive Exhibiting the property of spontaneously emitting alpha, beta, and gamma rays by disintegration of the nucleus.

radioactivity Spontaneous disintegration of an unstable atomic nucleus resulting in the emission of ionizing radiation.

radionuclide Unstable nucleus that transmutes by way of nuclear decay.

radiopharmaceutical Refers to a radioactive drug used for diagnosis or therapy.

rectilinear scanner Early imaging device that passed over the area of interest, moving in or forming a straight line.

scintillate To emit light photons.

scintillation camera See *gamma camera*.

scintillation detector Device that relies on the emission of light from a crystal subjected to ionizing radiation. The light is detected by a photomultiplier tube and converted to an electronic signal that can be processed further. An array of scintillation detectors are used in a gamma camera.

single photon emission tomography (SPECT) A nuclear medicine scanning procedure that measures conventional single photon gamma emissions (^{99m}Tc) with a specially designed rotating gamma camera.

tracer A radioactive isotope used to allow a biologic process to be seen. The tracer is introduced into the body, binds with a specific substance, and is followed by a scanner as it passes through various organs or systems in the body.

washout The end of the radionuclide procedure, during which time the radioactivity is eliminated from the body.

Selected bibliography

Bernier DR, Christian PE, Langan JK: *Nuclear medicine technology and techniques*, ed 4, St Louis, 1997, Mosby.

Cember H: *Introduction to health physics*, ed 3, New York, 1996, McGraw-Hill.

Chandra R: *Introductory physics of nuclear medicine*, ed 3, Philadelphia, 1987, Lea & Febiger.

Early PJ, Sodee DB: *Principles and practice of nuclear medicine*, ed 2, St Louis, 1995, Mosby.

O'Connor MK: *The Mayo Clinic manual of nuclear medicine*, New York, 1996, Churchill-Livingstone.

Saha GB: *Fundamentals of nuclear pharmacy*, ed 3, New York, 1992, Springer-Verlag.

Sandler MP et al: *Diagnostic nuclear medicine*, ed 3, Baltimore, 1996, Williams & Wilkins.

Shapiro J: *Radiation protection*, ed 3, Cambridge, Mass, 1990, Harvard University Press.

Steves AM: *Preparation for examinations in nuclear medicine technology*, Reston, Va,1997, Society of Nuclear Medicine.

Steves AM: *Review of nuclear medicine technology*, ed 2, Reston, Va, 1996, Society of Nuclear Medicine.

Stein E: *Electrocardiographic interpretation (a self-study approach to clinical electrocardiography)*, Philadelphia, 1991, Lea & Febiger.

39

BONE DENSITOMETRY

BARBARA A. BLUNT

RIGHT: DPA hip scan performed using a bone densitometer, mid-1980s.

(Courtesy Lunar Corp., Madison, Wis.)

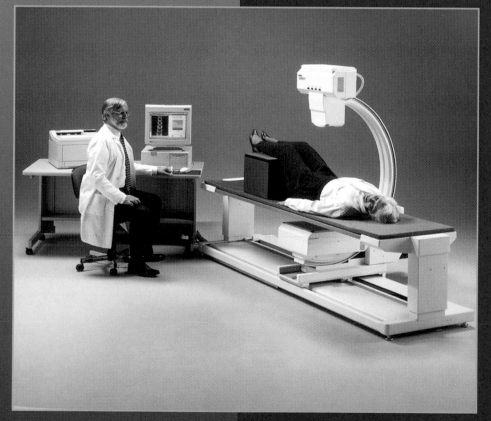

LEFT: DXA spine scan performed using a bone densitometer equipped with a C-arm, 1999.

(Courtesy Lunar Corp., Madison, Wis.)

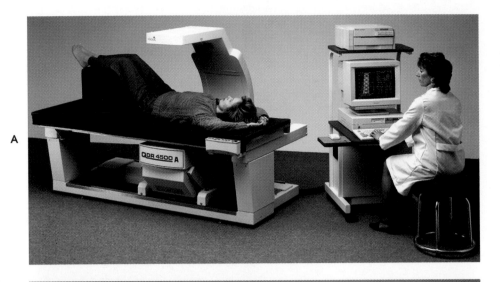

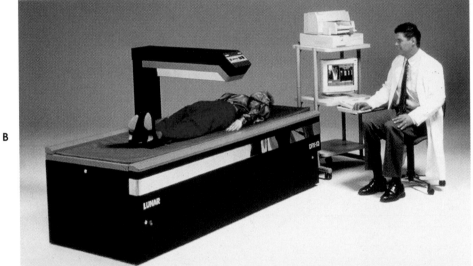

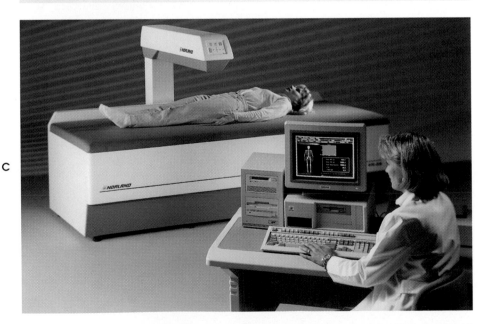

Principles of Bone Densitometry

*Bone densitometry** is a general term encompassing the art and science of measuring the bone mineral content and density of specific skeletal sites or the whole body. The bone measurement values are used to assess bone strength, diagnose diseases associated with low bone density (especially *osteoporosis*), monitor the effects of therapy for such diseases, and predict risk of future fractures.

Several techniques are available to perform bone densitometry using ionizing radiation or ultrasound. The most versatile and widely used technique is *dual x-ray absorptiometry (DXA)* (Fig. 39-1). This technique has the advantages of low radiation dose, wide availability, ease of use, short scan time, high-resolution images, good precision, and stable calibration. DXA is the focus of this chapter, but summaries of other techniques are also presented.

The introduction of new therapies for osteoporosis beyond the traditional estrogens has led to a rapid increase in the number of DXA scanners (Fig. 39-2). Over half of recent DXA installations have been in radiology offices.

---

*Almost all italicized terms are defined at the end of this chapter.

Fig. 39-1 A, DXA spine scan being performed on a Hologic model QDR 4500A. **B,** DXA hip scan being performed on a Lunar model DPX-IQ. **C,** DXA whole-body scan being performed on a Norland model XR-36.

(A, Courtesy Hologic, Inc., Waltham, Mass.; B, Courtesy Lunar Corp., Madison, Wis.; C, Courtesy Norland, Inc., Ft. Atkinson, Wis.)

DUAL X-RAY ABSORPTIOMETRY AND CONVENTIONAL RADIOGRAPHY

The differences between DXA and conventional radiography are as follows:

1. DXA is a *subtraction technique*. To quantitate *bone mineral density (BMD)* it is necessary to eliminate the contributions of soft tissue and measure the x-ray attenuation of bone alone. This is accomplished by scanning at two different x-ray photon energies (thus the term *dual x-ray)* and mathematically manipulating the recorded signal to take advantage of the differing attenuation properties of soft tissue and bone at the two energies. The density of the isolated bone is calculated based on the principle that denser, more mineralized bone attenuates (absorbs) more x-ray.

2. DXA scans provide images only for the purpose of confirming correct positioning of the patient and correct placement of the *regions of interest (ROI)*. Therefore the images may not be used for diagnosis. The bone density results are computed and printed by proprietary software. The referring and interpreting physicians must be skilled in interpreting the clinical and statistical aspects of the density results and relating them to the specific patient.

3. In conventional radiography, x-ray machines from different manufacturers are operated in essentially the same manner and produce identical images. This is not the case with DXA. There are three major DXA manufacturers in the United States (see Fig. 39-1), and technologists must be educated for the specific scanner model in their facility. The numeric bone density results cannot be compared among manufacturers without proper standardization. This chapter presents general scan positioning and analysis information, but the manufacturer's specific procedures must be used when actual scans are performed.

4. The effective radiation dose for DXA is considerably lower than that for conventional radiography. Thus, in many states and countries, scanning can be performed by personnel who are not radiologic technologists. The specific personnel requirements vary among states and countries. However, all bone density technologists should be instructed in core competencies, including radiation protection, patient care, history taking, basic computer operation, knowledge of scanner quality control, patient positioning, scan acquisition and analysis, and proper record keeping and documentation.

History of Bone Densitometry

Osteoporosis was an undetected and overlooked disease until the 1920s when the advent of x-ray film methods allowed the detection of markedly decreased density in bones. The first publications indicating an interest in *bone mass* quantification methods appeared in the 1930s, and much of the pioneering work was performed in the field of dentistry. *Radiographic absorptiometry (RA)* involved taking a radiograph of bone with a known standard placed in the field and optically comparing the densities. Interestingly, this technique has again gained popularity, with the comparison now automated by computer methods.

Radiogammetry was introduced in the 1960s, partly in response to the measurements of bone loss performed in astronauts. It is known that as bone loss progresses, the thickness of the outer shell of the small tubular bones (i.e., phalanges and metacarpals) decreases and the inner cavity enlarges. By measuring the inner and outer diameters and comparing them, indices of bone loss are established.

In the late 1970s, the emerging technique of computed tomography (CT) (see Chapter 33) was adapted, through the use of specialized software and reference phantoms, for quantitative measurement of the central area of the vertebral body, where early bone loss occurs. This technique, called *quantitative computed tomography (QCT)*, is still widely used.

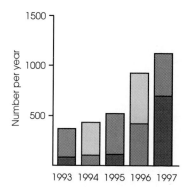

Fig. 39-2 Increased worldwide installation of Lunar axial densitometers over the fiscal years 1993–1997. North American installations are shown as hatched areas.

(Courtesy Lunar Corp., Madison, Wis.)

The 1970s and early 1980s brought the first scanners dedicated to bone densitometry. *Single photon absorptiometry (SPA)* (Fig. 39-3) and *dual photon absorptiometry (DPA)* (see chapter title page) are based on physical principles similar to those for DXA. The radiation source was a highly collimated beam from a radioisotope, usually iodine-125 for SPA and gadolinium-153 for DPA. The intensity of the attenuated beam was measured by a collimated *scintillation counter* and the bone mineral was then quantified.

The SPA approach was not a subtraction technique but relied on a water bath or other medium to eliminate the effects of soft tissue. It found application only in the peripheral skeleton. DPA used photons of two energies and was used to assess sites in the central skeleton (lumbar spine and proximal femur). Because of the radioisotope source, the scanners were often placed in nuclear medicine departments. As a result, bone densitometry became associated with nuclear medicine.

The first commercial DXA scanner was introduced in 1987. In this scanner the expensive, rare, and short-lived radioisotope source was replaced with an x-ray tube. Improvements over time have included the choice of *pencil-beam* or *fan-beam collimation*, a rotating C-arm to allow lateral spine imaging, shorter scan time, improved detection of low bone density, improved image quality, and enhanced computer power, multimedia, network, and modem capabilities.

In the late 1990s renewed attention has been given to smaller, more portable, less complex techniques for measuring the peripheral skeleton. This trend has been driven by the introduction of new therapies for osteoporosis and the resultant need for simple, inexpensive tests to identify persons with osteoporosis who are at increased risk for fracture. However, DXA of the hip and spine is still the most widely accepted method for measuring bone density, and it remains a superior technique for monitoring the effects of therapy.

Bone Biology and Remodeling

The skeleton serves several purposes:
- It supports the body and protects vital organs so that movement, communication, and life processes can be carried on.
- It manufactures red blood cells.
- It stores the minerals that are necessary for life, including calcium and phosphate.

The two basic types of bone are *cortical* and *trabecular* (or cancellous). Cortical bone forms the dense, compact outer shell of all bones as well as the shafts of the long bones. It supports weight, resists bending and twisting, and accounts for about 80% of the skeletal mass. Trabecular bone is the delicate, lattice-work structure within bones that adds strength without excessive weight. It supports compressive loading in the spine, hip, and calcaneus, and it is also found at the ends of long bones such as the distal radius.

Microscopically, cortical and trabecular bone have the same composition. In the central skeleton, 25% of bone volume is specific bone tissue and 75% is marrow and fat. The specific bone tissue is 40% organic matter (e.g., collagen) and 60% bone mineral. The bone mineral is deposited as hard, brittle crystals in the flexible collagen and gives bone its rigidity and strength. DXA measures the density of bone mineral in a given area of bone to quantify the strength of the bone.

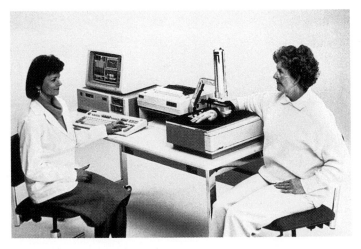

Fig. 39-3 SPA wrist scan being performed on a Lunar model SP2. This form of bone densitometry is now obsolete.

(Courtesy Lunar Corp., Madison, Wis.)

Bone is constantly going through a remodeling process in which old bone is replaced with new bone. With this bone-remodeling process (Fig. 39-4) the equivalent of a new skeleton is formed about every 7 years. Bone-destroying cells called *osteoclasts* break down and remove old bone, leaving pits. This part of the process is called *resorption*. Bone-building cells called *osteoblasts* fill the pits with new bone. This process is called *formation*. The comparative rates of resorption and formation determine whether bone mass increases (more formation than resorption), remains stable (equal resorption and formation), or decreases (more resorption than formation). Bone mass increases in youth until *peak bone mass* is reached at about 30 to 35 years of age. This is followed by a stable period in middle age. Then comes a period of decreasing bone mass starting at about age 50 in women and somewhat later in men. The decrease in bone mass becomes pronounced in women at menopause because of the loss of bone-preserving estrogen. If the peak bone mass is low and/or the resorption rate is excessive at menopause, osteoporosis may result (Fig. 39-5).

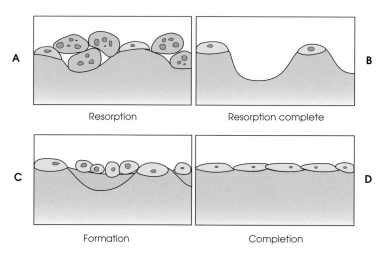

Fig. 39-4 The bone remodeling process. **A,** Osteoclasts break down bone in the process of resorption. **B,** Pits in the bone. **C,** Osteoblasts form new bone. **D,** With equal amounts of resorption and formation, the bone mass is stable.

(From *Boning up on osteoporosis,* Washington, D.C., 1997, National Osteoporosis Foundation.)

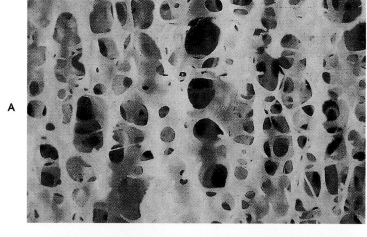

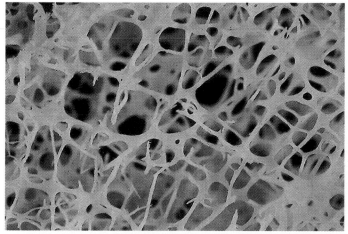

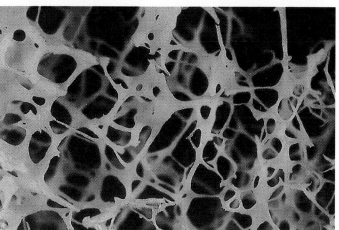

Fig. 39-5 Trabecular bone obtained from vertebrae. **A,** Normal bone. **B,** Osteoporotic bone. **C,** Severely osteoporotic bone. Note the progressive loss of trabecular continuity resulting from resorptive perforations in the severely osteoporotic subject.

(From Eriksen E: *Bone histomorphometry,* Philadelphia, 1994, Lippincott-Raven.)

Bone biology and remodeling

Osteoporosis

Osteoporosis is a disease characterized by a decrease in bone mass to a level that bones can no longer support the mechanical stress and loading of normal activity. As a result, the bones are at increased risk for *fragility fractures*. These nontraumatic fractures usually occur in the hip, spinal vertebrae, and wrist, but they can also occur in the proximal humerus, ribs, and other sites. Osteoporosis is a health threat for 25 million Americans (80% of whom are women), including 7 to 8 million with the disease and 17 million at increased risk of developing the disease because of *osteopenia* or low bone mass. Persons with osteoporosis may experience decreased quality of life from the pain, deformity, and disability of fragility fractures (especially at the hip and spine) and increased risk of morbidity and mortality, especially from hip fractures. In the United States, annual medical costs for the common fragility fractures have reached $4.5 billion.

The exact cause of osteoporosis is not known, but it is clearly a multifactorial disorder. Major contributors are genetics, aging, menopause, lifestyle, and factors regulating bone turnover. The following have been found to be risk factors for osteoporosis in women:
- Menopause
- Height of more than 5 feet, 6 inches (1.7 m).
- Thin, small-boned frame
- Family history of broken bones or stooped posture, especially on mother's side
- Natural or surgical menopause before the age of 45
- Abnormal absence of menstruation before menopause
- Advanced age
- Diet low in calcium
- Inactive lifestyle
- Caucasian or Asian heritage (others are at lower but significant risk)
- Cigarette smoking
- Anorexia nervosa or bulimia
- Gastrointestinal malabsorption problems
- Prolonged use of certain medications, including glucocorticoids for asthma or arthritis, certain anticancer drugs, excessive thyroid hormone, and some antiseizure medications

It is a common misconception that proper exercise and diet at menopause prevent bone loss associated with the decrease in estrogen. This is not true. Persons concerned about their risk of osteoporosis should consult their physician.

It is important to note that low bone mass determined by DXA does not automatically lead to a diagnosis of osteoporosis. Systemic or localized disturbances in bone mass are also associated with other diseases or disorders, including *osteomalacia*, primary hyperparathyroidism, rheumatoid arthritis, and systemic lupus erythematosus. These diseases must be ruled out before a final diagnosis of osteoporosis can be made.

Several prescription medications arrest bone loss and may increase bone mass. These include traditional estrogen or hormone replacement therapies and the newer bisphosphonates, selective estrogen receptor modulators (SERMs), and salmon calcitonin. Other therapies are in clinical trials and may be available in the future. The availability of therapies beyond the traditional estrogens has lead to the widespread use of DXA to diagnose osteoporosis.

Physical Principles of Dual X-ray Absorptiometry

PHYSICS

The measurement of bone density requires separation of the x-ray attenuating effects of soft tissue and bone. The mass attenuation coefficients of soft tissue and bone differ and also depend on the energy of the x-ray photons. The use of two different photon energies (dual x-ray) optimizes the differentiation. The Hologic scanners use an energy-switching system that synchronously switches the x-ray potential between 70 and 140 kVp and simultaneously calibrates the beam by passing it through a calibration wheel (Figs. 39-6 and 39-7). The Lunar and Norland scanners use a rare-earth filter to separate the x-ray distribution into effective energies of 40 and 70 keV and also use low- and high-energy pulse counting detectors (Figs. 39-6 and 39-8). Calibration is performed separately for filter systems.

The differing attenuation coefficients allow mathematic computations that cancel the soft tissue signals, thereby producing an image of the bone. Proprietary bone edge detection algorithms are next applied, and a two-dimensional area is calculated. The average BMD is calculated for all unit areas, and finally the *bone mineral content (BMC)* is calculated as BMC = BMD × area. Thus the three bone densitometry parameters reported on the DXA printouts are area in square centimeters (cm^2), BMC in grams (g), and BMD in g/cm^2.

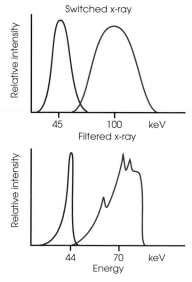

Fig. 39-6 Energy spectra (keV) for x-ray sources used in bone densitometry instruments.

(Courtesy Blake G, Wahner H, Fogelman I: *The evaluation of osteoporosis: dual energy x-ray absorptiometry and ultrasound in clinical practice,* London, 1998, Martin Dunitz.)

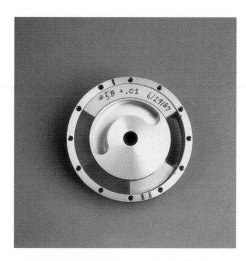

Fig. 39-7 Calibration wheel used as internal reference standard in Hologic instruments. The different segments represent a bone standard, a soft tissue standard, and an empty segment for air value.

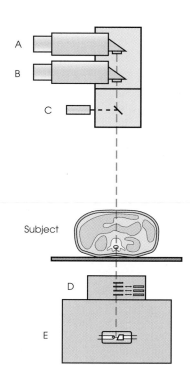

Fig. 39-8 Schematic drawing of a Norland model XR-36 illustrating the principle of operation of a rare-earth–filtered system. *A,* High-energy detector. *B,* Low-energy detector. *C,* Laser indicator. *D,* Samarium filter module (one fixed, three selectable). *E,* Ultra-stable 100 kV x-ray source.

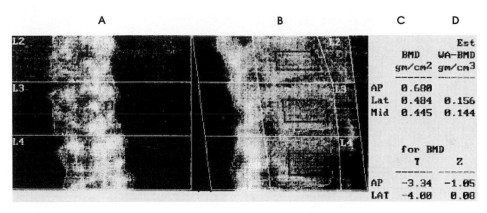

			BMD gm/cm²	Est VA-BMD gm/cm³
AP			0.680	
Lat			0.484	0.156
Mid			0.445	0.144
			for BMD	
			T	Z
AP			-3.34	-1.05
LAT			-4.00	0.00

Fig. 39-9 Partial printout for Hologic AP spine scans **(A)** and supine lateral spine scans **(B)**, showing scan images and BMD, T-scores, and Z-scores for areal densities **(C)** and volumetric **(D)** densities.

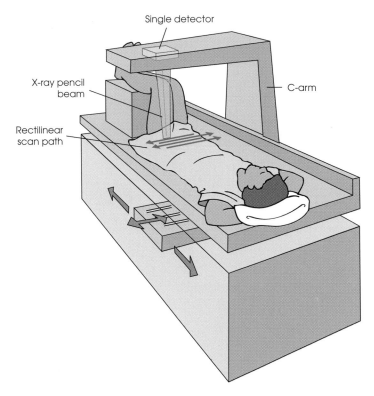

Fig. 39-10 DXA system using a pencil-beam single detector.

BMD is the most widely used parameter because it reduces the effect of body size. However, BMD is based on a two-dimensional area, not a three-dimensional volume, making DXA a *projectional,* or *areal, technique.* Techniques to estimate *volumetric density* from DXA scans have been developed but have not been shown to have any improved diagnostic sensitivity over traditional areal density. Fig. 39-9 shows the AP spine areal BMD and the lateral spine areal and volumetric BMDs.

BMD values from scanners made by different manufacturers cannot be directly compared. However, mathematical formulas have been developed for converting BMD from any manufacturer to *standardized BMD (sBMD)* values that can be compared.[1,2]

TYPES OF DETECTORS

The original DXA scanners employed a *pencil-beam* system. With this system a circular pinhole x-ray collimator produces a narrow (or pencil-beam) stream of x-ray photons that is received by a single detector. The pencil-beam of x-ray moves in a serpentine (or raster) fashion across or along the length of the body (Fig. 39-10). This system has good resolution and reproducibility, but the early scanners had relatively long scan times of 5 to 7 minutes. Furthermore, the system is not compatible with the newer C-arm design, which allows supine lateral lumbar spine scans. It should be noted that pencil-beam systems are very stable and are still in widespread use, with modern systems incorporating enhancements to improve image quality and achieve shorter scan times.

[1]Genant HK: Development of formulas for standardized DXA measurements, *J Bone Miner Res* 9:997, 1995.
[2]Genant HK et al: Universal standardization for dual x-ray absorptiometry: patient and phantom cross-calibration results, *J Bone Miner Res* 9:1503, 1994.

The *fan-beam* system has a narrow "slit" x-ray collimator and a multielement detector. Its action has been described as multiple pencil beams operating in parallel (Fig. 39-11). The scanning motion is reduced to only one direction, which greatly reduces scan time and permits supine lateral lumbar spine scans to be performed (Fig. 39-12). The fan-beam system introduces geometric magnification and a slight geometric distortion at the outer edges. Consequently, careful centering of the object of interest is necessary.

ACCURACY AND PRECISION

Bone densitometry differs from diagnostic radiology in that good image quality, which can tolerate variability in technique, is not the ultimate goal. Instead, the goal is accurate and precise quantitative measurement, which requires stable equipment and careful, consistent technique. Therefore, two important performance measures in bone densitometry are *accuracy* and *precision*. Accuracy relates

to the ability of the system to measure the true value of an object. Precision relates to the ability of the system to reproduce the same (but not necessarily accurate) results in repeat measurements of the same object. A target may be used to illustrate this point. In Fig. 39-13, *A,* the archer is precise but not accurate. In Fig. 39-13, *B,* the archer is accurate but not precise. Finally, in Fig. 39-13, *C,* the archer is both precise and accurate.

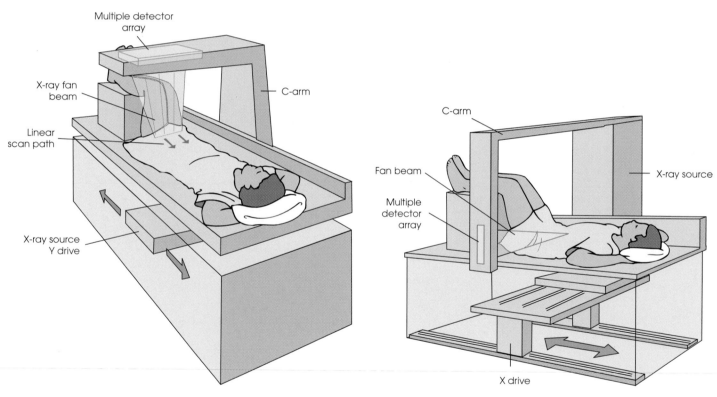

Fig. 39-11 DXA system using a fan-beam multiple detector.

Fig. 39-12 DXA system using a movable C-arm and fan-beam multiple detector to perform a lateral supine lumbar spine scan.

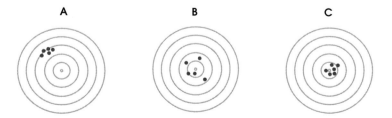

Fig. 39-13 Illustration of accuracy versus precision, assuming an archer is shooting for the center of the target. **A,** Precise but not accurate. **B,** Accurate but not precise. **C,** Accurate and precise.

In bone densitometry practice, precision is followed more closely than accuracy because it is easier to determine and is the most important performance measure in following a patient's BMD over time. Precision can be measured *in vitro* (in an inanimate object) or *in vivo* (in a live body). It is expressed as *percent coefficient of variation (%CV)*, and it measures the distance of the data points from their common average, expressed as a percent. A smaller percent coefficient of variation indicates better precision.

In vitro precision is the cornerstone of the quality control systems built into the scanners to detect drifts or jumps (variations) in calibration. Each manufacturer provides a unique phantom for this purpose, but a rule of thumb is that a Hologic *anthropomorphic* spine phantom measured at least 3 days a week over several months on any of the three manufacturers' scanners should have a percent coefficient of variation no greater than 0.5 to 0.7% CV. The Hologic quality control plot (Fig. 39-14) provides the percent coefficient of variation for the plotted BMD results.

In vivo precision has two main aspects in bone densitometry:
1. The variability within a patient that makes it easy or difficult to obtain similar BMD results from several scans on the same patient, on the same day, with repositioning between scans. (Patients with abnormal anatomy, very low bone mass, or thick bodies are known to have worse precision.)
2. The variability related to the skill of the technologist and how attentive they are to obtaining the best possible baseline scan and then reproducing the positioning, scanning parameters, and placement of ROI on all follow-up scans.

It is important that each clinic know its in vivo precision. This precision is used to determine the magnitude of change in BMD that must occur over a period of time to be certain that the change is not due solely to the in vivo precision error of the patient and the technologist. Calculating in vivo precision involves performing multiple scans on a number of patients and computing some statistical parameters.[1,2] Although this process is time-consuming, it is worth the effort involved. In vitro precision can never be substituted into a formula that requires in vivo precision.

[1]Bonnick SL: Bone densitometry in clinical practice: application and interpretation, Totowa, NJ, 1998, Human Press.
[2]Glüer CC et al: Accurate assessment of precision errors: how to measure the reproducibility of bone densitometry techniques, *Osteoporos Int* 5:262, 1995.

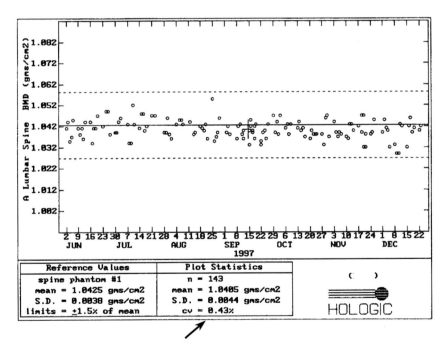

Fig. 39-14 Hologic spine phantom quality control plot. All plotted BMD points are within the control limits (*dotted lines*), which indicate ± 1.5% of the mean. The coefficient of variation (CV) (under Plot Statistics) is within acceptable limits at 0.43% (*arrow*).

REFERENCE POPULATIONS, Z-SCORES, T-SCORES, AND FRACTURE RISK

A BMD measurement from a patient is most useful when it can be compared statistically to an appropriate sex-matched *reference population*. The three DXA manufacturers have separately collected reference population databases and a large National Health and Nutrition Examination Survey (NHANES) hip reference database is widely used. These databases provide the average BMD at each age and the variability of the BMD about the average, as measured by the *standard deviation (SD)*. The *Z-score* indicates the number of SDs the patient's BMD is from the average BMD for the patient's respective age and sex groups. The *T-score* indicates the number of SDs the patient's BMD is from the average BMD of a young, normal, sex-matched individual with peak bone mass (see Fig. 39-9).

Large epidemiologic studies have investigated the clinical value of BMD in elderly women and have yielded information on the relationship of BMD and T-scores to fracture risk. A gradient of risk has been observed between BMD and fracture incidence, with lower BMD or T-score conferring increased risk of fracture. For each 1 SD decrease in T-score, the risk for fracture increases 1.5- to 2.5-fold. For example, a woman with a T-score of -2 has roughly twice the risk of fracture compared with a woman with a T-score of -1, all other factors being equal. This information helps clinicians explain the meaning of a bone density test to patients. Patients can then make informed decisions about the level of fracture risk they are willing to accept and whether to begin or continue therapy.

WORLD HEALTH ORGANIZATION CRITERIA FOR DIAGNOSIS OF OSTEOPOROSIS

Bone mass is normally distributed (i.e., has a bell-shaped curve) in the population, and no one exact cut point exists below which a person has osteoporosis. However, with the widespread availability of DXA and T-scores, there has been pressure to declare such a cut point. In 1994 the World Health Organization (WHO) recommended that the classifications presented in Table 39-1 be used in research studies.

The WHO classifications have become widely used in clinical practice. It is very important to note that the T-score is one important risk factor for osteoporosis, but the patient's history and other risk factors must also be considered in a complete clinical evaluation.

Core Competencies for Technologists

RADIATION PHYSICS, BIOLOGY, AND PROTECTION

Radiologic technologists receive extensive instruction in radiation physics, biology, and protection during their professional education. Practicing proper radiation protection and achieving the goal of ALARA (*As Low As Reasonably Achievable*) is relatively simple for DXA. The effective radiation dose in *sieverts (Sv)* for DXA scans is very low compared with conventional radiography doses and natural background radiation (Table 39-2). Some of the traditional technique factors (i.e., distance and time) are automated in DXA and do not require intervention from the technologist.

TABLE 39-1

World Health Organization classifications of bone density by T-score

Classification	Criteria
Normal	BMD or BMC T-score of ≥ -1
Low bone mass (osteopenia)	BMD or BMC T-score between -1 and -2.5
Osteoporosis	BMD or BMC T-score of < -2.5
Severe osteoporosis	BMD or BMC T-score of < -2.5 and one or more fragility fractures

BMD, bone mineral density; *BMC*, bone mineral content; *T-score*, the number of standard deviations a BMD is from the average BMD of a young, normal, sex-matched individual with peak bone mass.

TABLE 39-2

Bone densitometry radiation doses compared to other commonly acquired doses*

Type of radiation exposure	Effective dose (μSv)
Annual natural background radiation	2400
Round-trip air flight across the United States	60
Lateral lumbar spine radiograph	700
PA chest radiograph	50
QCT with localizer scan (from scanner offering low kV and mAs; may be up to 10 times higher for other scanners)	60
DXA scan (range allows for different anatomic sites; Lunar EXPERT-XL may be higher)	1–5
SXA scan	≤ 1
Quantitative ultrasound	0

PA, Posteroanterior; *QCT*, quantitive computed tomography; *kVp*, kilovolt (peak); *mAs*, milliampere-seconds; *DXA*, dual x-ray absorptiometry; *SXA*, single x-ray absorptiometry.
*From Kalender WA: Effective dose values in bone mineral measurements by photon absorptiometry and computed tomography, *Osteoporos Int* 2:82, 1992.

The following radiation protection guidelines will meet ALARA requirement for DXA:

- The technologist should wear individual dosimetry devices (film badge, thermoluminescent dosimeter [TLD]) and have it interpreted on a regular basis.
- The technologist should remain in the room during the scan but should sit at least 3 feet (about 1 m) from the scanner. The scan acquisition image should be monitored throughout the scan, allowing the scan to be aborted as soon as the need for repositioning and rescanning is obvious.
- The technologist should have adequate instruction and experience to minimize repositioning and repeated scans. For example, it is important to know how to prepare the patient to eliminate artifacts.
- The technologists should follow proper procedures to avoid scanning a pregnant patient.
- The technologist who is using a Lunar EXPERT-XL scanner must remember that this scanner employs higher levels of radiation and produces higher levels of scatter. Proper radiation protection procedures should be obtained from the manufacturer of this scanner.
- The technologists may use a lead glass shield on wheels, if available.

PATIENT CARE*

Typical DXA patients are ambulatory outpatients, but they may be frail and at increased risk for fragility fractures. Patient care and safety requires attention to the following points of courtesy and common sense:

- The technologist should maintain professionalism at all times by introducing self and other staff to the patient and explaining what is being done and why. It is important to listen to any concerns the patient may have about the actual scan and procedure and to be ready to answer questions about radiation exposure, the length of the examination, or the reporting system used by the facility.
- The technologist needs to consider certain aspects of patients' clothing. Some DXA laboratories have all patients undress and put on gowns to prevent external artifacts. However, it is possible to scan a patient who is wearing loose cotton clothing with no buttons, snaps, or zippers (i.e., "sweats"); in this situation, the brassiere must be undone, and all hooks and underwires must be removed from the scan field. Because shoes must be removed, a long-handled shoehorn should be available.
- The technologist should provide a simple explanation of the expected action of the scan-arm, the proximity of the scan-arm to the patient's face and head, the noise of the motor, and the length of time for the scan. This information may reduce the patient's anxiety.
- Although the scan tables are not more than 3 feet (about 1 m) in height, a steady footstool with a handle is recommended. All patients should be assisted on and off the table.
- At the end of the scan, the technologist should move the scan-arm to the foot of the table and have the patient sit upright for several seconds to regain stability.

*Appreciation is extended to JoAnn Caudill, R.T., for her work in the preparation of the patient care section.

PATIENT HISTORY*

Each bone density laboratory should develop a patient questionnaire customized for the types of patients referred to the laboratory and the needs of the referring and reporting physicians. The questionnaire should be directed at obtaining information in four basic categories:

1. Scanning information. Before scanning is performed, identify any information that could postpone or cancel the scan. Sample questions include the following:
   - Could you be pregnant?
   - Is it extremely painful for you to lie flat on your back?
   - Have you had a nuclear medicine, barium, or contrast x-ray done in the last week?
   - Have you have any previous fractures and/or surgeries in the hip, spine, abdomen, or forearm areas?
   - Do you have any other medical conditions affecting the bones, such as osteoporosis, curvature of the spine, or arthritis?
2. Patient information. This includes identifying information, referring physician, current height and weight, and medical history, including medications.
3. Insurance information. Because DXA scans are not universally covered by insurance, it is important to obtain information on the insurance carrier, the need for prior approval, and the information needed for ICD-9-CM coding.
4. Reporting information. The type and scope of the report that will be provided determines how much information is needed about the patient's risk factors for, and history of, low bone mass, fragility fractures, and bone diseases.

*Appreciation is extended to Peg Schmeer, C.D.T., for her work in the preparation of the patient history section.

REPORTING, CONFIDENTIALITY, RECORD KEEPING, AND SCAN STORAGE

Once the scan has been completed, the following guidelines should be observed:

- The technologist should end the examination by telling the patient when the scan results should be available to the referring physician. If a patient asks for immediate results, the technologist should explain that it is the physician's responsibility to interpret and explain DXA results.
- The technologist should remember that DXA scan results are confidential medical records and should be handled according to the institution's rules for such records. Results should not be discussed with other staff or patients, and printed results, whether on hard copy or a computer screen, should be shielded from inappropriate viewing.
- Complete records must be kept for each patient. If a patient returns in the future for *follow-up scans*, the positioning, acquisition parameters, and placement of the ROIs must be reproduced as closely as possible to the original scans. Thus the technologist should keep a log sheet with the patient's identifying information and date, the file name, and the archive location of each scan. The log should also identify any special information about why particular scans were or were not performed (e.g., the right hip was scanned because the left hip was fractured, or the forearm was not scanned because of the patient's severe arthritis) and any special procedures taken for positioning (e.g., the femur was not fully rotated because of pain) or scan analysis (e.g., the bone edge was manually placed for the radial ultradistal region). The patient questionnaire, log sheet, and complete scan printouts should be stored in an accessible location. All scan archive media must be clearly labeled and accessible.
- The general consensus is that DXA scan results should be kept indefinitely on file.

COMPUTER COMPETENCY

DXA scan acquisition, analysis, and archiving is controlled with a personal computer (PC). Therefore DXA technologists must be familiar with the basic PC components and how they work, such as the disk drives (hard, floppy, and optical), keyboard, monitor, printer, and mouse. Most DXA software currently runs on the DOS operating system, as opposed to Windows. Technologists working on DOS-based systems must know how to exit to DOS and use basic commands to change paths, check a directory, and copy files to disk. Technologists will need to upgrade their computer skills as DXA software and hardware are converted to Windows and are enhanced to allow communication between scanners and digital imaging systems via multimedia and networking capabilities.

ANATOMY, POSITIONING, AND ANALYSIS

Radiologic technologists receive extensive instruction in anatomy during their professional education. DXA scanning requires knowledge of specialized aspects of anatomy that relate to properly positioning the patient for scanning and the ROI for scan image analysis. The points presented in this section apply generally to all DXA scanners; however, instruction from the particular scanner's manufacturer is required before the scanner is used. The operator's manual that accompanies the equipment is the ultimate authority.

Like all technologies, DXA has operating limits. It may not be possible to obtain accurate and precise measurements if the bone mass is very low, the patient is too thick, or the anatomy is abnormal. The added value of experienced DXA technologists is that they can recognize and adapt to abnormal situations and they know the ultimate limits of the technology. All abnormalities that might compromise the scan results in an individual patient must be noted by the technologist and taken into consideration by the reporting physician.

It is also important to remember that DXA calculations are based on soft tissue as well as bone. Adequate amounts of artifact-free soft tissue are essential for valid results.

Core competencies for technologists

445

Follow-up scans

The BMD of a patient may be followed over time. Direct comparison of BMD results requires that follow-up scans be performed on the same scanner that was used for the baseline scans or at least on a scanner of the same manufacturer that has been calibrated to the baseline scanner. BMDs obtained by scanners from different manufacturers cannot be directly compared, nor can BMDs obtained using different technologies, such as DXA and QCT.

It is imperative that the patient positioning is exactly the same for the baseline and follow-up scans, that the same scan settings are used (i.e., field size, mode, or speed and current), and that the ROIs are placed identically on the images. These steps ensure that scan results are comparable over time. To accomplish this, the DXA technologist should have the baseline printouts available and should use the software's *compare feature*, if recommended by the manufacturer. All extraordinary measures taken for positioning and analysis for the baseline must be documented and available for use in performing follow-up scans.

Lumbar spine

Spine scans are most appropriate for predicting vertebral fracture risk in patients less than 65 years of age because degenerative changes in the elderly elevate spinal BMD, giving a false estimate of fracture risk. The following seven points can help in positioning patients for PA or AP lumbar spine DXA scans, analyzing the scan results, and evaluating the validity of the scans:

1. Degenerative changes in the spine, such as *osteophytosis*, scoliosis greater than 15 degrees (Fig. 39-15, *A*), overlying calcification, and compression fractures falsely elevate the BMD. Artifacts in the vertebral bodies (Fig. 39-15, *B*) or very dense artifacts in the soft tissue also affect the BMD. The supervising physician should set policies for dealing with these problems.
2. Generally the spine is centered in the scan field. In a patient with scoliosis, L5 may need to be off center so that adequate and relatively equal amounts of soft tissue are on either side of the spine throughout the scan.

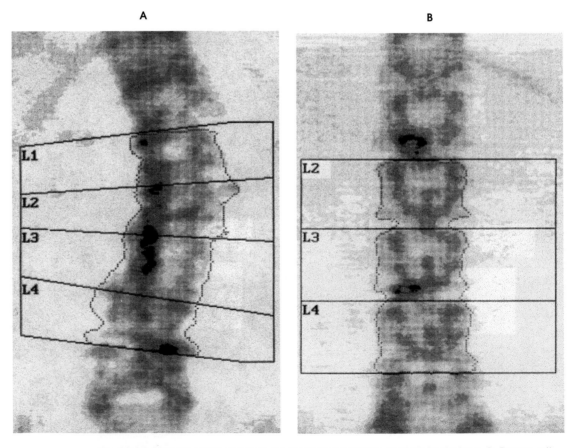

Fig. 39-15 DXA PA spine scans **A,** Scoliosis and scoliosis analysis technique. **B,** Dense artifacts in L1 and L3.

3. Several lines of iliac crest should be included in the scan. This ensures the inclusion of all of L4 and the iliac crest, which is an excellent landmark for consistent placement of the intervertebral markers at baseline and follow-up scanning.

4. The PA spine scan image displays primarily the vertebral posterior elements, which have characteristic shapes. These shapes can be used to place the intervertebral markers and label the vertebral levels when degenerative disease has obscured the intervertebral spaces. L1, L2, and L3 have a W or Y shape, L4 has an H or X shape, and L5 looks like a sideways I, or "dog bone." Other clues are that L3 commonly has the longest transverse processes and L4 is a little taller than the other vertebrae.

5. A small percentage of patients have four or six lumbar vertebrae rather than five, which is most commonly seen (Fig. 39-15, *C*). The vertebrae can be labeled by locating L5 and L4 based on their characteristic shapes and then counting up. The procedure of counting from the bottom superiorly biases towards a higher BMD and avoids including T12 without a rib, which significantly lowers the BMD. This procedure ensures a conservative diagnosis of low BMD.

6. Only if absolutely necessary should the bone edges be adjusted or the intervertebral markers angled. If used, these techniques should be performed in a manner that will be easy to reproduce at follow-up scanning.

7. A basic check list for a good PA or AP spine scan (Fig. 39-15, *D*) includes the following:
   - The spine is straight and centered in the scan field. Note that patients with scoliosis should have relatively equal amounts of soft tissue on either side of the spine.
   - The scan contains a few lines of the iliac crest and half of T12; the last set of ribs is shown.
   - The entire scan field is free of external artifacts.
   - The intervertebral markers are properly placed, and vertebral levels are properly labeled.
   - The bone edges are reasonably placed.

C

D

Fig. 39-15—cont'd C, Six lumbar vertebrae. Note that the vertebral labeling is done from the bottom to the top. **D,** Good patient positioning, scan acquisition, and scan analysis.

Core competencies for technologists

447

Proximal femur

The hip scan is perhaps the most important because it is the best predictor of future hip fracture, the most devastating of the fragility fractures. Compared with the spine scan, the hip scan is more difficult to perform properly and consistently because of variations in anatomy and the small ROIs. The following six points can help in positioning patients for hip DXA scans, analyzing the results and evaluating the validity of the scans:

1. Research has found no reason to support a preference for scanning the left hip over the right hip (or vice versa) in the normal individual. However, congenital scoliosis or unilateral osteoarthritis of the hip may cause left-right differences. All factors being equal, it is easier to position the left hip because it is on the side closest to the technologist. If arthritis is present, the less affected hip should be scanned. A fractured or replaced hip with orthopedic hardware should not be scanned.

2. With the patient in a supine position, the hip must be rotated 15 to 30 degrees medially to place the femoral neck parallel with the tabletop and perpendicular to the x-ray beam. A clue to successful rotation is the lesser trochanter is diminished in size and only slightly visible. All scanners come with positioning aids that should be used with the patient's shoes removed.

3. The body of the femur must be straight or, in other words, parallel with the long axis of the table. Because the lateral edge of the femoral body is not straight, it is best to imagine a straight line through the center of the body and verify that this line is parallel with the lateral edge of the scan field. Fig. 39-16, *A*, shows a poorly positioned femur with the body abducted.

4. No air should be present in the ROI because it will cause an incorrect soft tissue reading and thus affect the BMD. Air is a problem in small- to medium-size patients who do not have adequate soft tissue lateral to the greater trochanter. Scanner manufacturers handle the air problem differently; thus it is important to know the procedures for the equipment being used. If tissue equivalent bags are provided, they should be used properly and consistently. The Lunar femur scan in Fig. 39-16, *B*, was performed with air in the lateral scan field. Furthermore, the scan does not include several scan lines below the inferior edge of the ischium.

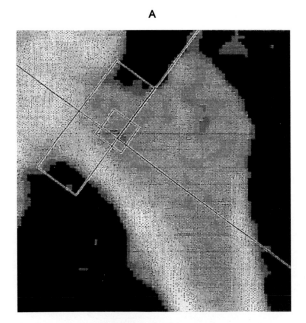

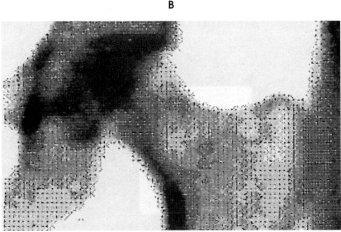

Fig. 39-16 DXA femur scans. **A,** Femoral body incorrectly abducted. **B,** Lunar scan with air in the lateral scan field.

5. The limits of the technology are taxed by patients with the following: extreme thinness or thickness, very low bone mass, very short femoral necks, and/or little to no space between the ischium and femoral neck. Short femoral neck and inadequate space between the neck and the ischium are easy to see on the image (Fig. 39-16, *C*). The first two problems are revealed by poor bone edge detection. Some images show the bone edges, and it is obvious when the proper edge cannot be detected. For images that do not show the bone edges, the area values must be checked and compared. A very large *Ward's triangle* area or a very small trochanter area is a clue that the bone edges are not being properly detected. The manufacturer's instructions and the operator's manual may not adequately cover all of these problems. It is the responsibility of the technologist to recognize the problems and query the manufacturer's applications department about the best ways to handle such difficulties. If a patient is deemed unsuitable for a DXA hip scan, a physician can suggest alternative scans at other anatomic sites using DXA or other technologies.

6. A basic checklist for a good DXA hip scan (Fig. 39-16, *D*) includes the following:
   - The midline of the femoral body is parallel to the lateral edge of the scan.
   - The proximal, distal, and lateral edges of the scan field are properly located.
   - Adequate space is present between the ischium and femoral neck.
   - No air is present in the scan field or ROI.

C

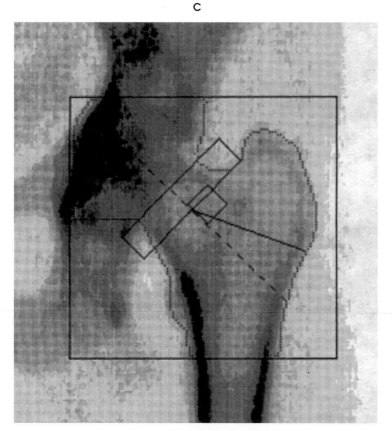

D

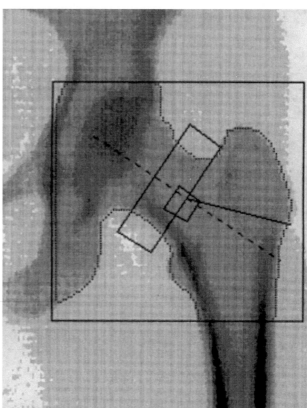

Fig. 39-16—cont'd C, Hologic scan showing a patient with a short femoral neck and inadequate space between the neck and ischium. The Hologic technique of manually changing the bone edge to "cut out" the ischium is demonstrated. **D,** Good patient positioning, scan acquisition, and scan analysis.

Forearm

Two important ROIs are present on the DXA forearm scan: the ultradistal region, which is the site of the common Colles' fracture; and the one-third region, which measures an area that is primarily cortical bone near the midforearm. Although the ulna is available for analysis, only the radius results are usually reported. The following six points can help in positioning patients for forearm DXA scans, analyzing the scan results, and evaluating the validity of the scans:

1. The left forearm is generally scanned because it is the nondominant arm for most people and therefore is expected to have slightly lower BMD than the right arm. A forearm should not be scanned in patients with a history of fracture, internal hardware, or severe deformity resulting from arthritis (Fig. 39-17, A). If the forearm is unsuitable for scanning, other anatomic sites should be considered.

2. At the time of the initial scan, the forearm should be measured according to the manufacturer's instructions. The measurement should be noted and then used again for follow-up scans. This ensures placing the one-third region at the same anatomic point on every scan. The directions for determining the starting and ending locations of the scan must be followed exactly (Fig. 39-17, B). A common problem is that a scan is too short in the proximal direction, which makes it impossible to place the one-third region properly.

3. The forearm must be straight and centered in the scan field (see Fig. 39-17, B). This is the only scan that requires adequate amounts of air in the scan field. Soft tissue must surround the ulna and radius, and several lines of air must be present on the ulnar side. If the forearm is very wide, the scan must be manually set for a wider scan region so that adequate air is included.

4. Motion is a common problem (see Fig. 39-17, B). Because scan time can be relatively long, the patient should be in a comfortable position so that the arm does not move during the scan. The hand and proximal forearm should be secured with straps or tape placed outside the scan field. Unnecessary conversation during the scan should be avoided to minimize movement.

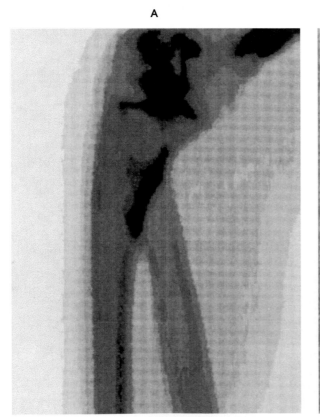

A

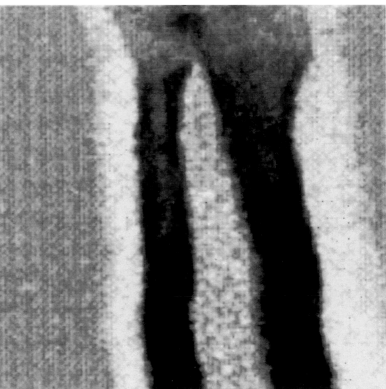

B

Fig. 39-17 A, DXA forearm scan showing severe arthritic deformity. This forearm is not suitable for bone densitometry, and another anatomic site should be chosen. **B,** This DXA forearm scan demonstrates several positioning and acquisition mistakes: the distal ends of the radius and ulna are cut off, indicating the scan was started too proximally; the forearm is not straight or centered in the scan field; and motion has occurred in the proximal radius and ulna.

5. Historically, the placement of the ultra-distal ROI has varied according to several different protocols. One popular method is to manually place the distal end of the ROI just below the radial endplate. This placement is easy to replicate on follow-up scans. The ultra-distal ROI is subject to low BMD, creating problems similar to low BMD at the hip. Questions about the accuracy and precision of the measurement should be reported, and measurements at other anatomic sites should be considered.

6. A basic checklist for a good DXA forearm scan (Fig. 39-17, *C*) includes the following:
   - The forearm is straight and centered in the scan field. Adequate amounts of soft tissue and air are included.
   - No motion occurs.
   - The proximal and distal ends of the scan field are properly placed.
   - No artifacts, such as watches or bracelets, are present in the scan field.

DXA SCANNER LONGITUDINAL QUALITY CONTROL

Longitudinal quality control procedures are performed on a regular basis, usually at least three times a week and always before the first patient scan of the day. These procedures have the common goal of ensuring that patients are scanned on properly functioning equipment with stable calibration. Unstable calibration can take the form of abrupt jumps or slow drifts in BMD, as seen on plots of phantom scan results (Fig. 39-18). These problems make the patient's BMD values too high or too low and prohibit a valid comparison between baseline and follow-up scans.

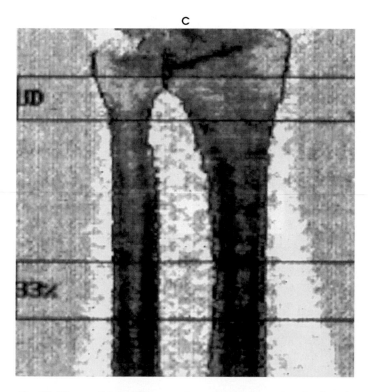

Fig. 39-17—cont'd C, This scan demonstrates good patient positioning, scan acquisition, and scan analysis.

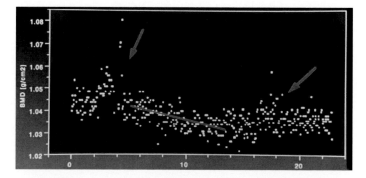

Fig. 39-18 Plot of spine phantom BMD and time (in months). The two *arrows* show abrupt jumps in BMD. The *straight line* shows a slow drift downwards in BMD. These indicate changes in scanner calibration.

Quality control procedures are unique to each manufacturer. Some systems use a scan of a calibration standard and print a report of the status of internal parameters. The technologist must note whether or not the system passed all tests (Fig. 39-19). Other systems use anthropomorphic or semianthropomorphic spine phantoms, which must be scanned, analyzed, and printed and for which the BMD must be plotted. The printouts and plots are then checked by the technologist for violation of statistical rules (i.e., %CV too high) and quality control rules (i.e., one BMD result more than 1.5 SD from the average) (see Fig. 39-14). When a result is found to be out of range, the quality control test should be repeated. If the second result falls within acceptable levels, the machine is functioning properly. However, when proper procedures have been followed and a problem is detected, the manufacturer should be contacted and no patients should be scanned until the equipment has been cleared for further use.

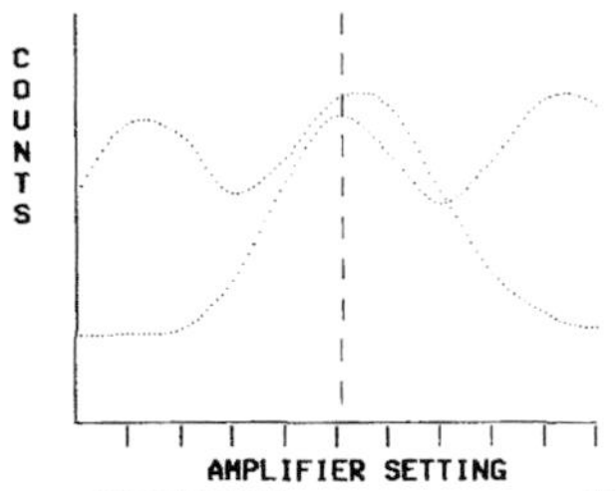

Inconsistent phantom scanning, analysis, and/or interpretation of the results may cause the calibration to appear unstable when it is actually stable. It is of utmost importance that the DXA technologist understand the quality control procedures and follow them consistently. Departments should have written procedures and documented instructions to ensure consistency within and among technologists.

Fig. 39-19 Lunar quality assurance report. This scanner passed all tests. At the bottom, values from the last five scans are averaged for calibration purposes.

(Courtesy Lunar Corp., Madison, Wis.)

Other Bone Densitometry Techniques

CENTRAL (OR AXIAL) SKELETAL MEASUREMENTS

Quantitative computed tomography (QCT) is an established method using cross-sectional CT images from commercial scanners (no special equipment needed other than QCT software) combined with a bone mineral reference standard. QCT has the unique ability to provide separate BMD measurements of trabecular and cortical bone and true volumetric density measurements in grams per cubic centimeter. QCT of the spine is used to assess vertebral fracture risk and age-related bone loss; it is also used for the follow-up of osteoporosis and other metabolic bone diseases and their therapies (Fig. 39-20). Current experimental uses of QCT involve measuring BMD at the hip and producing high-resolution three-dimensional images to analyze trabecular bone architecture.

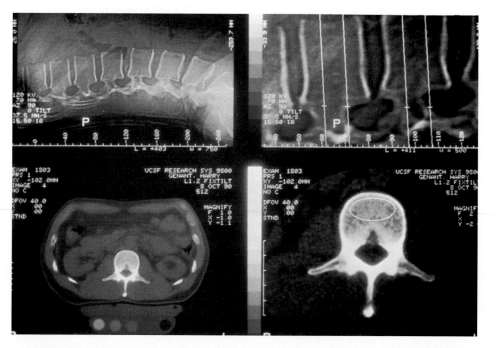

Fig. 39-20 Examples of various elements of a QCT examination: *upper left,* lateral scout image of lumbar spine; *upper right,* localizer lines for midvertebral slices through L1 and L2; *lower left,* CT slice showing the calibration phantom below the patient; *lower right,* elliptic ROI positioned in the trabecular bone of the vertebral body.

Lateral lumbar spine DXA scans can be performed with the patient in the supine position with scanners that have C-arms, (see Fig. 39-12). The decubitus lateral scans obtained with fixed-arm scanners are obsolete. Lateral spine DXA allows partial removal of the outer cortical bone and thus gives a truer measurement of the inner trabecular bone, which experiences earlier bone loss and is more responsive to therapy (see Fig. 39-9). However, lateral spine DXA is often confounded by superposition of the ribs and iliac crest with the vertebral bodies and has poorer precision than PA or AP spine DXA. Lateral DXA is not widely used in clinical practice.

Body composition can be measured as fat and fat-free mass in grams, percentage of body fat, and BMD of the total body and selected ROIs by performing a *DXA whole-body scan* (Fig. 39-21). Body composition data are useful for studying energy expenditure, energy stores, protein mass, skeletal mineral status, and relative hydration. DXA whole-body measurements have been used in research studies and clinical trials of, among others, osteoporosis therapies, obesity, fat distribution, and diabetes.

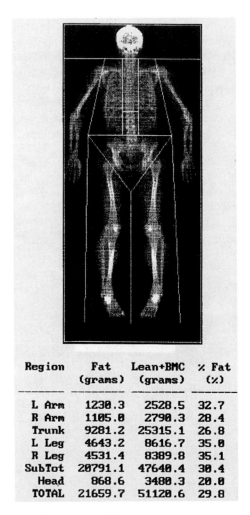

Region	Fat (grams)	Lean+BMC (grams)	% Fat (%)
L Arm	1230.3	2528.5	32.7
R Arm	1105.0	2790.3	28.4
Trunk	9281.2	25315.1	26.8
L Leg	4643.2	8616.7	35.0
R Leg	4531.4	8389.8	35.1
SubTot	20791.1	47640.4	30.4
Head	868.6	3480.3	20.0
TOTAL	21659.7	51120.6	29.8

Fig. 39-21 Hologic DXA whole-body scan with partial printout of body composition results. The percentage of body fat *(% Fat)* is reported at the lower right.

PERIPHERAL SKELETAL MEASUREMENTS

Peripheral bone density measurements include scans at the finger, wrist, forearm, and heel. Other skeletal sites are being investigated. The scanners are smaller, some even portable, making the scans more available to the public and less expensive than conventional DXA. Peripheral measurements can predict *overall risk of fragility fracture* to the same degree as measurements at central skeletal sites but are not generally accepted for following skeletal response to therapy.

Radiographic absorptiometry (RA) is a modern adaptation of the early bone density technique. It is a simple method that is gaining popularity in primary care offices. A hand radiograph containing an aluminum reference wedge is sent to a central reading facility where computerized image-processing tools read bone density (Fig. 39-22).

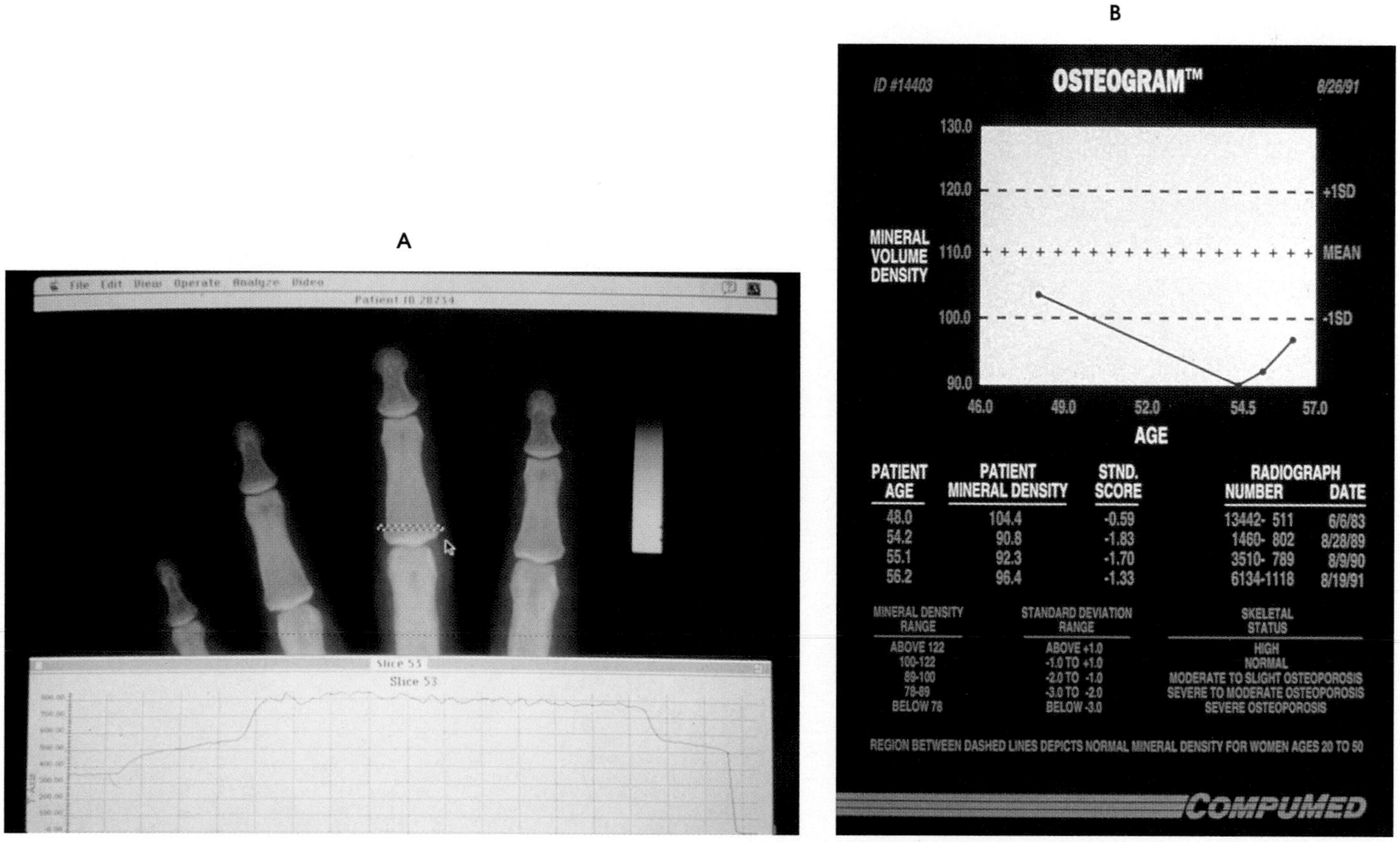

Fig. 39-22 A, Bone mineral measurements by radiographic absorptiometry: a bone mineral reading across the phalanx *(arrow)* of the left hand. **B,** Data summary from a longitudinal study of bone mineral at the phalanges by radiographic densitometry. The data were analyzed and reported by CompuMed, Inc.

(Courtesy Blake G, Wahner H, Fogelman I: *The evaluation of osteoporosis: dual energy x-ray absorptiometry and ultrasound in clinical practice,* London, 1998, Martin Dunitz; and CompuMed, Inc., Manhattan Beach, Calif.)

Single x-ray absorptiometry (SXA), peripheral dual x-ray absorptiometry (pDXA), and peripheral quantitative computed tomography (pQCT) are adaptations of DXA or QCT for measuring the thinner, easier-to-penetrate, peripheral skeletal sites. Most scanners measure the wrist (Figs. 39-23, 39-24, and 39-25, A) and/or the heel (Figs. 39-25, B, and 39-26).

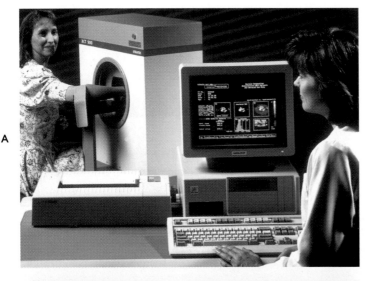

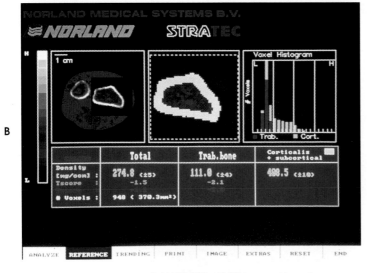

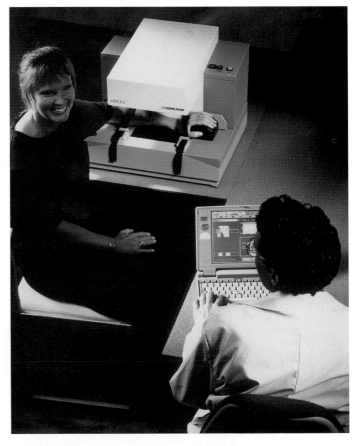

Fig. 39-23 A, Stratec model XCT-900 pQCT bone mineral analyzer for the wrist. **B,** pQCT wrist bone mineral report from Stratec model XCT-900.

(*A,* Courtesy Blake G, Wahner H, Fogelman I: *The evaluation of osteoporosis: dual energy x-ray absorptiometry and ultrasound in clinical practice,* London, 1998, Martin Dunitz; and Stratec GMBH, Pforzheim, Germany. *B,* Courtesy Stratec GMBH.)

Fig. 39-24 Norland model pDEXA performs pDXA bone mineral analysis of the wrist.

(Courtesy Norland, Inc., Ft. Atkinson, Wis.)

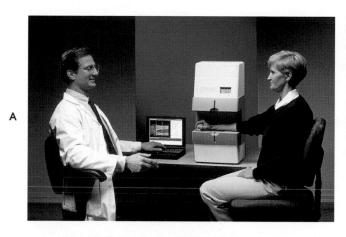

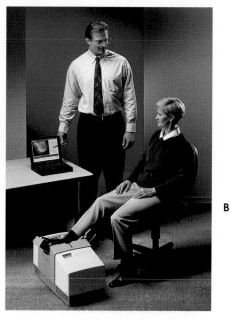

Fig. 39-25 Lunar model PIXI oriented to measure BMD of the wrist, **(A)** and the heel **(B)**.

(Courtesy Lunar Corp., Madison, Wis.)

A

B

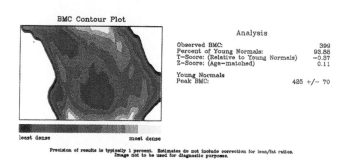

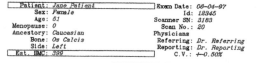

Osteoporosis Clinic
PATIENT CLINICAL REPORT

Patient: *Jane Patient*	Exam Date: *06-04-97*
Sex: *Female*	Id: *12345*
Age: *51*	Scanner SN: *3183*
Menopause: *0*	Scan No.: *20*
Ancestory: *Caucasian*	Physicians
Bone: *Os Calcis*	Referring: *Dr. Referring*
Side: *Left*	Reporting: *Dr. Reporting*
Est. BMC: *399*	C.V.: *+-0.50%*

% Change Compared To Previous Scan: *N/A*

PROJECTED BONE CHANGE CURVE

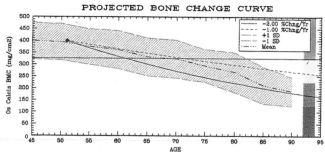

The projected bone change curve is based on the following assumptions
The patient begins losing bone mineral at age 51.
The loss rates per year are assumed to be −2.00% and −1.00%.
The projected bone change is not necessarily predictive of actual patient bone loss.

BMC Contour Plot

Analysis

Observed BMC:	399
Percent of Young Normals:	93.88
T-Score: (Relative to Young Normals)	−0.37
Z-Score: (Age-matched)	0.11
Young Normals	
Peak BMC:	425 +/− 70

least dense   most dense

Precision of results is typically 1 percent. Estimates do not include correction for lean/fat ratios.
Image not to be used for diagnostic purposes.

Fig. 39-26 A, Norland model OsteoAnalyzer performs SXA bone mineral analysis of the heel. **B,** Same model produces a bone mineral report.

(Courtesy Norland, Inc., Ft. Atkinson, Wis.)

The newest bone density measurement technique in the United States is *quantitative ultrasound (QUS)* of the heel (Fig. 39-27). Ultrasound waves are transmitted laterally through the calcaneus using either water or gel as a coupling medium. Bone affects the velocity and attenuation of ultrasound signals, permitting the assessment of QUS parameters that characterize the mechanical properties of bone relating to stiffness, strength, and consequently fracture risk. Other measurement sites under investigation include the finger, the tibia, the iliac crest, the vertebral arch and spinous processes, and the femoral neck and greater trochanter.

Summary

Bone densitometry is a rapidly growing field. Its main purpose is to assist in the diagnosis of osteoporosis by detecting low bone mass. DXA scans of the hip or spine are the most widely used techniques, but simpler, less expensive peripheral scans of the forearm, heel, and fingers are gaining in popularity. Osteoporosis is now a treatable disease, and people concerned about their risk of this disease should consult their physician for a complete evaluation.

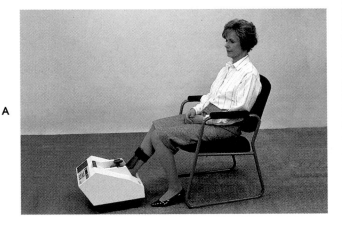
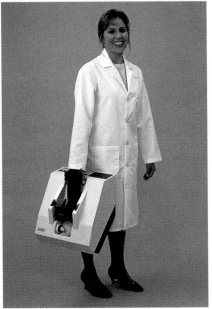

Fig. 39-27 A, Hologic model Sahara performs QUS of the heel. **B,** Hologic model Sahara portable QUS system for the heel.

(Courtesy Hologic, Inc., Waltham, Mass.)

Definition of Terms

accuracy Ability of system to measure the true value of an object.

anthropomorphic Simulating human form.

ALARA (As Low As Reasonably Achievable) Principle of reducing patient radiation exposure and dose to lowest reasonable amounts.

areal technique See *projectional technique.*

body composition Results from whole-body scans obtained by dual x-ray absorptiometry; reported as lean mass in grams, percent body fat, and bone mineral density of the total body and selected regions of interest.

bone densitometry Art and science of measuring the bone mineral content and density of specific anatomic sites or the whole body.

bone mass General term for the amount of mineral in a bone.

bone mineral content (BMC) Measure of bone mineral in the total area of a scan.

bone mineral density (BMD) Measure of bone mineral per unit area of a scan.

bone remodeling Process of bone resorption by osteoclasts, followed by bone formation by osteoblasts. The relative rates of resorption and formation determine whether bone mass increases, remains stable, or decreases.

compare feature Software feature of dual x-ray absorptiometry that replicates the size and placement of region of interest from the reference scan to the follow-up scan.

cortical bone Dense, compact outer shell of all bones and the shafts of the long bones; supports weight, resists bending and twisting, and accounts for about 80% of the skeletal mass.

dual photon absorptiometry (DPA) Obsolete method of measuring bone density at the hip or spine using a radioisotope source that produces two sources of photons; replaced by dual x-ray absorptiometry.

dual x-ray absorptiometry (DXA) Bone density measurement technique using an x-ray source separated into two energies. It has good accuracy and precision and can scan essentially any anatomic site, making it the most versatile of the bone density techniques.

fan-beam collimation Dual x-ray absorptiometry system that uses a narrow "slit" x-ray collimator and a multielement detector. The motion is in one direction only, which greatly reduces scan time and permits supine lateral spine scans. It introduces a slight geometric distortion at the outer edges, which necessitates careful centering of the object of interest.

follow-up scans Sequential scans, usually performed 18 to 24 months apart, to measure changes in bone density. Scans are best done on the same scanner or on a new scanner calibrated to the original scanner.

fragility fractures Nontraumatic fractures resulting from low bone mass, usually at the hip, spinal vertebrae, wrist, proximal humerus, or ribs.

in vitro Measurements taken in an inanimate object.

in vivo Measurements taken in a live body.

longitudinal quality control Manufacturer-defined procedures performed on a regular basis to ensure that patients are scanned on properly functioning equipment with stable calibration. Scanning must be postponed until identified problems are corrected.

osteoblasts Bone-building cells that fill the pits left by resorption with new bone.

osteoclasts Bone-destroying cells that break down and remove old bone, leaving pits.

osteomalacia Bone disorder characterized by variable amounts of uncalcified osteoid matrix.

osteopenia Reduction in bone mass, putting a person at increased risk of developing osteoporosis. By World Health Organization criteria, it is a bone mineral density or bone mineral content T-score between -1 and -2.5.

osteophytosis Form of degenerative joint disease resulting from mechanical stress that increases the measured spinal bone mineral density.

osteoporosis Systemic skeletal disease characterized by low bone mass and deterioration of the bone structure, resulting in decreased mechanical competence of bone and an increase in susceptibility to fracture. By World Health Organization criteria, it is a bone mineral density or bone mineral content T-score of less than -2.5.

overall risk of fragility fracture Risk of suffering an unspecified fragility fracture. The risk for hip fracture specifically is best measured at the hip.

peak bone mass Maximum bone mass, usually achieved between 30 and 35 years of age. Population peak bone mass is used as a reference point for the T-score.

pencil-beam collimation Dual x-ray absorptiometry system using a circular pinhole x-ray collimator that produces a narrow x-ray stream, that is received by a single detector. Its motion is serpentine (or raster) across or along the length of the body. Modern systems have improved scan time and image quality. Off-centering of the object does not cause geometric distortion.

percent coefficient of variation (% CV) Measure of the distance of the data points from their common average, expressed as a percent. A smaller % CV indicates better precision.

peripheral dual x-ray absorptiometry (pDXA) Dual x-ray absorptiometry system designed to scan only the peripheral skeleton; smaller and simpler to operate than DXA scanners.

peripheral quantitative computed tomography (pQCT) Dedicated QCT system designed to measure bone density on the peripheral skeleton, usually the forearm.

precision Ability of system to reproduce the same results in repeated measurements of the object.

projectional (or areal) technique Two-dimensional representation of a three-dimensional object.

quantitative computed tomography (QCT) System for quantitative CT measurements of bone density, allowing true measurement of volume and separation of trabecular and cortical bone; usually measured at spine or forearm.

quantitative ultrasound (QUS) Quantitative measurement of bone properties related to mechanical competence using ultrasound. The results are reported in terms of *broadband ultrasound attenuation (BUA), speed of sound (SOS),* and a nonstandardized mathematical combination of the two, called the *stiffness* or *Quantitative Ultrasound Index* (QUI). It predicts overall fracture risk without using ionizing radiation and is usually measured at the calcaneus.

radiogrammetry Older method of measuring bone loss by comparing the outer diameter and inner medullary diameter of small tubular bones, usually the finger phalanges, or metacarpals.

radiographic absorptiometry (RA) Bone density is calculated by computer from hand x-rays taken with a known standard in the exposure field.

reference population Large, sex-matched, community-based population used to determine the average bone mineral density and standard deviation at each age; used as reference base for T-scores and Z-scores; may also be matched on ethnicity and weight.

regions of interest (ROI) Defined portion of bone density scans where the bone mineral density is calculated; may be placed manually or automatically by computer software.

scintillation counter Counter employing a photomultiplier tube for the detection of radiation.

sievert (Sv) Measurement of effective radiation dose to a patient. Bone density doses are measured in microsieverts (μSv), which are 1 one millionth of a sievert.

single photon absorptiometry (SPA) Obsolete method of measuring bone density at the forearm using a single radioisotope source; replaced by single x-ray absorptiometry.

single x-ray absorptiometry (SXA) Bone density technique for the peripheral skeleton using a single energy x-ray source. Scanners are smaller and simpler to operate than dual x-ray absorptiometry scanners.

standard deviation (SD) Measure of the variability of the data points about their average value.

standardized BMD (sBMD) Result of converting bone mineral density values from any manufacturer to values that can be compared by applying mathematical formulas.

subtraction technique Removal of the density attributable to soft tissue so that the remaining density belongs only to bone.

T-score Number of standard deviations the individual's bone mineral density (BMD) is from the average BMD for sex-matched young normal peak bone mass.

trabecular bone Delicate, lattice-work structure within bones that adds strength without excessive weight; supports compressive loading at the spine, hip, and calcaneus and is also found in the ends of long bones such as the distal radius.

volumetric density Bone mineral density calculated by dividing by the true three-dimensional volume.

Ward's triangle Region on the proximal femur lying on the border of the femoral neck and greater trochanter; has low bone mineral density.

Z-score Number of standard deviations the individual's bone mineral density (BMD) is from the average BMD for sex and age-matched reference group.

Selected bibliography

Baran DT et al: Diagnosis and management of osteoporosis: guidelines for the utilization of bone densitometry, *Calcif Tiss Int* 61:433, 1997.

Blake G, Wahner H, Fogelman I: *The evaluation of osteoporosis: dual energy x-ray absorptiometry and ultrasound in clinical practice,* London, 1998, Martin Dunitz.

Blunt BA et al: Good clinical practice and audits for dual x-ray absorptiometry and x-ray imaging laboratories and quality assurance centers involved in clinical drug trials, private practice, and research, *J Clin Densitometry* 1:323, 1998.

Boning up on osteoporosis: a guide to prevention and treatment, Washington, DC, 1997, National Osteoporosis Foundation.

Bonnick SL: *Bone densitometry in clinical practice: application and interpretation,* Totowa, NJ, 1998, Humana Press.

Genant HK: Development of formulas for standardized DXA measurements, *J Bone Miner Res* 9:997, 1995.

Genant HK et al: Noninvasive assessment of bone mineral and structure: state of the art, *J Bone Miner Res* 11:707, 1996.

Genant HK et al: Universal standardization for dual x-ray absorptiometry: patient and phantom cross-calibration results, *J Bone Miner Res* 9:1503, 1994.

Genant HK, Guglielmi G, Jergas M: *Bone densitometry and osteoporosis,* New York, 1997, Springer-Verlag.

Glüer CC et al: Accurate assessment of precision errors: how to measure the reproducibility of bone densitometry techniques, *Osteoporos Int* 5:262, 1995.

Gowin W, Felsenberg D: Acronyms in osteodensitometry, *J Clin Densitometry* 1:137, 1998.

Kalender WA: Effective dose values in bone mineral measurements by photon absorptiometry and computed tomography, *Osteoporos Int* 2:82, 1992.

Kanis JA: *Osteoporosis,* London, 1997, Blackwell Healthcare Communications Ltd.

Kans JA: World Health Organization (WHO) Study Group: assessment of fracture risk and its application to screening for post menopausal osteoporosis: a synopsis of the WHO report, *Osteoporos Int* 4:368, 1994.

Miller PD, Bonnick SL, Rosen CJ: Consensus of an international panel on the clinical utility of bone mass measurements in the detection of low bone mass in the adult population, *Calcif Tissue Int* 58:207, 1996.

Mundy GR: *Bone remodeling and its disorders,* ed 2, London, 1997, Martin Dunitz.

Rosen CJ: *Osteoporosis: diagnostic and therapeutic principles,* Totowar, NJ, 1997, Humana Press.

Resources for Information and Instruction

Technologists must be properly informed about osteoporosis and prepared to perform bone density scans, ensure patient safety and well-being, and keep proper records. Information and/or instruction is available from the following sources:

American College of Radiology: *ACR Standard for the Performance of Adult Dual or Single X-Ray Absorptiometry (DXA/pDXA/SXA)*. Contact the Standards & Accreditation Department, American College of Radiology, 1891 Preston White Dr., Reston, VA 22091.

American Society of Radiologic Technologists: *Approved elective curriculum in bone densitometry for radiography programs*. Contact the American Society of Radiologic Technologists, 15000 Central Ave. SE, Albuquerque, NM 87123.

Association of Educators in Radiologic Sciences, Inc.: *Professional Curriculum for Dedicated Bone Densitometry Equipment*. Contact (web site) http://www.aers.org, or contact Association of Educators in Radiologic Sciences, Inc., Executive Office, 2021 Sprint Rd., Suite 600, Oak Brook, IL 60521.

International Society for Clinical Densitometry: Certification courses for technologists and physicians, site accreditation, and continuing education. The society newsletter, *SCAN,* provides a listing of domestic and international meetings and courses with relevant content for technologists. Contact International Society for Clinical Densitometry, 1200 19th St. NW, Suite 300, Washington, DC 20036-2422.

National Osteoporosis Foundation. Source of osteoporosis information and educational materials for staff and patients. National Osteoporosis Foundation, 1150 17th St. NW, Suite 500, Washington, DC 20036-4603.

Scanner manufacturers: source for technologist instruction and answers to scanner specific application questions. Refer to the operator's manual for contact information.

POSITRON EMISSION TOMOGRAPHY

RICHARD D. HICHWA

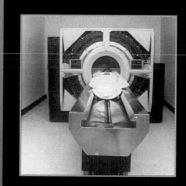

RIGHT: Early-prototype positron emission tomographic (PET) scanner.

(Courtesy CTI PET Systems, Inc.).

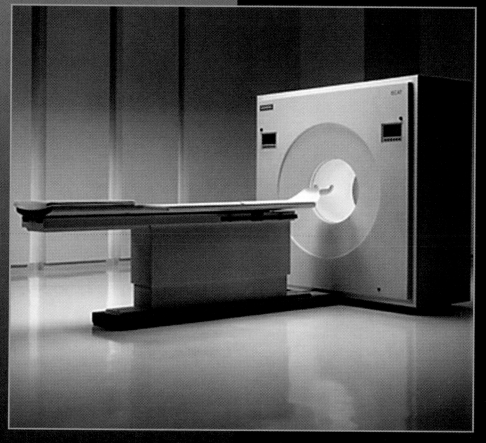

LEFT: State-of-the-art, high-resolution, dedicated PET scanner for brain and body imaging.

(Courtesy CTI PET Systems, Inc.)

Overview of Positron Emission Tomography

*Positron emission tomography (PET)** is a noninvasive nuclear imaging technique that involves the administration of a *radiopharmaceutical* and subsequent imaging of the distribution and *kinetics* of the radioactive material. PET imaging of the heart, brain, lungs, or other organs is possible if an appropriate radiopharmaceutical, also called a *radiotracer,* can be synthesized and administered to the patient.

Three important factors distinguish PET from all radiologic procedures and from other nuclear imaging procedures. First, the results of the data acquisition and analysis techniques yield an image related to a particular physiologic parameter such as blood flow or metabolism. The ensuing image is aptly called a *functional* or *parametric image.* Second, the images are created by the simultaneous detection of a pair of *annihilation* radiation that results from a *positron* decay (Fig. 40-1).

The third factor that distinguishes PET is the actual chemical and biologic form of the radiopharmaceutical. The radiotracer is specifically chosen for its similarity to naturally occurring biochemical constituents of the human body. Because very small amounts of the radiopharmaceutical are administered, equilibrium conditions within the body are not altered. If, for instance, the radiopharmaceutical is a form of sugar, it will behave very much like the natural sugar in the body. The kinetics of uptake and distribution of the radioactive sugar within the body are followed by using the PET scanner to measure the distribution of the *radioactivity concentration* as a function of time. From this measurement the distribution of metabolism of the sugar may be deduced by converting the many images that demonstrate the tracer kinetics into a single parametric image that indicates tissue function.

---

*Almost all italicized terms are defined at the end of this chapter.

Comparison with Other Modalities

PET is predominantly used to measure human cellular, organ, or system function. In other words, a parameter that characterizes a particular aspect of human physiology is determined from the measurement of the radioactivity emitted by a radiopharmaceutical in a given volume of tissue. In contrast, conventional radiography measures the structure, size, and position of organs or human anatomy by determining x-ray transmission through a given volume of tissue. X-ray attenuation by structures interposed between the x-ray source and the radiographic image receptor provides the contrast necessary to visualize an organ. Computed tomography (CT) creates cross-sectional images by computer reconstruction of multiple x-ray transmissions (see Chapter 33). The characteristics of PET and other imaging modalities are compared in Table 40-1.

Radionuclides used for conventional nuclear medicine (see Chapter 38) include ^{99m}Tc (technetium), ^{123}I (iodine), ^{131}I (iodine), ^{111}I (indium), ^{201}Tl (thallium), and ^{67}Ga (gallium). Labeled compounds with these high-atomic-weight radionuclides often do not mimic the physiologic properties of natural substances because of their size, mass, and distinctly different chemical properties.

Thus compounds labeled with conventional nuclear medicine radionuclides are poor radioactive *analogs* for natural substances. Imaging studies with these agents are qualitative and emphasize nonbiochemical properties. The elements hydrogen, carbon, nitrogen, and oxygen are the predominant constituents of natural compounds and have low atomic weight. Furthermore, nature has provided ^{11}C (carbon), ^{13}N (nitrogen), ^{15}O (oxygen), and ^{18}F (fluorine). These positron-emitting radionuclides can directly replace their stable counterparts in substrates, metabolites, drugs, and other biologically active compounds without disrupting normal biochemical properties. In addition, ^{18}F can replace hydrogen in many molecules, thereby providing an even greater assortment of biologic analogs that are useful PET radiopharmaceuticals.

Single photon emission computed tomography (SPECT) employs nuclear imaging techniques to determine tissue function (see Chapter 38). Because SPECT employs collimators and lower energy photons, it is less sensitive (by 10^1 to 10^5) and accurate than PET. In general, resolution is also less with SPECT. PET easily accounts for photon loss through attenuation by performing a *transmission scan.* This is difficult to achieve and not routinely done with SPECT imaging; however, significant effort is now being directed toward designing SPECT instrumentation that uses external radiation sources for the collection of attenuation information. Software approaches are also being investigated that assign known attenuation coefficients for specific tissues to *segmented regions* of images for analytic attenuation correction of SPECT data.

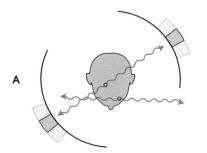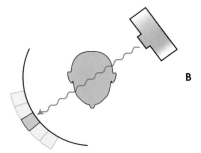

Fig. 40-1 A, PET relies on the simultaneous detection of a pair of annihilation radiations emitted from the body. **B,** In contrast, CT, depends on the detection of x-rays transmitted through the body.

The differences between the various imaging modalities can be highlighted using a study of blood flow within the brain as an example. Without an intact circulatory system, an IV-injected radiopharmaceutical cannot make its way into the brain for distribution throughout that organ's capillary network. If the circulatory system is not intact, a PET scan cannot be performed. For radiographic procedures such as CT, structures within the brain may well be intact but there may be no blood flow to and through the brain tissues. Under these circumstances the CT scan may appear almost normal. Brain studies using contrast materials require a working circulatory system for transport to the brain. The function of contrast media is to help define structures of interest by providing increased x-ray absorption.

The image-enhancing contrast agents used in many radiographic studies may cause a toxic reaction. The x-ray dose to the patient in these radiographic studies is greater than the radiation dose in nuclear imaging studies. The radiopharmaceuticals used in PET studies are similar to the body's own biochemical constituents and are administered in very small amounts. Biochemical compatibility of the tracers with the body minimizes the risks to the patient because the tracers are not toxic. Trace amounts minimize alteration of the body's *homeostasis.*

An imaging technique that augments both CT and PET is *magnetic resonance imaging (MRI)* (see Chapter 36). Images obtained with PET and MRI are shown in Fig. 40-2. MRI is used primarily to measure anatomy or morphology. Unlike CT, which derives its greatest image contrast from varying tissue densities (bone from soft tissue), MRI better differentiates tissues by their proton content and the degree to which the protons are bound in lattice structures. The tightly bound protons of bone make it virtually transparent to MRI.

TABLE 40-1

Comparison of imaging modalities

Modality information	Positron emission tomography	Single photon emission computer tomography	Magnetic resonance imaging	Computed tomography
Measures	Physiology	Physiology	Anatomy (physiology*)	Anatomy
Resolution	4.5 to 5 mm	8 to 10 mm	0.5 to 1 mm	1 to 1.5 mm
Technique	Positron annihilation	Gamma emission	Nuclear magnetic resonance	Absorption of x-ray transmissions
Harmful effects	Radiation exposure	Radiation exposure	None known	Radiation exposure
Use	Research and clinical	Clinical	Clinical (research*)	Clinical
Number of examinations per day	4 to 8	4 to 8	10 to 15	15 to 20

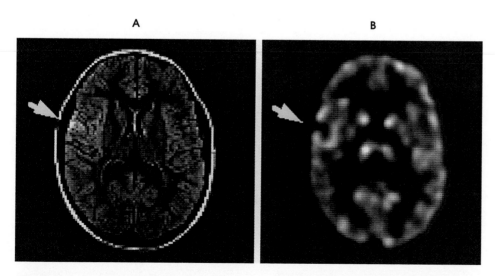

Fig. 40-2 Coregistered MRI and PET scans. The arrows indicate an abnormality on the anatomic image (**A,** MRI scan) and the functional image (**B,** PET scan). The ^{18}F-FDG PET image depicts hypometabolic area of seizure focus (*arrow*) in a patient diagnosed with epilepsy.

Advances in the spectroscopic imaging of fluorine, phosphorus, and other elements now permit, to some degree, the determination of organ and cellular function of relatively large tissue volumes. The image *resolution* obtained from spectroscopic techniques is poorer than that obtained from conventional proton MRI imaging. It is now possible to measure blood flow in both large vessels and capillaries. Paramagnetic contrast agents, improved MRI instrumentation, absolute quantification, and spectroscopy remain the major areas of MRI research. Functional MRI is rapidly advancing and is now capable of acquiring regional brain blood flow information similar to that acquired with PET, although at this time functional MRI is not completely validated against techniques of known accuracy.

It is important to note that CT, MRI, and other anatomic imaging modalities provide complementary information to PET. This imaging modality benefits from *image coregistration* with CT and MRI by pinpointing physiologic function from precise anatomic locations. Greater emphasis is being placed on multimodality image coregistration among PET, CT, SPECT, and MRI for brain research and for tumor localization throughout the body. PET remains unique in its ability to measure in vivo (i.e., within a living organism) physiology because its results are quantitative, rapidly repeatable, and validated against those of accurate but much more invasive techniques.

Historical Development

The use of positron-emitting radiopharmaceuticals for medical purposes was first conceived in the early 1930s by E.O. Lawrence, the inventor of the *cyclotron*. Simple compounds with positron-emitting radionuclides were synthesized, and Geiger counters were used to qualitatively measure the relative uptake in various parts of the body.

It was not until more suitable *scintillators*, such as sodium iodide (NaI), and more sophisticated nuclear counting electronics became available that positron coincidence localization was possible. F.W. Wrenn demonstrated the use of positron-emitting radioisotopes for the localization of brain tumors in 1951. G.L. Brownell further developed instrumentation for similar studies. The next major advance came in 1967, when G. Hounsfield demonstrated the clinical use of CT. The mathematics of PET image reconstruction are very similar to CT *reconstruction* techniques. Instead of x-rays from a point source traversing the body and being detected by a single detector, PET imaging uses two opposing detectors to count the resulting pairs of 0.511-MeV photons from the positron-electron annihilation.

From 1967 through 1974, significant developments occurred in computer technology, scintillator materials, and *photomultiplier tube (PMT)* design. In 1975 the first closed-ring transverse positron tomograph was built for PET imaging by M.M. Ter-Pogossian and M.E. Phelps.

Since 1975 developments on two fronts have accelerated the use of PET. First, scientists are nearing the theoretic limits (1 to 2 mm) of PET scan resolution by employing smaller, more efficient scintillators and PMTs. Microprocessors now tune and adjust the entire ring of *detectors* that surround the patient. Each ring may contain as many as 800 detectors. The second major area of development is in the design of new radiopharmaceuticals. Agents are being developed to measure blood flow, metabolism, protein synthesis, lipid content, receptor binding, and many other physiologic parameters.

During the mid 1980s, PET was used predominantly as a research tool; however, by the early 1990s, clinical PET centers had been established and PET was routinely used for diagnostic procedures on the brain, heart, and tumors. The middle to late 1990s saw the development of three-dimensional PET systems that eliminated the use of interdetector *septa*. This allowed the injected dose of the radiopharmaceutical to be reduced by approximately sixfold to tenfold. New image reconstruction methods were needed to better characterize the distribution of annihilation photons from these systems.

Principles and Facilities

The following sections discuss the major concepts of PET and the material and equipment used in this type of imaging. PET is a multidisciplinary technique involving four major processes: radionuclide production, radiopharmaceutical production, data acquisition, and a combination of image-reconstruction and image-processing. Particles called *positrons* are also briefly discussed.

> **BOX 40-1**
> Positron characteristics
>
> Definition: positively charged electron
> Origin: neutron-deficient nuclei
> Production: accelerators
> Nuclide decay: p = n + β^+ + neutrino
> Positron decay: annihilation to two 0.511-MeV photons
> Number: about 240 known
> Range: proportional to kinetic energy of β^+
> Routine PET nuclides: ^{11}C, ^{13}N, ^{15}O, ^{18}F, ^{68}Ga, ^{82}Rb

POSITRONS

Living organisms are composed primarily of compounds containing the elements hydrogen, carbon, nitrogen, and oxygen. In PET, radiotracers are made by synthesizing compounds with radioactive isotopes of these elements. Chemically the radioactive isotope is indistinguishable from its equivalent stable isotope. Neutron-rich (more neutrons than protons) radionuclides emit electrons or beta particles. (The effective range or distance traveled for a 1-MeV beta particle (β-) in human tissue is only 4 mm.) These radionuclides typically do not emit other types of radiation that can be easily measured externally with counters or scintillation detectors. The only *radioisotopes* of these elements that can be detected outside the body are positron-emitting nuclides. The stable and radioactive nuclides of several elements are depicted in Fig. 40-3.

Positron-emitting radionuclides have a neutron-deficient nucleus (i.e., the *nucleus* contains more protons than neutrons and thus is also called a *proton-rich* nucleus). Positrons (β^+) are identical in mass to electrons, but they possess positive instead of negative charge. The characteristics of positrons are given in Box 40-1. Positron decay occurs in unstable radioisotopes only if the nucleus possesses excess energy greater than the energy equivalent of two electron rest masses, or a total of 1.022 MeV. After a positron is emitted from the nucleus, it is rapidly slowed by interactions in the surrounding tissues until all of its kinetic energy is lost. At this point the positron combines momentarily with an electron. The combination of particles totally annihilates or disintegrates, and the combined positron-electron mass of 1.022 MeV is transformed into two equal-energy photons of 0.511 MeV, which are emitted at 180 degrees from each other (Fig. 40-4).

			F 17 64.5 s	F 18 1.83 h	F 19 100%	F 20 11 s
	O 14 70.6 s	O 15 122.2 s	O 16 99.76%	O 17 0.04%	O 18 0.2%	O 19 26.9 s
	N 13 9.97 m	N 14 99.63 m	N 15 0.37%	N 16 7.13 s		
C 11 20.3 m	C 12 98.9%	C 13 1.1%	C 14 5730 y	C 15 2.45 s		

Fig. 40-3 Excerpt from *The Chart of the Nuclides* showing the stable elements *(shaded boxes)*, positron emitters (to the left of the stable elements), and beta emitters (to the right of the stable elements). Isotopes farther from their stable counterparts have very short half-lives. The most commonly used PET nuclides are ^{11}C, ^{13}N, ^{15}O, and ^{18}F.

(From Walker FW et al: *The Chart of the Nuclides*, ed 13, San Jose, Calif, 1984, General Electric Company.)

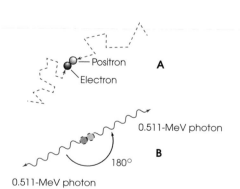

Fig. 40-4 Neutron-deficient nuclei decay by positron emission. A positron is ejected from the nucleus and loses kinetic energy by scattering (*erratic line* on **A**) until it comes to rest and interacts with a free electron. Two photons of 0.511 MeV ($E = m_oc^2$) result from the positron and electron annihilation (wavy line in **B**).

These annihilation photons behave like *gamma rays,* have sufficient energy to traverse the body tissues with only modest attenuation, and can be detected externally. Because two identical, or isoenergetic, photons are emitted at exactly 180 degrees from each other, the nearly simultaneous detection of both photons defines a line that passes through the body. The line is located precisely between the two scintillators that detected the photons. A simplified block diagram for a single coincidence circuit is shown in Fig. 40-5. The creation of images from coincidence detection is discussed in the data acquisition section in this chapter.

The positron annihilation photons from the positron-emitting radionuclides of carbon, nitrogen, and oxygen can be used for external detection. Table 40-2 depicts the positron ranges for three positron energies in tissue, air, and lead. Hydrogen has no positron-emitting radioisotope; however, ^{18}F is a positron (β^+) emitter that is used as a hydrogen substitute in many compounds. This substitution of radioactive fluorine for hydrogen is successfully accomplished because of its small size and strong bond with carbon.

RADIONUCLIDE PRODUCTION

Positron-emitting radionuclides are produced when a *nuclear particle accelerator* bombards appropriate nonradioactive *target* atoms with nuclei accelerated to high energies. The high energies are necessary to overcome the electrostatic and nuclear forces of the target nuclei so that a nuclear reaction can take place. An example is the production of ^{15}O. *Deuterons,* or heavy hydrogen ions, are accelerated to approximately 7 MeV. The target material is stable nitrogen gas in the form of an N_2 molecule. The resultant nuclear reaction yields a neutron and an ^{15}O atom, which can be written in the following form: $^{14}N(d,n)^{15}O$. The ^{15}O atom quickly associates with a stable ^{16}O atom that has been intentionally added to the target gas to produce a radioactive ^{15}O-^{16}O molecule in the form of O_2.

TABLE 40-2

Range (R) of positrons (β^+) in centimeters

E(MeV)*	R_{tissue}	R_{air}	R_{lead}
0.5	0.15	127	0.01
1.0	0.38	279	0.03
1.5	0.64	508	0.05

From *Radiological Health Handbook,* U.S. Dept. of Health, Education, and Welfare, Rockville, Md, 1970, Bureau of Radiological Health.
*The average positron energy is approximately one-third the maximum energy (see Fig. 40-7).

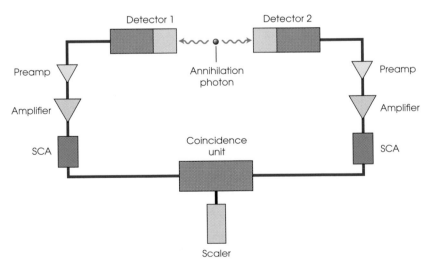

Fig. 40-5 Simplified coincidence electronics for one pair of detectors in a PET tomograph.

Statistically, it is very unlikely that two ^{15}O radionuclides will come together to form a doubly radioactive ^{15}O-^{15}O molecule because the total number of ^{15}O atoms created in the target is small compared with the number of intentionally added ^{16}O atoms. The unstable or radioactive ^{15}O atom emits a positron. This radioactive decay transforms a proton into a neutron. Hence upon decay the ^{15}O atom becomes a stable ^{15}N atom and the O_2 molecule breaks apart. This process is shown in Fig. 40-6, and the decay schemes for the four routinely produced PET radionuclides are depicted in Fig. 40-7. The common reactions used for the production of positron-emitting forms of carbon, nitrogen, oxygen, and fluorine are given in Table 40-3.

Because of the very short half-lives of the routinely used positron-emitting nuclides, nearby access to a nuclear particle accelerator is necessary to produce sufficient quantities of these radioactive materials. The most common device to achieve nuclide production within reasonable space (250 ft^2 [223 m^2]) and energy (150 kW) constraints is a compact medical cyclotron. This device is specifically designed for the following: (1) simple operation by the technologist staff, (2) reliable and routine operation with minimal downtime, and (3) computer-controlled automatic operation to reduce overall staffing needs.

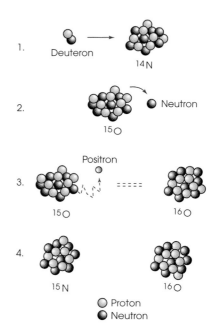

Principles and facilities

Fig. 40-6 Typical radionuclide production sequence. The ^{14}N(d,n)^{15}O reaction is used for making ^{15}O-^{16}O molecules. *1,* A deuteron ion is accelerated to high energy (7 MeV) by a cyclotron and impinges on a stable ^{14}N nucleus. *2,* As a result of the nuclear reaction, a neutron is emitted, leaving a radioactive nucleus of ^{15}O. *3,* The ^{15}O atom quickly associates with an ^{16}O atom to form an O_2 molecule. Sometime later the unstable ^{15}O atom emits a positron. *4,* As a result of positron decay (i.e., positron exits nucleus), the ^{15}O atom is transformed into a stable ^{15}N atom and the O_2 molecule breaks apart.

TABLE 40-3

Most common production reactions and target materials for the typical nuclides used in positron emission tomography

Nuclide	Half-life	Reaction(s) Proton	Reaction(s) Deuteron	Target material
^{11}C	20.4 min	^{14}N(p,α)^{11}C		N_2 (gas)
^{13}N	9.97 min	^{16}O(p,α)^{13}N		H_2O (liquid)
^{15}O	2.03 min	^{15}N(p,n)^{15}O	^{14}N(d,n)^{15}O	N_2 + 1% O_2 (gas)
^{18}F	109.8 min	^{18}O(p,n)^{18}F		95% ^{18}O - H_2O (liquid)
			^{20}Ne(d,α)^{18}F	Ne + 0.1% F_2 (gas)

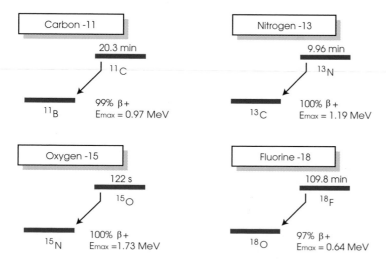

Fig. 40-7 Decay schemes for ^{11}C, ^{13}N, ^{15}O, and ^{18}F. Each positron emitter decays to a stable nuclide by ejecting a positron from the nucleus. *Emax* represents the maximum energy of the emitted positron. Electron capture is a competitive process with positron decay; hence positron decay is not always 100%.

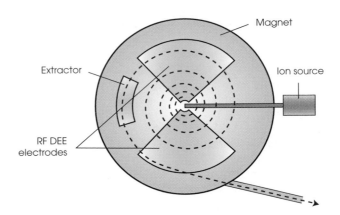

Fig. 40-8 Cyclotron schematic. The *dashed line* indicates the path of accelerated particles for a positive-ion cyclotron. Ions originate at the ion source, are constrained to circular paths by the magnetic field, are accelerated to higher energy and thus larger orbits by the RF applied to the DEE electrodes, and are finally directed toward the target by the extractor. For a negative-ion cyclotron with the magnetic field oriented in the same direction as the positive-ion cyclotron, the ions to be accelerated orbit clockwise rather than counterclockwise as shown in the figure.

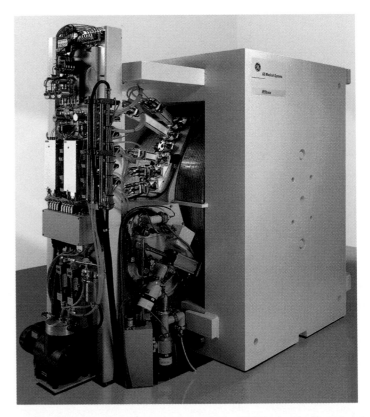

Fig. 40-9 Small cyclotron used for routine production of PET isotopes. The cyclotron can be located in a concrete vault, or it can be self-shielded. Particles are accelerated in vertical orbits and impinge on targets located near the top center of the machine. This is an example of a negative-ion cyclotron.

(Courtesy GE Medical Systems, Milwaukee, Wis.)

New linear accelerators have been developed that can also produce significant quantities of PET nuclides, but cyclotrons remain the most ubiquitous particle accelerator for PET applications.

A cyclotron consists of four major parts: the ion source, the magnet, the radiofrequency (RF) high-voltage acceleration system, and the extraction system (Fig. 40-8).

The ion source is used to create ions for acceleration from simple stable gases (e.g., protons from ionized hydrogen gas or deuterons from ionized deuterium gas). These ions are positive ions if their electrons have been stripped away and negative ions if an extra electron has been added. The ions are extracted from the ion source and accelerated toward the outer rim of the cyclotron magnet, which is used to constrain the charged particles or ions to move in circular orbits. As might be expected, particles with higher energy move with greater velocity and therefore travel in orbits of greater radii than particles with lower energy.

Fig. 40-9 shows a typical cyclotron used for radionuclide production. The cyclotron must be located in a thick concrete vault (a room with 5- to 6-foot [1.5- to 1.8-m] thick walls and ceiling), or it must have shielding material directly on all exterior surfaces (self-shielded cyclotron) to reduce the radiation levels to safe values when the cyclotron is in operation (less than 2 mR/hr on contact with shield).

Ions are accelerated by traversing the electric field gradient between the copper "dee" electrodes, whose shape somewhat resembles the capital letter D. The electric field gradient is created by charging the dees to a high voltage (30 to 50 kV), much as a large capacitor is charged. A positive ion is repelled by the positive polarity of one dee and attracted toward the negative polarity of the other dee. In this process, the ion gains kinetic energy and its velocity increases. Once an ion is enveloped by the conducting dee structure, it no longer experiences electrostatic forces and is constrained to move in a circular orbit toward the opposite dee by the magnetic field (1.4 to 1.8 tesla). During this time the polarity of the dees is automatically reversed. The alternating voltage cycle occurs at radio frequencies of 10 to 30 MHz. Therefore each time the ion traverses the gap between the two dees, it is accelerated by the respective attractive and repulsive electrostatic forces. It gains approximately twice the voltage difference between the two dees for every orbit or complete circular path. If the dee-to-dee voltage is 30 kV, a proton gains 60 keV per orbit and undergoes approximately 280 to 300 orbits to achieve the maximum output energy, which is 17 MeV for the cyclotron shown in Fig. 40-9. During this time the ion increases its orbital radius from the center of the cyclotron to near the outer edge of the main magnetic field by following an increasingly larger spiral path.

For positive-ion cyclotrons, a high-voltage electrostatic deflector operating at 20 to 50 kV is used to nudge positive ions from the edge of the magnetic field to a point where they can be extracted from the cyclotron. For negative-ion cyclotrons, negative ions are extracted by removing the added electrons by passing the ions through an extremely thin carbon foil (0.0025 mm thick). Because the overall charge on the ions was once negative (H^-) and is now positive (H+), the ions circulate in the opposite direction under the influence of the constant magnetic field produced by the large electromagnet of the cyclotron. Negative ions are more easily extracted from the cyclotron than positive ions. Furthermore, the electrostatic deflector becomes extremely radioactive under normal use, whereas the carbon foil extraction system does not. This difference is considered a significant advantage in favor of the negative-ion accelerator.

The ion source emits ions with every cycle of the RF voltage applied to the dees regardless of ion polarity. Therefore ions arrive at the extraction system in packets synchronized with the RF. These packets, or beams of particles (10 to 50 μA of protons or deuterons), are focused and directed toward the target material for the production of positron-emitting radioisotopes. The radioisotopes produced in the target may be solid, liquid, or gaseous, and they may be created continuously or in batches.

Proton-only cyclotrons produce nuclides by the reactions listed in Table 40-3 (see proton column). For cyclotrons that can produce both protons and deuterons, all of the reactions in Table 40-3 are possible; however, the $^{14}N(d,n)^{15}O$ deuteron reaction is used primarily to produce ^{15}O, whereas all other nuclides are typically produced with protons.

RADIOPHARMACEUTICAL PRODUCTION

Radiopharmaceuticals are synthesized from radionuclides derived from the target material. These agents may be very simple, like the ^{15}O-^{16}O molecules described earlier, or they may be very complex. Regardless of the chemical complexity of the radioactive molecule, all radiopharmaceuticals must be synthesized very rapidly. This entails specialized techniques not only to create the labeled substance but also to verify the purity (chemical, radiochemical, and radionuclidic) of the radiotracer.

Two important radiopharmaceuticals are presently used in many PET studies. The first is ^{15}O water (^{15}O-H_2O), which is produced continuously from the $^{14}N(d,n)^{15}O$ nuclear reaction or in batches from the $^{15}N(p,n)^{15}O$ nuclear reaction. As previously discussed, the radioactive oxygen quickly combines with a stable ^{16}O atom, which has been added to the stable N_2 target gas, to form an oxygen molecule (O_2). The ^{15}O-^{16}O molecule is reduced over a platinum catalyst with small amounts of stable H_2 and N_2 gas. Radioactive water vapor is produced and collected in sterile saline for injection. A typical bolus injection of ^{15}O-H_2O is approximately 30 to 50 mCi in a volume of 1 to 2 ml of saline for use in a two-dimensional PET scanner and approximately 3 to 8 mCi in the same volume of saline for a three-dimensional PET tomograph. A dose of radioactive water can be prepared every 2 to 5 minutes. Radioactive ^{15}O-H_2O is used primarily for the determination of *local cerebral blood flow (LCBF)*. PET LCBF images from one subject using two different techniques are shown in Fig. 40-10.

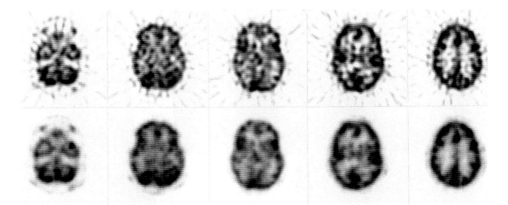

Fig. 40-10 PET LCBF images. The images in the top row were created using a standard filtered backprojection reconstruction technique. An iterative reconstructive method was used to create the images in the bottom row from the same raw data that are used for the upper images. In all images, dark areas correspond to high brain blood flow. There is about an 8-mm separation between each brain slice within a row.

The second major radiopharmaceutical used routinely in PET employs ^{18}F-labeled fluoride ions (F$^-$) to form a sugar analog called [^{18}F]-2-fluoro-2-deoxy-D-glucose, or ^{18}F-FDG. This agent is used to determine the *local metabolic rate of glucose utilization (LMRG)* in brain, heart, tumor, or other tissues that use glucose as a metabolic substrate. For example, the glucose obtained from food is metabolized by the brain to provide the adenosine triphosphate necessary for maintaining the membrane potential of neurons within the brain. The metabolism of glucose is proportional to the neural activity of the brain and thus brain metabolism. Radioactive ^{18}F-FDG and glucose enter the same biochemical pathways in the brain. However, unlike glucose, ^{18}F-FDG cannot be completely metabolized in the brain because its metabolism is blocked at the level of fluoro-deoxyglucose-6-phosphate ([^{18}F]-FDG-6-PO$_4$). Because ^{18}F-FDG follows the glucose pathway into the brain, the concentration of [^{18}F]-FDG-6-PO$_4$ within the brain cells is proportional to brain tissue metabolism. These pathways for glucose and ^{18}F-FDG are shown schematically in Fig. 40-11.

^{18}F-FDG is synthesized by displacing the triflate-leaving group of 1,3,4,6-tetra-O-acetyl-2-O-trifluoromethanesulfonyl-E1-D-mannopyranose with anhydrous ^{18}F-fluoride, obtained from drying ^{18}F-fluoride ions generated by proton bombardment of stable ^{18}O-H$_2$O (see Table 40-4). The intermediate is deacetylated by acid hydrolysis and purified chromatographically to give [^{18}F]-2-fluoro-2-deoxy-D-glucose, or ^{18}F-FDG. A standard dose of 5 to 10 mCi in a few milliliters of isotonic saline is administered intravenously. The total time for FDG production, which includes target irradiation (1 hour), radiochemical synthesis (30 minutes to 1 hour), and purity certification (15 minutes), is approximately 2 hours, depending on the exact synthesis method used.

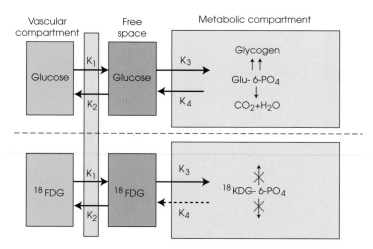

Fig. 40-11 Glucose compartmental model (above the *dashed line*) compared with the ^{18}F-FDG model (below the *dashed line*). Note that ^{18}F-FDG does not go to complete storage (glycogen) or metabolism (CO$_2$ + H$_2$O) as does glucose. The constants *(K)* refer to reaction rates for moving substances from one compartment to another. *Dashed arrow* refers to extremely small K value that can usually be neglected.

DATA ACQUISITION

The positron-electron annihilation photons are detected and counted with a PET scanner or tomograph (Fig. 40-12). In general, for neurologic PET scanners the distance between detector faces is approximately 70 cm (28 inches). This distance is increased to 90 to 100 cm (36 to 39 inches) for whole-body scanners. The radial field of view (FOV) for these scanners is approximately 24 cm (10 inches) and 55 cm (22 inches), respectively (Fig. 40-13). Typical scanners have 500 to 800 detectors per ring. A detector module consists of *BGO scintillators* organized into a matrix (6 × 6, 7 × 8, or 8 × 8) of small BGO cubes (3 to 6 mm long, 6 mm wide, and 20 to 30 mm deep), which are coupled to photomultiplier tubes.

Individual tubes are no longer mated to single scintillator crystals, as in the first PET scanners, but are arranged in an overlapping fashion similar to NaI crystals and photomultiplier tubes in conventional gamma cameras. Early scanners had only a single ring of detectors. Current tomographs are constructed of 18 to 24 rings. Not only are coincidence counts collected for detector pairs within each ring (direct-plane information), but data are also collected between adjacent rings (cross-plane information) as shown in Fig. 40-14. Therefore 35 to 47 tomographic slices (2 × number of rings−1) can be acquired simultaneously for 18- to 24-ring tomographs, which have a total of 10,000 to 20,000 detectors (BGO crystals). A new scintillator, lutetium orthosilicate ($Lu_2SiO_5:Ce$), also known as *LSO,* has a higher light output (approximately four times that of BGO) and faster photofluorescent decay (approximately 7.5 times that of BGO). LSO is being investigated as a replacement for BGO.

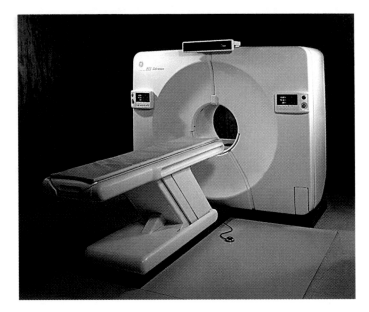

Fig. 40-12 Typical whole-body PET scanner. The bed is capable of moving in and out of the scanner to measure the distribution of PET radiopharmaceuticals throughout the body, and it adjusts to a very low position for easy patient access. Sophisticated computer workstations are required to view and analyze data.

(Courtesy GE Medical Systems, Milwaukee, Wis.)

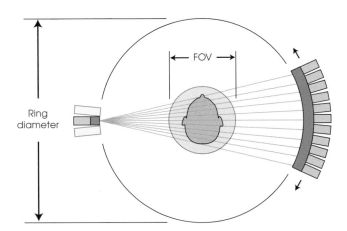

Fig. 40-13 Detector arrangement in neurologic PET ring (head-only scanner). Rays from opposed detector pairs (*lines* between detectors) depict possible coincidence events. The useful field of view *(FOV)* is delineated by the central circle.

The concept of PET scanner resolution can be explained using a bicycle wheel as an example. In the case of PET, *rays* between detectors correspond to the bicycle spokes. The highest density of spokes is located at the hub. At the rim of the wheel, the density of spokes is reduced. The same is true for the density between detectors. That is why the selected imaging FOV for these scanners is approximately the middle third of the distance from one detector face to the opposite detector face. Adequate ray density for the best resolution for image reconstruction is achieved only within this FOV.

The resolution within the image plane for PET scanners is between 4 and 6 mm full width at half maximum (FWHM). Thus an image of a point source of radioactivity appears to be 4 to 6 mm wide at one half the maximum intensity of the source image. The theoretical limit of resolution for PET tomographs is 1 to 2 mm FWHM and depends on the finite range of the positron in tissue for the particular radionuclide used. The resolution between tomographic planes or slices (i.e., along the z axis, which is the axis parallel to the PET scanner couch) is between 5 and 6 mm FWHM.

Further improvements in image resolution require that the number of rays between detectors be increased. This implies that the number of detectors in the tomograph must be increased. Some devices now being constructed will have more than 1000 detectors per ring. Of course, as the number of detectors in the tomograph increases, so does the complexity of acquiring and cataloging each annihilation event. The electronics systems, wiring, and heat loads generated from the associated electronics also increase. Previously, methods for improving resolution employed rotation of the detector array with respect to the patient. This achieved an increase in the number of rays used for image reconstruction. However, the complexity of detector rotation and the additional costs to engineer these systems limited the usefulness of this technique. Therefore increasing the number of detectors in the ring is the most effective way of improving image resolution, and it does so without detector motion.

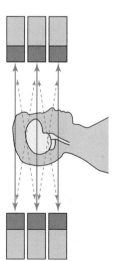

Fig. 40-14 Side-view schematic of a small portion of a multiring (three-ring) PET tomograph. The *darker green squares* indicate the scintillator-matrix, which is attached to multiple-photocathode PMTs. *Solid lines* indicate the direct planes, and *dashed lines* depict the cross planes. The X determined by the pair of cross planes forms a data plane located between direct planes. Improvements in PET scanner instrumentation not only permit cross-plane information between adjacent rings to be acquired but also allow for expansion to the second, third, fourth, and fifth near neighbor rings. This significantly enhances overall scanner sensitivity.

Not all photons emitted from the patient can be detected. Some of the pairs of 0.511-MeV photons from the positron annihilation impinge on detectors in the tomograph ring and are detected; most do not. The photon pairs are emitted 180 degrees from each other. The emission process is *isotropic,* which means that the annihilation photons are emitted with equal probability in all directions so that only a small fraction of the total number of photons emitted from the patient actually strike the tomograph detectors (Fig. 40-15).

PET scanners originally used ray information only from the nearest adjacent planes. However, with improvements in software reconstruction techniques and the elimination of septa between detector rings, the second, third, fourth, and even fifth adjacent plane can be used to produce three-dimensional PET images. With inclusion of the additional cross-plane information, PET scanner *sensitivity* is greatly increased. Hence the injected dose of radiopharmaceutical can be significantly reduced (50% to 90% less radioactivity given) to yield PET images with a quality equivalent to that of images obtained from the original dose levels used in two-dimensional PET scanners with septa.

When pairs of photons are detected, they are counted as valid events (i.e., true positron annihilation) only if they appear at the detectors within the resolving time for the coincidence electronics. For many PET tomographs this is typically 8 to 12 nsec. If one photon is detected and no other photon is observed during that time window, the original event is discarded. This is electronic collimation. No conventional lead collimators are used in PET scanners. PET detector systems must also be able to handle very high count rates with minimum *deadtime* losses.

Dual-headed coincidence SPECT systems are being developed that offer lower cost alternatives to conventional PET ring instrumentation. No collimators are used. The pair of gamma camera heads operate in coincidence, as with conventional ring detectors, but the pair of cameras revolve together about the patient to collect data from 180 degrees of rotation. At present, losses resulting from high count rate and poor sensitivity limit the effectiveness of the systems. FDG is the major pharmaceutical used for dual-headed coincidence systems.

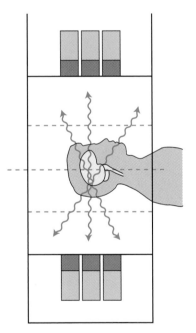

Fig. 40-15 Side view of PET scanner, illustrating possible photon directions. Only 15% of the total number of emitted photons from the patient can be detected in a whole-body tomograph (ring diameter: 100 cm (39 inches)). This is increased to 25% for a head tomograph (ring diameter: 60 cm (24 inches)). For these estimates, the z axis coverage was considered to be 15 cm (6 inches). The actual number of detected coincidences will be less than either the 15% or 25% estimate, because the detector efficiency is not 100% (typical efficiency: 30%).

For PET procedures, data acquisition is not limited to images of tomographic count rates. For example, the creation of *quantitative* parametric images of glucose metabolism requires that the blood concentrations of the radiopharmaceutical be measured. This is accomplished by discrete or continuous arterial sampling, discrete or continuous venous sampling, or *region of interest (ROI)* analysis of a sequential time series of major arterial vessels observed in reconstructed tomographic images. For arterial sampling, an indwelling catheter is placed in the radial artery. Arterial blood pressure forces blood out of the catheter for collection and radioactivity measurement. For venous sampling, blood is withdrawn through an indwelling venous catheter.

However, for obtaining *arterialized venous blood,* the patient's hand is heated to between 104°F and 108°F (40°C and 42.2°C). In this situation arterial blood is shunted directly to the venous system. If plasma radioactivity measurement is required in discrete samples, the red blood cells are separated from whole blood by centrifugation and the radioactivity concentration within plasma is determined by discrete sample counting in a gamma well counter. Continuous counting is performed on whole blood by directing the blood through a radiation detector via small-bore tubing. A peristaltic pump, a syringe pump, or the subject's arterial pressure is used for continuous or discrete blood sampling. For ROI analysis, the arterial blood curve is generated directly from each image of a multiple-frame time-series PET scan. An ROI is placed around the arterial vessel visualized in the PET images. The average number of counts for the ROI from each frame is plotted against time. Actual blood sampling is not usually required for ROI analysis.

A typical set of blood and tissue curves is given in Fig. 40-16. Curves created from plasma data, as well as other information (e.g., nonradioactive plasma glucose level), are supplied to a mathematic model that appropriately describes the physiologic process being measured (i.e., metabolic rate of glucose utilization in tissue). Parametric or functional images are created by applying the model to the original PET data.

IMAGE RECONSTRUCTION AND IMAGE PROCESSING

Images are created from raw data collected as rays corresponding to each detected annihilation event. A typical image (one slice) has 128×128 or 256×256 *pixels,* or *pi*cture *el*ements. Each pixel represents 2 *bytes* of information. The image storage requirement of a PET study can be computed by the following:

$$(\text{image size})^2 \times 2 \text{ bytes}$$
$$\times \text{ number of slices}$$
$$\times \text{ number of frames in a dynamic scan}$$

For an LCBF study, the image storage is calculated as follows:

$$(128 \text{ pixels})^2 \times 2 \text{ bytes}$$
$$\times 47 \text{ slices} \times 10 \text{ frames}$$
$$= 15 \text{ megabytes (MB)}$$

When multiple injections are contemplated for test/retest studies, the image storage requirements increase further.

An FOV of 15 to 20 cm (6 to 8 inches; axial direction) is required to adequately encompass the entire volume of the brain (from the top of the cerebral cortex to the base of the cerebellum) or the entire volume of the heart. Array processors are used to perform the filtered backprojection or maximum likelihood (iterative) reconstruction that converts the raw sinogram data into PET images. This technique is similar to that employed for CT image reconstruction. However, faster and less costly desktop computers are replacing array processor technology and thereby greatly simplifying software requirements for image reconstruction.

The disintegration of radionuclides follows Poisson statistics. As a result of this random process, photons from the different annihilation events may strike the tomograph detectors simultaneously. These are registered as true events because they occur within the coincidence time window. A simple approximation allows for the subtraction of the random events after image acquisition and is based on the individual count rates for each detector and the coincidence resolving time (8 to 12 nsec) of the tomograph electronics according to the following relationship:

$$N_R = N_1 N_2 2\tau$$

where *NR* is the random event rate, N_1 and *N2* are the photon counting rates for the individual detectors involved in the coincidence measurement, and τ is the resolving time of the electronics.

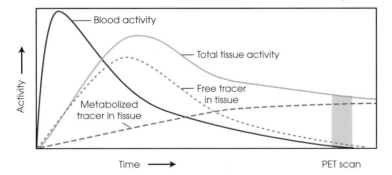

Fig. 40-16 Decay-corrected radioactivity curves for ^{18}F-FDG in tissue and blood (plasma). Injection occurs at the origin. The blood activity rapidly peaks after the injection. The metabolized tracer ((^{18}F)-FDG-6-PO$_4$) slowly accumulates in tissue. Typical static PET scanning occurs after an incorporation time of 40 to 60 minutes (as shown by the shaded box) in which the uptake of ^{18}F-FDG is balanced with the slow washout of the labeled metabolite.

Photons traversing biologic tissues also undergo absorption and scatter. As shown in Fig. 40-17, an attenuation correction is applied to account for those photons that should have been detected but were not. The correction is typically based on a transmission scan acquired under computer control using a radioactive rod or pin source of ⁶⁸Ge (germanium; 271-day half-life) that circumscribes the portion of the patient's body within the PET scanner. For brain studies, another attenuation correction technique is used, but it is less accurate. It approximates the outline of the skull with an ellipse and calculates the attenuation of photons based on the dimensions of the ellipse. A transmission scan measures the actual attenuation of photons based on the true cross-sectional area of head. The *attenuation coefficient* for 0.511-MeV photons in waterlike tissue is 0.096 cm²/g. In either case, the coincidence data for each image plane are multiplied by a matrix of numeric values (all greater than 1) within the boundaries of the skull to correct the observed sinogram to the true sinogram for losses that result from attenuation. The magnitude of the attenuation correction varies from approximately 4 in brain imaging to 32 or more in body imaging.

Count rates from the detectors are also corrected for deadtime losses. At high count rates the detector electronics cannot handle every incoming event; therefore some of these events are lost because the electronics are busy processing prior events. Measuring the tomograph response to known input count rates allows empirical formulations for the losses to be determined and applied to the image data. Valid corrections for deadtime losses can approach 100%.

Not every detector in the system responds exactly the same way to a uniform distribution of radioactivity. A calibration scan is performed to measure the count rate for each detector in the system from a homogeneous source. A correction mask is created from this calibration scan, and the raw data are multiplied by this mask to yield a uniform count rate image from the homogeneous (flood) source. This correction is then applied to all subsequent PET images.

For the creation of parametric images, the corrected PET scanner data and the blood radioactivity concentration data are used as input to the physiologic model. Each pixel in the parametric image is assigned a physiologic value for the volume represented by the pixel. As an example, pixels in an ¹⁸F-FDG metabolic rate image correspond to a value between 0 and 6 in units of mg of glucose utilization per minute per 100 g of tissue. For blood flow images, each pixel represents a value between 0 and 150 in units of milliliters of blood flow per minute per 100 g of tissue.

Once the raw data are converted to functional images, ROIs can be drawn on the images. Average values of counts/area or counts/pixel are determined for each ROI. The data analysis task then is to correlate the physiologic value obtained from the patient's PET image data with the normative data. Abnormalities are identified as either elevated or diminished values of function when compared with a standard database of similar pathology or normal subjects. Intrinsically, biologic parameters have approximately a 15% standard deviation. For a true intersubject difference to be observed, variations in LCBF and LCMRG values must be greater than 15%. Intrasubject variability from PET studies has been shown to be about 7%. Therefore, if a research or clinical protocol can be designed so that the patient also serves as the control, greater reliability and reduced errors are achieved.

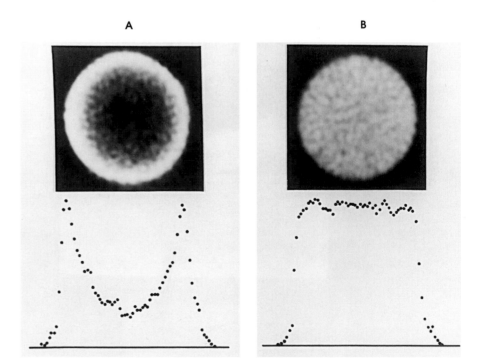

Fig. 40-17 A, Uncorrected image of a phantom homogeneously filled with a water-soluble PET nuclide of ⁶⁸Ga or ¹⁸F. **B,** Attenuation-corrected image of the same phantom. Cross-sectional cuts through the center of each image are shown in the lower panels. The attenuation correction for a phantom with a diameter of 20 cm (8 inches) can be as large as 70% in the center of the object.

Clinical Studies

PET imaging is relatively costly. It is best used for answering complex questions that involve tissue function (Figs. 40-18 and 40-19). It is unlikely that PET will be used as a broad-based clinical screening tool because it requires a relatively long imaging time (1 to 3 hours) compared with other imaging procedures.

It is important, then, that patients and normal volunteers be selected according to very stringent protocols. Before each imaging procedure, subjects typically receive a brief physical examination and laboratory blood tests. Certain external landmarks are measured. In brain imaging, for example, the measurements include the head diameter and the distance from the top of the head to an imaginary line passing from the lateral canthus of the eye to the meatus of the ear (the *CM line*). For quantitative studies, a radial artery is catheterized to obtain arterial blood samples, or heated hand techniques are used to obtain arterialized venous blood. Blood curves are collected and used as input functions for the physiologic models. Patients are oriented in the scanner in the supine position, either head or feet first.

The appropriate radiopharmaceutical is injected by IV bolus, IV infusion, or a combination of the two techniques. For dynamic studies, the injection is synchronized with the start of imaging. For quantitative studies, blood samples are collected according to established protocols. For ^{18}F-FDG studies, a decay-corrected plasma activity curve is constructed from blood samples (approximately 20×1 ml samples) acquired over the entire imaging procedure (1 to $1\frac{1}{2}$ hours) using discrete blood sampling techniques. For ^{15}O-H$_2$O studies, arterial samples are continuously withdrawn at a rate of 5 to 7 ml per minute for 2 minutes. Radioactivity detectors measure the whole-blood ^{15}O-H$_2$O concentration while the blood is being withdrawn. As much as 200 to 300 ml of blood may be drawn over a long study (5 to 10 injections of ^{15}O-H$_2$O).

^{18}F-FDG studies require a 40- to 60-minute period for incorporation of the radiopharmaceutical. Then 5- to 25-minute scans for each bed position are acquired to measure the almost static distribution of ^{18}F-FDG glucose metabolism in tissue. The scanning procedure, including the incorporation period, takes about $1\frac{1}{2}$ to $2\frac{1}{2}$ hours for a single injection of ^{18}F-FDG. The long half-life of ^{18}F (109.8 minutes) precludes multiple injections on the same day in most cases. Whole-body images are created by piecing together PET data acquired from several scans as the bed automatically moves out of the PET scanner. For safety reasons, bed operation is outward from the scanner when controlled by the computer in order to avoid contact between the PET scanner aperture and the patient's body (head, arms, or shoulders).

For ^{15}O-H$_2$O LCBF studies, a separate injection is necessary for each axial FOV (35 to 47 slices). For research studies, several injections are often administered; data are collected that show the differences in brain blood flow between each injection. The scanning procedure takes from 40 seconds to 6 minutes for blood flow studies and depends on specific imaging protocols. From one injection to the next, a total of 10 to 15 minutes is required for the ^{15}O radioactivity to decay to low enough levels to repeat the study.

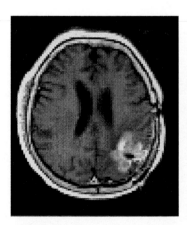 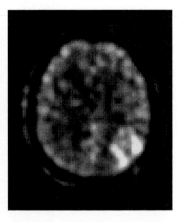

Fig. 40-18 Comparison of images obtained using transverse MRI *(left)* and PET *(right)* in a patient with recurrent brain tumor. PET depicts high ^{18}F-FDG metabolism at two locations, as indicated by the bright areas in the lower right portion of the image.

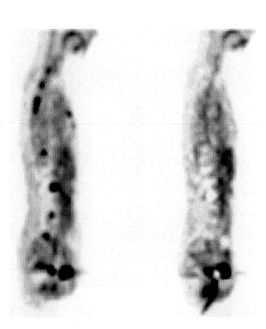

Fig. 40-19 Whole-body PET images. *Left,* ^{18}F-FDG sagittal image of patient with breast cancer metastasis. Numerous tumors (dark spots) are seen along the spine and sternum. *Right,* Image obtained after chemotherapy shows regression of the cancer.

After the scanning procedures are completed, the injection and arterial blood sampling catheters are removed, and the patient is permitted to leave the facility. Little residual radioactivity remains in the patient after ^{18}F-FDG imaging, especially after voiding, and practically none after ^{15}O-H$_2$O studies. Patients may immediately resume normal activities.

Clinically, PET is used primarily for diagnostic imaging of cancer, specifically cancer of the lung, breast, colon, and thyroid. ^{18}F-FDG is the radiopharmaceutical of choice. Qualitative imaging (no blood sampling) is routinely performed. Slow-growing brain tumors are not easily visualized with FDG imaging. PET plays an important role in differentiating benign from malignant processes, and it is also used for image guided biopsy. PET is an important modality for detecting cancer recurrence in patients who have undergone surgery or radiation treatments. Finally, PET is very effective in monitoring therapeutic interventions by rapidly yet noninvasively assessing the metabolic response of the tissues to drugs.

NORMAL VALUES

Normal volunteers studied using PET provide a database of normal values for comparison with patient data. Table 40-4 depicts local cerebral glucose metabolic rates and local cerebral blood flow rates for normal subjects. Three primary areas of brain LCMRG and LCBF are presented. The first area is associated with the control and coordination of voluntary muscle movements (cerebellum); the second area reflects the intact gray matter cortical regions (temporal cortex), which may be related to such functions as memory and fine motor movements; and the third region is responsible for decoding visual images (primary visual cortex). The visual cortex almost always shows the highest glucose utilization rates, and the cerebellum displays the lowest metabolic rates. The hemispheric averages do not differ significantly from each other or from the cerebellar values.

RADIATION DOSIMETRY

Image quality is related to the number of events detected by the PET scanner. By administering more radioactivity, better images are usually obtained. However, two constraints limit this action. First, the PET scanner deadtime losses and random coincidences increase as greater quantities of radioactivity are placed within the FOV of the PET tomograph. More importantly, regulations place maximum limits on the radiation *dose* a volunteer may receive during a PET study. The total dose (mrad) delivered to an organ is calculated by multiplying the specific value in Table 40-5 by the administered amount of radioactivity (mCi).

TABLE 40-4

LCMRG and LCBF rates in normal subjects

Parametric value	Cerebellum	Temporal cortex	Visual cortex	Left hemisphere	Right hemisphere	Whole brain
LCMRG	4.7	5.1	6.6	4.6	4.5	4.6
LCBF	60.8	65.3	82.7	54.5	55.3	54.8

LCMRG, Milligrams of glucose utilization per minute per 100 grams of tissue; *LCBF,* milliliters of blood flow per minute per 100 grams of tissue.

TABLE 40-5

Radiation dosimetry for PET studies

Organ	Absorbed dose (mrad/mCi) ^{15}O-H$_2$O*	^{18}F-FDG†
Bladder wall	—	440
Bone	1.42	37
Bone marrow (red)	1.98	41
Brain	6.13	96
Breast	4.59	41
GI tract—stomach	1.18	44
GI tract—small intestine	3.83	48
GI tract—large intestine	3.06	59
Heart	9.84	241
Kidneys	8.15	78
Lens of eye	0.24	41
Liver	3.62	44
Lung	3.77	41
Ovary	4.61	56
Testis	3.58	56
Thyroid	6.78	36

*From Narayana S et al: Dosimetry of (0-15) water: a physiologic approach, *Med Phys* 23:159, 1996.
†Fluorodeoxyglucose F 18 Systemic. In: *USP DI,* ed 17, Rockville, Md, 1997, United States Pharmacopeial Convention, Inc.

Future Studies

Considerable research has been conducted to study brain function with PET radiopharmaceuticals. Measurements of metabolism, blood flow, and receptor density are now considered routine. PET scanners have been specifically designed to acquire data from brain, heart, lung, organ transplants, and tumors. As the technology evolves, even greater emphasis will be placed on expanding clinical and research investigations of these tissues and organ systems.

Summary

PET is a very complex diagnostic imaging procedure. Consequently, it is both a clinical tool and a research tool. PET requires the multidisciplinary support of the physician, physicist, physiologist, chemist, engineer, and radiographer. This imaging procedure allows numerous biologic parameters in the working human body to be examined without disturbing normal-equilibrium physiology. PET measures regional function that cannot be determined by any other means, including CT and MRI.

Current PET studies involve the imaging of patients with epilepsy, Huntington's disease, stroke, schizophrenia, brain tumors, Alzheimer's disease, and other disorders of the brain. PET studies of the heart are providing routine diagnostic information on patients with coronary artery disease by identifying viable myocardium for revascularization. PET scanning is also used to evaluate organ transplant function, image tumors, determine the effects of therapeutic drug regimens, and differentiate necrosis from viable tumor. Human physiology will become better understood as the technology advances, yielding higher resolution instruments, new radiopharmaceuticals, and improved analysis of PET data.

Definition of Terms

analog PET radiopharmaceutical biochemically equivalent to a naturally occurring compound in the body.

annihilation Total transformation of matter into energy; occurs after the antimatter positron collides with an electron. Two photons are created; each equals the rest mass of the individual particles.

arterialized venous blood Arterial blood passed directly to the venous system by shunts in the capillary system after surface veins are heated to between 104°F and 108°F (40°C to 42.2°C). Blood gases from the vein under these conditions reflect near arterial levels of pO_2, pCO_2, and pH.

attenuation coefficient Number that represents the statistical reduction in photons that exit a material (N) from the value that entered the material (N_o). The reduced flux is the result of scatter and absorption, which can be expressed in the following equation: $N = N_o e^{-\mu x}$, where μ is the attenuation coefficient and χ is the distance traversed by the photons.

bit Term constructed from the words *bi*nary digi*t* and referring to a single digit of a binary number; for example, the binary of 101 is composed of 3 bits.

BGO scintillator bismuth germanate ($Bi_4Ge_3 O_{12}$) scintillator with an efficiency twice that of sodium iodide. BGO is used in nearly all commercially produced PET scanners.

byte Term used to define a group of bits, usually eight, being treated as a unit by the computer.

CM line Canthomeatal line defined by an imaginary line drawn between the lateral canthus of the eye and meatus of the ear.

cyclotron Cyclic particle accelerator used to increase the kinetic energy of nuclei, such as protons and deuterons, so that radioactive materials may be produced from the resultant nuclear reactions of the ions on stable materials.

deadtime Time when the system electronics are already processing information from one photon interaction with a detector and cannot accept new events to be processed from other detectors.

detector Device that is a combination of a scintillator and photomultiplier tube. It is used to detect x-rays and gamma rays.

deuteron Ionized nucleus of heavy hydrogen (deuterium), which contains one proton and one neutron.

dose Measure of the amount of energy deposited in a known mass of tissue from ionizing radiation. *Absorbed* dose is described in units of rads; 1 rad is equal to 10^{-2} joules/ kg or 100 ergs/g.

¹⁸F-FDG Radioactive analog of naturally available glucose. It follows the same biochemical pathways as glucose; however, unlike glucose, it is not totally metabolized to carbon dioxide and water.

fuctional image See *parametric image.*

gamma ray Electromagnetic radiation or photon emitted from the decay of a radioactive nucleus. Its energy is expressed in the equivalent energy of the photon in units of electron volts (eV) or millions of electron volts (MeV).

homeostasis State of equilibrium of the body's internal environment.

image coregistration Computer technique that permits realignment of images that have been acquired from different modalities and therefore have different orientations and magnifications. With realignment, the images possess the same orientation and size. The images can then be overlaid one on the other to demonstrate similarities and differences between the images.

isotropic Referring to uniform emission of radiation or particles in three dimensions.

kinetics Movement of materials into, out of, and through biologic spaces. A mathematical expression is often used to describe and quantify how substances traverse membranes or participate in biochemical reactions.

local cerebral blood flow (LCBF) Description of the parametric image of blood flow through the brain. It is expressed in units of milliliters of blood flow per minute per 100 g of brain tissue.

local metabolic rate of glucose utilization (LMRG) Units of milligrams of glucose utilization per minute per 100 g of tissue; used in conjunction with parametric images of tissues such as brain, heart, or tumor. LCMRG is specific to brain and corresponds to the local cerebral metabolic rate of glucose utilization.

magnetic resonance imaging (MRI) Technique of nuclear magnetic resonance (NMR) as it is applied to medical imaging. Magnetic resonance is abbreviated *MR.*

nuclear particle accelerator Device to produce radioactive material by accelerating ions (electrons, protons, deuterons, etc.) to high energies and projecting them toward stable materials. The list of accelerators includes linac, cyclotron, synchrotron, Van de Graaff accelerator, and betatron.

parametric image Image that relates anatomic position (the x and y position on an image) to a physiologic parameter such as blood flow (image intensity or color). It may also be referred to as a *functional image*.

photomultiplier tube (PMT) Vacuum tube that transforms visible light photons into minute electron currents that are subsequently amplified by a factor of approximately 10^6. Typically the output current is proportional to the energy of the incident photon.

pixel (*picture element*) Smallest indivisible part of an image matrix for display on a computer screen. Typical images may be 128 × 128, 256 × 256, or 512 × 512 pixels.

positron Positively charged particle emitted from neutron-deficient radioactive nuclei.

positron emission tomography (PET) Imaging technique that creates transaxial images of organ physiology from the simultaneous detection of positron annihilation photons.

quantitative Type of PET study in which the final images are not simply distributions of radioactivity but, rather, correspond to units of capillary blood flow, glucose metabolism, receptor density, etc. Studies between individuals and repeat studies in the same individual permit comparison of pixel values on an absolute scale.

radioactivity concentration Amount of radioactivity per unit volume. It can be expressed in units of mCi/ml (millicuries per milliliter).

radioisotope Synonym for *radioactive isotope*. Any isotope that is unstable undergoes decay with the emission of characteristic radiation.

radionuclide Nucleus of an atom that is unstable and will decay to a more stable configuration by the emission of a particle (e.g., positron, beta particle, alpha particle, etc.) or photon (gamma ray).

radiopharmaceutical Radioactive material that is inhaled, ingested, or injected into humans or animals; synonymous with *radiotracer.*

radiotracer Synonym for *radiopharmaceutical.*

ray Imaginary line drawn between a pair of detectors in the PET scanner or between the x-ray source and detector in a computed tomography (CT) scanner.

reconstruction Mathematic operation that transforms raw data acquired on a PET tomograph (sinogram) into an image with recognizable features.

region of interest (ROI) Area that circumscribes a desired anatomic location on a PET image. Image-processing systems permit drawing of ROIs on images. The average parametric value is computed for all pixels within the ROI and returned to the radiographer.

resolution Smallest separation of two point sources of radioactivity that can be distinguished for PET or single photon emission computed tomography imaging.

scintillator Organic or inorganic material that transforms high-energy photons such as x-rays or gamma rays into visible or nearly visible light (ultraviolet) photons for easy measurement.

segmented region Region of an image that has been defined and drawn based on simple intensity thresholding or other more complex mathematic expression.

sensitivity Ability to measure the total number of photons incident on a detector. In this case, the term is synonymous with *efficiency*. PET scanner sensitivity is often reported in units of counts per second per microcuries per milliliter in a 20-cm-diameter phantom homogeneously filled with ^{18}F, ^{68}Ge, or ^{68}Ga.

septa High-density metal collimators that separate adjacent detectors on a ring tomograph to reduce scattered photons from degrading image information.

single-photon emission computed tomography (SPECT) A nuclear medicine scanning procedure that measures conventional single photon gamma emissions (technetium-99m) with a specially designed rotating gamma camera.

target Device used to contain stable materials and subsequent radioactive materials during bombardment by high-energy nuclei from a cyclotron or other particle accelerator. The term is also applied to the material inside the device, which may be solid, liquid, or gaseous.

transmission scan Type of PET scan that is equivalent to a low-resolution CT scan. Attenuation is determined by rotating a rod of radioactive ^{68}Ge around the subject. Photons that traverse the subject either impinge on a detector and are registered as valid counts or are attenuated (absorbed or scattered). The ratio of counts with and without the attenuating tissue in place provides the factors to correct PET scans for the loss of counts from attenuation of the 0.511-MeV photons.

Selected bibliography

Bares R et al, editors: *Clinical PET,* Dordrecht, Netherlands, 1996, Kluwer Academic.

Barnes WE, editor: *Basic physics of radiotracers,* vols I and II, Boca Raton, Fla, 1983, CRC.

Beckers C et al: *Positron emission tomography in clinical research and clinical diagnosis,* Dordrecht, Netherlands, 1989, Kluwer Academic.

Bergmann SR, Sobel BE, editors: *Positron emission tomography of the heart,* Mount Kisco, NY, 1992, Futura.

Bergstrom M et al: Correction for scattered radiation in a ring detector positron camera by integral transformation of the projections, *J Comput Assist Tomogr* 7:42, 1983.

Brownell GL et al: New developments in positron scintigraphy and the application of cyclotron produced positron emitters, *Medical radioisotope scintigraphy,* Vol I, IAEA (Proceedings Series), Vienna, 1969.

Burns HD et al: (3-N-[^{11}C]Methyl) Spiperone, a ligand binding to dopamine receptors: radiochemical synthesis and biodistribution studies in mice, *J Nucl Med* 25:1222, 1984.

Bushberg JT et al: *The essential physics of medical imaging,* Baltimore, 1994, Williams & Wilkins.

Cho ZH et al: *Foundations of medical imaging,* New York, 1993, John Wiley & Sons.

Clark JC et al: Short-lived radioactive gases for clinical use, Boston, 1975, Butterworth.

Conte M et al: *An introduction to the physics of particle accelerators,* Singapore, 1991, World Scientific.

Daghighian F et al: PET imaging: an overview and instrumentation, *J Nucl Med Technol* 18:5, 1990.

Damasio H: *Human brain anatomy in computerized images,* New York, 1995, Oxford University Press.

Damasio H et al: A neural basis for lexical retrieval, *Nature* 380:486, 1996.

Diksic M et al, editors: *Radiopharmaceuticals and brain pathology studied with PET and SPECT,* Boca Raton, Fla, 1991, CRC.

Duhaylongsod FG et al: Detection of primary and recurrent lung cancer by means of F-18 fluorodeoxyglucose positron emission tomography (FDG PET), *J Thorac Cardiovasc Surg* 110:130, 1995.

Emran AM, editor: *Chemists' views of imaging centers,* New York, 1995, Plenum.

Frackowiak RSJ et al: Quantitative measurement of cerebral blood flow and oxygen metabolism in man using ^{15}O and positron emission tomography: theory, procedure and normal values, *J Comput Assist Tomogr* 4:727, 1980.

Freedman GS, editor: *Tomographic imaging in nuclear medicine,* New York, 1973, Society of Nuclear Medicine.

Frost JJ et al, editors: *Quantitative imaging: neuroreceptors, neurotransmitters, and enzymes,* New York, 1990, Raven.

Gilmore G et al: *Practical gamma-ray spectrometry,* Chichester, England, 1995, John Wiley & Sons.

Gose E et al: *Pattern recognition and image analysis,* Upper Saddle River, NJ, 1996, Prentice Hall.

Grabowski TJ et al: Neuroanatomical analysis of functional brain images: validation with retinotopic mapping, *Hum Brain Mapping* 2:134, 1995.

Greitz T et al, editors: *The metabolism of the human brain studied with positron emission tomography,* New York, 1985, Raven.

Heiss WD et al: Regional kinetic constants and cerebral metabolic rate for glucose in normal human volunteers determined by dynamic positron emission tomography of [^{18}F]-2-fluoro-deoxy-D-glucose, *J Cereb Blood Flow Metab* 4:212, 1984.

Helus F, editor: *Radionuclides production,* vols I and II, Boca Raton, Fla, 1983, CRC.

Hendee WR: *The physical principles of computed tomography,* Boston, 1983, Little, Brown.

Herman TG, editor: *Image reconstruction from projections: Implementation and applications,* New York, 1979, Springer-Verlag.

Hichwa RD et al: Design of target systems for production of positron nuclides, *Nucl Instr Methods Physics Res* B40/41:1110, 1989.

Hoffman EJ et al: Quantitation in positron emission computed tomography: 1. Effect of object size, *J Comput Assist Tomogr* 3:299, 1979.

Holman BL, editor: *Radionuclide imaging of the brain,* New York, 1985, Churchill Livingstone.

Hounsfield G: Computerized transverse axial scanning (tomography), *Br J Radiol* 46:1016, 1973.

Hubner KF et al: *Clinical positron emission tomography,* St Louis, 1992, Mosby.

Hubner KF et al: Characterization of chest masses by FDG positron emission tomography, *Clin Nucl Med* 20:293, 1995.

Hubner KF et al: *Clinical positron emission tomography,* St Louis, 1992, Mosby.

Hurtig RR et al: The effects of the timing and duration of cognitive activation of O-15 PET studies, *J Cereb Blood Flow Metab* 14:423, 1994.

Jahne B: *Practical handbook on image processing for scientific applications,* Boca Raton, Fla, 1997, CRC.

Jahne B: *Digital image processing: concepts, algorithms and scientific applications,* Berlin, 1995, Springer-Verlag.

Kantele J: *Handbook of nuclear spectrometry,* London, 1995, Academic.

Karp JS et al: Performance standards in positron emission tomography, *J Nucl Med* 32:2342, 1991.

Kember NF, editor: *Medical radiation detectors: fundamental and applied aspects,* Philadelphia, 1994, Institute of Physics.

Lawrence EO, Edlefsen NE: On the production of high speed protons, *Science* 72:376, 1930.

Lewis P et al: Whole-body 18F-fluorodeoxyglucose positron emission tomography in preoperative evaluation of lung cancer, *Lancet* 344:1265, 1994.

Livingood JJ: *Principles of cyclic particle accelerators,* Princeton, NJ, 1961, D Van Nostrand.

London ED, editor: *Imaging drug action in the brain,* Boca Raton, Fla, 1993, CRC.

Martin WH et al: A simplified intravenous glucose loading protocol for fluorine-18 fluorodeoxyglucose cardiac single-photon emission tomography, *Eur J Nucl Med* 24:1291, 1997.

Mazziotta JC et al: Tomographic mapping of human cerebral metabolism: normal unstimulated state, *Neurology* 31:503, 1981.

Matsuzawa T, editor: *Clinical PET in oncology,* River Edge, NJ, 1994, World Scientific.

Minton MA et al: Brain oxygen utilization measured with O-15 radiotracers and positron emission tomography, *J Nucl Med* 25:177, 1984.

Myers R et al: *Quantification of brain function using PET,* San Diego, 1996, Academic.

Patterson HW et al: *Accelerator health physics,* New York, 1973, Academic.

Phelps ME et al: A new computerized tomographic imaging system for positron-emitting radiopharmaceuticals, *J Nucl Med* 19:635, 1978.

Phelps ME et al: Tomographic measurements of local cerebral glucose metabolism rate in humans with (F-18)-2-fluoro-2-deoxy-D-glucose: validation of methods, *Ann Neurol* 6:371, 1979.

Phelps ME et al, editors: *Positron emission tomography and autoradiography: principles and applications for the brain and heart,* New York, 1986, Raven.

Phillis JW: *The regulation of cerebral blood flow,* Boca Raton, Fla, 1993, CRC.

Reivich M et al: The [^{18}F]fluorodeoxyglucose method for the measurement of local cerebral glucose utilization in man, *Circ Res* 44:127, 1979.

Riggs DS: *The mathematical approach to physiological problems,* Cambridge, Mass, 1963, Williams & Wilkins.

Rigo P et al: Oncological applications of positron emission tomography with fluorine-18 fluorodeoxyglucose, *Eur J Nucl Med* 231:1641, 1996.

Robertson JS, editor: *Compartmental distribution of radiotracers,* Boca Raton, Fla, 1983, CRC.

Schelbert HR et al: Regional myocardial perfusion assessed with N-13 labeled ammonia and positron emission computerized tomography, *Am J Cardiol* 43:209, 1979.

Sokoloff L et al: The 14C-deoxyglucose method for the measurement of local cerebral glucose utilization: theory, procedure and normal values in conscious and anesthetized albino rats, *J Neurochem* 28:879, 1977.

Ter-Pogossian MM et al: A positron-emission transaxial tomograph for nuclear imaging (PETT), *Radiology* 114:89,1975.

Toga AW: *Three-dimensional neuroimaging,* New York, 1990, Raven.

Toga AW et al: *Brain mapping: the methods,* San Diego, 1996, Academic.

Udupa JK et al: *3D imaging in medicine,* Boca Raton, Fla, 1991, CRC.

Wagner JG: *Pharmacokinetics for the pharmaceutical scientist,* Lancaster, Penn, 1993, Technomic.

Wolfe RR: *Radioactive and stable isotope tracers in biomedicine: principles and practice of kinetic analysis,* New York, 1992, Wiley-Liss.

Wollenweber SD et al: A simple on-line arterial time-activity curve for [O-15] water PET studies, *IEEE Trans Nucl Sci* 44:1613, 1997.

Zeki S: *A vision of the brain,* Oxford, England, 1993, Blackwell Scientific.

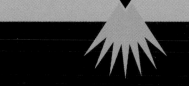

RADIATION ONCOLOGY

LEILA A. BUSSMAN

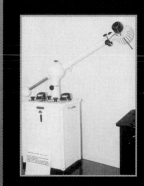

RIGHT: Grenz x-ray device for superficial therapy treatments, approximately 1940.

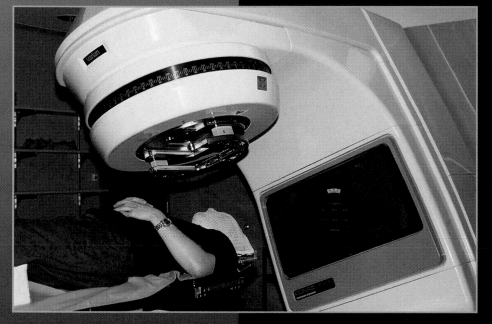

LEFT: A 1999 linear accelerator equipped with a multileaf collimator and asymmetric jaws.

Principles of Radiation Oncology

*Radiation oncology,** or *radiation therapy,* is one of three principal modalities used in the treatment of cancer. The others are surgery and chemotherapy. In radiation therapy for malignancies, *tumors* or *lesions* are treated with *cancericidal doses* of ionizing radiation as prescribed by a *radiation oncologist,* a physician specialized in the treatment of malignant disease with radiation. The goals of the treatment are to precisely deliver a cancericidal dose of radiation to the tumor but to limit as much as possible the dose of radiation received by normal, noncancerous tissues. These dual tasks make this form of treatment complex and often challenging. Input from all members of the radiation oncology team is crucial in developing the optimum treatment plan or approach for a patient.

Cancer treatment requires a multidisciplinary approach. First, diagnostic radiologic studies such as radiographs, computed tomographic (CT) scans, and/or sonograms are obtained to acquire information about the location and anatomic extent of the tumor. Second, a tissue specimen *(biopsy)* is removed surgically. A *pathologist* then examines the tissue to determine whether the lesion is cancerous. Once cancer is diagnosed, the plan for the best treatment is determined through consultation with various *oncology* specialists (e.g., surgical *oncologist,* radiation oncologist, and/or medical oncologist).

Although radiation oncology may be used as the only method of treatment for malignant disease, a more common approach is to use radiation in conjunction with surgery, chemotherapy, or both. Some cancer patients may be treated only with surgery or chemotherapy; however, approximately 75% of all diagnosed cancer patients are treated with radiation. The choice of treatment can depend on a number of patient variables such as the patient's overall physical and emotional

condition, the histologic type of the disease, and the extent and anatomic position of the tumor. If a tumor is small and its margins are well defined, a surgical approach alone may be prescribed. If the disease is *systemic,* a chemotherapeutic approach may be chosen. Most tumors, however, exhibit degrees of size, invasion, and spread and require variations in the treatment approach that in all likelihood will include radiation treatments administered as an adjunct to or in conjunction with surgery or chemotherapy.

Radiation is generally used after surgery when a patient is deemed to be at high risk for tumor recurrence in the *surgical bed.* The risk of recurrence is considered to be increased in the following situations:

- When the surgical margin between normal tissue and cancerous tissue is minimal (less than 2 cm)
- When the margin is positive for cancer, (i.e., when cancerous tissue is not completely removed)
- When the tumor is incompletely resected because of it large size and/or its relationship with normal vital structures
- When the cancer has spread to adjacent lymph nodes

Thus the radiation can be used as definitive (primary) cancer treatment or adjuvant treatment (i.e., in combination with another form of therapy). It can also be used for *palliation.*

Radiation treatments most often are delivered on a daily basis, Monday through Friday, for 2 to 8 weeks. The length of time and the total dose of radiation delivered depend on the type of cancer being treated and the purpose of treatment *(cure* or palliation). Prescribed dosages of radiation can range from 2000 centigray (cGy) for palliation to 7600 cGy for curative intent (total doses). The delivery of a small amount of radiation per day (180 to 200 cGy) for a certain number of treatments, instead of one large dose, is termed *fractionation.* Because these smaller doses of radiation are more easily tolerated by normal tissue, fractionation can help minimize the acute toxic effect a patient experiences during treatment as well as the possible long-term side effects of treatment.

The precision and accuracy necessary to administer high doses of radiation to tumors while not harming normal tissue require the combined effort of all members of the radiation oncology team. Members of this team include the radiation oncologist, a physicist, dosimetrists, radiation therapists, and oncology nurses.

The radiation oncologist prescribes the quantity of radiation and determines the anatomic region(s) to be treated. The *medical physicist* is responsible for calibration and maintenance of the radiation-producing equipment. The physicist also advises the physician about dosage calculations and complex treatment techniques. The *medical dosimetrist* devises a plan for delivering the treatments in a manner to best meet the physician's goals of irradiating the tumor while protecting vital normal structures. The *radiation therapist* is responsible for obtaining radiographs that localize the area to be treated, administering the treatments, keeping accurate records of the dose delivered each day, and monitoring the patient's physical and emotional well-being. Educating patients about potential radiation side effects and assisting patients with the management of these side effects are often the responsibilities of the oncology nurse.

The duties and responsibilities of the radiation therapist are more thoroughly described elsewhere in this chapter. In addition, more information is provided about the circumstances in which radiation is used to treat cancer. The steps necessary to prepare a patient for treatment are also described. These steps include (1) simulation, (2) evolution of the optimum treatment plan in dosimetry, and (3) treatment delivery. Current techniques and future trends are also discussed.

---

*Almost all italicized terms are defined at the end of this chapter.

Historical Development

Ionizing radiation was originally used to obtain a radiographic image of internal anatomy for diagnostic purposes. The resultant image depended on many variables, including the energy of the beam, the processing techniques, the material on which the image was recorded, and most importantly the amount of energy absorbed by the various organs of the body. The transfer of energy from the beam of radiation to the biologic system and the observation of the effects of this interaction became the foundation of radiation oncology.

Two of the most obvious and sometimes immediate biologic effects observed during the early diagnostic procedures were epilation (loss of hair) and erythema (reddening of the skin). Epilation and erythema resulted primarily from the great amount of energy absorbed by the skin during radiographic procedures. These short-term radiation-induced effects afforded radiographic practitioners an opportunity to expand the use of radiation to treat conditions ranging from relatively benign maladies such as hypertrichosis (excessive hair), acne, and boils to grotesque and malignant diseases such as lupus vulgaris and skin cancer.

Ionizing radiation was first applied for the treatment of a more in-depth lesion on Jan. 29, 1896, when Dr. Émile H. Grubbé is reported to have irradiated a woman with carcinoma of the left breast. This event occurred only 3 months after the discovery of x-rays by Dr. W.K. Röntgen (Table 41-1). Although Dr. Grubbé neither expected nor observed any dramatic results from the irradiation, the event is significant simply because it occurred.

The first reported curative treatment using ionizing radiation was performed by Dr. Clarence E. Skinner of New Haven, Connecticut, in January 1902. Dr. Skinner treated a woman who had a diagnosed malignant fibrosarcoma. Over the next 2 years and 3 months the woman received a total of 136 applications of the x-rays. In April 1909, 7 years after initial application of the radiation, the woman was free of disease and considered "cured."

As data were collected, the interest in radiation therapy grew. More sophisticated equipment, a greater understanding of the effects of ionizing radiation, an appreciation for time-dose relationships, and a number of other related medical breakthroughs gave impetus to the interest in radiation therapy that led to the evolution of a distinct medical specialty—radiation oncology.

Cancer

Cancer is a disease process that involves an unregulated, uncontrolled replication of cells; put more simply, the cells do not know when to stop dividing. These abnormal cells grow without regard to normal tissue. They invade adjacent tissues, destroy normal tissue, and create a mass of tumor cells. Cancerous cells can further spread by invading the lymph or blood vessels that drain the area. When tumor cells invade the lymphatic or vascular system, they are transported by that system until they become caught or lodged within a lymph node or an organ such as the liver or lungs, where secondary tumors form. The spread of cancer from the original site to different, remote parts of the body is termed *metastasis*. Once cancer has spread to a distant site via bloodborne metastasis, the patient is considered incurable. Therefore early detection and diagnosis are the keys to curing cancer.

An estimated 1,228,600 persons in the United States were diagnosed with cancer in 1998. This number does not include basal and squamous cell skin cancers, which have high cure rates. These types of cancer are the most common malignant diseases, with more than 900,000 cases diagnosed in 1998. *The overall lifetime risk of developing cancer is 50% for men and about 33% for women. Cancer can occur in persons of any age, although the majority of patients are diagnosed after the age of 50 years.*

TABLE 41-1

Significant developments in radiation therapy

Dates	Persons	Events
1895	W.K. Röntgen	Discovery of x-rays
1896	É. Grubbé	First use of ionizing radiation in treatment of cancer
	A.H. Becquerel	Discovery of radioactive emissions by uranium compounds
1898	M. and P. Curie	Discovery of radium
1902	C.E. Skinner	First documented case of cancer "cure" using ionizing radiation
1906	J. Bergonié and L. Tribondeau	Postulation of first law of radiosensitivity
1932	E.O. Lawrence	Invention of cyclotron
1934	F. Joliot and I. Joliot-Curie	Production of artificial radioactivity
1939	E.O. Lawrence and R.S. Stone	Treatment of cancer patient with neutron beam from cyclotron
1940	D.W. Kerst	Construction of betatron
1951		Installation of first cobalt-60 teletherapy units
1952		Installation of first linear accelerator (Hammersmith Hospital, London)

The most common cancers that occur in the United States are lung, prostate, breast, and colorectal cancer. Prostate cancer is the most common malignancy in men; for women, breast cancer is the most common. In both men and women, the second and third most common cancers are lung and colorectal cancer (Table 41-2).

Cancer is the second only to heart disease as the leading cause of death in the United States. Lung cancer is the leading cause of cancer deaths for both men and women. In 1998 an estimated 32% of cancer deaths in men and 25% in women were due to lung cancer. The next most common types of terminal cancer are prostate cancer and breast cancer, which respectively account for 13% and 16% of cancer deaths in the United States.

TABLE 41-2

Top five most common cancers in men and women

Men	Women
1. Prostate	Breast
2. Lung and bronchus	Lung and bronchus
3. Colon and rectum	Colon and rectum
4. Bladder	Uterus (endometrium)
5. Non-Hodgkin's lymphomas	Ovary

RISK FACTORS
External factors

Many factors can contribute to a person's potential for the development of a *malignancy*. These factors can be external exposure to chemicals, viruses, or radiation within the environment or internal factors such as hormones, genetic mutations, and disorders of the immune system. Cancer commonly is the result of exposure to a *carcinogen,* which is a substance or material that causes cells to undergo malignant transformation and become cancerous. Some of the known carcinogenic agents are listed in Table 41-3. Cigarettes and other tobacco products are the principal cause of cancers of the lung, esophagus, oral cavity/pharynx, and bladder. Cigarette smokers are 10 times more likely to develop lung cancer than are nonsmokers. Occupational exposure to chemicals such as chromium, nickel, or arsenic can also cause lung cancer. A person who smokes and also works with chemical carcinogens is at even greater risk for developing lung cancer than is a nonsmoker. In other words, risk factors can have an additive effect, acting together to initiate or promote the development of cancer.

Another carcinogen is *ionizing radiation.* It was responsible for the development of osteogenic sarcoma in radium-dial painters in the 1920s and 1930s, and it caused the development of skin cancers in pioneer radiologists. Early radiation therapy equipment used in the treatment of cancer often induced a second malignancy in the bone. The low-energy x-rays produced by this equipment were within the photoelectric range of interactions with matter, resulting in a 3:1 preferential absorption in bone compared to soft tissue.

Therefore some breast cancer patients who were irradiated developed an osteosarcoma of their ribs after a 15- to 20-year latency period. With the advances in diagnostic and therapeutic equipment and improved knowledge of radiation physics, radiobiology, and radiation safety practices, radiation-induced malignancies have become relatively uncommon, although the potential for their development still exists. In keeping with standard radiation safety guidelines, any dose of radiation, no matter how small, significantly increases the chance of a genetic mutation.

Internal factors

Internal factors are causative factors over which persons have no control. Genetic mutations on individual genes and *chromosomes* have been identified as predisposing factors for the development of cancer. Mutations can be sporadic or hereditary, as in colon cancer. Chromosomal defects have also been identified in other cancers, such as leukemia, Wilms' tumor, retinoblastoma, and breast cancer. Because of their familial pattern of occurrence, breast, ovarian, and colorectal cancer are three major areas currently under study to obtain earlier diagnosis, which increases the cure rate. For example, patients with a family history of breast or ovarian cancer can be tested to see whether they have inherited the altered *BRCA-1* and *BRCA-2* genes. Patients with these altered genes are at a significantly higher risk for developing breast and ovarian cancer. Women identified as carriers of the altered genes can benefit from more intensive and early screening programs in which breast cancer may be diagnosed at a much earlier and thus more curable stage. These patients also have the option of *prophylactic surgery* to remove the breasts or ovaries. Some women, however, still develop cancer in the remaining tissue after surgery.

TABLE 41-3

Carcinogenic agents and the cancers they cause

Carcinogen	Resultant cancer
Cigarette smoking	Cancers of lung, esophagus, bladder, and oral cavity/pharynx
Arsenic, chromium, nickel, hydrocarbons	Lung cancer
Ultraviolet light	Melanoma and nonmelanomatous skin cancers
Benzene	Leukemia
Ionizing radiation	Sarcomas of bone and soft tissue, skin cancer, and leukemia

Familial adenomatous polyposis

Familial adenomatous polyposis (FAP) is a hereditary condition in which the lining of the colon becomes studded with hundreds to thousands of polyps by late adolescence. A mutation in a gene identified as the adenomatous polyposis coli (APC) gene is considered the cause of this abnormal growth of polyps. Virtually all patients with this condition eventually develop colon cancer. Furthermore, they develop cancer at a much earlier age than the normal population. Treatment involves removal of the entire colon and rectum.

Hereditary nonpolyposis colorectal cancer

Hereditary nonpolyposis colorectal cancer (HNPCC) syndrome is a cancer that develops in the proximal colon in the absence of polyps or with fewer than five polyps. It has a familial distribution, occurring in three first-degree relatives in two generations, with at least one person being diagnosed before the age of 50 years. HNPCC has also been associated with the development of cancers of the breast, endometrium, pancreas, and biliary tract.

Familial cancer research

Current research to identify the genes responsible for cancer will assist in detecting cancers at a much earlier stage in high-risk patients. Many institutions have familial cancer programs to provide genetic testing and counseling for persons with strong family histories of cancer. Experts assist in educating persons about their potential risk for developing cancer and the importance of screening and early detection. Genetic testing remains the patient's option, and many patients prefer not to be tested.

TISSUE ORIGINS OF CANCER

Cancers may arise in any human tissue. However, tumors are usually categorized under six general headings according to their tissue of origin (Table 41-4). Ninety percent of cancers arise from *epithelial tissue* and are classified as *carcinomas*. Epithelial tissue lines the free internal and external surfaces of the body. Carcinomas are further subdivided into squamous cell carcinomas and adenocarcinomas based on the type of epithelium from which they arise. For example, a squamous cell carcinoma arises from the surface (squamous) epithelium of a structure. Examples of surface epithelium include the oral cavity, pharynx, bronchus, skin, and cervix. An adenocarcinoma is a cancer that develops in glandular epithelium such as that in the prostate, colon/rectum, lung, breast, or endometrium.

To facilitate the exchange of patient information from one physician to another, a system of classifying tumors based on anatomic and histologic considerations was designed by the International Union Against Cancer and the American Joint Committee for Cancer Staging and End Results Reporting. The TNM classification (Table 41-5) describes a tumor according to the size of the primary lesion (T), the involvement of the regional lymph nodes (N), and the occurrence of metastasis (M).

TABLE 41-4

Categorization of cancers by tissue of origin

Tissue of origin	Type of tumor
Epithelium	
Surface epithelium	Squamous cell carcinoma
Glandular epithelium	Adenocarcinoma
Connective tissue	
Bone	Osteosarcoma
Fat	Liposarcoma
Lymphoreticular-hematopoietic tissue	
Lymph nodes	Lymphoma
Plasma cells	Multiple myeloma
Blood cells/ bone marrow	Leukemia
Nerve tissue	
Glial tissue	Glioma
Neuroectoderm	Neuroblastoma
Tumors of more than one tissue	
Embryonic kidney	Nephroblastoma
Tumors that do not fit into above categories	
Testis	Seminoma
Thymus	Thymoma

TABLE 41-5

Application of the TNM classification system*

Classification	Description of tumor
Stage 0 $T_0N_0M_0$	Occult lesion; no evidence clinically
Stage I $T_1N_0M_0$	Small lesion confined to organ of origin with no evidence of vascular and lymphatic spread or metastasis
Stage II $T_2N_1M_0$	Tumor of less than 5 cm invading surrounding tissue and first-station lymph nodes but no evidence of metastasis
Stage III $T_3N_2M_0$	Extensive lesion greater than 5 cm with fixation to deeper structure and with bone and lymph invasion but no evidence of metastasis
Stage IV $T_4N_3M_+$	More extensive lesion than above with distant metastasis

*Although variations of the TNM classification system exist, the general description of the tumor does not change, that is, a T1 lesion is confined to the organ of origin regardless of whether it is 0.5 or 1.5 cm in diameter.

Theory

The biologic effectiveness of ionizing radiation in living tissue is dependent partially on the amount of energy that is deposited within the tissue and partially on the condition of the biologic system. The terms used to describe this relationship are *linear energy transfer (LET)* and *relative biologic effectiveness (RBE).*

LET values are expressed in thousands of electron volts deposited per micron of tissue (keV/μm) and will vary depending on the type of radiation being considered. Particles, because of their mass and possible charge, tend to interact more readily with the material through which they are passing and therefore have a greater LET value. For example, a 5-MeV alpha particle has an LET value of 100 keV/μm in tissue; nonparticulate radiations such as 250-kilovolt (peak) (kVp) x-rays and 1.2-MeV gamma rays have much lower LET values: 1.5 and 0.3 keV/μm, respectively.

RBE values are determined by calculating the ratio of the dose from a standard beam of radiation to the dose required of the radiation beam in question to produce a similar biologic effect. The standard beam of radiation is 250-kVp x-rays, and the ratio is set up as follows:

$$RBE = \frac{\text{Standard beam dose to obtain effect}}{\text{Similar effect using beam in question}}$$

As the LET increases, so does the RBE. Some RBE and LET values are listed in Table 41-6.

The effectiveness of ionizing radiation on a biologic system depends not only on the amount of radiation deposited but also on the state of the biologic system. One of the first laws of radiation biology, postulated by Bergonié and Tribondeau, stated in essence that the *radiosensitivity* of a tissue is dependent on the number of *undifferentiated* cells in the tissue, the degree of mitotic activity of the tissue, and the length of time that cells of the tissue remain in active proliferation. Although exceptions exist, the preceding is true in most tissues. The primary target of ionizing radiation is the DNA molecule, and the human cell is most radiosensitive during mitosis. Current research tends to indicate that all cells are equally radiosensitive; however, the manifestation of the radiation injury occurs at different time frames (i.e., acute versus late effects).

Because tissue cells are composed primarily of water, most of the *ionization* occurs with water molecules. These events are called *indirect effects* and result in the formation of free radicals such as OH, H, and HO$_2$. These highly reactive free radicals may recombine with no resultant biologic effect, or they may combine with other atoms and molecules to produce biochemical changes that may be deleterious to the cell. The possibility also exists that the radiation may interact with an organic molecule or atom, which may result in the inactivation of the cell; this reaction is called the *direct effect.* Because ionizing radiation is nonspecific (i.e., it interacts with normal cells as readily as with tumor cells), cellular damage will occur in both normal and abnormal tissue. The deleterious effects, however, are greater in the tumor cells because a greater percentage of these cells are undergoing mitosis; tumor cells also tend to be more poorly *differentiated.* In addition, normal cells have a greater capability for repairing sublethal damage than do tumor cells. Thus greater cell damage occurs to tumor cells than to normal cells for any given increment of dose. The effects of the interactions in either normal or tumor cells may be expressed by the following descriptions:

- Loss of reproductive ability
- Metabolic changes
- Cell transformation
- Acceleration of the aging process
- Cell mutation

Certainly the greater the number of interactions that occur, the greater the possibility of cell death.

The preceding information leads to a categorization of tumors according to their radiosensitivity:

- Very radiosensitive
  1. Gonadal germ cell tumors (seminoma of testis, dysgerminoma of ovary)
  2. Lymphoproliferative tumors (Hodgkin's disease, lymphoma)
  3. Embryonal tumors (Wilms' tumor of the kidney, retinoblastoma)
- Moderately radiosensitive
  1. Epithelial tumors (squamous and basal cell carcinomas of skin)
  2. Glandular tumors (adenocarcinoma of prostate)
- Relatively radioresistant
  1. Mesenchymal tumors (sarcomas of bone, connective tissue, and muscle)
  2. Nerve tumors (glioma, melanoma)

Many concepts that originate in the laboratory have little practical application, but some are beginning to influence the selection of treatment modalities and the techniques of radiation oncology. As cellular function and the effects of radiation on the cell are increasingly understood, attention is being focused on the use of drugs, or simply oxygen, to enhance the effectiveness of radiation treatments.

TABLE 41-6

Relative biologic effectiveness (RBE) and linear energy transfer (LET) values for certain forms of radiation

Radiation	RBE	LET
250-kV x-rays	1	2.0
^{60}Co gamma rays	0.85	0.3
14-MeV neutrons	12	75
5-MeV alpha particles	20	100

Technical Aspects

EXTERNAL-BEAM THERAPY AND BRACHYTHERAPY

Two major categories for the application of radiation for cancer treatment are external-beam therapy and brachytherapy. For *external-beam treatment,* the patient lies underneath a machine that emits radiation or generates a beam of x-rays. This technique is also called *teletherapy,* or long-distance treatment. Most cancer patients are treated in this fashion. However, some patients may also be treated with *brachytherapy,* a technique in which the radioactive material is placed within the patient.

The theory behind brachytherapy is to deliver low-intensity radiation over an extended period to a relatively small volume of tissue. Brachytherapy may be accomplished in any of the following ways:

1. Mould technique—placement of a *radioactive* source or sources on or in close proximity to the lesion
2. Intracavitary implant technique—placement of a radioactive source or sources in a body cavity
3. Interstitial implant technique—placement of a radioactive source or sources directly into the tumor site and adjacent tissue

The majority of brachytherapy applications tend to be temporary in that the sources are left in the patient until a designated tumor dose has been attained (a period of possibly 3 to 4 days). A radioactive nuclide commonly used for intracavitary implants is cesium-137. Gynecologic tumors are treated with this type of implant. Iridium-192 is used for interstitial implants. After being sterilized or disinfected, the nuclides may be reused.

Permanent implant therapy may also be accomplished. An example of a permanent implant nuclide is iodine-125 seeds. Permanent implant nuclides have *half-lives* of hours or days and are left in the patient essentially forever. The amount and distribution of the radionuclide implanted in this manner depends on the total dose that the radiation oncologist is trying to deliver. Early stage prostate cancer is commonly treated with this technique. In most if not all cases of brachytherapy implantation, the implant is applied as part of the patient's overall treatment plan and may be preceded by or followed by additional external beam radiation therapy or possibly surgery.

EQUIPMENT

Most radiation oncology departments have available some or all of the following units:

- 120-kVp superficial x-ray unit for treating lesions on or near the surface of the patient
- 250-kVp orthovoltage x-ray unit for moderately superficial tissues
- Cobalt-60 *gamma ray* source with an average energy of 1.25-MeV
- 35-MeV *linear accelerator* or *betatron* to serve as a source of high-energy (megavoltage) electrons and x-rays

The dose depositions of these units are compared in Fig. 41-1.

The penetrability, or energy, of an x-ray or gamma ray is totally dependent on its wavelength: the shorter the wavelength, the more penetrating the photon; conversely, the longer the wavelength, the less penetrating the photon. A low-energy beam (120 kVp or less) of radiation tends to deposit all or most of its energy on or near the surface of the patient and thus is suitable for treating lesions on or near the skin surface. In addition, with the low-energy beam a greater amount of absorption or dose deposition takes place in bone than in soft tissue.

A high-energy beam of radiation (1 MeV or greater) tends to deposit its energy throughout the entire volume of tissue irradiated, with a greater amount of dose deposition occurring at or near the entry port than at the exit port. In this energy range the dose is deposited about equally in soft tissue and bone. The high-energy (megavoltage) beam is most suitable for tumors deep beneath the body surface.

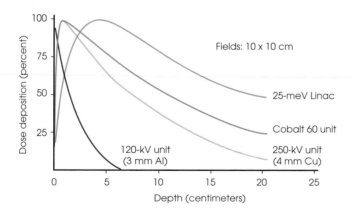

Fig. 41-1 Plot of the percent of dose deposition in relation to the depth in centimeters of tissue for various energies of photon beams.

The *skin-sparing* effect, a phenomenon that occurs as the energy of a beam of radiation is increased, is of value from a therapeutic standpoint. In the superficial and orthovoltage energy range, the maximum dose occurs on the surface of the patient, and deposition of the dose decreases as the beam traverses the patient. As the energy of the beam increases into the megavoltage range, the maximum dose absorbed by the patient occurs at some point below the skin surface. The skin-sparing effect is of importance clinically because the skin is a radiosensitive organ and excessive dose deposition to the skin may compromise the treatment dose to a tumor that is at some depth within the patient. The greater the energy of the beam, the more deeply the maximum dose will be deposited (Fig. 41-2).

Cobalt-60 units

The *cobalt-60* unit was the first skin-sparing machine. It replaced the orthovoltage unit in the early 1950s because of its greater ability to treat tumors located deeper within tissues. ^{60}Co is an artificially produced *isotope* formed in a nuclear *reactor* by the bombardment of stable cobalt-59 with neutrons. ^{60}Co emits two gamma ray beams with an energy of 1.17 and 1.33 MeV. The unit was known as a "workhorse" because it was extremely reliable, mechanically simple, and had little downtime. It was the first radiation therapy unit to rotate 360 degrees around a patient. A machine that rotates around a fixed point, or axis, and maintains the same distance from the source of radiation is called an *isocentric machine*. All modern therapeutic units are isocentric machines. This type of machine allows the patient to remain in one position, lessening the chance for patient movement during treatment. Isocentric capabilities also assist in directing the beam precisely at the tumor while sparing normal structures.

Because ^{60}Co is a radioisotope, it constantly emits radiation as it decays in an effort to return to a stable state. It has a half-life $T_{1/2}$ of 5.26 years (i.e., its activity is reduced by 50% at the end of 5.26 years). Because the source *decays* at a rate of 1% per month, the radiation treatment time must be adjusted, resulting in longer treatment times as the source decays.

The use of cobalt units has declined significantly since the 1980s. This decline has been basically attributed to the introduction of the more sophisticated linear accelerator (linac), which has greater skin-sparing capabilities and more sharply defined radiation *fields*. The radiation beam, or field, from a cobalt unit also has large penumbra, which results in fuzzy field edges, another undesirable feature.

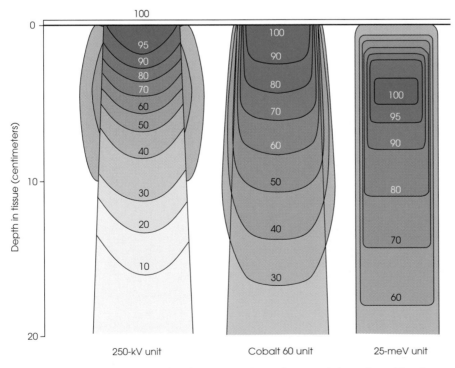

Fig. 41-2 Three isodose curves showing comparison of percent dose deposition from three x-ray units of different energies. As the energy of the beam is increased, the percentage of dose deposited on surface of patient decreases.

Linear accelerators

Linear accelerators are the most commonly used machines for cancer treatment. The first linear accelerator was developed in 1952, and first used clinically in the United States in 1956. A linear accelerator is capable of producing high-energy beams of photons (x-rays) or electrons in the range of 4 million to 35 million volts. These megavoltage photon beams allow a better distribution of dose to deep-seated tumors with better sparing of normal tissues than their earlier counterparts—the orthovoltage or cobalt units.

The photon beam is produced by accelerating a stream of electrons toward a target. When the electrons hit the target, a beam of x-rays is produced. By removing the target, the linac can also produce a beam of electrons of varying energies.

Linear accelerators can now be purchased with a single photon energy or a dual-photon machine with two x-ray beams. Typically a dual-photon energy machine consists of one low-energy (6-MeV) and one high-energy (18-MV) photon beam plus a range of electron energies (Fig. 41-3). The dual-photon energy machine gives the radiation oncologist more options in prescribing radiation treatments. As the energy of the beam increases, so does its penetrating power. Put simply, a lower-energy beam is used to treat tumors in thinner parts of the body, whereas high-energy beams are prescribed for tumors in thicker parts of the body. For example, a brain tumor or a tumor in a limb would most likely be treated with a 6-MeV beam; conversely, a pelvic malignancy would be better treated with an 18-MeV beam. Thus a small oncology center can serve its patients well by purchasing one dual-photon linear accelerator for a cost of approximately $1.2 million to $1.5 million, instead of having to purchase two single-energy 6- and 18-MeV machines for almost $2 million.

Electrons are advantageous over photons in that they are a more superficial form of treatment. Electrons are energy dependent, which means that they deposit their energy within a given depth of tissue and go no deeper, depending on the energy selected. For example, an 18-MeV beam has a total penetration depth of 9 cm. Any structure located deeper than 9 cm would not be appreciably affected. This is important when the radiation oncologist is trying to treat a tumor that overlies a critical structure.

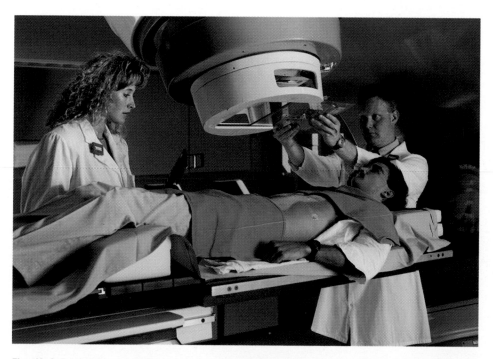

Fig. 41-3 Radiation therapists shown aligning patient and shielding block in preparation for treatment using a modern linear accelerator. X-ray beams of between 6 and 25 million volts may be produced to treat tumors in the body.

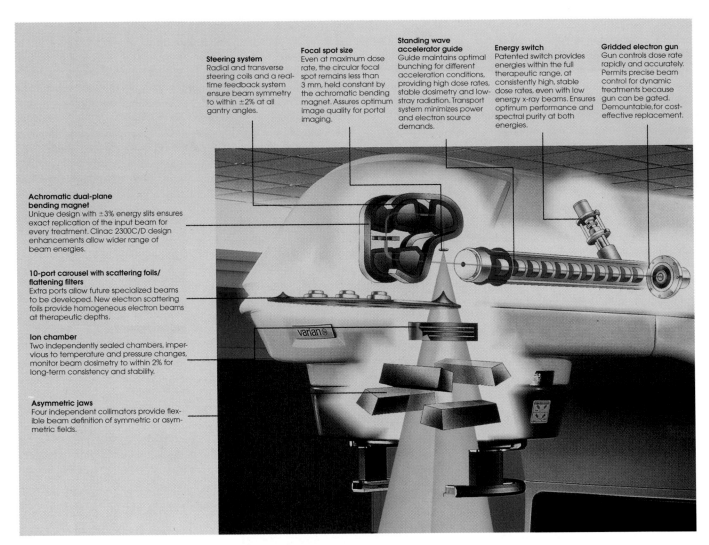

Steering system
Radial and transverse steering coils and a real-time feedback system ensure beam symmetry to within ±2% at all gantry angles.

Focal spot size
Even at maximum dose rate, the circular focal spot remains less than 3 mm, held constant by the achromatic bending magnet. Assures optimum image quality for portal imaging.

Standing wave accelerator guide
Guide maintains optimal bunching for different acceleration conditions, providing high dose rates, stable dosimetry and low-stray radiation. Transport system minimizes power and electron source demands.

Energy switch
Patented switch provides energies within the full therapeutic range, at consistently high, stable dose rates, even with low energy x-ray beams. Ensures optimum performance and spectral purity at both energies.

Gridded electron gun
Gun controls dose rate rapidly and accurately. Permits precise beam control for dynamic treatments because gun can be gated. Demountable, for cost-effective replacement.

Achromatic dual-plane bending magnet
Unique design with ±3% energy slits ensures exact replication of the input beam for every treatment. Clinac 2300C/D design enhancements allow wider range of beam energies.

10-port carousel with scattering foils/flattening filters
Extra ports allow future specialized beams to be developed. New electron scattering foils provide homogeneous electron beams at therapeutic depths.

Ion chamber
Two independently sealed chambers, impervious to temperature and pressure changes, monitor beam dosimetry to within 2% for long-term consistency and stability.

Asymmetric jaws
Four independent collimators provide flexible beam definition of symmetric or asymmetric fields.

Fig. 41-4 Dualing asymmetric jaws. Note the four independent collimators.

(Courtesy Varian Associates, Palo Alto, Calif.)

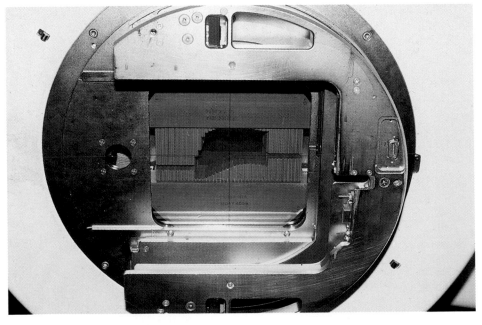

Fig. 41-5 Multileaf collimation system on the treatment head.

As with a diagnostic x-ray machine, the irradiated field of a linear accelerator is defined by a light field projected onto the patient's skin. This corresponding square or rectangle equals the length and width setting of the x-ray *collimators*. Today's modern linac is equipped with dualing *asymmetric (independent) jaws;* this allows each of the four collimator blades that define length or width to move independently (Fig. 41-4). For instance, the jaw that defines the superior extent of the field may be 7 cm from the central axis, whereas the inferior region may be at 10 cm. The total length would equal 17 cm, but it is not divided equally as it is in a diagnostic x-ray collimator. This allows the radiation oncologist to design a field that optimally covers the area of interest while sparing normal tissue. Independent collimation can also assist in reducing the total weight of lead shielding blocks normally constructed to protect normal tissues.

Multileaf collimation

Multileaf collimation (MLC) is the newest and most complex beam-defining system. From 45 to 80 individual collimator blades, about $3/8$ to $3/4$ inch (1 to 2 cm) wide, are located within the head of the linac and can be adjusted to shape the radiation field to conform to the target volume (Fig. 41-5). The design of the field is digitized from a radiograph into a computer software program, which is transferred to the treatment room. The MLC machine receives a code that tells it how to position the individual leaves for the treatment field. Before MLC, custom-made lead blocks, or *cerrobend blocks,* were constructed to shape radiation fields and shield normal tissues from the beam of radiation. Heavy cerrobend blocks were placed within the head of the linac for each treatment field. Linacs equipped with the MLC package now receive a custom-designed field at the stroke of a computer keyboard.

Steps in Radiation Oncology
SIMULATION

The first step of radiation therapy involves determining the volume of tissue that needs to be encompassed within the radiation field. This is done with a *simulator,* which is a diagnostic quality x-ray machine that has the same geometric and physical characteristics as a treatment unit. During simulation, the radiation oncologist uses the patient's radiographic images or the CT or MRI scan to determine the tumor's precise location and to design a treatment volume, or area. The treatment volume often includes the tumor plus a small margin, the draining lymphatics that are at risk for involvement, and a rim of normal tissue to account for patient movement.

Using fluoroscopy, the radiation therapist determines the field dimensions (length and width) and depth of isocenter as specified by the radiation oncologist. The *treatment field* outline and positioning marks are placed on the patient's skin surface (Fig. 41-6). A radiographic image is then taken of all treatment fields to facilitate treatment planning, block fabrication, and document the anatomic regions to be treated.

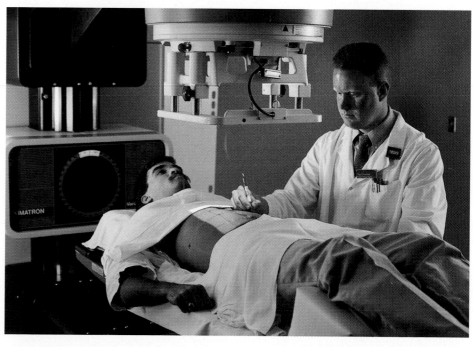

Fig. 41-6 The radiation therapist places skin marks on the patient's skin surface for alignment of the radiation beam during treatment.

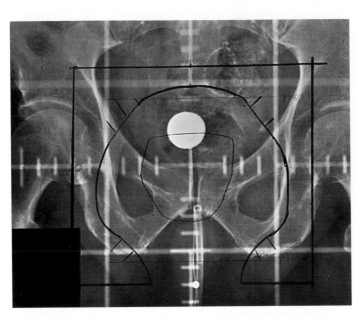

Fig. 41-7 AP pelvic radiograph demonstrating contrast in the bladder and its relationship to the prostate gland.

Precise measurements and details about the field dimensions, machine position, and patient positioning are recorded in the treatment chart. In some centers the treatment parameters, such as field length, width, couch, and gantry positions, are electronically captured and transferred to the treatment unit. Recording of this information is crucial so that the therapist performing the treatment can precisely reproduce the exact information.

Contrast material is often administered during a simulation to localize the area that needs to be treated or to identify vital normal structures that are to be shielded. For example, a small amount of barium is injected into the rectum of a patient with rectal cancer to assist in localizing the rectum on the simulation images. In Fig. 41-7, bladder contrast is used to assist in localizing the prostate gland, which lies directly inferior to the bladder. The rectal contrast is used to demonstrate the relationship of the rectum to the prostate in an effort to monitor and minimize the dose the rectum receives (Fig. 41-8).

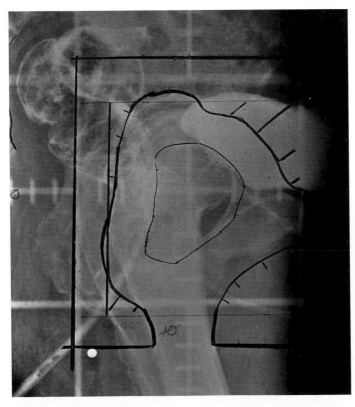

Fig. 41-8 Lateral radiograph demonstrating contrast in the rectum and its relationship to the prostate gland.

Immobilization devices are also constructed as part of the simulation. One goal of simulation is to position the patient in a manner that is stable and reproducible for each of the 28 to 40 radiation treatments. It is important for a patient to hold still and maintain the same position. If the patient does not maintain the planned position, critical normal tissues may be irradiated or the tumor may not be irradiated. Immobilization devices greatly assist the therapist in correctly aligning the patient for each treatment, and many patients feel more secure when supported by these devices. Immobilization devices can be constructed for any part of the body but are most important for more mobile parts, such as the head and neck region or the limbs. Many different types of immobilization systems exist. Fig. 41-9 shows a thermoplastic device that secures the head and neck against rotation or flexion/extension.

DOSIMETRY

Dosimetry refers to the measurement of radiation dose, and it demonstrates how the radiation is distributed or *attenuated* throughout the patient's body (absorbing medium). The dosimetrist devises a treatment plan that best fulfills the physician's prescription for the desired dose to the *tumor/target volume* while minimizing the amount of radiation to critical normal structures or tissues.

Each organ of the body has a tolerance dose to radiation that limits the amount it can receive and still function normally. If an organ receives an excess of the tolerance dose, the organ can fail, resulting in a fatal complication. For example, the kidneys are one of the more radiosensitive structures of the body (Table 41-7). A dose in excess of 2500 cGy can result in fatal radiation nephritis. The spinal cord has a higher tolerance dose, but many tumors require even higher doses for treatment to be effective.

TABLE 41-7

Tolerance doses to radiation

Structure	Tolerance dose
Testes	500cGy
Ovary	500cGy
Lung (whole lung)	1800 cGy
Kidney (whole organ)	2300 cGy
Liver (whole organ)	3500 cGy
Spinal cord (5 cm³)	4500 cGy

Precise localization of dose-limiting structures and their relationship with the target volume is critical for adequate planning. The dosimetrist must devise a plan that delivers a homogeneous dose to the tumor while not exceeding the tolerance dose of a specific organ. This task can be quite challenging. For instance, the radiation oncologist might prescribe 6000 cGy to treat lung cancer located in the mediastinum directly over the spine but must limit the spinal cord dose to 4500 cGy to prevent irreparable damage, which could result in paralysis. The dosimetrist must then devise a plan that enables combined treatment and protection to be accomplished.

The first step in dosimetry is to obtain a contour or CT scan of the patient in treatment position. A *contour* is an outline of the external surface of the patient's body at the level of the central axis (center of treatment field). This is typically performed in the transverse plane, but other planes may be used. Then the tumor volume and critical dose limiting internal structures are transferred from the simulation radiographs and drawn onto the contour (Fig. 41-10). With CT scanning, the tumor and internal structures and their relationships are directly visible. These images are then interfaced with the treatment-planning computer system for development of the plan. To obtain an even distribution of radiation to the target volume, radiation is delivered from various angles, all focused on the area of interest.

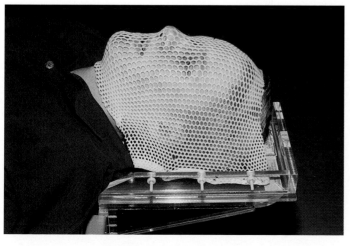

Fig. 41-9 Aquaplast mask.

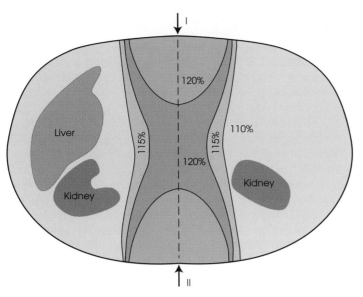

The standard approach for a tumor located in the pelvis, such as prostate or rectal cancer, is the use of four fields—AP, PA, and right and left lateral. Using the treatment parameters established in the simulator, the dosimetrist enters this information into the treatment-planning computer and obtains an isodose distribution, which demonstrates how the radiation is being deposited. An *isodose line/curve* is a summation of areas of equal radiation dosage and may be stated as percentages of the total prescribed dose (see Fig. 41-10) or as actual radiation dosages in *gray (Gy)* (Fig. 41-11).

Fig. 41-10 Opposing AP-PA ports. Summated isodose lines represent equal dose contributions from fields I and II.

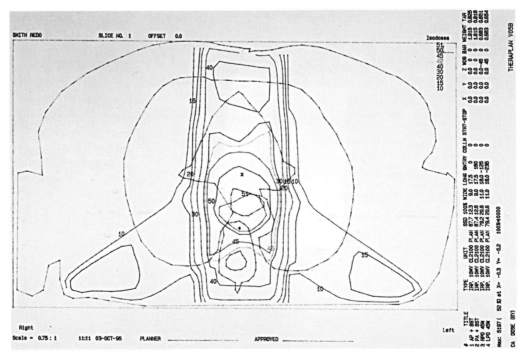

Fig. 41-11 AP and two posterior oblique treatment fields are used to avoid the spinal cord *(arrow)* but treat the centrally located tumor. Isodose lines are expressed in the unit of radiation absorbed dose, the gray (45 gray = 4500 cGy).

The dosimetrist optimizes the plan by eliminating any areas of dose inhomogeneity such as "hot spots." A hot spot is an area of excessive radiation dose. One method to adjust for hot spots is to add a *wedge filter*. This wedge-shaped device is made of lead and is placed within the radiation beam to preferentially absorb the radiation, altering the shape of the isodose curve (Fig. 41-12). Another method of reducing hot spots is to change the weighting of the radiation beams by, for example, delivering a greater dose of radiation from the anterior field than from the posterior field.

Another major task of the dosimetrist is to monitor the dose that critical structures are receiving and to keep the dose within the established guidelines dictated by the physician. To avoid treating the spinal cord in the aforementioned example, the dosimetrist may angle the entry points of the radiation beams to include the target volume while not irradiating the spinal cord. The resultant fields might be right anterior oblique and left posterior oblique (RAO/LPO) fields or an anterior treatment field with two posterior obliques (see Fig. 41-10). These changes would require another simulation of the patient to document these oblique fields. The final plan directs the radiation therapist, who will treat the patient, on how to proceed. For the example presented previously (i.e., lung cancer in the mediastinum directly over the spine), the plan might consist of the following:

1. 20 treatments AP or PA fields
2. Begin off-cord obliques, 5 treatments RAO and LPO, 30 degrees off vertical
3. Reduce field size to 12 long, 5 more RAO/LPO treatments

Once the plan is complete, treatment of the patient can commence.

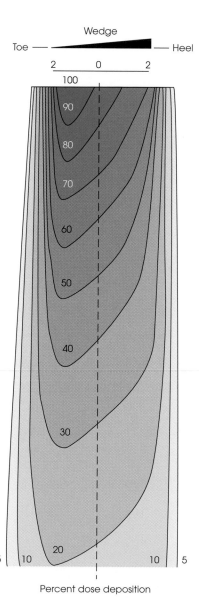

Fig. 41-12 Isodose curve obtained from cobalt-60 unit, with wedge placed between source and absorbing material.

TREATMENT

On completion of the planning stage, including simulation and dosimetry, patient treatment can begin. The radiation therapist positions the patient and aligns the skin marks according to what was recorded in the treatment chart at the time of simulation. Accuracy and attention to detail are critical for precise administration of the radiation to the patient. The therapist is responsible for interpreting the radiation oncologist's prescription and calculating the correct monitor units, or timer setting, to achieve a desired dose of radiation for each treatment field. This also involves recording the daily administration of the radiation and the cumulative dose to date.

Precision in positioning the machine, accurate placement of cerrobend blocks or wedges, and the implementation of any change in a patient's treatment plan are critical for ensuring optimum treatment. Failure to do any of these may result in an overdose to normal tissue, causing long-term side effects, or underexposure of the tumor, reducing the patient's chance for cure. Verification images, called *port films* or *images,* are taken on a weekly basis to ensure accuracy and consistent application of the radiation treatments. These port images are not of diagnostic quality because of the high-energy photon beams of the accelerator, but they are of enough detail to be compared with the simulation radiographs to verify accurate alignment of the field and blocks (Fig. 41-13).

The radiation therapist is also responsible for monitoring the patient's physical and emotional well-being. The therapist is generally the only member of the radiation oncology team who sees the patient on a daily basis. The therapist monitors the patient's progress and assists in the management of any side effects. Acting as a liaison between the patient and the physician, the therapist must know when to withhold treatment and when to refer the patient to be seen by the physician or oncology nurse for further evaluation. The daily interaction with the patient is the most rewarding aspect of the therapist's job. Putting the patient at ease and making a cancer diagnosis and subsequent treatment a less traumatic experience is a satisfying aspect of this career. Patients often express their gratitude to the therapists for their care and support.

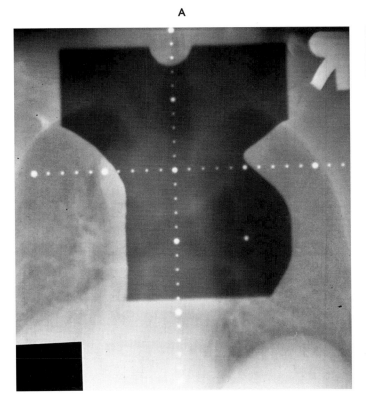
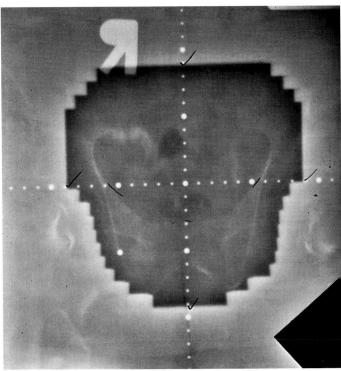

Fig. 41-13 A, AP lung image with cerrobend blocking. **B,** AP pelvis port image with multileaf collimation beam shaping.

Clinical Applications

The amount of radiation prescribed depends on the type of tumor and the extent of the disease. The following are brief summaries of radiation therapy treatment techniques used in the management of some of the more common forms of cancer.

LUNG CANCER

Treatment varies by type and stage. Radiation therapy is often used in conjunction with surgery and chemotherapy. A dose of 5000 to 6000 cGy of 10-MeV photons is often applied via a combination of AP, PA, and off-cord oblique fields. The primary tumor plus draining lymphatics are generally included in the treatment volumes (Fig. 41-14).

PROSTATE CANCER

Definitive radiation therapy is a standard treatment for prostate cancer. Surgical removal of the prostate gland is another common approach to the management of this disease. A four-field technique of AP, PA, and right and left lateral ports using a megavoltage beam of 10 MV or more is often used to deliver a dose of 7000 cGy to the prostate gland.

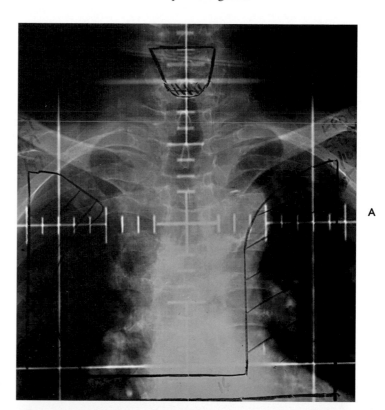

A

Fig. 41-14 A, AP lung-field simulation radiograph. **B,** Off-cord oblique simulation radiograph. The striped lines in **A** and **B** indicate areas to be shielded. **C,** Off-cord oblique port radiograph.

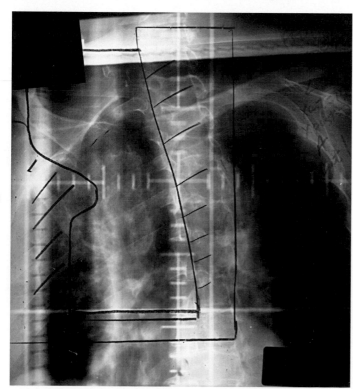

B

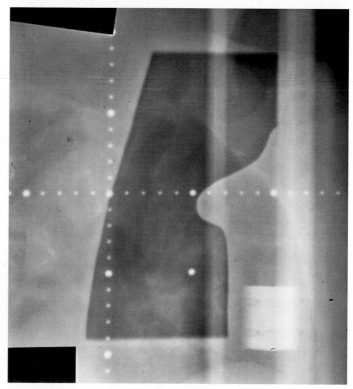

C

ORAL CAVITY CANCER

A number of approaches may be used, depending on the size and the extent of a tumor in the oral cavity. An intraoral cone may be used to deliver 6000 cGy in 4 weeks, with an orthovoltage beam used for small lesions. Larger lesions may be treated with irradiation through opposing lateral ports from a megavoltage unit, possibly followed by brachytherapy.

CERVICAL CANCER

Early diagnosed cervical cancers can be treated with either surgery or radiation therapy. A four-field technique of AP, PA, and right and left lateral ports using a megavoltage unit, preferably 10 MV or greater, delivers 4500 to 5000 cGy in 5 weeks to an area of the primary and regional lymph nodes (Fig. 41-15). An intracavitary implant is also included in the standard treatment of cervical cancer.

HODGKIN'S DISEASE

The age of the patient and extent of the disease may determine the prognosis for Hodgkin's disease. Extended field therapy includes the lymphatic chain above and/or below the diaphragm and is applied by a megavoltage unit that delivers 4000 to 4500 cGy through AP-PA ports. Chemotherapy may also be indicated for more advanced cases.

BREAST CANCER

Using two tangential fields to the chest wall or intact breast, megavoltage radiation delivers 5000 cGy in 5 weeks (Fig. 41-16). An electron boost to the site of initial lumpectomy adds an additional 1000 cGy. Chemotherapy may also be indicated for the treatment of breast cancer.

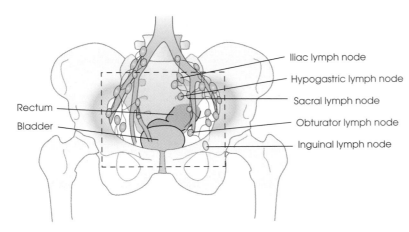

Iliac lymph node
Hypogastric lymph node
Sacral lymph node
Obturator lymph node
Inguinal lymph node
Rectum
Bladder

Fig. 41-15 Field used for irradiation of primary tumor and adjacent lymph nodes.

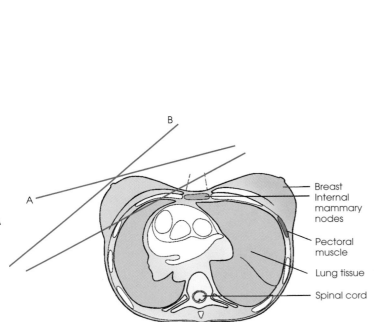
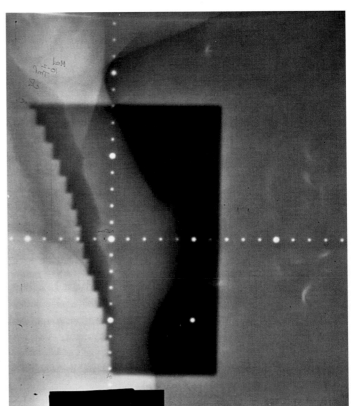

A
B

Breast
Internal mammary nodes
Pectoral muscle
Lung tissue
Spinal cord

Fig. 41-16 A, Cross section of thorax showing field arrangements to tangentially irradiate the intact breast while sparing the lung *(lines A and B).* **B,** Port image of tangential breast field. Note sparing of lung tissue.

LARYNGEAL CANCER

Cancer of the larynx is best treated with megavoltage radiation. Tumors that are confined to the true vocal cord, with normal cord mobility, have a 90% 5-year cure rate; in addition, the voice remains useful. The method of treatment is usually accomplished by using opposing lateral wedged fields of $1\frac{3}{4} \times 2$ inches (4×5 cm) or 2×2 inches (5×5 cm) and delivering a dose of 6500 cGy over a 6-week period.

SKIN CANCER

Carcinomas of the skin are usually squamous cell or basal cell lesions and are may be treated with superficial radiation or surgery. Cure rates tend to run between 80% and 90%, and basal cell lesions less than $\frac{3}{8}$ inch (1 cm) in diameter have a cure rate of almost 100%. The method of treatment is usually a single-field approach with attention given to shielding the uninvolved skin and delivering 5000 cGy in a 4-week period.

MEDULLOBLASTOMA

Children with medulloblastoma are usually referred to the radiation oncology department after a biopsy and shunt procedure. The tumor is radiosensitive, and patients who have had treatment of the entire cerebrospinal axis have a 5-year cure rate of 40% to 50%. The therapeutic approach tends to be complicated because the entire brain is irradiated with 4500 cGy, the spinal cord receives a dose of between 3500 and 4500 cGy, and the cerebellum receives an additional 1000 cGy (Fig. 41-17). This irradiation is usually accomplished with parallel opposed fields to the cranial vault and an extended single field to the spinal cord. A megavoltage unit is often used, with extreme care given to any areas of abutting fields.

Clinical applications

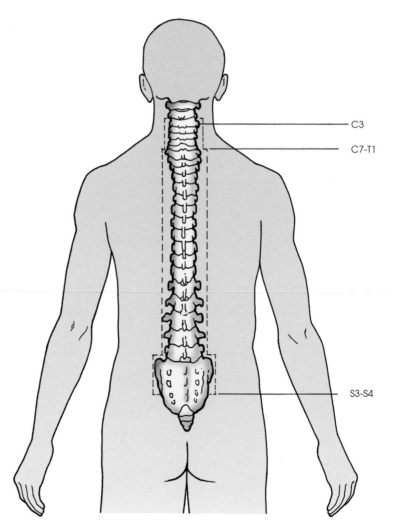

C3

C7-T1

S3-S4

Fig. 41-17 Spinal treatment portal for medulloblastoma.

503

Future Trends

Radiation therapy has entered the electronic age. Many institutions already use computer-interfaced accelerators with treatment verification software packages to ensure accurate treatment. Paperless treatment charting and filmless departments are becoming the standard design of a facility.

Advances in computer software and equipment will result in the routine implementation of three-dimensional treatment planning systems and more three-dimensional *conformal radiation* and virtual simulations. Three-dimensional treatment planning allows for the design of a beam that exactly conforms to the shape of the tumor at any plane within the body. The computer can digitally reconstruct the anatomy, which allows the dosimetrist to manipulate the image to view the tumor from any angle or plane. Such a system allows the dosimetrist to plan and design beams that are non-coplanar. The current standard method is two-dimensional planning in which the isodoses are planned from a transverse plane, as in a CT scan. The beam's eye view obtained by three-dimensional beams allows higher doses of radiation to be more safely administered by treating the cancer through multiple fields (more than four) on different planes, which reduces the amount of dose that normal tissues receive.

Three-dimensional conformal radiation uses the same principles mentioned in the previous paragraph. With this technique, the linac gantry, the couch, and the MLCs are synchronized and programmed to move as the treatment is being delivered. The collimators are programmed to automatically adjust to the treatment volume as it would be visualized from each angle or plane. This technique is currently being used in the treatment of brain tumors at a few major cancer centers and is being researched for use in other sites.

Standard planning to determine the volume of tissue that needs to be irradiated starts by taking localizing radiographs in the simulator. A CT scan with the patient in treatment position is then obtained in diagnostic radiology. The CT information is then interfaced into the radiation oncology treatment-planning computer for development of the treatment plan. Virtual simulation is performed with the use of a specially modified CT scanner. It combines the two aforementioned steps into one. First, CT scan images necessary to plan the treatment are obtained. Second, digitally reconstructed images that depict the anatomy, as in standard simulation radiographs, are processed; then the traditional marks to be placed on the patient are marked with the unit's sophisticated patient-marking system. This system enables a more accurate design of treatment fields and facilitates the implementation of three-dimensional treatment planning.

Summary

From a somewhat questionable beginning, radiation therapy has emerged as one of the primary modalities used in the treatment of malignant disease. Radiation therapy departments are currently examining and treating approximately 75% of all newly diagnosed cancer patients. Radiation oncologists and radiation therapists are integral members of the health care team that discusses and selects the appropriate treatment regimens for all cancer patients.

As the factors that initiate cellular change, growth, and spread become better understood, the radiation treatments for cancer will become even more effective. The irradiation techniques presently used may change dramatically based on this new information. In addition, new, more sophisticated radiation-producing equipment is currently under design and may lead to the reevaluation of presently accepted therapeutic techniques and dose levels. Finally, new chemotherapeutic agents are being produced that, when used by themselves or with other drugs, may enhance tumor sensitivity when used in conjunction with irradiation.

Definition of Terms

absorbed dose Amount of ionizing radiation absorbed per unit of mass of irradiated material.

accelerator (particle) Device that accelerates charged subatomic particles to great energies. These particles or rays may be used for direct medical irradiation and basic physical research. Medical units include linear accelerators, betatrons, and cyclotrons.

asymmetric jaws Four independent x-ray collimators that are used to define the radiation treatment field.

attenuation Removal of energy from a beam of ionizing radiation when it traverses matter, accomplished by disposition of energy in matter and by deflection of energy out of the beam.

betatron Electron accelerator that uses magnetic induction to accelerate electrons in circular path; also capable of producing photons.

biopsy Removal of a small piece of tissue for examination under the microscope.

brachytherapy Placement of radioactive nuclide(s) in or on a neoplasm to deliver a cancericidal dose.

cancer Term commonly applied to malignant disease; abnormal growth of cells; neoplasm (new growth) or *-oma* (tumor).

cancericidal dose Dose of radiation that results in the death of cancer cells.

carcinogen Any cancer-producing substance or material, such as nicotine, radiation, or ingested uranium.

carcinoma Cancer that arises from epithelial tissue—either glandular or squamous epithelium.

cerrobend block Beam-shaping device made of a lead alloy that attenuates the x-ray beam, preventing exposure of normal tissue.

chromosome Unit of genetic information that guides cytoplasmic activities of the cell and transmits hereditary information.

cobalt-60 Radioisotope with half-life of 5.26 years, average gamma ray energy of 1.25 MeV (range: 1.17 to 1.33 MeV), and ability to spare skin with buildup depth in tissue of 0.5 cm.

collimator Diaphragm or system of diaphragms made of radiation-absorbing material that defines dimension and direction of beam.

conformal radiation Treatment designed to deliver radiation to the exact target volume as seen on any plane (e.g., transverse, sagittal, vertex views); requires a three-dimensional treatment planning system.

contour Reproduction of an external body shape typically in the transverse plane at the level of the central axis of the beam; facilitates planning of radiation treatment. Other planes of interest may also be obtained.

cure Usually a 5-year period after completion of treatment during which time the patient exhibits no evidence of disease.

decay or disintegration Transformation of radioactive nucleus, resulting in emission of radiation.

differentiation Acquisition of cellular function/structure that differs from function/structure of original cell type.

direct effect Radiation that interacts with an organic molecule such as DNA, RNA, or a protein molecule. This interaction may inactivate the cell.

dosimetry Measurement of radiation dose in an absorbing medium.

epithelial tissue Cells that line the surfaces of serous and mucous membranes, including the skin.

etiology Study of causes of diseases.

external-beam treatment Delivery of radiation to a patient from a unit such as a linear accelerator in which the radiation enters the patient from the external surface of the body.

field Geometric area defined by collimator or radiotherapy unit at skin surface.

fractionation Division of total planned dose into a number of smaller doses to be given over longer period. Consideration must be given to biologic effectiveness of smaller doses.

gamma ray Electromagnetic radiation that originates from radioactive nucleus and causes ionization in matter; identical in properties to x-ray.

gray (Gy) International unit for the quantity of radiation received by the patient; previously rad. 1 cGy = 1 rad.

grenz rays X-rays generated at 20 kVp or less.

half-life Time (specific for each radioactive substance) required for radioactive material to decay to half its initial activity; types are biologic and physical.

half-value layer Thickness of attenuating material inserted in beam to reduce beam intensity to half of the original intensity.

independent jaws X-ray collimator with four individual blades that can be moved independently of one another (see *asymmetric jaws*).

indirect effect Interaction of radiation with water molecules within the cell; results in the formation of free radicals OH, H, and HO_2, which can damage the cell.

ionization Process in which one or more electrons are added to or removed from atoms, creating ions; can be caused by high temperatures, electrical discharges, or nuclear radiations.

ionizing radiation Energy emitted and transferred through matter that results in the removal of orbital electrons (e.g., x-rays or gamma rays).

isocentric Referring to rotation about a fixed point.

isodoseline-curve Curve or line drawn to connect points of identical amounts of radiation in a given field.

isotope Atoms that have the same atomic number but different mass number.

lesion Morbid change in tissue; mass of abnormal cells.

linear accelerator Device for accelerating charged particles, such as electrons, to produce high-energy electron or photon beams.

linear energy transfer (LET) Rate at which energy is deposited as it travels through matter.

malignancy Cancerous tumor or lesion.

medical dosimetrist Person responsible for calculation of the proper radiation treatment dose who assists the radiation oncologist in designing individual treatment plans.

medical physicist A specialist in the study of the laws of ionizing radiation and their interactions with matter.

metastasis Transmission of cells or groups of cells from primary tumor to site(s) elsewhere in body.

multileaf collimator Individual collimator rods within the treatment head of the linear accelerator that can slide inward to shape the radiation field.

oncologist Doctor of medicine specializing in the study of tumors.

oncology Study of tumors.

palliation To relieve symptoms; not for cure.

pathologist A specialist in the study of the microscopic nature of disease.

prophylactic surgery Preventive surgical treatment.

radiation oncologist Doctor of medicine specializing in use of ionizing radiation in the treatment of disease.

radiation oncology Medical specialty involving the treatment of cancerous lesions using ionizing radiation.

radiation therapist Person trained to assist and take directions from radiation oncologist in the use of ionizing radiation for the treatment of disease.

radiation therapy Older term used to define medical specialty of treatment with ionizing radiation.

radioactive Pertaining to atoms of elements that undergo spontaneous transformation, resulting in emission of radiation.

radiocurable Susceptibility of neoplastic cells to cure (destruction) by ionizing radiation.

radiosensitivity Responsiveness of cells to radiation.

radium (ra) Radionuclide (atomic number, 88; atomic weight, 226; half-life, 1622 years) used clinically for radiation therapy. In conjunction with its subsequent transformations, radium emits alpha and beta particles and gamma rays. In encapsulated form it is used for various intracavitary radiation therapy applications such as that for cancer of cervix.

reactor Cubicle in which isotopes are artificially produced.

relative biologic effectiveness (RBE) Compares radiation beams with different LETs and their ability to produce a specific biologic response. Dose in gray from 250 kVp beam of x-rays/dose from another type of radiation to produce the same effect.

simulator A diagnostic x-ray machine that has the same geometric and physical characteristics as a radiation therapy treatment unit.

skin sparing In megavoltage beam therapy, reduced skin injury per centigray (cGy) exposure because electron equilibrium occurs below skin; occurs from $1/4$ inch to 2 inches (0.6 cm to 5 cm) deep, depending on energy.

surgical bed Area of excision and adjacent tissues manipulated during surgery.

systemic Throughout the human body.

teletherapy Radiation therapy technique for which source of radiation is at some distance from patient.

treatment field Anatomic area outlined for treatment (e.g., AP or RL pelvis).

tumor/target volume Portion of anatomy that includes tumor and adjacent areas of invasion.

undifferentiation Lack of resemblance of cells to cells of origin.

wedge filter Wedge-shaped beam attenuating device used to preferentially absorb the beam to alter the shape of the isodose curve.

windows The perpendicular interface that allows the transducer to send and receive sound waves without interference.

Selected bibliography

Bentel GC et al: *Treatment planning and dose calculation in radiation oncology,* ed 3, New York, 1982, Pergamon.

Bentel GC: *Radiation therapy planning,* New York, ed 2, 1996, Macmillan.

Brenner DJ: Dose, volume, and tumor-control predictions in radiotherapy, *J Radiat Oncol Biol Phys* 26:171, 1993.

Cancer facts and figures—1997, Atlanta, 1997, American Cancer Society.

Cooper JS et al: *Concepts in cancer care,* Philadelphia, 1983, Lea & Febiger.

Dische S: Radiotherapy in the nineties: increase in cure, decrease in morbidity, *Acta Oncol* 31:501, 1992.

Grabowski CM, Unger JA, Potish RA: Factors predictive of completion of treatment and survival after palliative radiation therapy, *Radiology* 184:329, 1992.

Jessup JM et al: Diagnosing colorectal carcinoma: clinical and molecular approaches, *CA Cancer J Clin* 47:70, 1997.

Landis SH et al: Cancer statistics, 1998, *CA Cancer J Clin* 48:6, 1998.

Lipa LA, Mesina CF: Virtual simulation in conjunction with 3-D conformal therapy, *Radiat Therapist,* 2:99, 1995.

Marks JE, Armbruster JS: Accreditation of radiation oncology in the U.S., *Int J Radiat Oncol Biol Phys* 24:863, 1992.

Morgan HM: Quality assurance of computer controlled radiotherapy treatments, *Br J Radiol* 65:409, 1992.

Moss WT et al: *Radiation oncology rationale, technique, and results,* ed 5, St Louis, 1979, Mosby.

Genetic testing for breast cancer risk: it's your choice, Washington, DC, 1997, National Cancer Institute.

Order SE: Training in systemic radiation therapy, *Int J Radiat Oncol Biol Phys* 24:895, 1992.

Perez CA: Quest for excellence: ultimate goal of the radiation oncologist: astro gold medal address 1992.

Perez CA, *Int J Radiat Oncol Biol Phys* 26:567, 1993.

Roberge SL: Virtual reality: radiation therapy treatment planning of tomorrow, *Radiat Therapist* 2:113, 1996.

Stanton R, Stinson D: *Applied physics for radiation oncology,* Madison, Wis, 1996, Medical Physics.

Travis EL: *Primer of radiobiology,* ed 2, St Louis, 1989, Mosby.

Wagner LK: Absorbed dose in imaging: why measure it? *Radiology,* 178:622, 1991.

Washington CM, Leaver DT: *Principles and practice of radiation therapy: introduction to radiation therapy,* St Louis, 1996, Mosby.

Washington CM, Leaver DT: *Principles and practice of radiation therapy: physics, simulation,* and *treatment planning,* St Louis, 1996, Mosby.

Washington CM, Leaver DT: *Principles and practice of radiation therapy: practical applications,* St Louis, 1996, Mosby.

Varmus H, Weinberg R: *Genes and the biology of cancer,* New York, 1993, Scientific American Library.

INTRODUCTION TO RADIOGRAPHIC QUALITY ASSURANCE

WILLIAM F. FINNEY III

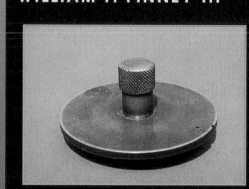

RIGHT: Early quality assurance consisted primarily of checking timer accuracy using a top that had to be spun by hand.

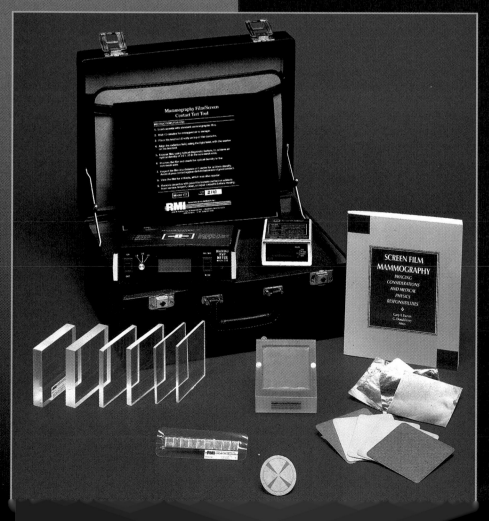

Quality assurance kit, 1999.

(Courtesy Gammex RMI.)

Principles of Radiographic Quality Assurance

A medical diagnostic radiographic imaging system contains numerous sources of variability. If these sources are not controlled, image quality may be adversely affected. Subquality radiographs most often require repeat examinations, resulting in additional radiation exposure to the patient and increased cost to the department. A systematic and structured mechanism to control these variables is the foundation on which radiographic *quality assurance** is built.

---

*Almost all italicized terms are defined at the end of this chapter.

This chapter provides an overview of the radiographic quality assurance concepts. It is not designed to be a procedures manual for the various *quality control* tests. Additional information on the topics discussed in this chapter is provided in the works cited in the selected bibliography at the end of the chapter.

The information in this chapter draws heavily from the quality assurance series developed and published by the *Center for Devices and Radiological Health (CDRH),* previously known as *NCDRH,* and from material by *Radiation Measurements Incorporated (RMI),* now known as *Gammex RMI.* These organizations have been active in promoting quality assurance and have been instrumental in creating a practical approach to quality assurance that allows its concepts to be realized by *diagnostic radiology facilities* regardless of size (Figs. 42-1 and 42-2).

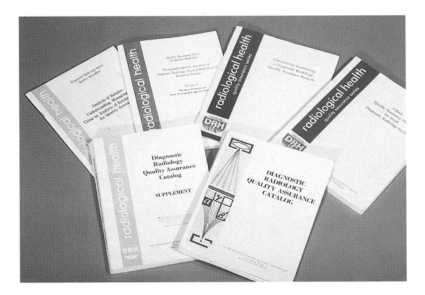

Fig. 42-1 CDRH quality assurance publications.

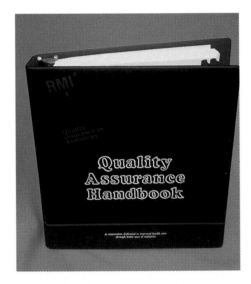

Fig. 42-2 Gammex RMI specializes in quality control test tools for radiology.

Quality Assurance and Quality Control

The terms *radiographic quality assurance* and *radiographic quality control* are often used synonymously. Both refer to concepts that define a mechanism used to enhance the quality of the services and products rendered. Their main difference is the scope of their intent.

One concept of radiographic quality assurance encompasses the total picture of radiographic care delivery, with the primary objective being enhancement of patient care. Patient selection parameters, management techniques, departmental policies and procedures, technical effectiveness and efficiency, and inservice education are some of the elements that are included. The Joint Commission for Accreditation of Healthcare Organizations (JCAHO) uses this quality assurance concept in its accreditation process.

The CDRH's concept of radiographic quality assurance focuses primarily on the enhancement of radiographic image quality and the reduction of unnecessary patient exposure by using *quality administrative procedures* and quality control techniques.

As applied by the CDRH, quality control deals with the techniques used in the monitoring and maintenance of the technical elements of the system that affect the quality of the image. Although the idea of "control" is basic to this concept, the goal of optimizing the performance and ensuring the accuracy of these elements must not be forgotten. This chapter uses the terms *radiographic quality assurance* and *radiographic quality control* in the context as defined by the CDRH.

Historical Development

Quality assurance in diagnostic radiology is not new. Many radiography departments have been systematically monitoring their equipment since long before "quality assurance and control" became buzzwords. This interest in radiographic quality assurance can be traced to actions taken by the federal government.

In 1968 the Radiation Control for Health and Safety Act was passed. This act required the U.S. Department of Health, Education and Welfare (HEW)—now Health and Human Services (HHS)—to conduct a radiation control program through the development and administration of standards to reduce human exposure to radiation from electronic products. The Bureau of Radiological Health (BRH)—now the CDRH—was given the responsibility of carrying out this act.

In 1974 the BRH set forth regulatory action to control the manufacture and installation of medical/dental diagnostic x-ray equipment to reduce the production of useless radiation. This action—the X-ray Equipment Standard—was designed to regulate the *performance* of *x-ray systems,* not the *use* of such systems.

Another approach to help realize the goal of reducing the patient's exposure to unnecessary radiation was the development of facility-based *quality assurance programs.* Support for this concept came from numerous studies, which pointed out that many diagnostic radiology facilities were producing subquality images and delivering unnecessary amounts of radiation during patient examinations. It was believed that the best way to discourage such practices was to educate the radiologic community about the concept of radiographic quality assurance. In 1976 the professional community was made aware of the BRH's intent to develop recommendations concerning quality assurance programs. The professional community was solicited for input in the development of quality assurance recommendations, and in 1978 the proposed Recommendation for Quality Assurance Programs in Diagnostic Radiology Facilities was published. Comments on the proposal were solicited, and in 1979 the recommendation was published in its final form in the *Federal Register.*

The Consumer-Patient Radiation Health and Safety Act of 1981 established guidelines for further reducing unnecessary patient exposure to radiation. This act addressed issues such as unnecessary repeat examinations, quality assurance techniques, radiation exposure, referral criteria, and unnecessary mass screening programs. In addition, the act established minimum standards for the accreditation of educational programs in the radiologic sciences and for the certification of radiographic equipment operators.

Benefits of a Quality Assurance Program

A well-administered radiographic quality assurance program has numerous benefits. Use of such a program is one of the methods that can minimize unnecessary radiation to patients in diagnostic radiology facilities. Studies have demonstrated that the number of repeated radiographs, which result in additional radiation exposure to patients, can be reduced with the implementation of quality assurance procedures. Although the reduction in unnecessary patient exposure is significant, these programs can also improve the overall efficiency of radiologic service delivery, increasing patient satisfaction.

The radiology facility is also the beneficiary of quality assurance. Improvement of radiographic image quality is achievable, as is increased consistency of image production. Quality control procedures can increase the reliability, efficiency, and cost-effectiveness of the equipment used by the facility. These are important gains, considering the current emphasis on cost containment in health care delivery. Although increased overall departmental efficiency in itself is a major advantage, the betterment of personnel morale resulting from such improvements may be the most important benefit in the long run.

Facilities engaged in quality assurance are certain to improve their effectiveness. Efficiency of the radiologic services delivered, which includes the reduction of unnecessary radiation delivered to patients, is also achieved. With the proper planning, design, and management of a quality assurance program, these benefits are easily achievable.

Center for Devices and Radiological Health: Quality Assurance Program Recommendation

The CDRH's recommendation for establishing quality assurance programs in diagnostic radiology facilities was based on research, empiric data, and feedback from the professional community. Although the recommendation is not mandatory, the CDRH strongly believes that the establishment of quality assurance programs helps to achieve the goals of reducing unproductive patient radiation, minimizing unnecessary costs, and improving the consistency of quality images.

The CDRH's recommendation includes 10 elements that are considered essential for a viable program:

- Responsibility
- Evaluation
- Purchase specifications
- Standards for image quality
- Monitoring and maintenance
- Education
- Committee
- Records
- QA manual
- Review

All facilities do not have to have an approach to quality assurance as comprehensive as that recommended. Instead, the CDRH suggests that the size, objectives, and available resources of a facility should determine the extent to which each element needs to be implemented. The CDRH recommendation provides some valuable insight into the concepts of quality assurance. A brief description of each element follows.

ESSENTIAL ELEMENTS

Responsibility

Although quality assurance is the responsibility of the entire staff of the diagnostic radiographic facility, an efficient and effective quality assurance program requires accountability. Therefore distinct and documented assignments of *responsibility* for the program and its components are essential for success. The size of the facility, scope of the program, and available resources are some of the factors that dictate the levels to which these responsibilities are assigned. (A physicist, a field or in-house service engineer, a chief radiographer, supervisory personnel, a staff radiographer, and a consultant are examples of the individuals who have quality assurance responsibilities.) Regardless of facility size, the facility's owner or the practitioner in charge has the primary responsibility for quality assurance.

Evaluation

The element of *evaluation* within a quality assurance program should be addressed at different levels. First, the performance of the facility should be evaluated. This information can be used to determine the scope and design of a quality assurance program for the facility and/or to provide data that can be used for comparison with data generated at future points in time. These comparison evaluations demonstrate the effectiveness of the quality assurance program. The most often applied procedure used to evaluate facility performance is the analysis of rejected radiographs, commonly known as *reject analysis*. On another level, equipment monitoring results should be evaluated to assess the need for corrective action or to determine trends that may indicate that preventive maintenance is required.

Purchase specifications

When new equipment is purchased, the facility should determine the desired performance criteria for the equipment. These performance criteria are then reflected in the *purchase specifications*. Before final acceptance, the equipment should be tested to ensure that the actual performance meets the criteria requested in the purchase specifications. The future monitoring and testing of the equipment can be compared with the equipment performance criteria to determine whether the equipment is continuing to perform at the acceptable level.

Standards for image quality

Standards for image quality should be established for the performance parameters of the x-ray system that are of interest to the facility. The creation of these standards should, when possible, *objectively* indicate the amount of performance variation that can be accepted before the quality of the image is affected. A *subjective* determination of the standards is often used when objective standards cannot be defined. If the equipment monitoring results show that the equipment does not meet the acceptance limits of the standard, then corrective actions should be taken.

Monitoring and maintenance

Monitoring and maintenance is sometimes referred to as the *quality control portion of the program*. Equipment monitoring and maintenance is the center of a quality assurance program. The CDRH suggests that every facility consider monitoring the following system components:

- Wet chemical film/image processing
- Performance of radiographic/fluoroscopic units
- Cassettes and grids
- Illuminators
- Darkroom

The system component parameters that should be monitored vary from facility to facility, depending on factors such as program goals, available resources, and cost. The CDRH includes a listing of parameters for all system components in its recommendation (Box 42-1). A maintenance program that includes both the preventative and corrective aspects of equipment maintenance is an important aspect of any quality assurance program.

Education

A plan for educating personnel in quality assurance responsibilities is recommended. A mechanism for the continuing education of these individuals should also be included. A subtle but important aspect of this element is instructing the facility's staff about the importance, design, and goals of the quality assurance program. The real strength of a quality assurance program is based on the support and commitment of the entire staff.

BOX 42-1

X-ray system component parameters

I. Film processing
  A. Index of speed
  B. Index of contrast
  C. Base plug fog
  D. Solution temperatures
  E. Film artifact identification
II. Fluoroscopic x-ray units
  A. Tabletop exposure rates
  B. Centering alignment
  C. Collimation
  D. kVp accuracy and reproducibility
  E. mA accuracy and reproducibility
  F. Exposure time accuracy and reproducibility
  G. Reproducibility of x-ray output
  H. Focal spot size consistency
  I. Half-value layer
  J. Representative entrance skin exposures
III. Image intensification systems
  A. Resolution
  B. Focusing
  C. Distortion
  D. Glare
  E. Low-contrast performance
  F. Physical alignment of camera and collimating lens
IV. Radiographic x-ray units
  A. Reproducibility of x-ray output
  B. Linearity and reproducibility of mA stations
  C. Reproducibility and accuracy of timer stations
  D. Reproducibility and accuracy of kVp stations
  E. Accuracy of source-to-image receptor distance (SID) indicators
  F. Light/x-ray field congruence
  G. Half-value layer
  H. Focal spot size consistency
  I. Representative entrance skin exposures
V. Automatic exposure control devices (AEC)
  A. Reproducibility
  B. kVp compensation
  C. Field sensitivity matching
  D. Minimum response time
  E. Back-up timer verification

VI. Cassettes and grids
  A. Cassettes
    1. Film-screen contact
    2. Screen condition
    3. Light leaks
    4. Artifact identification
    5. Uniformity of screen speed
  B. CR/DR image receptor
    1. Cassette integrity
    2. Storage phosphor plate
  C. Grids
    1. Alignment and focal distance
    2. Artifact identification
VII. Illuminators
  A. Consistency of light output with time
  B. Consistency of light output from one illuminator to another
  C. Illuminator surface conditions
VIII. Darkrooms
  A. Darkroom integrity
  B. Safelight conditions
IX. Tomographic systems
  A. Accuracy of depth and cut indicator
  B. Thickness of cut plane
  C. Exposure angle .
  D. Completeness of tomographic motion
  E. Flatness of tomographic field
  F. Resolution
  G. Continuity of exposure
  H. Flatness of cassette
  I. Representative entrance skin exposures
X. Computed tomography
  A. Precision (noise)
  B. Contrast scale
  C. High-contrast and low-contrast resolution
  D. Alignment
  E. Representative entrance skin exposures

kVp, Kilovolt (peak); mA, millampere.

Committee

The *committee* element might better be described as *communication.* Large facilities may require a quality assurance committee structure for planning, review, and evaluation purposes. Smaller facilities may not require a formal committee but instead may rely on input directly from the staff. The intent of this element is to emphasize the importance of maintaining open communication among all participants in the quality assurance program.

Records

The *documentation* of equipment monitoring results, maintenance actions, and other such activities should be included in a quality assurance program. A regular and systematic method of collecting and recording data is the foundation on which the review and evaluation elements of the program are based.

QA manual

A quality assurance program should develop and maintain a complete, comprehensive, and up-to-date *manual,* which should serve as a source document or guide for all elements of the program. The manual should include items such as quality assurance personnel, monitoring procedures, monitoring schedules, monitoring evaluations, corrective actions, and service records.

Review

Periodic *review* is necessary to determine the status of the quality assurance program. A look at the entire program can determine whether it is operating at its maximum effectiveness or whether changes must be made. Inspection of the important program elements reveals their currentness, appropriateness, consistency, regularity, and effectiveness in achieving the goals of the program.

Quality Assurance Program Design

Every radiographic facility is a unique entity. Although the mission of various facilities may be the same, the process and environment of each are different. With this in mind, a facility must custom-fit quality assurance to its own situation. A review of the quality assurance literature provides valuable guidance for the design of a program. A systematic approach to fitting a quality assurance program to the needs of a facility makes such a seemingly large task manageable. A facility begins by planning an assessment of its performance. This information may reveal areas that should be attended to first, and may also provide documentation for supporting the program plan.

One method of assessing the facility's performance is reject analysis. This is a planned, systematic procedure in which rejected subquality radiographs are collected, analyzed, and categorized according to cause, which may be related to the competence of technical personnel, equipment problems, specific difficulties associated with the examination, or some combination of these elements. The analysis of rejected radiographs is an effective method of identifying equipment performance problems. A reject analysis program as a routine part of the quality assurance program acts as a link between a department's quality assurance efforts and the consistency of its image quality. It may be used to evaluate problems leading to poor image quality; it may also serve as a self-improvement tool for the staff, a management database, or an excellent method of evaluating the impact of the quality assurance program on the quality of the radiographic images.

Organizing the program plan is the next step. Instructing personnel, establishing image quality standards, developing and documenting monitoring procedures, and procuring the necessary monitoring equipment are some of the aspects of the organization phase.

Implementation of the plan is next, followed by an evaluation of the program's impact, which can be assessed by repair records, monitoring results, reject analysis results, or subjective methods. The feedback from the evaluation phase provides input to the original planning steps and should be used to make necessary adjustments so that the program becomes more effective and more efficient.

BASIC QUALITY CONTROL TESTS

The quality control tests used to monitor x-ray system components usually require some type of device to measure the parameter being evaluated. Quality control tools range from simple homemade devices to sophisticated microprocessors (Fig. 42-3). Gammex RMI manufactures a comprehensive line of quality control test tools that are relatively inexpensive and easy to use. These tools can be purchased individually or as a complete quality control kit (Fig. 42-4). The multiple test cassette, which tests several x-ray unit parameters with a single exposure, is especially popular in smaller facilities (Fig. 42-5). Also available are multiple-function digital meters that display digital readouts of the measurements for the tested parameters, including exposure time, kilovolt (peak) (kVp), and milliroentgen (mR) output. The decision of what quality control tools to use depends on factors such as cost, ease of use, accuracy, and dependability. Most vendors of x-ray supplies carry a variety of quality control test tools. To familiarize the reader with some examples of quality control test tools, the following section briefly reviews some of the basic tests for quality control.

AUTOMATIC FILM PROCESSING

Film processors are one of the biggest contributors of variability in an x-ray system that uses a film and fluorescent intensifying screen. Most authorities suggest in-house sensitometric monitoring of the film processor. This approach provides a quantitative means of recording processor variability. Sensitometric monitoring requires the use of a *sensitometer* and a *densitometer* (Fig. 42-6). In addition, a dependable thermometer should be used to accurately measure developer temperature, and one specific box of radiographic film should be reserved for use as control film in the testing procedure.

The sensitometer is used to deliver a graduated series of controlled light intensities to a piece of radiographic control film. The exposed control film is then processed, producing a series of graduated, or stepped, densities and is known as a sensitometric *control strip* (Fig. 42-7).

A densitometer is used to quantitatively measure the densities of the developed sensitometric control strip. Normally only three measurements are needed. A midrange step, which is close to having an optical density of 1, is known as the *speed step*. The optical density of the second step above the speed step is measured. The difference between this step and the speed step is known as the *density difference,* or *contrast.* The gross, or *base plus fog,* should also be measured. It is good practice to also measure the developer temperature, using an accurate thermometer, at the time the sensitometric control strip is processed.

The data generated are then plotted on a processor control chart (Fig. 42-8). This procedure should be performed at least daily. Charting these processing characteristics allows operating conditions to be interpreted on a daily basis. Data trends pointing to possible future problems may also be detected. The measurements should fall within the facility's film processing standards for image quality (speed, contrast, base plus fog), which are established when the processor is considered to be operating in an optimum fashion. If the measurements fall outside the standards, the situation should be analyzed and immediately corrected. The CDRH recommends the following processing standards of quality: base plus fog ± 0.05 optical density units; contrast ± 0.10 optical density units; and speed ± 0.10 optical density units.

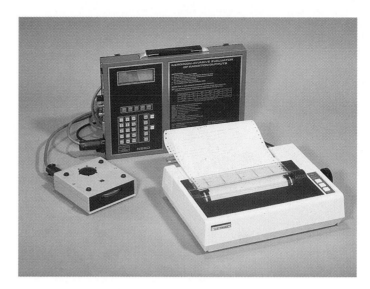

Fig. 42-3 NERO is a microprocessor that can be programmed to acquire and analyze exposure data, providing quality control test results for numerous parameters.

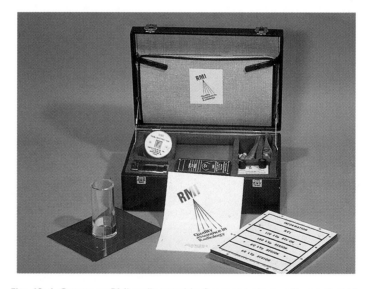

Fig. 42-4 Gammex RMI radiographic-fluoroscopic quality control kit.

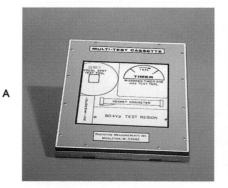
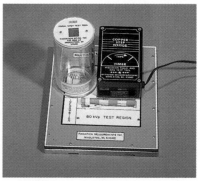

Fig. 42-5 Gammex RMI multiple test cassette. **A,** Cassette only. **B,** Cassette with quality control tools in place.

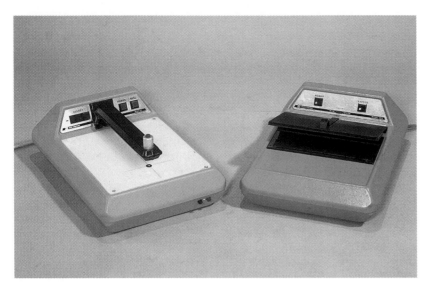

Fig. 42-6 Processor quality control program requires a sensitometer *(right)* and a densitometer *(left)*.

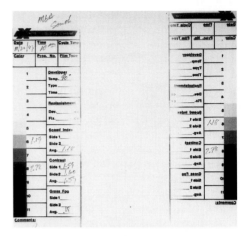

Fig. 42-7 Sensitometric control strip. Both sides of the control film emulsion are sensitometrically exposed. The densitometer measurements of both sides are averaged and recorded on the control strip.

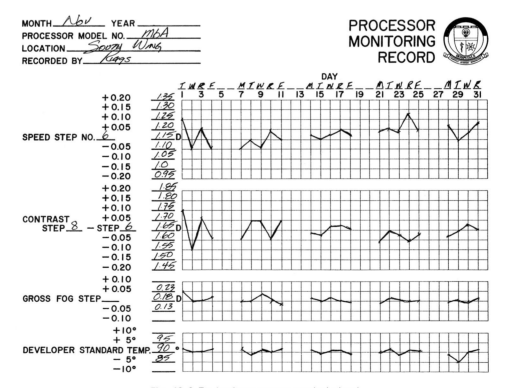

Fig. 42-8 Typical processor control chart.

The integrity and condition of the darkroom should also be tested periodically. For this test the darkroom is visually inspected for light leaks and the safelights are tested to determine the level of fog they may contribute to the radiographic film.

RADIOGRAPHIC X-RAY UNITS

Numerous radiographic x-ray unit parameters can be monitored. A few of the more basic tests are described in the following sections.

Beam alignment and beam–light field congruence

The centering and perpendicularity of the beam must be checked, and the *congruence,* or *alignment,* of the collimator light field and the x-ray beam field must be determined. This testing is important because a great deal of unproductive radiation can be delivered to the patient if the system is misaligned.

Radiographing straightened paper clips aligned with the edges of the collimator light field is a quick, simple, and inexpensive method of evaluating the accuracy of beam–light field alignment. A tool specifically designed to test these parameters is shown in Fig. 42-9. Light field–x-ray beam alignment is measured by exposing the collimator template. Beam alignment and perpendicularity are assessed by the plastic cylinder, which has a small metallic bead enclosed in each end. The cylinder is centered to the template and exposed. These tests are usually performed on the tabletop and can be used to test both the manual and automatic collimator modes.

Beam–light field alignment should be within ± 2% of the source-to-image receptor distance (SID). Beam perpendicularity is acceptable if both beads are projected within the center ring (Fig. 42-10).

Exposure time

A test of exposure time determines whether the x-ray unit is delivering the same time of exposure as indicated by the control panel's radiographic exposure time. A manually operated spinning top is appropriate for testing single-phase generators, but evaluating three-phase and high-frequency generators requires a motorized synchronous top (Fig. 42-11).

The radiopaque face of the synchronous motor device contains a radius slit aperture. An exposure is made of the rotating top. As the slit rotates, it allows radiation to pass, producing an arc of density on the image receptor. By measuring the angle of the arc, the time of exposure can be calculated and compared with the time selected on the control panel. This calculation is simplified by using a template to determine the actual exposure time (Fig. 42-12).

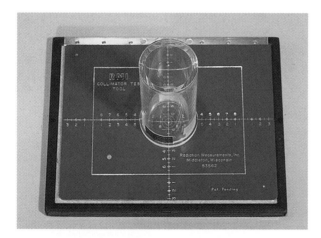

Fig. 42-9 Beam perpendicularity and beam-light field alignment test tools.

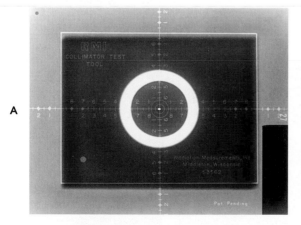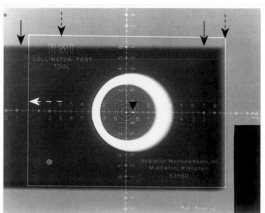

Fig. 42-10 A, Acceptable beam perpendicularity and beam–light field alignment. **B,** Unacceptable beam perpendicularity and beam–light field alignment. Radiation beam *(arrows)* does not agree with collimator light field *(broken arrows).* Perpendicularity is out of alignment. Note top bead is shifted to the right *(arrowhead).*

Digital x-ray exposure timer test tools can be used to test single-phase, three-phase, and high-frequency generators.

When exposed, these meters measure the x-ray exposure time and display it as a direct digital readout on the face of the meter (Fig. 42-13).

Beam quality

The quality of the primary x-ray beam refers to the energy of the x-ray photons that comprise it and is generally described by the *half-value layer (HVL)*. The HVL is a measurement of the x-ray beam quality or average energy. It is an indication of the total equivalent filtration in the path of the x-ray beam (it is not a direct measure of the total filtration). Total equivalent filtration includes the filtration properties of the x-ray glass envelope, the mirror and plastic underside of the collimator, and any added filtration at the port of the x-ray tube. Added filtration is used to increase the *beam hardness,* or average beam energy, by removing more low-energy than high-energy photons from the beam. Ad-

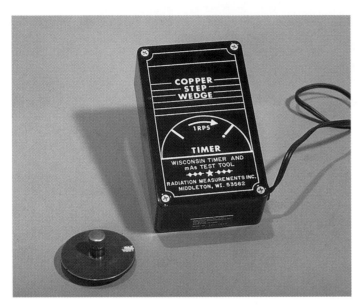

Fig. 42-11 Hand-spun spinning top *(left)* and Gammex RMI motorized synchronous top *(right).*

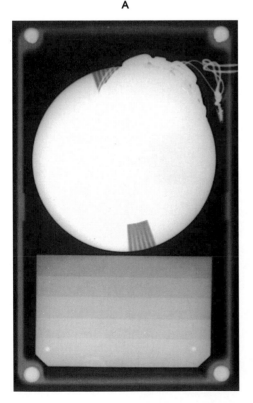

A

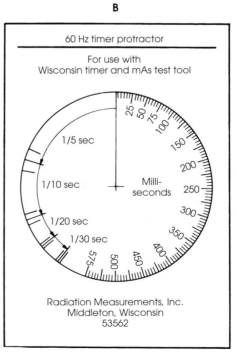

B

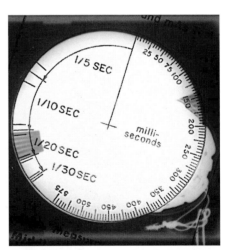

C

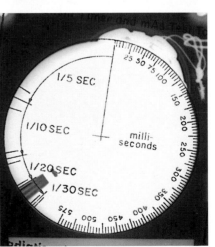

D

Fig. 42-12 A, Radiograph produced at 200-mA and $\frac{1}{20}$-second exposure. **B,** RMI protractor template. **C,** Radiograph A with template showing acceptable results for a $\frac{1}{20}$-second exposure. **D,** Radiograph produced at 300 mA and $\frac{1}{30}$ second showing unacceptable results.

ditional filtration is an important radiation protection consideration, since low-energy x-ray photons are absorbed more readily by the patient.

The *beam quality* test verifies that the beam's HVL is sufficient to reduce the patient's exposure to low-energy radiation. The HVL is determined by plotting the thickness of aluminum *attenuators* (Fig. 42-14, *A*) that are added to the beam compared to the resultant exposures that are measured with a dosimeter (Fig. 42-14, *B*). The acceptable HVL for a single-phase generator 80-kVp beam is 2.3 mm of aluminum. An HVL less than this indicates that the total filtration of the beam must be increased (Fig. 42-14, *C*), assuming that the kVp is accurate. Inaccurate HVL values may also indicate inaccurate kVp calibration or tube problems.

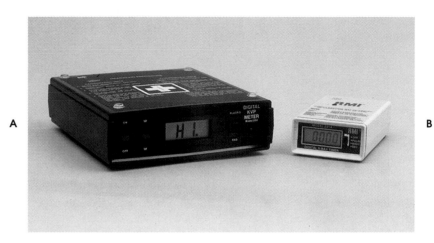

Fig. 42-13 A, Digital kVp meter. **B,** Digital x-ray timer.

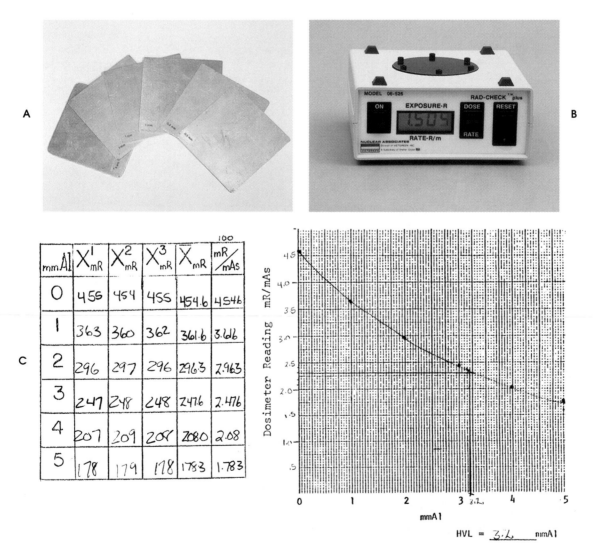

mmAl	X^1_{mR}	X^2_{mR}	X^3_{mR}	X_{mR}	mR/mAs
0	455	454	455	454.6	4546
1	363	360	362	361.6	3.66
2	296	297	296	296.3	2.963
3	247	248	248	247.6	2.476
4	207	209	208	208.0	2.08
5	178	179	178	178.3	1.783

HVL = __3.2__ mmAl

Fig. 42-14 A, Set of aluminum attenuators of various thicknesses. **B,** Digital dosimeter used to measure exposure output. **C,** Half-value layer (HVL) is calculated by plotting the average output of exposure in mR/mAs vs. thickness of added aluminum attenuator. Graph shows acceptable results.

Kilovolt (peak)

The maximum kVp, or peak electric potential, across the x-ray tube affects the radiation intensity reaching the image receptor and the subject contrast of the final image. Radiographic density and contrast can be adversely affected by inaccurate kVp calibration. Noninvasive electronic digital kVp meters are available that accurately measure kVp and provide a digital readout of the measured kVp in a fast, convenient manner (see Fig. 42-13, *A*).

Another device used to test the accuracy of kVp settings is the kVp test cassette (Fig. 42-15, *A*). The cassette works on the principle that kVp can be determined by the amount of attenuation that occurs in a filtered beam. The specially designed cassette contains a copper filter, a series of *step wedges,* and an optical attenuator built into the cassette. The cassette works on the principle that the effective kVp defines the step of the wedge that attenuates the radiation equal to the attenuation of the intensifying screen light by the optical attenuator. The attenuation effects are recorded as radiographic densities on an image receptor that has been exposed in the cassette at a given kVp setting (Fig. 42-15, *B*). By matching the step density produced by the step wedge attenuator to the density produced by the optical attenuator, the effective kVp can be determined from a calibration curve supplied with the cassette. The measured effective kVp should be within ± 4 kVp of the kVp setting tested.

Exposure reproducibility and linearity

Predictable radiographic exposures are essential for consistent radiographic images. The test for *exposure reproducibility* (repeatability) determines whether the same results are attained every time the same technique factors are used. *Linearity* (reciprocity) tests are performed to determine that the same exposure is obtained at a given milliampere-second (mAs) selection, without regard to the combination of milliampere (mA) and exposure time selections chosen to achieve the mAs setting.

The reproducibility-linearity test can be accomplished qualitatively by repeatedly exposing a step wedge or penetrometer with the same mA-exposure time combination to determine the exposure reproducibility. Exposure linearity can be tested by repeatedly exposing the step wedge using the same total mAs but different mA-exposure time combinations. By matching the radiographic densities of the step wedge images, the accuracy of the parameters can be evaluated (Fig. 42-16). A dosimeter can also be used to record the output of the exposures that are compared quantitatively to determine their accuracy.

An x-ray unit should produce reproducible exposures to within 5% of their average. Exposure linearity should not exceed 10%.

Focal spot size

The *recorded detail* in a radiographic image is partially dependent on the size of the x-ray tube's focal spot. As the size of the focal spot increases, the ability to define small structures is diminished. In addition, a change in focal spot size over time may be symptomatic of the x-ray tube's deterioration. A *slit camera* is used to measure the physical size of the focal spot. This device is used by physicists or other appropriately educated individuals to obtain accurate, quantitative focal spot measurements.

An easy test to determine changes in focal spot size over time is to periodically evaluate its resolving capability. A *resolution* test pattern (Fig. 42-17, *A*), which is composed of groups of different-sized bar patterns (line pairs), is radiographed using a direct exposure technique (Fig. 42-17, *B*). The radiograph of the test pattern is evaluated to determine the smallest group of line pairs that can be seen clearly (Fig. 42-17, *C* and *D*). Tables are available that equate the effective focal spot size to the smallest pattern resolved. The star test pattern is another type of resolution test pattern that is often used (Fig. 42-18). This pattern provides more accurate information but is more difficult to use. Determining the resolving capability of a focal spot should be considered a qualitative test because of its inability to accurately measure the true physical size of the focal spot.

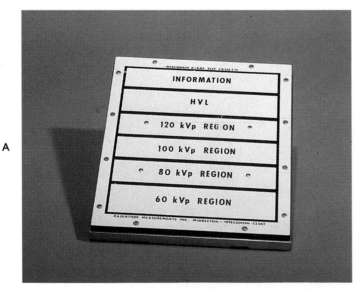

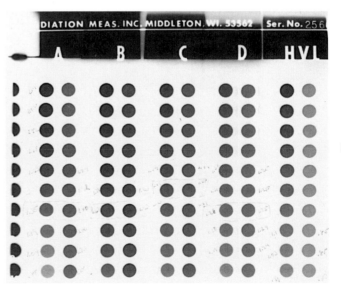

Fig. 42-15 A, Gammex RMI 8 × 10 inch (20 × 24 cm) kVp test cassette. This cassette can be used to measure the accuracy of 60-, 80-, 100-, and 120-kVp settings. The cassette can also be used to measure HVL. **B,** A kVp test radiograph. By measuring the densities of the adjacent dots with a densitometer, an accuracy of ± 2 kVp can be achieved.

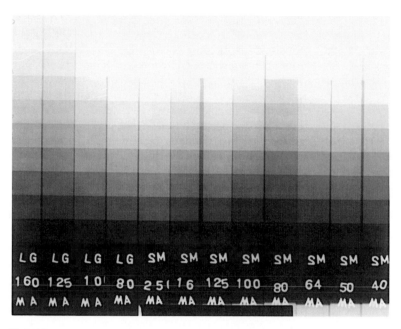

Fig. 42-16 Step wedge exposures of various mA time combinations can be used to check linearity. Density should not vary more than one step between exposures.

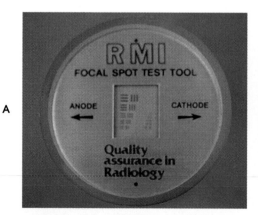

A

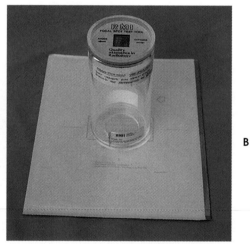

B

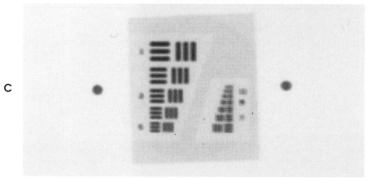

C

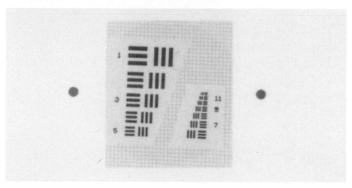

D

Fig. 42-17 **A,** Gammex RMI resolution test pattern used to measure focal spot size. **B,** Set-up of focal spot test tool. **C,** Test results on a large focal spot, showing the effective size to be 1.4 mm. **D,** Test results on a small focal spot, showing the effective size to be 0.6 mm.

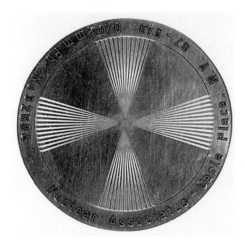

Fig. 42-18 Star resolution test pattern.

IMAGE RECEPTORS

The image receptor referred to in this chapter and most commonly used in diagnostic radiology is a cassette containing intensifying screens and radiographic film. This cassette is a rigid, lightproof holder that compresses the screens and film together when closed. The care and condition of the image receptor have a direct bearing on radiographic image quality.

Cassettes

Loss of film-screen cassette integrity may produce unsharp or fogged images. Cassettes should be physically inspected periodically for wearing of the latches and hinges, warping of the cassette frame, and deterioration of the foam or felt compression material. Testing for light leaks should also be part of the inspection process. Cassettes should be repaired or replaced if they do not pass such inspections.

Computed radiography system cassettes also must be physically inspected. The cassette used in a computed radiography system is similar in external appearance to a film-screen cassette; however, the primary function of the computed radiography cassette is to physically protect the photostimulable imaging plate as compared to protecting a radiographic film from light in a film-screen cassette. (For additional information on computed radiography; see Chapter 34.)

Intensifying screens

Dirty and worn intensifying screens can cause radiographic artifacts. It is important to visually inspect the screens for wear, abrasions, and stains and to clean them on a routine basis. Screens should be cleaned with a soft cloth and either a recommended screen cleaner or a mild soap-and-water solution. The screens must be thoroughly dry before they are returned to service.

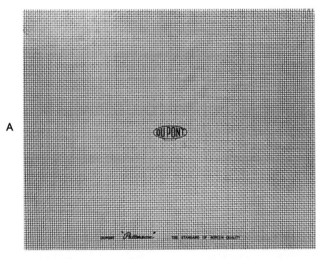

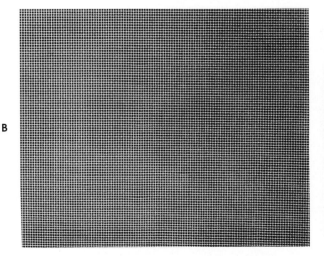

Fig. 42-19 A, Wire mesh test tool. **B,** Test radiograph exhibiting acceptable film-screen contact. **C,** Test radiograph exhibiting unacceptable film-screen contact.

The speed (sensitivity) of similar types of intensifying screens may vary as they age or as new cassettes and screens are added to service. This lack of uniformity results in radiographic density variations. In testing for screen-speed uniformity, the following steps are taken:

- Use a reliable generator and the appropriate exposure technique to produce a radiographic density of approximately 1.5.
- Identify all similar screened cassettes in service with lead markers.
- Expose each cassette using the same technique.
- Use a densitometer to measure the density of each of the radiographs. The measured density variation between the radiographs should not exceed ± 0.2.

Film-screen contact

Poor contact between the intensifying screens and the radiographic film reduces the contrast and recorded detail in the radiographic image. Radiographic cassettes should be periodically tested for poor film-screen contact. A wire-mesh test object is used for this purpose (Fig. 42-19, *A*). The test object is placed on top of the cassette and radiographed. The radiographic image of the wire mesh should have a uniform radiographic density. Any areas that appear darker indicate poor contact (Fig. 42-19, *B* and *C*). Cassettes that exhibit areas of poor contact in the central portion of the cassette should be repaired or replaced.

GRIDS

Misaligned grids attenuate an increased portion of the primary radiation beam, resulting in an increase in patient radiation and a reduction in radiographic image quality. The loss of image quality caused by improper grid alignment can be subtle and is often attributed to other causes. A simple test to evaluate grid alignment requires radiographing a 35 × 43 cm (14 × 17 inch) homogeneous phantom such as water, aluminum, or fiberboard. The following steps are observed:

- Expose the phantom crosswise on the radiographic table.
- Place a 35 × 43 cm (14 × 17 inch) cassette crosswise in the Bucky tray. Select an exposure technique that will produce a radiographic density of approximately 1.5.

A properly aligned grid will produce an even density across the radiograph. An uneven density indicates the need for corrective maintenance.

ILLUMINATORS

An important but often overlooked aspect of radiographic quality control is the evaluation of illuminator performance. Illuminator variations affect radiographic density and contrast. Output changes as the illuminator ages, and output intensity is affected by the type of light source used. Illuminators with a reduced light output increase the visual appearance of the density of the radiograph being viewed. Lack of uniformity between illuminators may cause radiographs to appear underexposed when one illuminator is used and overexposed when another is used, resulting in reduced contrast in both situations. A photographic or optical light meter can measure illuminator intensity and can check for variation among illuminators. Gross mismatches should be corrected.

VISUAL INSPECTIONS

Periodically, but at least annually, the radiographic and fluoroscopic equipment and accessory devices should undergo a thorough visual inspection to assess their mechanical integrity and safety. Some of the more important visual checks include the following:

Overhead tube cranes: Inspect their stability, movement, detent operation, and lock function; the SID and angulation indicator function; the Bucky center light and light localizer brightness and accuracy; and the condition of the high-tension cables.

Radiographic table: Check for the proper functioning of the Bucky tray and cassette locks, the power-top and angulation switches, and the table angulation indicator. Also inspect the stability and function of foot and shoulder braces.

Control panel: Check for the proper functioning of the panel lights/meters and switches, the overload protection indicator, and the tube heat sensors; the availability and currentness of technique charts; and an unobstructed view of the exposure room through the control panel window.

Fluoroscopic systems: Check for the proper functioning of fluoroscopic lights, meters, switches, locks, and Bucky slot cover; the presence and integrity of lead tower drapes; and the smoothness of movement of the power assist.

Protective lead apparel: Radiograph or fluoroscopically view lead aprons and gloves, and document the results to determine whether any cracks are present. When not in use, protective apparel should be stored on appropriate hangers to prevent cracks from forming. Check the lead sheets used to mask cassettes for multiple exposures in the same manner.

Miscellaneous: Examine positioning aids for foreign substances that could produce artifacts on radiographs, such as barium stains on sponges. These items should be either radiographed or viewed fluoroscopically to rule out any such contamination. Check the mechanical integrity of additional equipment such as footstools, IV stands, and upright support devices.

Mammography Quality Assurance

In 1992 the federal government passed the *Mammography Quality Standards Act (MQSA)*. This legislation requires mammography facilities to establish an ongoing quality assurance program. Mammography quality assurance programs are similar to those used in conventional radiography, but quality control tests are required to be performed more frequently than what is recommended for conventional diagnostic equipment. The MQSA requires evaluation of the entire imaging chain via the demonstration of acceptable image quality of phantom-generated images on a monthly basis.

IMAGING EQUIPMENT QUALITY CONTROL

Radiographic equipment used for mammography imaging must be dedicated for this purpose only. The parameters of the equipment must be tested by a certified health physicist on a semiannual basis. Equipment parameters tested include the following:

- Exposure timer accuracy and reproducibility
- mR-mAs linearity
- kVp accuracy and reproducibility
- Beam quality (HVL)
- Entrance skin exposure measurements
- Focal spot size
- Beam restriction
- Automatic exposure control (AEC) device performance
- Screen speed uniformity
- Artifact evaluation and image quality
- Overall equipment integrity and operation

DARKROOM AND FILM PROCESSOR QUALITY CONTROL

The mammographer or quality assurance technologist is usually responsible for performing and documenting tests dealing with film processing and image quality. On a daily basis, the processing is tested sensitometrically and the darkroom countertops and processor feed tray are cleaned before films are processed. A more thorough cleaning, including a complete dusting and mopping of the floor and countertops, should be done on a weekly basis. The darkroom should be tested for fog at least twice each year. Fixer retention tests, performed on a quarterly basis, determine the quantity of residual fixer retained in the film. Excess residual fixer reduces the stability of the image over time (archival quality) and is an indication of inadequate washing of the film.

IMAGE QUALITY CONTROL

Illuminator surfaces and intensifying screens must be cleaned on a weekly basis to remove dust particles that may produce artifacts. Film-screen contact tests are also performed semiannually to ensure that recorded detail is not degraded because of poor film-screen contact.

Mammography test phantom images must be obtained on a monthly basis (Fig. 42-20). Because the phantom images are used to evaluate the overall imaging chain in regard to maintaining a consistent level of image quality, the tests must be performed and evaluated using strict controls. These controls include using the same cassette, the same technical factors, the same phantom position, and the same illuminator and viewing conditions each time the test is performed. One individual should be responsible for the performance and evaluation of the phantom test film. Visual inspections of the mammography equipment should also be performed monthly to ensure the working integrity of the equipment.

The analysis of repeated mammograms is instrumental in identifying problem areas in the mammography examination. Every 3 months a repeat analysis should be conducted in which the number and cause of repeated examinations are evaluated against the total examinations done during a specified time period. A test unique to mammography is the *compression test,* which is done semiannually. This test ensures that the compression device delivers adequate compression to the breast, which reduces scatter radiation, motion effects, and exposure dose. All mammography quality assurance tests must be performed at the specified frequencies, must be adequately documented, and must meet established acceptance criteria to maintain their compliance with the MQSA.

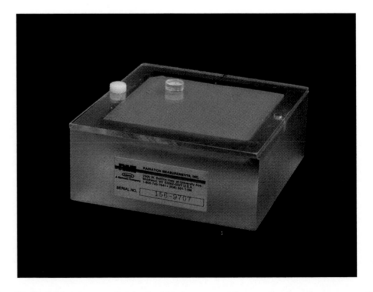

Fig. 42-20 Mammography test phantom used for evaluating image quality.

(Courtesy Kevin D. Evans.)

Conclusion

The quality control tests described in this chapter can be considered basic tests for monitoring film processors, radiographic units, and image quality. Similar quality control tests should be used to monitor fluoroscopic equipment and mobile radiographic units. Quality control tests are also designed for image intensifiers, tomographic equipment, AEC devices, computed tomography, magnetic resonance imaging, and sonography units. Quality control should also be extended to include nuclear medicine and radiation therapy facilities.

Radiographic quality assurance programs can play a major role in the improvement of patient care, the reduction of unnecessary radiation to both personnel and patients, and the containment of costs for radiologic health care delivery. Although this chapter has dealt primarily with quality assurance in the context of the technical elements of the radiographic system, medical radiography personnel must remember that their responsibilities to the patient extend beyond the technical aspects of image production.

Definition of Terms

alignment Closeness of agreement of the centers and edges of the x-ray beam and collimator light fields.

attenuator Object that reduces the intensity of an x-ray beam.

base plus fog Density of unexposed processed radiographic film resulting from opacity of film base and density inherent to film emulsion.

beam hardening Increasing the mean energy the x-ray beam spectrum by removing of the low-energy photons.

beam quality Energy of an x-ray beam.

Center for Devices and Radiological Health (CDRH) Federal agency responsible for ensuring the safety and effectiveness of medical devices and eliminating unnecessary human exposure to man-made radiation from medical, occupational, and consumer products; previously called the *National Center for Devices and Radiological Health (NCDRH) and the Bureau of Radiological Health (BRH)*.

congruence Closeness of agreement in position and size of x-ray beam and collimator light fields.

compression test Test designed to determine the adequacy of compression delivered to the breast by the compression system of mammographic imaging equipment.

control strip Radiographic film that has been exposed by a sensitometer or radiation passing through a stepwedge.

densitometer Device used to measure the optical density of photographic film.

diagnostic radiology facility Any establishment using an x-ray system in procedures involving irradiation of the human body for the purpose of diagnosis or visualization.

exposure reproducibility Ability to obtain the same exposure output using the same milliamperage and exposure time from one exposure to the next.

film processor Machine that transports exposed radiographic film through developing, fixing, washing, and drying sections to produce a finished radiograph.

half-value layer (HVL) Thickness of an absorber that will reduce the intensity of an x-ray beam by one half.

linearity Ability to obtain the same exposure for the same mAs, regardless of the milliamperage and exposure time used.

Mammography Quality Standards Act (MQSA) Federal law passed in 1992, designed to ensure a minimum uniform quality standard for mammography in the United States.

NCDRH Old term for National Center for Devices and Radiological Health, previously called the Bureau of Radiological Health (BRH) (see *CDRH*).

objective standards Standards of image quality that relate to aspects that can be directly measured.

penetrometer See *step wedge*.

performance criterion The standard or measurement of operation by which a piece of equipment functions.

purchase specification A description of the details and operating characteristics of specific equipment in preparation to acquire the equipment in exchange for payment.

quality administrative procedures Management procedures that provide for the organization of the quality assurance program.

quality assurance (QA) Planned and organized efforts within a diagnostic radiology facility to ensure the production of consistent optimum-quality images with minimum radiation exposure and cost to the patient.

quality assurance program Distinct organized structure designed to furnish quality assurance for a diagnostic radiology facility.

quality control (QC) Methods and procedures used in the testing and maintenance of the components of an x-ray system.

recorded detail Sharpness of the structural lines as recorded in the radiographic image.

reject analysis Study of repeated radiographs to determine the cause for their being discarded.

resolution Ability to record separate images of small objects that are placed close together.

Radiation Measurements Incorporated (RMI) Now Gammex RMI; a company that designs and manufactures quality control products for diagnostic radiology.

sensitometer Device designed to give precise, reproducible, and graduated light exposures to photographic film.

slit camera Device used to measure the effective focal spot size.

speed step The step on a sensitometric strip that has a net optical density closest to 1.

step wedge Device used to put a series of increasing exposures on a radiographic film when exposed by a radiographic beam.

subjective standards Standards of image quality that are expressed by the feelings, perceptions, and thoughts of the observer rather than by direct measurement.

x-ray system Collection of components for the production, recording, and viewing of radiographic images.

Selected bibliography

American College of Radiology Committee on Quality Assurance in Mammography: *Mammography quality control manual,* Reston, Va, 1994, American College of Radiology.

Andolina VF, Lille S, Willison KM: *Mammographic imaging: a practical guide,* Philadelphia, 1992, Lippincott.

Barber TC et al: *Radiologic quality control manual,* Reston, Va, 1984, American College of Radiology.

Basic quality control in diagnostic radiology. Report No. 4, Chicago, 1978, American Association of Physicists in Medicine.

Burkhart RL: *A basic quality assurance program for small diagnostic radiology facilities.* HHS Pub No (FDA) 83-8218, Washington, DC, 1983, US Department of Health and Human Services.

Burkhart RL: *Checklist for establishing a diagnostic radiology quality assurance program.* HHS Pub No (FDA) 83-8219, Washington, DC, 1983, US Department of Health and Human Services.

Burkhart RL: *Diagnostic radiology quality assurance catalog.* HEW Pub No (FDA) 77-8028, Washington, DC, 1977, US Department of Health, Education and Welfare.

Burkhart RL: *Diagnostic radiology quality assurance catalog: supplement.* HEW Pub No (FDA) 78-8028, Washington, DC, 1978, US Department of Health, Education and Welfare.

Burkhart RL: *Quality assurance programs for diagnostic radiology facilities.* HEW Pub No (FDA) 80-8110, Washington, DC, 1980, US Department of Health, Education and Welfare.

Burns B: Achieving darkroom and processing quality control in mammography: a step beyond minimum recommendations, *Semin Radiol Technol* 3:68, 1995.

Carlton R: Establishing a total quality assurance program in diagnostic radiology, *Radiol Technol* 35:23, 1980.

Farria DM et al: Mammography quality assurance from A to Z, *Radiographics* 14:371, 1994.

Goldman LW: *Analysis of retakes: understanding, managing and using an analysis of retakes program for quality assurance.* HEW Pub No (FDA) 79-8097, Washington, DC, 1979, US Department of Health, Education and Welfare.

Gray JE: *Photographic quality assurance in diagnostic radiology, nuclear medicine, and radiation therapy, vol 1. The basic principles of daily photographic quality assurance.* HEW Pub No (FDA) 76-8043, Washington, DC, 1976, US Department of Health, Education and Welfare.

Gray JE: *Photographic quality assurance in diagnostic radiology, nuclear medicine and radiation therapy, vol 2. Photographic processing, quality assurance and the evaluation of photographic materials.* HEW Pub No (FDA) 77-8018, Washington, DC, 1977, US Department of Health, Education and Welfare.

Gray JE et al: *Mammography quality control: radiologic technologist's manual,* Reston, Va, 1992, American College of Radiology and the American Cancer Society.

Gray JE et al: *Quality control in diagnostic imaging,* Baltimore, 1983, University Park Press.

Hauss AG, Jaskulski SM: *The basics of film processing in medical imaging,* Madison, Wis, 1997, Medical Physics.

Hendee WR et al: *Quality assurance for conventional tomographic x-ray units.* HEW Pub No (FDA) 80-8096, Washington, DC, 1980, US Department of Health, Education and Welfare.

Hendee WR et al: *Quality assurance for fluoroscopic x-ray units and associated equipment.* HEW Pub No (FDA) 80-8095, Washington, DC, 1980, US Department of Health, Education and Welfare.

Hendee WR et al: *Quality assurance for radiographic x-ray units and associated equipment.* HEW Pub No (FDA) 79-8094, Washington, DC, 1979, US Department of Health, Education and Welfare.

Mammography: a user's guide. NCRP Report No 85, Bethesda, Md, 1986, National Council on Radiation Protection and Measurements.

Lawrence DJ: A simple method of processor control, *Med Radiogr Photogr* 49:2, 1973.

Mammography quality assurance manual: in accordance with the requirements of the Mammography Quality Standards Act (21 CFR 900), Victor, NY, 1995, Upstate Medical Physics, Inc.

McKinney WE: *Radiographic processing and quality control,* Philadelphia, 1988, Lippincott.

McLemore JM: *Quality assurance in diagnostic radiology,* St Louis, 1981, Mosby.

Nelson RE et al: Economic analysis of a comprehensive quality assurance program, *Radiol Technol* 49:129, 1977.

Neyes RS: The economics of quality assurance, *RNM Mag* 10:7, 1980.

Papp J: *Quality management in the imaging sciences,* St Louis, 1998, Mosby.

Quality assurance for diagnostic imaging equipment, NCRP Report No. 99, Bethesda, Md, 1988, National Council on Radiation Protection and Measurements.

Quality assurance in diagnostic radiology and nuclear medicine—the obvious decision, HHS Pub No (FDA) 81-8141, Washington, DC, 1981, US Department of Health and Human Services.

Quality assurance programs for diagnostic radiology facilities, final recommendation, *Fed Register* 44:71728, 1979.

Tortorici M: *Concepts in medical radiographic imaging,* Philadelphia, 1992, WB Saunders.

Wentz G: *Mammography for radiologic technologists,* ed 2, New York, 1997, McGraw Hill.

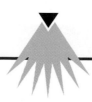

INDEX

Index

Index

Index

Heart—cont'd
  projections of—cont'd
    PA oblique, **1:**532-535
      in RAO and LAO positions, **1:**532-535
      in right or left position, **1:**528-531
      in RPO or LPO positions, **1:**536-537
    sectional anatomy of, **3:**111
Heart rate, **3:**23
Helium-neon laser, definition of, **3:**320
Hematologic depression, secondary to radiation exposure, **1:**36
Hematoma, definition of, **3:**90, **3:**258
Hemidiaphragm, sectional anatomy of, **3:**113
Hemodynamics, definition of, **3:**258
Hemostasis, definition of, **3:**90, **3:**258
Henschen method, for petromastoid portion imaging, **2:**386, **2:**388
Hepatic artery, **2:**37
  arteriograms of, **3:**39
  sectional anatomy of, **3:**117
Hepatic ducts, **2:**38
Hepatic veins, **2:**37
  sectional anatomy of, **3:**113
Hepatic venography, **3:**45
Hepatopancreatic ampulla, **2:**38
Hernia, **2:**118-119
Herniated nucleus pulposus, **1:**372
Heterogenous, definition of, **3:**407
Hiatal hernia, Wolf method for imaging of, **2:**118-119
Hickey method
  for hip, **1:**344-345
  for mastoid process imaging, **2:**404-405
High-resolution scans, definition of, **3:**304
Hill-Sachs defect, **1:**168, **1:**185
Hilum, **1:**510, **2:**160
Hindbrain, **3:**2
Hinge joint, **1:**66, **1:**67
Hip
  Clements-Nakayama modification for, **1:**348-349
  congenital dislocation of, **1:**341
  contrast arthrography of
    in adults, **1:**566-567
    in children, **1:**566
    dislocations, **1:**561
    indications, **1:**566
    subtraction technique, **1:**566-567
  Danelius-Miller method for, **1:**346-347
  Hickey method for, **1:**344-345
  Hsieh method, **1:**354-355
  Lauenstein method for, **1:**344-345
  Lilienfeld method, **1:**356-357
  projections for
    AP, **1:**320-321, **1:**342-343
    axiolateral
      using Clements-Nakayama method, **1:**348-349
      using Danelius-Miller method, **1:**346-347
      using Friedman method, **1:**352-353
      using Leonard-George method, **1:**350-351
    lateral, **1:**344-345
    mediolateral oblique, **1:**356-357
    overview, **1:**324t
    PA, **1:**354-355
    in RAO and LAO positions, **1:**354-357
  tomography of, **3:**199t, **3:**204
Hip bone, anatomy of
  description of, **1:**325
  ilium, **1:**325

Hip bone, anatomy of—cont'd
  ischium, **1:**326
  pubis, **1:**326
Hip joint
  axial projection of, **1:**336-337
    Chassard-Lapiné method, **1:**336-337
  palpation of, **1:**329
Hirtz modification, for petromastoid portion imaging, **2:**402
Histogram, definition of, **3:**320
Hodgkin's disease, radiation therapy for, **3:**502
Holmblad method, for intercondylar fossa, **1:**300-301
Homeostasis, definition of, **3:**481
Homogenous, definition of, **3:**407
Hook of hamate, **1:**86
Horizontal plane, **1:**52, **1:**53
Horizontal ray method, for double-contrast arthrography of knee, **1:**564-565
Horn, definition of, **1:**68
Host computer, definition of, **3:**305
Hounsfield units, **3:**289, **3:**305
Hughston method, for patella and patellofemoral joint, **1:**311
Humeral condyle, **1:**88
Humeroradial joint, **1:**90
Humeroulnar joint, **1:**90
Humerus
  anatomy of, **1:**88, **1:**157
  distal
    anatomy of, **1:**88
    projections for
      acute flexion, **1:**138
      AP, **1:**136, **1:**138
      overview, **1:**84t
      PA axial, **1:**142
      partial flexion, **1:**136
  projections for, **1:**205, **1:**209
    AP, **1:**144, **1:**146
    lateral, **1:**145, **1:**148-149
    lateromedial lateral recumbent, **1:**148-149
    lateromedial recumbent, **1:**147
    lateromedial upright, **1:**145
    recumbent, **1:**146
    upright, **1:**144
  proximal
    anatomy of, **1:**88, **1:**157
    Blackett-Healy method
      for subscapular insertion, **1:**189
      for teres minor insertion, **1:**188
    Fisk modification, **1:**186
    Lawrence method, **1:**150-151
    overview, **1:**154t
    projections of
      AP, **1:**189
      AP axial, **1:**185
      PA, **1:**188
      transthoracic lateral, **1:**150-151
    Stryker notch method for, **1:**185
    teres minor insertion, **1:**188
Hydronephrosis, **2:**175
  definition of, **3:**90
Hyoid bone
  anatomy of, **2:**16, **2:**249
  sectional anatomy of, **3:**99
Hyperechoic, definition of, **3:**407
Hyperextension, **1:**80
Hyperflexion, **1:**80
Hypersthenic body habitus, **1:**58, **1:**59
Hypocycloidal motion, **3:**182

Hypodermic needles, **2:**203
Hypoechoic, definition of, **3:**407
Hypoglossal canal
  Miller method, **2:**420-421
  projections of
    in anterior profile, **2:**420-421
    axiolateral oblique, **2:**420-421
    overview, **2:**378t
Hypophyseal fossa, **3:**97
  radiologic imaging of, **2:**261
Hypophysis cerebri, **2:**239, **3:**2, **3:**97
  sectional anatomy of, **3:**102
Hyposthenic body habitus, **1:**58, **1:**59
Hypotonic duodenography, **2:**105
Hysterosalpingography, **2:**218-219

I

Iatrogenic, definition of, **3:**90
Identification, of radiograph, **1:**22-23, **1:**23
Ileocecal valve, **2:**90
Ileum, anatomy of, **2:**89
Iliac crest, **1:**333
Iliacus, sectional anatomy of, **3:**121, **3:**127
Iliopsoas, sectional anatomy of, **3:**123
Ilium
  anatomy of, **1:**325
  AP and PA oblique projections, **1:**364-365
  radiologic imaging of, **1:**343
  sectional anatomy of, **3:**121, **3:**127
Illuminator; *see* Viewbox
Image coregistration, definition of, **3:**481
Image intensifier, definition of, **3:**333
Image plate reader, **3:**311
  definition of, **3:**320
Image processor, **3:**326
  definition of, **3:**333
Image reader, for computed radiography images, **1:**32
Image receptor
  body habitus and, **1:**57
  definition of, **1:**3
  for patient protection, **1:**45
  placement, **1:**24, **1:**25
Imaging plate, definition of, **3:**320
Incus, **2:**245
Independent jaws, definition of, **3:**505
Indirect effect, definition of, **3:**505
Indium, radiopharmaceutical use, **3:**415t
Infant; *see also* Children; Neonate; Pediatric imaging
  foreign body localization
    aspirated objects, **1:**589
    swallowed objects, **1:**590
Infection, nuclear medicine imaging of, **3:**429
Inferior, definition of, **1:**69
Inferior mesenteric artery, arteriograms of, **3:**41
Inferior nasal conchae, **2:**247
Inferior orbital sulci
  anatomy of, **2:**289
  Bertel method, **2:**298-299
  projections of
    overview, **2:**232t
    PA axial, **2:**298-299
Inferior vena cava
  anatomy of, **3:**21
  cavography of, **3:**44
  filter placement, **3:**78-80
  sectional anatomy of, **3:**108, **3:**113, **3:**115, **3:**117, **3:**119
Infraorbital foramen, **2:**246

Index

Index

Xiphisternal joint
  anatomy of, **1**:469t
  description of, **1**:470
Xiphoid process, **1**:468
X-ray beam, collimation of, **1**:28, **1**:29
X-ray diffraction unit, **1**:39
X-ray grids, patient instructions regarding, **1**:19
X-rays
  discovery of, **1**:36
  early injuries associated with, **1**:36
X-ray units, quality assurance of
  beam alignment, **3**:515
  beam/light field congruence, **3**:515
  beam quality, **3**:516-517
  exposure reproducibility and linearity, **3**:518
  exposure time, **3**:515-516
  focal spot size, **3**:518
  kilovolts, **3**:518

Z

Zonography
  abdominal structures evaluated using, **3**:193
  definition of, **3**:179, **3**:205
Zoom, definition of, **3**:333
Z-scores, **3**:443, **3**:460
Zygapophyseal joints
  anatomy of, **1**:372, **1**:382
  of cervical vertebrae, **1**:375
  of lumbar region, **1**:379
  projections of
    AP oblique, **1**:423-425, **1**:434-435
    overview, **1**:369t
    PA oblique, **1**:423-425, **1**:436-437
    positioning rotations for, **1**:375t
    in RAO and LAO positions, **1**:423-425, **1**:436-437

Zygapophyseal joints—cont'd
  projections of—cont'd
    in recumbent position, **1**:424-425
    in RPO and LPO positions, **1**:423-425, **1**:434-435
  of thoracic vertebrae, **1**:377
Zygomatic arch
  description of, **2**:247
  May method, **2**:330-331
  modified Titterington method, **2**:332-333
  modified Towne method, **2**:334-335
  projections of
    AP axial, **2**:334-335
    overview, **2**:310t
    tangential, **2**:326-331
Zygomatic bones, **2**:247
Zygomatic process, **2**:242
Zygote, **2**:215

ISBN 0-8151-2653-0

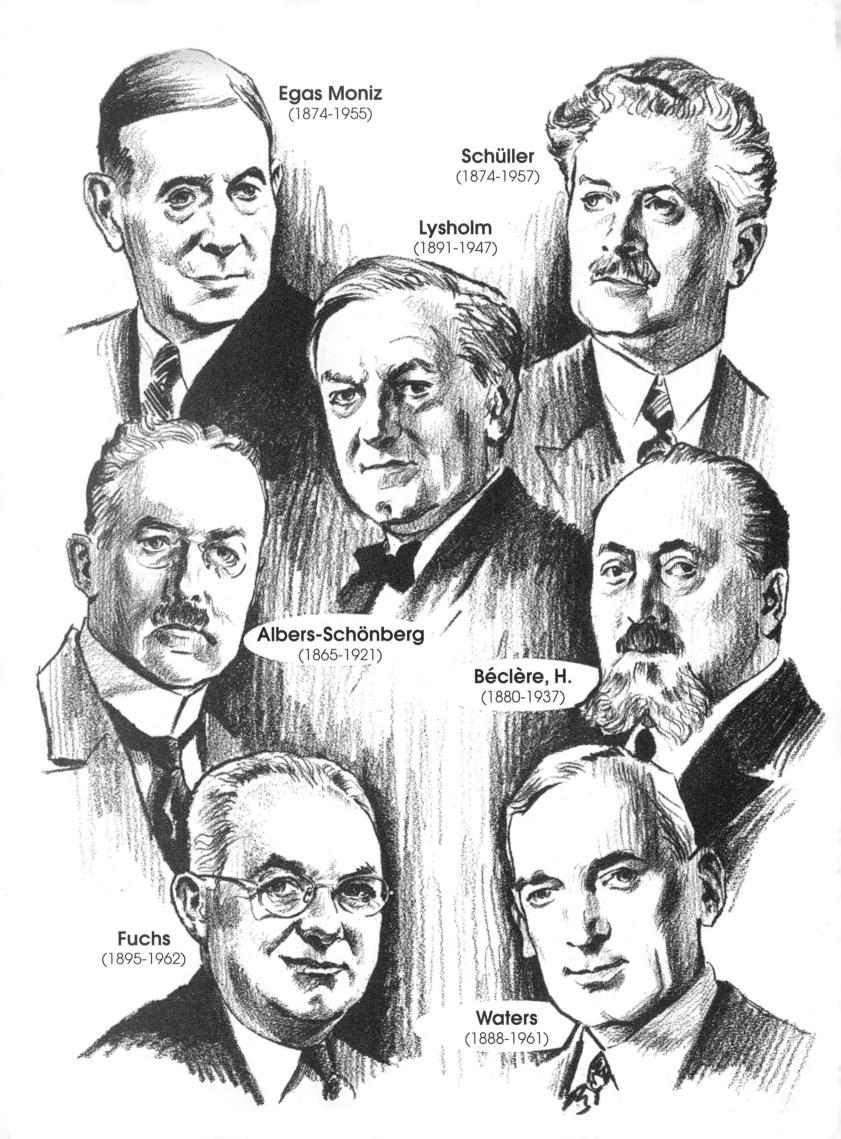

Egas Moniz
(1874-1955)

Schüller
(1874-1957)

Lysholm
(1891-1947)

Albers-Schönberg
(1865-1921)

Béclère, H.
(1880-1937)

Fuchs
(1895-1962)

Waters
(1888-1961)